ANTIBIOTIC ESSENTIALS

Edited by

Burke A. Cunha, M.D.

Chief, Infectious Disease Division
Winthrop-University Hospital
Mineola, New York
Professor of Medicine
State University of New York
School of Medicine
Stony Brook, New York

2004

PHYSICIANS' PRESS

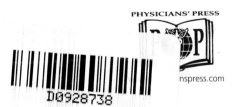

nspress.com

D0928738

ABOUT THE EDITOR

Burke A. Cunha, MD, is Chief, Infectious Disease Division at Winthrop-University Hospital, Mineola, New York; Professor of Medicine, State University of New York School of Medicine, Stony Brook, New York; and one of the world's leading authorities on the treatment of infectious diseases. During his 30-year career, he has contributed more than 800 articles, 150 book chapters, and 12 books on infectious diseases to the medical literature. He has received numerous teaching awards, including the prestigious Aesculapius Award for outstanding teaching. He also serves on the editorial boards of more than two dozen medical journals, is Editor-in-Chief of *Infectious Disease Practice* and *Antibiotics for Clinicians*, and is Infectious Disease Editor-in-Chief for eMedicine on-line. Dr. Cunha is a Fellow of the Infectious Disease Society of America, American Academy of Microbiology, American College of Clinical Pharmacology, and American College of Chest Physicians. He has had a life-long interest in antimicrobial therapy in normal and compromised hosts, antibiotic pharmacokinetics/pharmacodynamics, pharmacoeconomics, and antibiotic resistance. Dr. Cunha is a Master of the American College of Physicians, awarded for achievements as a master clinician and teacher.

Copyright © 2002, 2003, 2004
Physicians' Press

Be sure to visit www.physicianspress.com for a complete listing of medical titles, along with topical reviews, self-assessment questions, and other clinical information. Feel free to contact us by e-mail with comments or suggestions.

Additional copies of *Antibiotic Essentials* may be obtained at medical bookstores, or you may contact us directly at:

Physicians' Press
620 Cherry Avenue
Royal Oak, Michigan, 48073
Tel: (248) 616-3023
Fax: (248) 616-3003
www.physicianspress.com

Printed in the United States of America

ISBN: 1–890114–53–7

TABLE OF CONTENTS

CONTRIBUTORS

Burke A. Cunha, MD
Chief, Infectious Disease Division
Winthrop-University Hosptial
Mineola, New York
Professor of Medicine
SUNY School of Medicine
Stony Brook, New York
All chapters except HIV Infection

Demary Castanheira, PharmD
Clinical Pharmacy Specialist
Winthrop-University Hospital
Mineola, New York
Assistant Clinical Professor of Pharmacy
College of Pharmacy, St. John's University
Queens, New York
Antimicrobial Drug Summaries

Pierce Gardner, MD
John E. Fogarty International Center for
Advanced Study in the Health Sciences
Senior Advisor, Clinical Research and Training
National Institutes of Health
Bethesda, Maryland
Prophylaxis and Immunization

Mark H. Kaplan, MD
Director, Center for AIDS Research and
Treatment
North Shore University Hospital
Manhasset, New York
Jane and Dayton Brown Professor of Clinical
Medicine
New York University School of Medicine
New York, New York
HIV Drug Summaries

Christy Owens, PharmD
Department of Medical and Scientific Affairs
Novartis
South Freeport, Maine
Antimicrobial Drug Interactions

Robert C. Owens, Jr., PharmD
Clinical Specialist, Infectious Disease
Maine Medical Center
Portland, Maine
Clinical Instructor
University of Vermont College of Medicine
Burlington, Vermont
Antimicrobial Drug Interactions

John H. Rex, MD
Vice-President and Medical Director for Infection
AstraZeneca Pharmaceuticals
Macclesfield, United Kingdom
Adjunct Professor of Medicine
University of Texas Medical School–Houston
Houston, Texas
Antifungal Therapy

Paul E. Sax, MD
Director, HIV Program
Brigham and Women's Hospital
Assistant Professor of Medicine
Harvard Medical School
Boston, Massachusetts
HIV Infection

Paul E. Schoch, PhD
Director, Clinical Microbiology Laboratory
Winthrop-University Hospital
Mineola, New York
Medical Microbiology

Kenneth F. Wagner, DO
Attending Physician, Infectious Disease
Consultant
National Naval Medical Center
Associate Professor of Medicine
Uniformed Services
University of the Health Sciences
F. Edward Hebert School of Medicine
Bethesda, Maryland
Parasites, Fungi, Unusual Organisms

ACKNOWLEDGMENTS

To accomplish the task of presenting the data compiled in this reference, a small, dedicated team of professionals was assembled. This team focused their energy and discipline for many months into typing, revising, designing, illustrating, and formatting the many chapters that make up this text. I wish to acknowledge Monica Crowder-Kaufmann, Lisa Lusardi, and Rebecca Smith for their important contribution. I would also like to thank the many contributors who graciously contributed their time and energy, Mark Freed, MD, President and Editor-in-Chief of Physicians' Press, for his vision, commitment, and guidance, Norman Lyle for cover design, and the staff at Dickinson Press for their printing expertise.

Burke A. Cunha, MD

NOTICE

for
Marie

"Grace in her steps,
Heaven in her eye,
In every gesture, dignity and love"
Milton

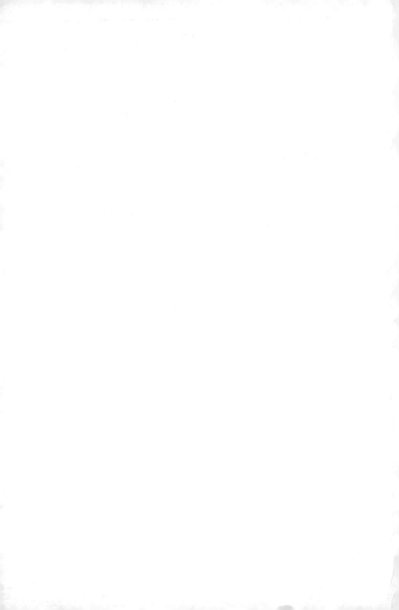

ABBREVIATIONS

A-V	atrio-ventricular	ENT	ear, nose, throat
AAC	antibiotic associated colitis	Enterobacteriaceae:	Citrobacter, Edwardsiella,
AAD	antibiotic associated diarrhea		Enterobacter, E. coli, Klebsiella,
ABE	acute bacterial endocarditis		Proteus, Providencia, Salmonella,
ABM	acute bacterial meningitis		Serratia, Shigella
AFB	acid fast bacilli	ESBLs	extended spectrum β-lactamases
ANA	antinuclear antibody	esp	especially
ARC	AIDS-related complex	ESR	erythrocyte sedimentation rate
ARDS	adult respiratory distress syndrome	ESRD	end-stage renal disease
ASD	atrial septal defect	ET	endotracheal
AV	arteriovenous	FTA-ABS	fluorescent treponemal antibody
β-lactams	penicillins, cephalosporins, cephamycins		absorption test
	(not monobactams or carbapenems)	FUO	fever of unknown origin
BAL	bronchoalveolar lavage	g	gram
BMT	bone marrow transplant	G6PD	glucose-6-phosphate dehydrogenase
CAB	catheter associated bacteriuria	GC	gonococcus/gonorrhea
CABG	coronary artery bypass grafting	GI	gastrointestinal
CAH	chronic active hepatitis	gm	gram
CAP	community acquired pneumonia	GU	genitourinary
CCU	critical care unit	HAV	Hepatitis A virus
CD₄	CD_4 T-cell lymphocyte	HBcAb	hepatitis B core antibody
CE	California encephalitis virus	HBsAg	hepatitis B surface antigen
CIE	counter-immunoelectrophoresis	HAV	Hepatitis A virus
CLL	chronic lymphocytic leukemia	HBV	Hepatitis B virus
CMV	Cytomegalovirus	HCV	Hepatitis C virus
CNS	central nervous system	HDCV	human diploid cell vaccine
CPH	chronic persistent hepatitis	HDV	Hepatitis D virus
CPK	creatine phosphokinase	HEENT	head, eyes, ears, nose, throat
CrCl	creatinine clearance	HEV	Hepatitis E virus
CSD	Cat Scratch Disease	HFV	Hepatitis F virus
CSF	cerebrospinal fluid	HGE	human granulocytic ehrlichiosis
CT	computerized tomography	HHV-6	human Herpes virus 6
CVA	costovertebral angle	HLA	histocompatibility antigen
CXR	chest x-ray	HME	human monocytic ehrlichiosis
D & C	dilatation and curettage	HPV	human papilloma virus
DFA	direct fluorescent antibody	HRIG	human rabies immune globulin
DI	diabetes insipidus	HSV	Herpes simplex virus
DIC	disseminated intravascular coagulation	I & D	incision and drainage
DM	diabetes mellitus	IBD	inflammatory bowel disease
DNA	deoxyribonucleic acid	IFA	immunofluorescent antibody
e.g.	for example	IgA	immunoglobulin A
EBV	Ebstein-Barr virus	IgG	immunoglobulin G
EEE	Eastern equine encephalitis virus	IgM	immunoglobulin M
EEG	electroencephalogram	INH	isoniazid
EIA	enzyme immunoassay	IT	intrathecal
ELISA	enzyme-linked immunosorbent assay	ITP	idiopathic thrombocytopenic purpura
EM	erythema migrans	IUD	intrauterine device
EMB	ethambutol	IV/PO	IV or PO

IV	intravenous	PMN	polymorphonuclear leucocytes
IVDA	intravenous drug abuser	PO	oral
kg	kilogram	PPNG	penicillinase-producing N. gonorrhoeae
L	liter	PVD	peripheral vascular disease
LCM	lymphocytic choriomeningitis	PVE	prosthetic valve endocarditis
LDH	lactate dehydrogenase	PZA	pyrazinamide
LFT	liver function test	q__h	every __ hours
LGV	lymphogranuloma venereum	q__d	every __ days
LLQ	left lower quadrant	qmonth	once a month
LUQ	left upper quadrant	qweek	once a week
MAI	Mycobacterium avium-intracellulare	RBC	red blood cells
mcg	microgram	RLQ	right lower quadrant
mcL	microliter	RMSF	Rocky Mountain spotted fever
mg	milligram	RNA	ribonucleic acid
mL	milliliter	RUQ	right upper quadrant
MIC	minimum inhibitory concentration	RVA	rabies vaccine absorbed
min	minute	SBE	subacute bacterial endocarditis
MMR	measles, mumps, rubella	SGOT/SGPT liver function test	
MRI	magnetic resonance imaging	SLE	systemic lupus erythematosus
MRSA	methicillin-resistant S. aureus	SOT	solid organ transplant
MRSE	methicillin-resistant S. epidermidis	sp.	species
MSSA	methicillin-sensitive S. aureus	SPEP	serum protein electrophoresis
MSSE	methicillin-sensitive S. epidermidis	SQ	subcutaneous
MTT	methlyletrathiazolethiol	STD	sexually transmitted diseases
MVP	mitral valve prolapse	TAH/BSO	total abdominal hysterectomy/bilateral
NCCLS	National Committee for Clinical		salpingoopherectomy
	Laboratory Standards	TB	tuberculosis
NNRTI	non-nucleoside reverse transcriptase	TEE	transesophageal echocardiogram
	inhibitor	TID	three times per day
NP	nosocomial pneumonia	TMP	trimethoprim
NRTI	nucleoside reverse transcriptase	TMP-SMX	trimethoprim-sulfamethoxazole
	inhibitor	TRNG	tetracycline-resistant N. gonorrhoeae
NS	neurosurgical	TST	tuberculin skin test
NSAIDS	nonsteroidal anti-inflammatory drugs	TTE	transthoracic echocardiogram
OI	opportunistic infection	TURP	transurethral resection of prostate
PBS	protected brush specimen	UTI	urinary tract infection
PCEC	purified chick embryo cells	VA	ventriculoatrial
PCN	penicillin	VP	ventriculoperitoneal
PCP	Pneumocystis carinii pneumonia	VAP	ventilator-associated pneumonia
PCR	polymerase chain reaction	VCA	viral capsid antigen
PDA	patent ductus arteriosus	VEE	Venezuelan equine encephalitis virus
PEP	post-exposure prophylaxis	VRE	vancomycin-resistant enterococci
PI	protease inhibitor	VZV	Varicella zoster virus
PML	progressive multifocal	WBC	white blood cells
	leukoencephalopathy	WNE	Western Nile encephalitis virus
		yrs	years

Chapter 1

Overview of Antimicrobial Therapy

Burke A. Cunha, MD

Overview of Antimicrobial Therapy

Infectious diseases are the leading cause of morbidity and mortality worldwide. The ability of bacteria, viruses, mycobacteria, fungi, protozoa, chlamydiae, mycoplasmas, spirochetes, rickettsia, and helminths to cause infection is a balance between inoculum size, virulence, and the adequacy of host defenses. Despite the ability of antimicrobial therapy to augment normal host defenses and prevent/control infection, prescribing errors are common, including treatment of colonization, suboptimal empiric therapy, inappropriate combination therapy, dosing and duration errors, and mismanagement of apparent antibiotic failure. Inadequate consideration of antibiotic resistance potential, tissue penetration, drug interactions, side effects, and cost also limits the effectiveness of antimicrobial therapy. *Antibiotic Essentials* is a concise, practical, and authoritative guide to the treatment and prevention of infectious diseases commonly encountered in adults.

FACTORS IN ANTIBIOTIC SELECTION

A. **Spectrum.** Antibiotic spectrum refers to the range of microorganisms an antibiotic is usually effective against, and is the basis for empiric antibiotic therapy (Chapter 2).

B. **Tissue Penetration**. Antibiotics that are effective against a microorganism in-vitro but unable to reach the site of infection are of little or no benefit to the host. Antibiotic tissue penetration depends on properties of the antibiotic (e.g., lipid solubility, molecular size) and tissue (e.g, adequacy of blood supply, presence of inflammation). Antibiotic tissue penetration is rarely problematic in acute infections due to increased microvascular permeability from local release of chemical inflammatory mediators. In contrast, chronic infections (e.g., chronic pyelonephritis, chronic prostatitis, chronic osteomyelitis) and infections caused by intracellular pathogens often rely on chemical properties of an antibiotic (e.g., high lipid solubility, small molecular size) for adequate tissue penetration. Antibiotics cannot be expected to eradicate organisms from areas that are difficult to penetrate or have impaired blood supply, such as abscesses, which usually require surgical drainage for cure. In addition, implanted foreign materials associated with infection usually need to be removed for cure, since microbes causing infections associated with prosthetic joints, shunts, and intravenous lines produce a slime/glycocalyx on plastic/metal surfaces that permits organisms to survive despite antimicrobial therapy.

C. **Antibiotic Resistance.** Bacterial resistance to antimicrobial therapy can be natural or acquired, and relative or absolute. Pathogens not covered by the usual spectrum of an antibiotic are *naturally* resistant (e.g., 25% of S. pneumoniae are naturally resistant to macrolides); *acquired* resistance occurs when a previously sensitive pathogen is no longer as sensitive to an antibiotic (e.g., ampicillin-resistant H. influenzae). Organisms with *intermediate level (relative)* resistance manifest increases in minimum inhibitory concentrations (MICs), but they remain susceptible to the antibiotic at achievable serum/tissue concentrations (e.g., penicillin-resistant S. pneumoniae). In contrast, organisms with *high level (absolute)* resistance manifest a sudden increase in MICs during therapy, and cannot be overcome by higher-than-usual antibiotic doses (e.g., gentamicin-resistant P. aeruginosa).

Most acquired antibiotic resistance is *agent-specific*, not a class phenomenon, and is usually limited to one or two species. Resistance is *not* related, per se, to volume or duration of use. Some antibiotics have little resistance potential even when used in high volume; other antibiotics can induce resistance with little use. Successful antibiotic resistance control strategies include eliminating antibiotics from animal feeds, microbial surveillance to detect resistance problems early, infection control precautions to limit/contain spread of clonal resistance, restricted hospital formulary (i.e., controlled use of high resistance potential antibiotics), and preferential use of low resistance potential antibiotics by clinicians. Unsuccessful strategies include rotating formularies, restricted use of certain antibiotic classes (e.g., 3rd generation cephalosporins, fluoroquinolones), and use of combination therapy. In choosing between similar antibiotics, try to select an antibiotic with low resistance potential. Some antibiotics (e.g., ceftazidime) are associated with increased prevalence of methicillin-resistant S. aureus (MRSA); other antibiotics (e.g., vancomycin) are associated with increased prevalence of vancomycin-resistant enterococci (VRE).

D. Safety Profile. Whenever possible, avoid antibiotics with serious/frequent side effects.

E. Cost. Switching early from IV to PO antibiotics is the single most important cost saving strategy in hospitalized patients, as the institutional cost of IV administration (~$10/dose) may exceed the cost of the antibiotic itself. Antibiotic costs can also be minimized by using antibiotics with long half-lives, and by choosing monotherapy over combination therapy. Other factors adding to the cost of antimicrobial therapy include the need for an obligatory second antimicrobial agent, antibiotic side effects (e.g., diarrhea, cutaneous reactions, seizures, phlebitis), and outbreaks of resistant organisms, which require cohorting and prolonged hospitalization.

FACTORS IN ANTIBIOTIC DOSING

Usual antibiotic dosing assumes normal renal and hepatic function. Patients with significant renal insufficiency and/or hepatic dysfunction may require dosage reduction in antibiotics metabolized/eliminated by these organs (Table 1). Specific dosing recommendations based on the degree of renal and hepatic insufficiency are detailed in Chapter 7.

A. Renal Insufficiency. Since most antibiotics eliminated by the kidneys have a wide "toxic-to-therapeutic ratio," dosing strategies are frequently based on formula-derived estimates of creatinine clearance (Table 1), rather than precise quantitation of glomerular filtration rates. Dosage adjustments are especially important for antibiotics with narrow toxic-to-therapeutic ratios (e.g., aminoglycosides), and for patients who are receiving other nephrotoxic medications or have preexisting renal disease.

1. **Loading and Maintenance Dosing in Renal Insufficiency.** For drugs eliminated by the kidneys, the loading dose (if required) is left unchanged, and the maintenance dose and dosing interval are modified in proportion to the degree of renal insufficiency. For moderate renal insufficiency (CrCl ~ 40-60 mL/min), the maintenance dose is usually cut in half and the dosing interval is left unchanged. For severe renal insufficiency (CrCl ~ 10-40 mL/min), the maintenance dose is usually cut in half and the dosing interval is doubled. Dosing adjustment problems in renal insufficiency can be circumvented by selecting an antibiotic with a similar spectrum that is eliminated by the hepatic route.

2. **Aminoglycoside Dosing.** Aminoglycosides have a narrow toxic-to-therapeutic ratio and high nephrotoxic potential, and are of particular concern for patients with renal insufficiency. Single daily dosing—adjusted for the degree of renal insufficiency after the loading dose is administered—has virtually eliminated the nephrotoxic potential of aminoglycosides, and is recommended for all patients, including the critically ill. (A possible exception is enterococcal endocarditis, where gentamicin dosing every 8 hours may be preferable.) Aminoglycoside-induced tubular dysfunction is best assessed by quantitative renal tubular cast counts in urine, which more accurately reflect aminoglycoside nephrotoxicity than serum creatinine.

B. **Hepatic Insufficiency.** Antibiotic dosing for patients with hepatic dysfunction is problematic, since there is no hepatic counterpart to the serum creatinine to accurately assess liver function. In practice, antibiotic dosing is based on clinical assessment of the severity of liver disease. For practical purposes, dosing adjustments are usually not required for mild or moderate hepatic insufficiency. For severe hepatic insufficiency, dosing adjustments are usually made for antibiotics with hepatotoxic potential (Chapter 7). Relatively few antibiotics depend solely on hepatic inactivation/elimination, and dosing adjustment problems in these cases can be circumvented by selecting an appropriate antibiotic eliminated by the renal route.

C. **Combined Renal and Hepatic Insufficiency.** There are no good dosing adjustment guidelines for patients with hepatorenal insufficiency. If renal insufficiency is worse than hepatic insufficiency, antibiotics eliminated by the liver are often administered at half the total daily dose. If hepatic insufficiency is worse than renal insufficiency, antibiotics eliminated by the kidneys are usually administered and dosed in proportion to renal function.

Table 1. Dosing Strategies in Hepatic/Renal Insufficiency*

Hepatic Insufficiency
- Decrease total daily dose of hepatically-eliminated antibiotic by 50% in presence of clinically severe liver disease
- Alternative: Use antibiotic eliminated/inactivated by the renal route in usual dose

Renal Insufficiency
- If creatinine clearance ~ 40-60 mL/min, decrease dose of renally-eliminated antibiotic by 50% and maintain the usual dosing interval
- If creatinine clearance ~10-40 mL/min, decrease dose of renally-eliminated antibiotic by 50% and double the dosing interval
- Alternative: Use antibiotic eliminated/inactivated by the hepatic route in usual dose

Major Route of Elimination			
Hepatobiliary		**Renal**	
Chloramphenicol	Quinupristin/dalfopristin	Most β-lactams	Gatifloxacin
Cefoperazone	Nafcillin	Aminoglycosides	Vancomycin
Doxycycline	Linezolid	TMP-SMX	Nitrofurantoin
Minocycline	INH/Pyrazinamide	Monobactams	Fluconazole
Moxifloxacin	Rifampin	Carbapenems	Acyclovir
Macrolides	Itraconazole	Polymyxin B	Valacyclovir
Telithromycin	Caspofungin	Ciprofloxacin	Famciclovir
Clindamycin	Ketoconazole	Ofloxacin	Tetracycline
Metronidazole	Voriconazole	Levofloxacin	Flucytosine

* See individual drug summaries in Chapter 7 for specific dosing recommendations
Creatinine clearance (CrCl) is used to assess renal function, and can be estimated by the following formula: CrCl (mL/min) = [(140 – age) x weight (kg)] / [72 x serum creatinine (mg/dL)]. Multiply by 0.85 if female. It is important to recognize that due to age-dependent declines in renal function, elderly patients with "normal" serum creatinines may have CrCls requiring dosage adjustment. For example, a 70-year-old, 50-kg female with a serum creatinine of 1.2 mg/dL has an estimated CrCl of 34 mL/min

---

MICROBIOLOGY AND SUSCEPTIBILITY TESTING

A. Overview. In-vitro susceptibility testing provides information about microbial sensitivities of a pathogen to various antibiotics and is useful in guiding therapy. Proper application of microbiology and susceptibility data requires careful assessment of the in-vitro results to determine if they are consistent with the clinical context; if not, the clinical impression usually should take precedence.

B. Limitations of Microbiology Susceptibility Testing
  1. **In-vitro data do not differentiate between colonizers and pathogens.** Before treating a culture report from the microbiology laboratory, it is important to determine whether the organism is a pathogen or a colonizer in the clinical context. As a rule, colonization should not be treated.

2. **In-vitro data do not necessarily translate into in-vivo efficacy.** Reports which indicate an organism is "sensitive" or "resistant" to a given antibiotic in-vitro do not necessarily reflect in-vivo activity. Table 2 lists antibiotic-microorganism combinations for which susceptibility testing is usually unreliable.

3. **In-vitro susceptibility testing is dependent on the microbe, methodology, and antibiotic concentration.** In-vitro susceptibility testing by the microbiology laboratory *assumes* the isolate was recovered from *blood,* and is being exposed to *serum* concentrations of an antibiotic given in the *usual* dose. Since some body sites (e.g., bladder, urine) contain higher antibiotic concentrations than found in serum, and other

Table 2. Antibiotic-Organism Combinations for Which In-Vitro Susceptibility Testing Is Unreliable[1]

Antibiotic	"Sensitive" Organism
Penicillin	H. influenzae, Yersinia pestis
TMP-SMX	Klebsiella, Enterococci, Bartonella
Polymyxin B	Proteus, Salmonella
Imipenem	Stenotrophomonas maltophilia[2]
Gentamicin	Mycobacterium tuberculosis
Vancomycin	Erysipelothrix rhusiopathiae
Aminoglycosides	Streptococci, Salmonella, Shigella
Clindamycin	Fusobacteria, Clostridia, enterococci, Listeria
Macrolides	P. multocida
1st, 2nd generation cephalosporins	Salmonella, Shigella, Bartonella
3rd, 4th generation cephalosporins[4]	Enterococci, Listeria, Bartonella
All antibiotics except vancomycin, minocycline, quinupristin/dalfopristin, linezolid	MRSA[3]

1. In-vitro susceptibility *does not* predict in-vivo activity; susceptibility data cannot be relied upon to guide therapy for antibiotic-organism combinations in this table
2. Formerly Pseudomonas
3. In spite of apparent in-vitro susceptibility of many antibiotics against MRSA, only vancomycin, quinupristin/dalfopristin, linezolid, and minocycline are effective in-vivo
4. Cefoperazone is the only cephalosporin with clinically useful anti-enterococcal activity (E. faecalis, not E. faecium [VRE])

body sites (e.g., CSF) contain lower antibiotic concentrations than found in serum, in-vitro data may be misleading for non-bloodstream infections. For example, a Klebsiella pneumoniae isolate obtained from the CSF may be reported as "sensitive" to cefazolin even though cefazolin does not penetrate the CSF. Likewise, E. coli and Klebsiella urinary isolates are often reported as "resistant" to ampicillin/sulbactam despite in-vivo efficacy, due to high antibiotic concentrations in the urinary tract. Antibiotics should be prescribed at the usual recommended doses; attempts to lower cost by reducing dosage may decrease antibiotic efficacy (e.g., cefoxitin 2 gm IV inhibits ~ 85% of B. fragilis isolates, whereas 1 gm IV inhibits only ~ 20% of strains).

4. **Unusual susceptibility patterns.** Organisms have predictable susceptibility patterns to antibiotics. When an isolate has an unusual susceptibility pattern (i.e., isolate of a species demonstrates the reverse of the usual susceptibility pattern) (Table 3), further testing should be performed by the microbiology laboratory to verify the identity of the isolate and characterize the mechanism of resistance. Expanded susceptibility testing is also warranted.

C. **Susceptibility Breakpoints for Streptococcus pneumoniae.** Because antibiotic susceptibility is, in part, concentration related, the National Committee for Clinical Laboratory Standards (NCCLS) has revised its breakpoints for S. pneumoniae susceptibility testing, which differentiate between meningeal and non-meningeal sites of pneumococcal infection (Table 4).

D. **Summary.** In-vitro susceptibility testing is useful in most situations, but should not be followed blindly. Many factors need to be considered when interpreting in-vitro microbiologic data, and infectious disease consultation is recommended for all but the most straightforward susceptibility interpretation problems. Since susceptibility is concentration-dependent, IV-to-PO switch changes using antibiotics of the same class is best made when the oral antibiotic can achieve similar blood/tissue levels as the IV antibiotic. For example, IV-to-PO switch from cefazolin 1 gm (IV) to cephalexin 500 mg (PO) may not be effective against all pathogens at all sites, since cephalexin 500 mg (PO) achieves much lower serum concentrations compared to cefazolin 1 gm (IV) (16 mcg/mL vs. 200 mcg/mL).

Table 3. Unusual Susceptibility Patterns Requiring Further Testing

Organism	Unusual Susceptibility Patterns	Usual Susceptibility Patterns
Neisseria meningitidis	Penicillin resistant	Penicillin susceptible
Staphylococci	Vancomycin/clindamycin resistant; erythromycin susceptible	Vancomycin susceptible
Enterococci	Vancomycin intermediate/resistant	Vancomycin susceptible
Viridans streptococci	Vancomycin intermediate/resistant	Vancomycin susceptible
Streptococcus pneumoniae	Vancomycin intermediate/resistant	Vancomycin susceptible
Beta-hemolytic streptococci	Penicillin intermediate/resistant	Penicillin susceptible
Enterobacteriaceae	Imipenem resistant	Imipenem susceptible
E. coli, P. mirabilis, Klebsiella	Cefoxitin/cefotetan resistant	2nd generation cephalosporin susceptible
Enterobacter, Serratia	Ampicillin/cefazolin susceptible	Ampicillin/cefazolin resistant
Morganella, Providencia	Ampicillin/cefazolin susceptible	Ampicillin/cefazolin resistant
Klebsiella	Cefotetan susceptible; ceftazidime resistant	Cefotetan resistant; ceftazidime susceptible
Pseudomonas aeruginosa	Amikacin resistant; gentamicin/tobramycin susceptible	Amikacin susceptible; gentamicin/tobramycin resistant
Stenotrophomonas maltophilia	TMP-SMX resistant; imipenem susceptible	TMP-SMX susceptible

Isolates with unusual susceptibility patterns require further testing by the microbiology laboratory to verify the identity of the isolate and characterize resistance mechanism. Expanded susceptibility testing is indicated.

Table 4. NCCLS Susceptibility Breakpoints for Streptococcus pneumoniae*

Antibiotic	MIC (mcg/mL)		
	Sensitive	Intermediate	Resistant
Amoxicillin (non-meningitis)	≤ 2	4	≥ 8
Amoxicillin-clavulanic acid (non-meningitis)	≤ 2/1	4/2	≥ 8/4
Penicillin	≤ 0.06	0.12-1	≥ 2
Azithromycin	≤ 0.5	1	≥ 2
Clarithromycin/erythromycin	≤ 0.25	0.5	≥ 1
Doxycycline/tetracycline	≤ 2	4	≥ 8
Telithromycin	≤ 1	2	≥ 4
Cefaclor	≤ 1	2	≥ 4
Cefdinir/cefpodoxime	≤ 0.5	1	≥ 2
Cefprozil	≤ 2	4	≥ 8
Cefuroxime axetil (oral)	≤ 1	2	≥ 4
Loracarbef	≤ 2	4	≥ 8
Cefepime (non-meningitis)	≤ 1	2	≥ 4
Cefepime (meningitis)	≤ 0.5	1	≥ 2
Cefotaxime (non-meningitis)	≤ 1	2	≥ 4
Cefotaxime (meningitis)	≤ 0.5	1	≥ 2
Ceftriaxone (non-meningitis)	≤ 1	2	≥ 4
Ceftriaxone (meningitis)	≤ 0.5	1	≥ 2
Imipenem	≤ 0.12	0.25–0.5	≥ 1
Meropenem	≤ 0.25	0.5	≥ 1
Vancomycin	≤ 1	–	–
Gatifloxacin/moxifloxacin	≤ 1	2	≥ 4
Levofloxacin	≤ 2	4	≥ 8
TMP-SMX	≤ 0.5/9.5	1/19 – 2/38	≥ 4/78
Chloramphenicol	≤ 4	–	≥ 8
Clindamycin	≤ 0.25	0.5	≥ 1
Linezolid	≤ 2	–	–
Rifampin	≤ 1	2	≥ 4

NCCLS = National Committee for Clinical Laboratory Standards (2002)
* *Testing Conditions:* Medium: Mueller-Hinton broth with 2.5% lysed horse blood (cation-adjusted). Inoculum: colony suspension. Incubation: 35°C (20-24 hours)

OTHER CONSIDERATIONS IN ANTIMICROBIAL THERAPY

A. **Bactericidal vs. Bacteriostatic Therapy.** For most infections, bacteriostatic and bactericidal antibiotics inhibit/kill organisms at the same rate, and should not be a factor in antibiotic selection. Bactericidal antibiotics have an advantage in certain infections, such endocarditis, meningitis, and febrile leukopenia, but there are exceptions even in these cases.

B. **Monotherapy vs. Combination Therapy**. Monotherapy is preferred to combination therapy, and is possible for most infections. In addition to cost savings, monotherapy results in less chance of medication error and fewer missed doses/drug interactions. Combination therapy may be useful for drug synergy or for extending spectrum beyond what can be obtained with a single drug. However, since drug synergy is difficult to assess and the possibility of antagonism always exists, antibiotics should be combined for synergy only if synergy is likely based on experience or actual testing. Combination therapy is not effective in preventing antibiotic resistance, except in very few situations (Table 5).

C. **Intravenous vs. Oral Switch Therapy.** Patients admitted to the hospital are usually started on IV antibiotic therapy, then switched to equivalent oral therapy after clinical improvement/defervescence (usually within 72 hours). Advantages of early IV-to-PO switch programs include reduced cost, early hospital discharge, less need for home IV therapy, and virtual elimination of IV line infections. Drugs well-suited for IV-to-PO switch or for treatment entirely by the oral route include doxycycline, minocycline, clindamycin, metronidazole, chloramphenicol, amoxicillin, trimethoprim-sulfamethoxazole, quinolones, and linezolid. Only some penicillins and cephalosporins are useful for IV-to-PO switch programs, due to limited bioavailability.

Table 5. Combination Therapy and Antibiotic Resistance

Examples of Antibiotic Combinations That Prevent Resistance
Anti-pseudomonal penicillin (carbenicillin) + aminoglycoside (gentamicin, tobramycin, amikacin)
Rifampin + other TB drugs (INH, ethambutol, pyrazinamide)
5-flucytosine + amphotericin B

Examples of Antibiotic Combinations That Do Not Prevent Resistance*
TMP-SMX
Most other antibiotic combinations

* These combinations are often prescribed to prevent resistance when, in actuality, they do not

Most infectious diseases should be treated orally unless the patient is critically ill, cannot take antibiotics by mouth, or there is no equivalent oral antibiotic. If the patient is able to take/absorb oral antibiotics, there is no difference in clinical outcome using equivalent IV or PO antibiotics. It is more important to think in terms of antibiotic spectrum, bioavailability and tissue penetration, rather than route of administration. Nearly all non-critically ill patients should be treated in part or entirely with oral antibiotics. When switching from IV to PO therapy, the oral antibiotic chosen ideally should achieve the same blood and tissue levels as the equivalent IV antibiotic (Table 6).

D. Duration of Therapy. Most bacterial infections in normal hosts are treated with antibiotics for 1-2 weeks. The duration of therapy may need to be extended in patients with impaired immunity (e.g., diabetes, SLE, alcoholic liver disease, neutropenia, diminished splenic function, etc.), chronic bacterial infections (e.g., endocarditis, osteomyelitis), chronic viral and fungal infections, or certain bacterial intracellular pathogens (Table 7). Infections such as HIV and CMV in compromised hosts usually require life-long suppressive therapy. Antibiotic therapy should ordinarily not be continued for more than 2 weeks, even if low-grade fevers persist. Prolonged therapy offers no benefit, and increases the risk of adverse side effects, drug interactions, and superinfections.

Table 6. Bioavailability of Oral Antimicrobials

Bioavailability	Antimicrobials		
Excellent[1]	Amoxicillin	TMP	Minocycline
	Clindamycin	TMP-SMX	Linezolid
	Quinolones	Doxycycline	Fluconazole
	5-Flucytosine	Chloramphenicol	Voriconazole
	Rifampin	Metronidazole	Itraconazole (solution)
Good[2]	Most beta-lactams	Acyclovir	
	Most 1st,2nd,3rd gen.	Valacyclovir	
	oral cephalosporins	Famciclovir	
	Macrolides	Telithromycin	
Inadequate[3]	Vancomycin		

1. Oral administration results in equivalent blood/tissue levels as the same dose given IV (PO = IV)
2. Oral administration results in lower blood/tissue levels than the same dose given IV (PO < IV)
3. Oral administration results in inadequate blood/tissue levels

Table 7. Infectious Diseases Requiring Prolonged Antimicrobial Therapy

Duration of Therapy	Infectious Diseases
3 weeks	Lymphogranuloma venereum (LGV), syphilis (late latent)
4 weeks	Chronic otitis media, chronic sinusitis, acute osteomyelitis, chronic pyelonephritis, brain abscess, SBE (viridans streptococci), Legionella
6 weeks	Acute bacterial endocarditis (S. aureus, enterococcal), H. pylori
3 months	Chronic prostatitis, lung abscess[1]
6 months	Pulmonary TB, extrapulmonary TB, Actinomycosis[2], Nocardia[3], chronic osteomyelitis[4]
12 months	Whipple's disease
> 12 months	Bartonella, chronic suppressive therapy for Pneumocystis carinii pneumonia (PCP), cytomegalovirus (CMV), HIV, prosthetic-related infections[5]

1. Treat until resolved or until chest x-ray is normal/nearly normal and remains unchanged
2. May require longer treatment; treat until resolved
3. May require longer treatment in compromised hosts
4   Adequate surgical debridement is required for cure
5. Implanted foreign materials associated with infection (prosthetic valves, vascular grafts, joint replacements, hemodialysis shunts) should be removed as soon as possible after diagnosis. If removal is not feasible, then chronic suppressive therapy may be attempted, although clinical failure is the rule

EMPIRIC ANTIBIOTIC THERAPY

Microbiology susceptibility data are not ordinarily available prior to initial treatment with antibiotics. Empiric therapy is based on directing coverage against the most likely pathogens, and takes into consideration drug allergy history, hepatic/renal function, possible antibiotic side effects, resistance potential, and cost. If a patient is moderately or severely ill, empiric therapy is usually initiated intravenously. Patients who are mildly ill, whether hospitalized or ambulatory, may be started on oral antibiotics with high bioavailability. Cultures of appropriate clinical specimens (e.g., sputum, urine) should be obtained prior to starting empiric therapy to provide bacterial isolates for in-vitro susceptibility testing. Empiric therapy for common infectious diseases is described in Chapter 2.

ANTIBIOTIC FAILURE

There are many possible causes of *apparent* antibiotic failure, including drug fever, antibiotic-unresponsive infections, and febrile non-infectious diseases. The most common error in the management of apparent antibiotic failure is changing/adding additional antibiotics instead of determining the cause (Tables 8, 9).

Table 8. Causes of Apparent/Actual Antibiotic Failure

In-vitro susceptibility but inactive in-vivo
Antibiotic tolerance with gram-positive cocci
Inadequate coverage/spectrum
Inadequate antibiotic blood levels
Inadequate antibiotic tissue levels
    Undrained abscess
    Foreign body-related infection
    Protected focus (e.g., cerebrospinal fluid)
    Organ hypoperfusion/diminished blood supply (e.g., chronic osteomyelitis in diabetics)
Drug-induced interactions
    Antibiotic inactivation
    Antibiotic antagonism
Decreased antibiotic activity in tissue
Fungal superinfection
Treating colonization, not infection
Non-infectious diseases
    Medical disorders mimicking infection (e.g., SLE)
    Drug fever (Table 9)
Antibiotic-unresponsive infectious diseases
    Most viral infections

Table 9. Clinical Features of Drug Fever

History
    Many but not all individuals are atopic
    Patients have been on a sensitizing medication for days or years "without a problem"
Physical exam
    Fevers may be low- or high-grade, but usually range between 102°-104°F and may exceed 106°F
    Relative bradycardia*
    Patient appears "inappropriately well" for degree of fever
Laboratory tests
    Elevated WBC count (usually with left shift)
    Eosinophils almost always present, but eosinophilia is uncommon
    Elevated erythrocyte sedimentation rate in majority of cases
    Early, transient, mild elevations of serum transaminases (common)
    Negative blood cultures (excluding contaminants)

* Relative bradycardia refers to heart rates that are inappropriately slow relative to body temperature (pulse must be taken simultaneously with temperature elevation). Applies to adult patients with temperature ≥ 102°F; does not apply to patients with second/third-degree heart block, pacemaker-induced rhythms, or those taking beta-blockers.
Appropriate Temperature-Pulse Relationships

Pulse (beats/min)	Temperature
150	41.1°C (106°F)
140	40.6°C (105°F)
130	40.7°C (104°F)
120	39.4°C (103°F)
110	38.9°C (102°F)

PITFALLS IN ANTIBIOTIC PRESCRIBING

- Use of antibiotics to treat non-infectious or antibiotic-unresponsive infectious diseases (e.g., viral infections) or colonization

- Overuse of combination therapy. Monotherapy is preferred over combination therapy unless compelling reasons prevail, such as drug synergy or extended spectrum beyond what can be obtained with a single drug. Monotherapy reduces the risk of drug interactions and side effects, and is usually less expensive

- Use of antibiotics for persistent fevers. For patients with persistent fevers on an antimicrobial regimens that appears to be failing, it is important to reassess the patient rather than add additional antibiotics. Causes of prolonged fevers include undrained septic foci, non-infectious medical disorders, and drug fevers. Undiagnosed causes of leukocytosis/low-grade fevers should not be treated with prolonged courses of antibiotics

- Inadequate surgical therapy. Infections involving infected prosthetic materials or fluid collections (e.g., abscesses) often require surgical therapy for cure. For infections such as chronic osteomyelitis, surgery is the only way to cure the infection; antibiotics are useful only for suppression or to prevent local infectious complications

- Home IV therapy. There is less need to use home IV therapy given the vast array of excellent oral antibiotics (e.g., linezolid)

REFERENCES AND SUGGESTED READINGS

Cunha BA. Strategies to control the emergence of resistant organisms. Sem Respir Infect 17:250-258, 2002.

Cunha BA. Strategies to control antibiotic resistance. Semin Respir Infect 17:250-8, 2002.

Cunha BA. Pseudomonas aeruginosa: Resistance and therapy. Semin Respir Infect 17:231-9, 2002.

Cunha BA. Antimicrobial side effects. Medical Clinics of North America 85:149-185, 2001.

Cunha BA. Intravenous to oral antibiotic switch therapy. Drugs for Today 37:311-319, 2001.

Cunha BA. Effective antibiotic resistance and control strategies. Lancet 357:1307-1308, 2001.

Cunha BA. Clinical relevance of penicillin-resistant Streptococcus pneumoniae. Semin Respir Infect 17:204-14, 2002.

Cunha BA. Factors in Antibiotic selection for hospital formularies (part I). Hospital Formulary 33:558-572, 1998.

Cunha BA. Factors in antibiotic selection for hospital formularies (part II). Hospital Formulary 33:659-662, 1998.

Cunha BA. The significance of antibiotic false sensitivity testing with in vitro infections. J Chemother 9:25-33, 1997.

Cunha BA, Ortega A. Antibiotic failure. Medical Clinics of North America 79:663-672, 1995.

Cunha BA. Drug fever. Postgraduate Medicine 80:123-129, 1986.

Cunha BA. Antibiotic pharmacokinetic considerations in pulmonary infections. Sem Respir Infect 6:168-182, 1991.

Empey KM, Rapp RP, Evans ME. The effect of an antimicrobial formulary change on hospital resistance patterns. Pharmacotherapy 22:81-7, 2002.

Johnson DH, Cunha BA. Drug fever. Infectious Disease Clinics of North America 10:85-91, 1996.

NCCLS. 2002. Performance standards for antimicrobial susceptibility testing: twelfth informational supplement M100-S12. NCCLS, Wayne, PA.

TEXTBOOKS

Amabile-Cuevas CF (ed). Antibiotic Resistance From Molecular Basics to Therapeutic Options. R.G. Landes Company, Austin, 1996.

Ambrose P, Nightingale AT (eds). Principles of Pharmacodynamics. Marcel Dekker, Inc., New York, 2001.

Anaissie EJ, McGinnis MR, Pfaller MA (eds). Clinical Mycology. Churchill Livingstone, New York, 2003.

Chadwick DJ, Goode J (eds). Antibiotic Resistance: Origins, Evolution, Selection and Spread. John Wiley & Sons, New York, 1997.

Cunha BA (ed). Medical Clinics of North America Antimicrobial Therapy. W.B. Saunders Company, Philadelphia, PA, 1982.

Cunha BA (ed). Medical Clinics of North America Antimicrobial Therapy I. W.B. Saunders Company, Philadelphia, PA, 1995.

Cunha BA (ed). Medical Clinics of North America Antimicrobial Therapy II. W.B. Saunders Company, Philadelphia, PA, 1995.

Cunha BA (ed). Medical Clinics of North America Antimicrobial Therapy I. W.B. Saunders Company, Philadelphia, PA, 2000.

Cunha BA (ed). Medical Clinics of North America Antimicrobial Therapy II. W.B. Saunders Company, Philadelphia, PA, 2001.

Kaye D (ed). Infectious Disease Clinics of North America Pharmacology, New Agents. W.B. Saunders Company, Philadelphia, PA, 1997.

Kaye D (ed). Infectious Disease Clinics of North America Pharmacology, New Agents. W.B. Saunders Company, Philadelphia, PA, 2000.

Mandell GL, Bennett JE, Dolin R (eds). Mandell, Douglas and Bennett's Principles and Practice of Infectious Disease, 5th Edition. Churchill Livingstone, Philadelphia, PA, 2000.

O'Grady F, Lambert HP, Finch RG, Greenwood D (eds). Antibiotic and Chemotherapy, 2nd Edition. Churchill, Livingstone, New York, 1997.

Scholar EM Pratt WB (eds). The Antimicrobial Drugs, 2nd edition, Oxford University Press, New York, 2000.

Chapter 2

Empiric Therapy Based on Clinical Syndrome

Burke A. Cunha, MD
John H. Rex, MD

This chapter is organized by clinical syndrome, patient subset, and in some cases, specific organism. Clinical summaries immediately follow each treatment grid.

Therapeutic recommendations are based on antimicrobial effectiveness, reliability, cost, safety, and resistance potential. Switching to a more specific/narrow spectrum antimicrobial is not more effective than well-chosen empiric/initial therapy and usually results in increased cost and more side effects/drug interactions. The antimicrobial dosages in this section represent the usual dosages for normal renal and hepatic function. ***For any treatment category (i.e., preferred IV therapy, alternate IV therapy, PO therapy), recommended drugs are equally effective and not ranked by priority.*** Dosage adjustments, side effects, drug interactions, and other important prescribing information is described in the individual drug summaries in Chapter 7.

"IV-to-PO Switch" in the last column of the shaded title bar in each treatment grid indicates the clinical syndrome should be treated either by IV therapy alone or IV followed by PO therapy, but *not* by PO therapy alone. "PO Therapy or IV-to-PO Switch" indicates the clinical syndrome can be treated by IV therapy alone, PO therapy alone, or IV followed by PO therapy (unless otherwise indicated in the footnotes under each treatment grid). Most patients on IV therapy able to take PO medications should be switched to PO equivalent therapy after clinical improvement.

Empiric Therapy of CNS Infections

Acute Bacterial Meningitis (ABM)

Subset	Usual Pathogens	Preferred IV Therapy	Alternate IV Therapy	IV-to-PO Switch
Normal host	N. meningitidis H. influenzae S. pneumoniae	Ceftriaxone 2 gm (IV) q12h x 2 weeks	Meropenem 2 gm (IV) q8h x 2 weeks **or** Cefotaxime 3 gm (IV) q6h x 2 weeks **or** Ceftizoxime 3 gm (IV) q6h x 2 weeks	Chloramphenicol 500 mg (PO) q6h x 2 weeks
Elderly or malignancy	Listeria monocytogenes plus usual meningeal pathogens in normal hosts	<u>Before culture results</u> Ceftriaxone 2 gm (IV) q12h x 2 weeks **plus** Ampicillin 2 gm (IV) q4h x 2 weeks <u>After culture results</u> <u>*Listeria present*</u> Ampicillin 2 gm (IV) q4h x 2 weeks <u>*Listeria not present*</u> Treat as normal host	<u>After culture results</u> <u>*Listeria present*</u> TMP-SMX 5 mg/kg (IV) q6h x 2 weeks **or** Chloramphenicol 500 mg (IV) q6h x 2 weeks <u>*Listeria not present*</u> Treat as for normal host, above	<u>For Listeria meningitis only</u> TMP-SMX 5 mg/kg (PO) q6h x 2 weeks **or** Chloramphenicol 500 mg (PO) q6h x 2 weeks <u>For usual meningeal pathogens</u> Chloramphenicol 500 mg (PO) q6h x 2 weeks
CNS shunt infections (VA shunts) (Treat initially for MSSA; if later identified as MRSA, MSSE, or MRSE, treat accordingly)	S. aureus S. epidermidis (coagulase-negative staphylococci)	<u>MSSA/MSSE</u> Cefotaxime 3 gm (IV) q6h* **or** Ceftizoxime 3 gm (IV) q6h* <u>MRSA/MRSE</u> Linezolid 600 mg (IV) q12h*	<u>MSSA/MSSE</u> Cefepime 2 gm (IV) q8h* **or** Meropenem 2 gm (IV) q8h* <u>MRSA/MRSE</u> Vancomycin 1 gm (IV) q12h* plus 20 mg (IT) q24h until shunt removal	<u>MSSE/MRSE</u> Linezolid 600 mg (PO) q12h* <u>MSSA/MRSA</u> Minocycline 100 mg (PO) q12h* **or** Linezolid 600 mg (PO) q12h*

MSSA/MRSA = methicillin-sensitive/resistant S. aureus; MSSE/MRSE = methicillin-sensitive/resistant S. epidermidis.
Duration of therapy represents total time IV or IV + PO. Most patients on IV therapy able to take PO meds should be switched to PO therapy after clinical improvement
* Treat for 1 week after shunt removal

Acute Bacterial Meningitis (ABM) (cont'd)

Subset	Usual Pathogens	Preferred IV Therapy	Alternate IV Therapy	IV-to-PO Switch
CNS shunt infections (VP shunts)	E. coli K. pneumoniae Enterobacter S. marcescens	Ceftriaxone 2 gm (IV) q12h x 2 weeks after shunt removal **or** Ceftizoxime 3 gm (IV) q6h x 2 weeks after shunt removal	Cefotaxime 3 gm (IV) q6h x 2 weeks after shunt removal **or** TMP-SMX 5 mg/kg (IV) q6h x 2 weeks after shunt removal	TMP-SMX 5 mg/kg (PO) q6h x 2 weeks after shunt removal

Duration of therapy represents total time IV or IV + PO. Most patients on IV therapy able to take PO meds should be switched to PO therapy after clinical improvement

Clinical Presentation: Abrupt onset of fever, headache, stiff neck
Diagnosis: CSF gram stain/culture

Acute Bacterial Meningitis (Normal Hosts)

Diagnostic Considerations: Gram stain of centrifugated CSF is still the best diagnostic test. CSF antigen/CIE are unhelpful in establishing the diagnosis (many false-negatives). Blood cultures are positive for ABM pathogen in 80-90%. Typical CSF findings include a WBC count of 100-5000 cells/mm^3, elevated opening pressure, elevated protein and lactic acid levels (> 4-6 mmol/L), and a positive CSF gram stain. If the WBC is extremely high (> 20,000 cells/mm^3), suspect brain abscess with rupture into the ventricular system, and obtain a CT/MRI to confirm. S. pneumoniae meningitis is associated with cranial nerves abnormalities, mental status changes, and neurologic sequelae. With H. influenzae or S. pneumoniae meningitis, obtain a head CT/MRI to rule out other CNS pathology

Pitfalls: If ABM is suspected, always perform lumbar puncture (LP) *before* obtaining a CT scan, since early antibiotic therapy is critical to prognosis. A CT/MRI should be obtained before LP *only* if a mass lesion/suppurative intracranial process is of primary concern, after blood cultures have been drawn. A stiff neck on physical examination has limited diagnostic value in the elderly, since nuchal rigidity may occur without meningitis (e.g., cervical arthritis) and meningitis may occur without nuchal rigidity. Recurrence of fever during the first week of H. influenzae meningitis is commonly due to subdural effusion, which usually resolves spontaneously over several days. Meningococcal meningitis may occur with or without meningococcemia. On gram stain, S. pneumoniae may be mistaken for H. influenzae, and Listeria may be mistaken for S. pneumoniae

Therapeutic Considerations: Do not reduce meningeal antibiotic dosing as the patient improves. Repeat LP only if the patient is not responding to antibiotics after 48 hours; lack of response may be due to therapeutic failure, relapse, or a non-infectious CNS disorder. For S. pneumoniae meningitis, obtain penicillin MICs on all CSF isolates; nearly all penicillin-resistant strains have relatively low MICs (2-5 mcg/mL) and are susceptible to meningeal doses of beta-lactam antibiotics (e.g., ceftriaxone). All but the most highly penicillin-resistant pneumococci are still effectively treated with meningeal doses of beta-lactams. Highly resistant pneumococcal strains (rare in the CSF) may be treated for 2 weeks with meropenem 2 gm (IV) q8h, cefepime 2 gm (IV) q8h, linezolid 600 mg (IV) q12h, or vancomycin (IV/IT). Dexamethasone 0.15 mg/kg (IV) q6h x 4 days may be given to children with ABM to reduce the incidence/severity of neurologic sequelae, although the value of steroids in adult ABM is unclear; if used, give dexamethasone 30 minutes before the initial antibiotic dose

Prognosis: Uniformly fatal without treatment. Case-fatality rates in treated adults are 10-20%. Neurological deficits on presentation are associated with a poor prognosis. Permanent neurological deficits are more frequent with S. pneumoniae than H. influenzae, even with prompt therapy. In meningococcal meningitis with meningococcemia, prognosis is related to the number of petechiae, with few or no neurological deficits in survivors

Acute Bacterial Meningitis (Elderly Patients/Malignancy)

Diagnostic Considerations: Diagnosis by CSF gram stain/culture. ABM pathogens include usual pathogens in normal hosts plus Listeria monocytogenes, a gram-positive, aerobic, bacillus. Listeria is the most common ABM pathogen in patients with malignancies, and is a common pathogen in the elderly. With Listeria meningitis, CSF cultures are positive in 100%, but CSF gram stain is negative in 50%. Meningeal carcinomatosis is suggested by multiple cranial nerve abnormalities

Pitfalls: "Diphtheroids" isolated from CSF should be speciated to rule out Listeria. Listeria are motile and hemolytic on blood agar plate, diphtheroids are not

Therapeutic Considerations: Elderly patients and cancer patients with ABM require empiric coverage of Listeria plus other common pathogens in normal hosts (N. meningitidis, H. influenzae, S. pneumoniae). Specific monotherapy can be administered once the organism is known. Third-generation cephalosporins are not active against Listeria

Prognosis: Related to underlying health of host

Acute Bacterial Meningitis (CNS Shunt Infections)

Diagnostic Considerations: Diagnosis by CSF gram stain/culture. S. epidermidis meningitis usually occurs only with infected prosthetic implant material (e.g., CNS shunt/plate)

Pitfalls: Blood cultures are usually negative for shunt pathogens

Therapeutic Considerations: 15% of S. epidermidis strains are resistant to nafcillin/clindamycin. In addition to systemic antibiotics in meningeal doses, adjunctive intraventricular/intrathecal antibiotics are sometimes given to control shunt infections before shunt removal

Prognosis: Good if prosthetic material is removed

Acute Non-Bacterial Meningitis/Chronic Meningitis

Subset	Usual Pathogens	IV Therapy	IV-to-PO Switch
Viral (aseptic)	EBV, VZV, LCM, Enteroviruses, WNE	Not applicable	Not applicable
	HSV-1 HSV-2	Acyclovir 10 mg/kg (IV) q8h x 14-21 days	Acyclovir 400 mg (PO) 5x/day x 14-21 days **or** Valacyclovir 500 mg (PO) q8h x 14-21 days **or** Famciclovir 500 mg (PO) q8h x 14-21 days
Primary amebic meningo-encephalitis (PAM)	Naegleria fowleri	Amphotericin B deoxycholate 1 mg/kg (IV) q24h until cured **plus** Amphotericin B deoxycholate 1 mg into ventricles via Ommaya reservoir q24h until cured	Not applicable

Acute Non-Bacterial Meningitis/Chronic Meningitis (cont'd)

Subset	Usual Pathogens	Preferred IV Therapy	Alternate IV Therapy	PO Therapy or IV-to-PO Switch
Granulomatous amebic meningoencephalitis	Acanthamoeba	No proven treatment (amphotericin B, fluconazole, ketoconazole, itraconazole, flucytosine, rifampin, isoniazid, aminoglycosides, sulfonamides, pentamidine mostly with little success. Success reported in transplant recipient with IV pentamidine followed by itraconazole, and in AIDS patient with ketoconazole plus flucytosine)		
TB	M. tuberculosis	IV Therapy Not applicable	PO Therapy INH 300 mg (PO) q24h x 6-9 months **plus** Rifampin 600 mg (PO) q24h x 6-9 months If multiresistant TB strain likely, also add: EMB 15 mg/kg (PO) q24h x 6-9 months **plus** PZA 25 mg/kg (PO) q24h x 6-9 months	
Fungal *Non-HIV*	Cryptococcus neoformans	Amphotericin B deoxycholate 0.7-1 mg/kg (IV) q24h x 2-6 weeks* **plus** Flucytosine 25 mg/kg (PO) q6h x 6 weeks*, **followed by** Fluconazole 800 mg (IV or PO) x 1 dose, then 400 mg (PO) q24h x 10 weeks*	Liposomal amphotericin B (AmBisome) 6 mg/kg (IV) q24h x 6-10 weeks† **or** Fluconazole 800 mg (IV or PO) x 1 dose, then 400 mg (PO) q24h x 10 weeks	PO therapy alone Not applicable
HIV	Cryptococcus neoformans	See p. 249		
Chronic meningitis	M. tuberculosis, Brucella, Leptospirosis, Listeria, T. pallidum, Cryptococcus, Coccidioidomycosis, Histoplasmosis, Toxoplasmosis, Toxocariasis, CMV, Neurocysticercosis, Neuroborreliosis, Enteroviruses			Treat specific pathogen after confirming diagnosis. Do not treat empirically

Duration of therapy represents total time PO (for TB), IV, or IV + PO

* The 6-week amphotericin B deoxycholate plus flucytosine regimen is the classical approach to achieving a durable cure. Anecdotal data suggest that a shorter course followed by fluconazole x 10 weeks (or longer) may be successful. Expert consultation is advised

† Other lipid-associated amphotericin B formulations at 3-5 mg/kg (IV) q24h may also be used (p. 297)

Viral (Aseptic) Meningitis

Clinical Presentation: Headache, low-grade fever, mild meningismus, photophobia

Diagnostic Considerations: Diagnosis by specific serological tests/viral culture. HSV-2 genital infections are often accompanied by mild CNS symptoms, which usually do not require anti-viral therapy. HSV-1 causes a variety of CNS infections, including meningitis, meningoencephalitis, and encephalitis (most common; see p. 24). HSV meningitis is indistinguishable clinically from other causes of viral meningitis. EBV meningitis is usually associated with clinical/laboratory features of EBV infectious mononucleosis; suspect the diagnosis in a patient with a positive monospot and unexplained meningoencephalitis. VZV meningitis is typically associated with cutaneous vesicular lesions (H. zoster), and usually does not require additional therapy beyond that given for shingles. LCM meningitis begins as a "flu-like" illness usually in the fall after hamster contact, and may have low CSF glucose. Enterovirus meningitis is often associated with a maculopapular rash, non-exudative pharyngitis, diarrhea, and rarely low CSF glucose

Pitfalls: Consider NSAIDs and IV immunoglobulin as non-infectious causes of aseptic meningitis

Therapeutic Considerations: Treat specific pathogen

Prognosis: Without neurological deficits, full recovery is the rule

Primary Amebic Meningoencephalitis (PAM) (Naegleria fowleri)

Clinical Presentation: Acquired by freshwater exposure containing the protozoa, often by jumping into a lake/pool. Affects healthy children/young adults. Organism penetrates cribriform plate and enters CSF. Symptoms occur within 7 days of exposure and are indistinguishable from fulminant bacterial meningitis, including headache, fever, anorexia, vomiting, signs of meningeal inflammation, altered mental status, coma. May complain of unusual smell/taste sensations early in infection. CSF has RBCs and very low glucose

Diagnostic Considerations: Diagnosis by demonstrating organism in CSF. Worldwide distribution. Free-living freshwater amoeba flourish in warmer climates. Key to diagnosis rests on clinical suspicion based on history of freshwater exposure in previous 1-2 weeks

Pitfalls: CSF findings resemble bacterial meningitis, but RBCs present

Therapeutic Considerations: Often fatal despite early treatment

Prognosis: Almost always fatal

Granulomatous Amebic Meningoencephalitis (Acanthamoeba)

Clinical Presentation: Insidious onset with focal neurologic deficits ± mental status changes, seizures, fever, headache, hemiparesis, meningismus, ataxia, visual disturbances. May be associated with Acanthamoeba keratoconjunctivitis, skin ulcers, or disseminated disease. Usually seen only in immunocompromised/debilitated patients

Diagnostic Considerations: Diagnosis by demonstrating organism in brain biopsy specimen. CT/MRI shows mass lesions. "Stellate cysts" characteristic of Acanthamoeba vs. "round cysts" of Naegleria. Worldwide distribution. Strong association with extended wear of contact lenses

Pitfalls: Not associated with freshwater exposure, unlike primary amebic meningoencephalitis (Naegleria fowleri). Resembles subacute/chronic meningitis. No trophozoites in CSF. Skin lesions may be present for months before onset of CNS symptoms

Therapeutic Considerations: No proven treatment. Often fatal despite early treatment

Prognosis: Usually fatal

TB Meningitis (Mycobacterium tuberculosis)

Clinical Presentation: Subacute onset of non-specific symptoms. Fever usually present ± headache, nausea, vomiting. Acute presentation and cranial nerve palsies uncommon

Diagnostic Considerations: Diagnosis by CSF AFB smear/culture; PCR of CSF is sensitive/specific. CSF may be normal, but often shows low glucose, increased protein, RBCs, and increased lactic acid. May find characteristic "pellicle" in CSF after 12 hours. Look for TB elsewhere

Pitfalls: CSF may have PMN predominance early, before developing typical lymphocytic predominance. Eosinophils in CSF is not a feature of TB, and should suggest another diagnosis

Therapeutic Considerations: Dexamethasone 4 mg (IV or PO) q6h x 2-4 weeks is useful to reduce CSF inflammation if given early

Prognosis: Poor prognostic factors include delay in treatment, neurologic deficits, or hydrocephalus. Proteinaceous TB exudates may obstruct ventricles and cause hydrocephalus, which is diagnosed by CT/MRI and may require shunt

Fungal (Cryptococcal) Meningitis (Cryptococcus neoformans)

Clinical Presentation: Insidious onset of non-specific symptoms. Headache most common. Chronic cases may have CNS symptoms for weeks to months with intervening asymptomatic periods. Acute manifestations are more common in AIDS, chronic steroid therapy, lymphoreticular malignancies. 50-80% of patients are abnormal hosts

Diagnostic Considerations: C. neoformans is the most common cause of fungal meningitis, and the only encapsulated yeast in the CSF to cause meningitis. Diagnosis by CSF India ink cryptococcal latex antigen/culture. Rule out HIV and other underlying immunosuppressive diseases

Pitfalls: CSF latex antigen titer may not return to zero. Continue treatment until titers decline/do not decrease further, and until CSF culture is negative for cryptococci. India ink smears of CSF are useful for initial infection, but should not be relied on to diagnose recurrent episodes, since smears may be positive despite negative CSF cultures (dead cryptococci may remain in CSF for years). Diagnosis of recurrences rests on CSF culture

Therapeutic Considerations: Treat until CSF is sterile or initial CSF latex antigen titer is zero or remains near zero on serial lumbar punctures. After patient defervesces on deoxycholate/5FC, switch to oral fluconazole x 10 weeks. Lipid-associated formulations of amphotericin B may be used if amphotericin B deoxycholate cannot be tolerated (p. 297). HIV patients require life-long suppressive therapy with fluconazole 200 mg (PO) q24h

Prognosis: Good. Poor prognostic factors include no CSF pleocytosis, many organisms in CSF, and altered consciousness on admission

Chronic Meningitis

Clinical Presentation: Same as acute meningitis, but signs/symptoms less prominent and clinical presentation is subacute (> 1 month)

Diagnostic Considerations: Differential diagnosis is too broad for empiric treatment. Subacute/chronic clinical presentation allows time for complete diagnostic work-up. Culture CSF and obtain CSF/serum tests to identify a specific pathogen, then treat

Pitfalls: If infectious etiology is not found, consider NSAIDs, SLE, meningeal carcinomatosis, sarcoidosis, etc. Chronic CMV or enterococcal meningitis should prompt search for underlying host defense defects/immunosuppression

Therapeutic Considerations: If suspicion of TB meningitis is high, empiric anti-TB treatment is warranted. Otherwise, treat only after diagnosing specific infection

Prognosis: Related to underlying health of host

Encephalitis

Subset	Usual Pathogens	IV-to-PO Switch
Herpes	HSV-1	Acyclovir 10 mg/kg (IV) q8h x 14-21 days. If able to take oral medications after 7 days of IV therapy, can complete 14-21 days of total therapy with acyclovir 400 mg (PO) 5x/day *or* valacyclovir 1 gm (PO) q8h *or* famciclovir 500 mg (PO) q8h
Arbovirus	<u>Usual Pathogens</u> California encephalitis (CE), Western equine encephalitis (WEE), Venezuelan equine encephalitis (VEE), Eastern equine encephalitis (EEE), St. Louis encephalitis (SLE), Japanese encephalitis (JE), West Nile encephalitis (WNE) <u>IV/PO Therapy</u> Not applicable	

Encephalitis (cont'd)

Subset	Usual Pathogens	Preferred IV Therapy	Alternate IV Therapy	IV-to-PO Switch
Mycoplasma	M. pneumoniae	Doxycycline 200 mg (IV) q12h x 3 days, then 100 mg (IV) q12h x 2-4 weeks	Minocycline 100 mg (IV) q12h x 2-4 weeks	Doxycycline 200 mg (PO) q12h x 3 days, then 100 mg (PO) q12h x 2-4 weeks* **or** Minocycline 100 mg (PO) q12h x 2-4 weeks
Solid organ transplants, HIV/AIDS	CMV T. gondii	For organ transplants, see pp. 125-126. For HIV/AIDS, see p. 249		

Duration of therapy represents total time IV or IV + PO. Most patients on IV therapy able to take PO meds should be switched to PO therapy after clinical improvement
* *Loading dose is not needed PO if given IV with the same drug*

Herpes Encephalitis (HSV-1)

Clinical Presentation: Acute onset of fever and change in mental status without nuchal rigidity

Diagnostic Considerations: EEG is best early (< 72 hours) presumptive test, showing unilateral temporal lobe abnormalities. Brain MRI is abnormal before CT scan, which may require several days before a temporal lobe focus is seen. Definitive diagnosis is by CSF PCR for HSV-1 DNA. Usually presents as encephalitis or meningoencephalitis; presentation as meningitis alone is uncommon. Profound decrease in sensorium is characteristic of HSV meningoencephalitis. CSF may have PMN predominance and low glucose levels, unlike other viral causes of meningitis

Pitfalls: Rule out non-infectious causes of encephalopathy

Therapeutic Considerations: HSV is the only treatable common cause of viral encephalitis in normal hosts. Treat as soon as possible, since neurological deficits may be mild and reversible early on, but severe and irreversible later

Prognosis: Related to extent of brain injury and early antiviral therapy

Arboviral Encephalitis

Clinical Presentation: Acute onset of fever, headache, change in mental status days to weeks after inoculation of virus through the bite of an infected insect (e.g., mosquito/tick). May progress over several days to stupor/coma

Diagnostic Considerations: Diagnosis by specific arboviral serology

Pitfalls: Usually occurs in summer/fall. Diagnosis suggested by arboviral contact/travel history. Electrolyte abnormalities due to syndrome of inappropriate antidiuretic hormone (SIADH) may occur

Therapeutic Considerations: Only supportive therapy is available at present

Prognosis: Permanent neurological deficits are common, but not predictable. May be fatal

Mycoplasma Encephalitis

Clinical Presentation: Acute onset of fever and change in mental status without nuchal rigidity

Diagnostic Considerations: Diagnosis suggested by CNS and extra-pulmonary manifestations—sore throat, otitis, E. multiforme, soft stools/diarrhea—in a patient with community-acquired pneumonia, elevated IgM mycoplasma titers, and very high (≥ 1:1024) cold agglutinin titers. CSF shows mild mononucleosis/pleocytosis and normal/low glucose

Pitfalls: CNS findings may overshadow pulmonary findings

Therapeutic Considerations: Macrolides will treat pulmonary infection, but not CNS infection (due to poor CNS penetration)
Prognosis: With early treatment, prognosis is good without neurologic sequelae

CMV Encephalitis (see pp. 125-126, 249)

Toxoplasma Encephalitis (see p. 249)

Brain Abscess/Subdural Empyema/Cavernous Vein Thrombosis/Intracranial Suppurative Thrombophlebitis

Subset	Usual Pathogens	Preferred IV Therapy	Alternate IV Therapy	IV-to-PO Switch
Brain Abscess (Single Mass Lesion)				
Open trauma	S. aureus Entero-bacteriaceae P. aeruginosa	Cefepime 2 gm (IV) q8h x 2 weeks	Meropenem 2 gm (IV) q8h x 2 weeks	Not applicable
Neurosurgical procedure (Treat initially for MSSA; if later identified as MRSA, MSSE or MRSE, treat accordingly)	S. aureus S. epidermidis	<u>MSSA/MSSE</u> Nafcillin 2 gm (IV) q4h x 2 weeks **or** Cefepime 2 gm (IV) q8h x 2 weeks **or** Ceftizoxime 3 gm (IV) q6h x 2 weeks <u>MRSA/MRSE</u> Linezolid 600 mg (IV) q12h x 2 weeks		<u>MSSA/MRSA</u> Linezolid 600 mg (PO) q12h x 2 weeks
Mastoid/ otitic source	Enterobacter Proteus	Cefepime 2 gm (IV) q8h x 2 weeks	Meropenem 2 gm (IV) q8h x 2 weeks	Not applicable
Dental source	Oral anaerobes Actinomyces	Ceftizoxime 3 gm (IV) q6h x 2 weeks	Ceftriaxone 2 gm (IV) q12h x 2 weeks **plus** Metronidazole 1 gm (IV) q24h x 2 weeks	Not applicable
Subdural empyema/ sinus source	Oral anaerobes H. influenzae	Ceftizoxime 3 gm (IV) q6h x 2 weeks	Ceftriaxone 2 gm (IV) q12h x 2 weeks **plus** Metronidazole 1 gm (IV) q24h x 2 weeks	Not applicable

Brain Abscess/Subdural Empyema/Cavernous Vein Thrombosis/Intracranial Suppurative Thrombophlebitis (cont'd)

Subset	Usual Pathogens	Preferred IV Therapy	Alternate IV Therapy	IV-to-PO Switch
Brain Abscess (Multiple Mass Lesions)				
Cardiac source (ABE; right-to-left shunt)	S. aureus S. pneumoniae H. influenzae	Cefepime 2 gm (IV) q8h x 2 weeks	Cefotaxime 3 gm (IV) q6h x 2 weeks **or** Meropenem 1 gm (IV) q8h x 2 weeks	Not applicable
Pulmonary source	Oral anaerobes Actinomyces	Ceftizoxime 3 gm (IV) q6h x 2 weeks	Ceftriaxone 2 gm (IV) q12h x 2 weeks **plus** Metronidazole 1 gm (IV) q24h x 2 weeks	Not applicable

MSSA/MRSA = methicillin-sensitive/resistant S. aureus; MSSE/MRSE = methicillin-sensitive/resistant S. epidermidis. Duration of therapy represents total time IV or IV + PO. Most patients on IV therapy able to take PO meds should be switched to PO therapy after clinical improvement

Clinical Presentation: Variable presentation, with fever, change in mental status, cranial nerve abnormalities ± headache

Diagnostic Considerations: Diagnosis by CSF gram stain/culture. If brain abscess is suspected, obtain head CT/MRI. Lumbar puncture may induce herniation

Pitfalls: CSF analysis is negative for bacterial meningitis unless abscess ruptures into ventricular system

Therapeutic Considerations: Treatment with meningeal doses of antibiotics is required. Large single abscesses may be surgically drained; multiple small abscesses are best treated medically

Prognosis: Related to underlying source and health of host

Brain Abscess (Mastoid/Otitic Source)

Diagnostic Considerations: Diagnosis by head CT/MRI demonstrating focus of infection in mastoid

Pitfalls: Rule out associated subdural empyema

Therapeutic Considerations: ENT consult for possible surgical debridement of mastoid

Prognosis: Good. May require mastoid debridement for cure

Brain Abscess (Dental Source)

Diagnostic Considerations: Diagnosis by panorex x-rays/gallium scan of jaw demonstrating focus in mandible/erosion into sinuses

Pitfalls: Apical root abscess may not be apparent clinically

Therapeutic Considerations: Large single abscess may be surgically drained. Multiple small abscesses are best treated medically. Treat until lesions on CT/MRI resolve or do not become smaller on therapy

Prognosis: Good if dental focus is removed

Brain Abscess (Subdural Empyema/Sinus Source)

Diagnostic Considerations: Diagnosis by sinus films/CT/MRI to confirm presence of sinusitis/bone erosion (cranial osteomyelitis/epidural abscess). Usually from paranasal sinusitis

Pitfalls: Do not overlook underlying sinus infection, which may need surgical drainage
Therapeutic Considerations: Obtain ENT consult for possible surgical debridement of sinuses
Prognosis: Good prognosis if sinus is drained

Brain Abscess (Cardiac Source; Acute Bacterial Endocarditis)
Diagnostic Considerations: Diagnosis by blood cultures positive for acute bacterial endocarditis (ABE) pathogen and multiple brain lesions on head CT/MRI
Pitfalls: Do not overlook right-to-left cardiac shunt (e.g., patent foramen ovale, atrial septal defect) as source of brain abscess. Cerebral embolization results in aseptic meningitis in SBE, but septic meningitis/brain abscess in ABE (due to high virulence of pathogens)
Therapeutic Considerations: Multiple lesions suggest hematogenous spread. Use sensitivity of blood culture isolates to determine coverage. Meningeal doses are the same as endocarditis doses
Prognosis: Related to location/size of CNS lesions and extent of cardiac valvular involvement

Brain Abscess (Pulmonary Source)
Diagnostic Considerations: Diagnosis suggested by underlying bronchiectasis, empyema, cystic fibrosis, or lung abscess in a patient with a brain abscess
Pitfalls: Brain abscesses are associated with chronic suppurative lung disease (e.g., bronchiectasis, lung abscess/empyema), not chronic bronchitis
Therapeutic Considerations: Lung abscess may need surgical drainage
Prognosis: Related to extent/location of CNS lesions, drainage of lung abscess/empyema, and control of lung infection

Empiric Therapy of HEENT Infections

Facial/Periorbital Cellulitis

Subset	Usual Pathogens	Preferred IV Therapy	Alternate IV Therapy	PO Therapy or IV-to-PO Switch
Facial cellulitis	Group A streptococci H. influenzae	Ceftriaxone 1 gm (IV) q24h x 2 weeks **or** Cefotaxime 2 gm (IV) q6h x 2 weeks **or** Ceftizoxime 2 gm (IV) q8h x 2 weeks	Quinolone* (IV) q24h x 2 weeks	Any oral 2nd or 3rd gen. cephalosporin x 2 weeks **or** Quinolone* (PO) q24h x 2 weeks

Duration of therapy represents total time IV, PO, or IV + PO. Most patients on IV therapy able to take PO meds should be switched to PO therapy soon after clinical improvement (usually < 72 hours)
* *Gatifloxacin 400 mg or levofloxacin 500 mg or moxifloxacin 400 mg*

Clinical Presentation: Acute onset of warm, painful, facial rash without discharge, swelling, pruritus
Diagnostic Considerations: Diagnosis by clinical appearance. May spread rapidly across face. Purplish hue suggests H. influenzae
Pitfalls: If periorbital cellulitis, obtain head CT/MRI to rule out underlying sinusitis/CNS involvement
Therapeutic Considerations: May need to treat x 3 weeks in compromised hosts (chronic steroids, diabetics, SLE, etc.)
Prognosis: Good with early treatment; worse if underlying sinusitis/CNS involvement

Sinusitis

Subset	Usual Pathogens	IV Therapy (Hospitalized)	PO Therapy or IV-to-PO Switch (Ambulatory)
Acute *Adults*	S. pneumoniae H. influenzae M. catarrhalis	Ceftriaxone 1 gm (IV) q24h x 2 weeks **or** Quinolone[†] (IV) q24h x 2 weeks **or** Doxycycline 200 mg (IV) q12h x 3 days, then 100 mg (IV) q12h x 11 days	Amoxicillin/clavulanic acid XR 2 tablets (PO) q12h x 10 days **or** Quinolone[†] (PO) q24h x 2 weeks **or** Telithromycin 800 mg (PO) q24h x 2 weeks **or** Doxycycline 200 mg (PO) q12h x 3 days, then 100 mg (PO) q12h x 11 days* **or** Cephalosporin[‡] (PO) x 2 weeks **or** Clarithromycin XL 1 gm (PO) q24h x 2 weeks
Children	S. pneumoniae H. influenzae M. catarrhalis	Ceftriaxone 25 mg/kg (IV) q12h x 1-2 weeks	Amoxicillin/clavulanic acid ES-600[§] 90 mg/kg/day (PO) in 2 divided doses x 10 days **or** Clarithromycin 7.5 mg/kg (PO) q12h x 2 wks **or** Cephalosporin[¶] (PO) x 2 weeks
Chronic	Same as acute + oral anaerobes	Requires prolonged antimicrobial therapy (2-4 weeks)	

Duration of therapy represents total time IV, PO, or IV + PO. Most patients on IV therapy able to take PO meds should be switched to PO therapy soon after clinical improvement (usually < 72 hours)
* *Loading dose is not needed PO if given IV with the same drug*
† *Moxifloxacin 400 mg or levofloxacin 500 mg or gatifloxacin 400 mg*
‡ *Adults: cefdinir 300 mg q12h or cefditoren 400 mg q12h or cefixime 400 mg q12h or cefpodoxime 200 mg q12h*
§ *ES-600 = 600 mg amoxicillin/5 mL*
¶ *Children: cefprozil 15 mg/kg (PO) q12h or cefuroxime axetil 15 mg/kg (PO) q12h or cefdinir 7 mg/kg (PO) q12h or 14 mg/kg (PO) q24h or cefpodoxime 5 mg/kg (PO) q12h*

Acute Sinusitis

Clinical Presentation: Nasal discharge and cough frequently with headache, facial pain, and low-grade fever lasting > 10-14 days. Can also present acutely with high fever (≥ 104° F) and purulent nasal discharge ± intense headache lasting for ≥ 3 days. Other manifestations depend on the affected sinus: maxillary sinus: percussion tenderness of molars; maxillary toothache; local extension may cause osteomyelitis of facial bones with proptosis, retroorbital cellulitis, ophthalmoplegia; direct intracranial extension is rare; frontal sinus: prominent headache; intracranial extension may cause epidural/brain abscess, meningitis, cavernous sinus/superior sagittal sinus thrombosis; orbital extension may cause periorbital cellulitis; ethmoid sinus: eyelid edema and prominent tearing; extension may cause retroorbital pain/periorbital cellulitis and/or cavernous sinus/superior sagittal sinus thrombosis; sphenoid sinus: severe headache; extension into cavernous sinus may cause meningitis, cranial nerve paralysis [III, IV, VI], temporal lobe abscess, cavernous sinus thrombosis. Cough and nasal discharge are prominent in children

Diagnostic Considerations: Diagnosis by sinus x-rays or CT/MRI showing complete sinus opacification, air-fluid levels, mucosal thickening. Consider sinus aspiration in immunocompromised hosts or treatment failures. In children, acute sinusitis is a clinical diagnosis; imaging studies are not routine

Pitfalls: May present as periorbital cellulitis (obtain head CT/MRI to rule out underlying sinusitis). If

CT/MRI demonstrates "post-septal" involvement, treat as acute bacterial meningitis. In children, transillumination, sinus tenderness to percussion, and color of nasal mucus are not reliable indicators of sinusitis

Therapeutic Considerations: Treat for full course to prevent relapses/complications. Macrolides and TMP-SMX may predispose to drug-resistant S. pneumoniae (DRSP), and 25% of S. pneumoniae are naturally resistant to macrolides

Prognosis: Good if treated for full course. Relapses may occur with suboptimal treatment. For frequent recurrences, consider radiologic studies and ENT consultation

Chronic Sinusitis

Clinical Presentation: Generalized headache, fatigue, nasal congestion, post-nasal drip lasting > 3 months with little/no sinus tenderness by percussion. Local symptoms often subtle. Fever is uncommon

Diagnostic Considerations: Sinus films and head CT/MRI are less useful than for acute sinusitis (chronic mucosal abnormalities may persist after infection is treated). Many cases of chronic maxillary sinusitis are due to a dental cause; obtain odontogenic x-rays if suspected

Pitfalls: Clinical presentation is variable/non-specific. Malaise and irritability may be more prominent than local symptoms. May be mistaken for allergic rhinitis. Head CT/MRI can rule out sinus tumor

Therapeutic Considerations: Therapeutic failure/relapse is usually due to inadequate antibiotic duration, dose, or tissue penetration. Treat for full course. If symptoms persist after 4 weeks of therapy, refer to ENT for surgical drainage procedure

Prognosis: Good

Keratitis

Subset	Pathogens	Topical Therapy
Bacterial	S. aureus M. catarrhalis P. aeruginosa	Antibacterial eyedrops (ciprofloxacin, ofloxacin, or tobramycin/bacitracin/polymyxin B) hourly while awake x 2 weeks
Viral	HSV-1	Trifluridine 1% solution 1 drop hourly while awake x 2 days, then 1 drop q6h x 14-21 days **or** viral ophthalmic topical ointment (e.g., vidarabine) at bedtime x 14-21 days
Amebic	Acanthamoeba	Propamidine (0.1%), neomycin, gramicidin, or polymyxin B eyedrops hourly while awake x 1-2 weeks **or** polyhexamethylene biguanide (0.02%) eyedrops hourly while awake x 1-2 weeks **or** chlorhexidine (0.02%) eyedrops hourly while awake x 1-2 weeks

Clinical Presentation: Corneal haziness, infiltrates, or ulcers
Diagnosis: Appearance of corneal lesions/culture

Bacterial Keratitis

Diagnostic Considerations: Usually secondary to eye trauma. Always obtain ophthalmology consult
Pitfalls: Be sure to culture ulcer. Unusual organisms are common in eye trauma
Therapeutic Considerations: Treat until lesions resolve. Ointment easier/lasts longer than solutions. Avoid topical steroids
Prognosis: Related to extent of trauma/organism. S. aureus, P. aeruginosa have a worse prognosis

Viral Keratitis (HSV-1)

Diagnostic Considerations: "Dendritic" corneal ulcers characteristic. Obtain ophthalmology consult
Pitfalls: Small corneal ulcers may be missed without fluorescein staining
Therapeutic Considerations: Treat until lesions resolve. Oral acyclovir is not needed. Avoid ophthalmic steroid ointment
Prognosis: Good if treated early (before eye damage is extensive)

Amebic Keratitis (Acanthamoeba)
Diagnostic Considerations: Usually associated with extended use of soft contact lenses. Corneal scrapings are positive with calcofluor staining. Acanthamoeba keratitis is painful with typical circular, hazy, corneal infiltrate. Always obtain ophthalmology consult
Pitfalls: Do not confuse with HSV-1 dendritic ulcers. Avoid topical steroids
Therapeutic Considerations: If secondary bacterial infection, treat as bacterial keratitis
Prognosis: No good treatment. Poor prognosis

Conjunctivitis

Subset	Usual Pathogens	PO/Topical Therapy
Bacterial	M. catarrhalis H. influenzae S. pneumoniae	Antibacterial eyedrops (ciprofloxacin, ofloxacin, or tobramycin/bacitracin/polymyxin B) q12h x 1 week plus antibacterial ointment (same antibiotic) at bedtime x 1 week
Viral	Adenovirus	Not applicable
	VZV	Famciclovir 500 mg (PO) q8h x 10-14 days *or* Valacyclovir 1 gm (PO) q8h x 10-14 days
Chlamydial	C. trachomatis C. psittaci	Doxycycline 100 mg (PO) q12h x 1-2 weeks *or* Azithromycin 1 gm (PO) x 1 dose

Bacterial Conjunctivitis
Clinical Presentation: Profuse, purulent exudate from conjunctiva
Diagnostic Considerations: Reddened conjunctiva; culture for specific pathogen
Pitfalls: Do not confuse with allergic conjunctivitis, which itches and has a clear discharge
Therapeutic Considerations: Obtain ophthalmology consult. Ointment lasts longer in eye than solution. Do not use topical steroids without an antibacterial
Prognosis: Excellent when treated early, with no residual visual impairment

Viral Conjunctivitis
Adenovirus
Clinical Presentation: Reddened conjunctiva, watery discharge, negative bacterial culture
Diagnostic Considerations: Diagnosis by cloudy/steamy cornea with negative bacterial cultures. Clue is punctate infiltrates with a cloudy cornea. Extremely contagious; careful handwashing is essential. Obtain viral culture of conjunctiva for diagnosis
Pitfalls: Pharyngitis a clue to adenoviral etiology (pharyngoconjunctival fever)
Therapeutic Considerations: No treatment available. Usually resolves in 1-2 weeks
Prognosis: Related to degree of corneal haziness. Severe cases may take weeks to clear

VZV Ophthalmicus
Diagnostic Considerations: Vesicles on tip of nose predict eye involvement
Pitfalls: Do not miss vesicular lesions in external auditory canal in patients with facial palsy (Ramsey-Hunt Syndrome)
Therapeutic Considerations: Obtain ophthalmology consult. Topical steroids may be used if given with anti-VZV therapy
Prognosis: Good if treated early with systemic antivirals

Chlamydial Conjunctivitis
Diagnostic Considerations: Diagnosis by direct fluorescent antibody (DFA)/culture of conjunctiva
Pitfalls: Do not confuse bilateral, upper lid, granular conjunctivitis of Chlamydia with viral/bacterial conjunctivitis, which involves both upper and lower eyelids
Therapeutic Considerations: Ophthalmic erythromycin treatment is useful for neonates
Prognosis: Excellent with early treatment

Chorioretinitis

Subset	Usual Pathogens	Preferred IV Therapy	Alternate IV Therapy	PO Therapy or IV-to-PO Switch
Viral	CMV	See p. 253		
Fungal†	Candida albicans	Fluconazole 800 mg (IV) x 1 dose, then 400 mg (IV) q24h x 2 weeks **or** Caspofungin 70 mg (IV) x 1 dose, then 50 mg (IV) q24h x 2 weeks	Amphotericin B deoxycholate 0.6 mg/kg (IV) q24h for total of 1 gm **or** Lipid-associated formulation of amphotericin B (p. 297) (IV) q24h x 3 weeks	Fluconazole 800 mg (PO) x 1 dose, then 400 mg (PO) q24h x 2 weeks*
Protozoal	Toxoplasma gondii	<u>IV Therapy</u> Not applicable	<u>PO Therapy</u> Pyrimethamine 75 mg (PO) x 1 dose, then 25 mg (PO) q24h x 6 weeks **plus either** Sulfadiazine 1 gm (PO) q6h x 6 weeks **or** Clindamycin 300 mg (PO) q8h x 6 weeks	

Duration of therapy represents total time IV, PO, or IV + PO. Most patients on IV therapy able to take PO meds should be switched to PO therapy after clinical improvement
† *Treat only IV or IV-to-PO switch*
* *Loading dose is not needed PO if given IV with the same drug*

CMV Chorioretinitis (see p. 253)

Candida Chorioretinitis
Clinical Presentation: Small, raised, white, circular lesions on retina
Diagnostic Considerations: Fundus findings similar to white, raised colonies on blood agar plates
Pitfalls: Candida endophthalmitis signifies invasive/disseminated candidiasis
Therapeutic Considerations: Treat as disseminated candidiasis
Prognosis: Good with early treatment

Toxoplasma Chorioretinitis
Clinical Presentation: Grey/black pigmentation of macula
Diagnostic Considerations: Diagnosis by IgM IFA toxoplasmosis titers
Pitfalls: Unilateral endophthalmitis usually indicates acquired toxoplasmosis; congenital toxoplasmosis is usually bilateral
Therapeutic Considerations: Obtain ophthalmology consult. Treat only acute/active toxoplasmosis with visual symptoms; do not treat chronic chorioretinitis. Add folinic acid 10 mg (PO) q24h to prevent folic acid deficiency
Prognosis: Related to degree of immunosuppression

Endophthalmitis

Subset	Usual Pathogens	Preferred IV Therapy	Alternate IV Therapy	PO Therapy or IV-to-PO Switch
Bacterial (Treat initially for MSSA; if later identified as MRSA or S. epidermidis, treat accordingly)	Streptococci H. influenzae S. aureus (MSSA)	Intravitreal injection: Cefepime 2.25 mg/0.1 mL sterile saline x 1 dose; repeat x 1 if needed in 2-3 days **plus** Subconjunctival injection: Cefepime 100 mg/0.5 mL sterile saline q24h x 1-2 weeks		
	S. aureus (MRSA) S. epidermidis	Intravitreal injection: Vancomycin 1 mg/0.1 mL sterile saline x 1 dose; repeat x 1 if needed in 2-3 days **plus** Subconjunctival injection: Vancomycin 2.5 mg/0.5 mL sterile saline q24h x 1-2 weeks		
TB	M. tuberculosis	<u>IV Therapy</u> Not applicable	<u>PO Therapy</u> INH 300 mg (PO) q24h x 6-12 months **plus** Rifampin 600 mg (PO) q24h x 6-12 months <u>If multiresistant TB strain likely, also add</u> EMB 15 mg/kg (PO) q24h x 6-12 months **plus** PZA 25 mg/kg (PO) q24h x 6-12 months	
Infected lens implant* (Treat initially for MSSA; if later identified as MRSA, treat accordingly)	Entero-bacteriaceae S. aureus (MSSA)	Meropenem 1 gm (IV) q8h x 2 weeks **or** Imipenem 500 mg (IV) q6h x 2 weeks	Cefepime 2 gm (IV) q8h x 2 weeks **or** Chloramphenicol 500 mg (IV) q6h x 2 weeks	Chloramphenicol 500 mg (PO) q6h x 2 weeks
	S. aureus (MRSA)	Linezolid 600 mg (IV) q12h x 2 weeks	Minocycline 100 mg (IV) q12h x 2 weeks	Linezolid 600 mg (PO) q12h x 2 weeks **or** Minocycline 100 mg (PO) q12h x 2 weeks

EMB = ethambutol; INH = isoniazid; MSSA/MRSA = methicillin-sensitive/resistant S. aureus; PZA = pyrazinamide. Duration of therapy represents total time IV, PO, or IV + PO. Most patients on IV therapy able to take PO meds should be switched to PO therapy after clinical improvement (usually < 72 hours)
* Treat only IV or IV-to-PO switch

Bacterial Endophthalmitis
Clinical Presentation: Ocular pain/sudden vision loss
Diagnosis: Post-op endophthalmitis occurs 1-7 days after surgery. Hypopyon seen in anterior chamber
Pitfalls: Delayed-onset endophthalmitis may occur up to 6 weeks post-op. White intracapsular plaque is characteristic
Therapeutic Considerations: Use steroids (dexamethasone 0.4 mg/0.1 mL intravitreal and 10 mg/

1 mL subconjunctival) with antibiotics in post-op endophthalmitis. Also use systemic antibiotics for severe cases. Vitrectomy is usually necessary
Prognosis: Related to pathogen virulence

Tuberculous (TB) Endophthalmitis
Clinical Presentation: Raised retinal punctate lesions ± visual impairment
Diagnostic Considerations: Signs of extraocular TB are usually present. Confirm diagnosis of miliary TB by liver/bone biopsy
Pitfalls: TB endophthalmitis is a sign of disseminated TB
Therapeutic Considerations: Treat as disseminated TB. Systemic steroids may be used if given with anti-TB therapy
Prognosis: Related to degree of immunosuppression

Infected Lens Implant
Diagnostic Considerations: Diagnosis by clinical appearance and culture of anterior chamber. Obtain ophthalmology consult
Pitfalls: Superficial cultures are inadequate. Anterior chamber aspirate may be needed for culture
Therapeutic Considerations: Infected lens must be removed for cure
Prognosis: Good with early lens removal and recommended antibiotics

External Otitis

Subset	Usual Pathogens	Preferred IV Therapy	Alternate IV Therapy	Topical Therapy or IV-to-PO Switch
Benign	P. aeruginosa	Not applicable	Not applicable	Use otic solutions only (ofloxacin 0.3%, tobramycin, polymyxin B); apply ear drops q6h x 1 week
Malignant	P. aeruginosa	**One "A" drug + one "B" drug:** **"A" drugs** Cefepime 2 gm (IV) q8h x 4-6 weeks **or** Piperacillin/tazobactam 4.5 gm (IV) q8h x 4-6 weeks **"B" drugs** Ciprofloxacin 400 mg (IV) q12h x 4-6 weeks **or** Gentamicin 120 mg (IV) q24h x 4-6 weeks	Aztreonam 2 gm (IV) q8h x 4-6 weeks **plus either** Gentamicin 120 mg (IV) q24h x 4-6 weeks **or** Amikacin 1 gm (IV) q24h x 4-6 weeks	Ciprofloxacin 750 mg (PO) q12h x 4-6 weeks **or** Levofloxacin 750 mg (PO) q24h x 4-6 weeks

Duration of therapy represents total time topically (benign), or IV + PO (malignant). Most patients on IV therapy able to take PO meds should be switched to PO therapy soon after clinical improvement (usually < 72 hours)

Benign External Otitis (Pseudomonas aeruginosa)

Clinical Presentation: Acute external ear canal drainage without perforation of tympanic membrane or bone involvement

Diagnostic Considerations: Diagnosis suggested by external ear drainage after water exposure. Usually acquired from swimming pools ("swimmers ear"). Not an invasive infection

Pitfalls: Be sure external otitis is not associated with perforated tympanic membrane, which requires ENT consultation and systemic antibiotics

Therapeutic Considerations: Treat topically until symptoms/infection resolve

Prognosis: Excellent with topical therapy

Malignant External Otitis (Pseudomonas aeruginosa)

Clinical Presentation: External ear canal drainage with bone involvement

Diagnostic Considerations: Diagnosis by demonstrating P. aeruginosa in soft tissue culture from ear canal plus bone/cartilage involvement on x-ray. Usually affects diabetics. CT/MRI of head shows bony involvement of external auditory canal

Pitfalls: Rare in non-diabetics

Therapeutic Considerations: Requires surgical debridement plus antibiotic therapy for cure

Prognosis: Related to control of diabetes mellitus

Acute Otitis Media

Subset	Usual Pathogens	IM Therapy	PO Therapy
Initial uncomplicated bacterial infection	S. pneumoniae H. influenzae M. catarrhalis	Ceftriaxone 50 mg/kg (IM) x 1 dose	Amoxicillin 30 mg/kg (PO) q8h x 10 days **or** Clarithromycin 7.5 mg/kg (PO) q12h x 10 days **or** Azithromycin 10 mg/kg (PO) x 1 dose, then 5 mg/kg (PO) q24h x 4 days
Treatment failure or resistant organism*	DRSP Beta-lactamase positive H. influenzae	Ceftriaxone 50 mg/kg (IM) q24h x 3 doses	Amoxicillin/clavulanic acid ES-600 90 mg/kg/day (PO) in 2 divided doses x 10 days[†] **or** Cephalosporin[†] (PO) x 10 days

DRSP = drug-resistant S. pneumoniae. Pediatric doses are provided; acute otitis media is uncommon in adults. For chronic otitis media, prolonged antimicrobial therapy is required

* Treatment failure = persistent symptoms and otoscopy abnormalities 48-72 hours after starting initial antimicrobial therapy. For risk factors for DRSP, see Therapeutic Considerations (top next page)

† ES-600 = 600 mg amoxicillin/5 mL. Cephalosporins: cefuroxime axetil 15 mg/kg (PO) q12h or cefdinir 7 mg/kg (PO) q12h or 14 mg/kg (PO) q24h or cefpodoxime 5 mg/kg (PO) q12h may be used

Acute Otitis Media

Clinical Presentation: Fever, otalgia, hearing loss. Nonspecific presentation is more common in younger children (irritability, fever). Key to diagnosis is examination of the tympanic membrane. Uncommon in adults

Diagnostic Considerations: Diagnosis is made by finding an opaque, hyperemic, bulging tympanic membrane with loss of landmarks and decreased mobility on pneumatic otoscopy

Pitfalls: Failure to remove cerumen (inadequate visualization of tympanic membrane) and reliance on history of ear tugging/pain are the main factors associated with overdiagnosis of otitis media. Otitis media with effusion (i.e., tympanic membrane retracted or in normal position with decreased mobility or mobility with negative pressure; fluid present behind the drum but normal in color) usually resolves spontaneously and should not be treated with antibiotics

Therapeutic Considerations: Risk factors for infection with drug-resistant S. pneumoniae (DRSP) include antibiotic therapy in past 30 days, failure to respond within 48-72 hours of therapy, day care attendance, and antimicrobial prophylaxis. Macrolides and TMP-SMX may predispose to DRSP, and 25% of S. pneumoniae are naturally resistant to macrolides

Prognosis: Excellent, but tends to recur. Chronic otitis, cholesteatomas, mastoiditis are rare complications. Tympanostomy tubes/adenoidectomy for frequent recurrences of otitis media are the leading surgical procedures in children

Mastoiditis

Subset	Usual Pathogens	Preferred IV Therapy	Alternate IV Therapy	PO Therapy or IV-to-PO Switch
Acute	S. pneumoniae H. influenzae S. aureus	Ceftriaxone 1-2 gm (IV) q24h x 2 weeks **or** Cefotaxime 2 gm (IV) q6h x 2 weeks **or** Cefepime 2 gm (IV) q12h x 2 weeks	Gatifloxacin 400 mg (IV) q24h x 2 weeks **or** Levofloxacin 500 mg (IV) q24h x 2 weeks **or** Moxifloxacin 400 mg (IV) q24h x 2 weeks	Gatifloxacin 400 mg (PO) q24h x 2 weeks **or** Levofloxacin 500 mg (PO) q24h x 2 weeks **or** Moxifloxacin 400 mg (PO) q24h x 2 weeks
Chronic	S. pneumoniae H. influenzae P. aeruginosa S. aureus Oral anaerobes	Cefepime 2 gm (IV) q8h x 4-6 weeks **or** Meropenem 1 gm (IV) q8h x 4-6 weeks	Quinolone* (IV) x 4-6 weeks	Quinolone* (PO) x 4-6 weeks

Duration of therapy represents total time IV, PO, or IV + PO. Most patients on IV therapy able to take PO meds should be switched to PO therapy soon after clinical improvement (usually < 72 hours)

* Ciprofloxacin 400 mg (IV) or 750 mg (PO) q12h or gatifloxacin 400 mg (IV or PO) q24h or levofloxacin 750 mg (IV or PO) q24h or moxifloxacin 400 mg (IV or PO) q24h

Acute Mastoiditis

Clinical Presentation: Pain/tenderness over mastoid with fever

Diagnostic Considerations: Diagnosis by CT/MRI showing mastoid involvement

Pitfalls: Obtain head CT/MRI to rule out extension into CNS presenting as acute bacterial meningitis

Prognosis: Good if treated early

Chronic Mastoiditis

Clinical Presentation: Subacute pain/tenderness over mastoid with low-grade fever

Diagnostic Considerations: Diagnosis by CT/MRI showing mastoid involvement

Pitfalls: Obtain head CT/MRI to rule out CNS extension

Therapeutic Considerations: Usually requires surgical debridement for cure. Should be viewed as chronic osteomyelitis

Prognosis: Progressive without surgery. Poor prognosis with associated meningitis/brain abscess

Suppurative Parotitis

Subset	Usual Pathogens	Preferred IV Therapy	Alternate IV Therapy	PO Therapy or IV-to-PO Switch
Parotitis	S. aureus Entero-bacteriaceae Oral anaerobes	Meropenem 1 gm (IV) q8h x 2 weeks **or** Ceftriaxone 1 gm (IV) q24h x 2 weeks **or** Piperacillin/ tazobactam 4.5 gm (IV) q8h x 2 weeks	Clindamycin 600 mg (IV) q8h x 2 weeks **plus** Quinolone* (IV) q24h x 2 weeks **or monotherapy with** Ceftizoxime 2 gm (IV) q8h x 2 weeks	Clindamycin 300 mg (PO) q8h x 2 weeks **plus** Quinolone* (PO) q24h x 2 weeks

Duration of therapy represents total time IV, PO, or IV + PO. Most patients on IV therapy able to take PO meds should be switched to PO therapy soon after clinical improvement (usually < 72 hours)
* *Gatifloxacin 400 mg or levofloxacin 500 mg or moxifloxacin 400 mg*

Clinical Presentation: Unilateral parotid pain/swelling with discharge from Stensen's duct ± fever
Diagnostic Considerations: Diagnosis by clinical presentation, ↑ amylase, CT/MRI demonstrating stone in parotid duct/gland involvement
Pitfalls: Differentiate from unilateral mumps by purulent discharge from Stensen's duct
Therapeutic Considerations: If duct is obstructed, remove stone
Prognosis: Good with early therapy/hydration

Pharyngitis/Chronic Fatigue Syndrome (CFS)

Subset	Usual Pathogens	PO Therapy
Bacterial	Group A streptococci	Amoxicillin 1 gm (PO) q8h x 7-10 days **or** Cefprozil 500 mg (PO) q12h x 7-10 days **or** Clindamycin 300 mg (PO) q8h x 7-10 days **or** Clarithromycin XL 1 gm (PO) q24h x 7-10 days **or** Azithromycin 500 mg (PO) x 1 dose, then 250 mg (PO) q24h x 4 days
Viral	Respiratory viruses EBV, CMV, HHV-6	Not applicable. EBV/CMV do not cause primary pharyngitis, but pharyngitis is part of the infectious mono syndrome, along with hepatitis and lymph node involvement. See viral hepatitis (p. 75)
Other	M. pneumoniae C. pneumoniae	Quinolone* (PO) q24h x 1 weeks **or** Doxycycline 100 mg (PO) q12h x 1 weeks **or** Clarithromycin XL 1 gm (PO) q24h x 1 weeks **or** Azithromycin 500 mg (PO) x 1 dose, then 250 mg (PO) q24h x 4 days

Chronic fatigue syndrome. Pathogen not known (not EBV). See therapeutic considerations (p. 39)

* *Gatifloxacin 400 mg or levofloxacin 500 mg or moxifloxacin 400 mg*

Bacterial Pharyngitis

Clinical Presentation: Acute sore throat with fever, bilateral anterior cervical adenopathy, and elevated ASO titer. No hoarseness

Diagnostic Considerations: Diagnosis of Group A streptococcal pharyngitis by elevated ASO titer after initial sore throat and positive throat culture. Rapid strep tests unnecessary, since delay in culture results (~1 week) still allows adequate time to initiate therapy and prevent acute rheumatic fever. Group A streptococcal pharyngitis is rare in adults > 30 years

Pitfalls: Gram stain of throat exudate differentiates Group A streptococcal colonization (few or no PMNs) from infection (many PMNs) in patients with a positive throat culture or rapid strep test. Neither throat culture nor rapid strep test alone differentiates colonization from infection

Therapeutic Considerations: Benzathine penicillin 1.2 mu (IM) x 1 dose can be used as an alternative to oral therapy. Penicillin, erythromycin, and ampicillin fail in 15% of cases due to poor penetration into oral secretions or beta-lactamase producing oral organisms

Prognosis: Excellent. Treat within 10 days to prevent acute rheumatic fever

Viral Pharyngitis

Clinical Presentation: Acute sore throat. Other features depend on specific pathogen

Diagnostic Considerations: Most cases of viral pharyngitis are caused by respiratory viruses, and are frequently accompanied by hoarseness, but not high fever, pharyngeal exudates, palatal petechiae, or posterior cervical adenopathy. Other causes of viral pharyngitis (EBV, CMV, HHV-6) are usually associated with posterior cervical adenopathy and ↑ SGOT/SGPT. EBV mono may present with exudative or non-exudative pharyngitis, and is diagnosed by negative ASO titer with a positive mono spot test or elevated EBV IgM viral capsid antigen (VCA) titer. Before mono spot test turns positive (may take up to 8 weeks), a presumptive diagnosis of EBV mono can be made by ESR and SGOT, which are elevated in EBV and normal in Group A streptococcal pharyngitis. If EBV mono spot is negative, retest weekly x 8 weeks; if still negative, obtain IgM CMV/toxoplasmosis titers to diagnose the cause of "mono spot negative" pharyngitis

Pitfalls: 30% of patients with viral pharyngitis have Group A streptococcal colonization. Look for viral features to suggest the correct diagnosis (leukopenia, lymphocytosis, atypical lymphocytes)

Therapeutic Considerations: Symptomatic care only. Short-term steroids should only be used in EBV infection if airway obstruction is present/imminent. Since 30% of patients with viral pharyngitis are colonized with Group A streptococci, do not treat throat cultures positive for Group A streptococci if non-streptococcal pharyngitis features are present (e.g., bilateral posterior cervical adenopathy)

Prognosis: Related to extent of systemic infection. Post-viral fatigue is common. CMV may remain active in liver for 6-12 months with mildly elevated serum transaminases

Mycoplasma/Chlamydia Pharyngitis

Clinical Presentation: Acute sore throat ± laryngitis. Usually non-exudative

Diagnostic Considerations: Diagnosis by elevated IgM M. pneumoniae or C. pneumoniae titers. Consider diagnosis in patients with non-exudative pharyngitis without viral or streptococcal pharyngitis. Mycoplasma pharyngitis is often accompanied by otitis/bullous myringitis

Pitfalls: Patients with C. pneumoniae frequently have laryngitis, which is not a feature of EBV, CMV, Group A streptococcal, or M. pneumoniae pharyngitis

Therapeutic Considerations: Treatment of C. pneumoniae laryngitis results in rapid (~ 3 days) return of normal voice, which does not occur with viral pharyngitis

Prognosis: Excellent

Chronic Fatigue Syndrome (CFS)

Clinical Presentation: Fatigue > 1 year with cognitive impairment ± mild pharyngitis

Diagnostic Considerations: Rule out other causes of chronic fatigue (cancer, adrenal/thyroid disease, etc.) before diagnosing CFS. HHV-6/Coxsackie B titers are usually elevated. Some have ↓ natural kill (NK) cells/activity. ESR ~ 0. Crimson crescents in the posterior pharynx are common

Pitfalls: ↑ VCA IgG EBV titers is common in CFS, but EBV does not cause CFS. Do not confuse CFS with fibromyalgia, which has muscular "trigger points" and no cognitive impairment. CFS and fibromyalgia may coexist

Therapeutic Considerations: No specific therapy is available. Patients with ↓ NK cells may benefit from beta-carotene 50,000 U (PO) q24h x 3 weeks. Patients with ↑ C. pneumoniae titers may benefit from doxycycline 100 mg (PO) q24h x 2 weeks or azithromycin 250 mg (PO) q24h x 2 weeks

Prognosis: Cyclical illness with remissions and flares (precipitated by exertion). Avoid exercise

Thrush (Oropharyngeal Candidiasis)

Subset	Usual Pathogens	PO Therapy
Fungal	C. albicans	Fluconazole 200 mg (PO) x 1 dose, then 100 mg (PO) q24h x 1-2 weeks **or** Itraconazole 200 mg (PO) solution q24h x 1-2 weeks **or** Clotrimazole 10 mg troches (PO) 5x/day x 2 weeks
	Fluconazole-unresponsive infection	Itraconazole 100 mg (PO) solution q12h x 1-2 weeks **or** Voriconazole 200 mg (PO) q12h x 1-2 weeks **or** Caspofungin 70 mg (IV) x 1, then 50 mg (IV) q24h x 1-2 weeks

Thrush (Oropharyngeal Candidiasis)

Clinical Presentation: White coated tongue or oropharynx. White adherent plaques may be on any part of the oropharynx

Diagnostic Considerations: Gram stain/culture of white plaques demonstrates yeasts (Candida). Culture and susceptibility testing of causative fungus is useful in analyzing failure to respond to therapy

Pitfalls: Lateral, linear, white, striated tongue lesions may resemble thrush but are really hairy leukoplakia. Hairy leukoplakia should suggest HIV/AIDS. Thrush may occur in children, alcoholics, diabetics, those receiving steroids/antibiotic therapy, HIV/AIDS

Therapeutic Considerations: Almost all infections are caused by C. albicans, a species that is usually sensitive to fluconazole. Fluconazole-unresponsive infections may be caused by infection with fluconazole-resistant C. albicans (most common explanation), infection with a fluconazole-resistant non-albicans species (rare), noncompliance with therapy (common), or drug interactions (e.g., concomitant usage of rifampin, which markedly reduced azole blood levels). For suspected fluconazole-resistance, a trial with another azole is appropriate as cross-resistance is not universal

Prognosis: Non-HIV/AIDS patients respond well to therapy, particularly when the predisposing factor is eliminated/decreased (i.e., antibiotics discontinued, steroids reduced, etc.). HIV/AIDS patients may require longer courses of therapy and should be treated until cured. Relapse is frequent in HIV/AIDS patients, and institution of effective antiretroviral therapy is the most effective general strategy

Mouth Ulcers/Vesicles

Subset	Usual Pathogens	Preferred IV Therapy	Alternate IV Therapy	PO Therapy or IV-to-PO Switch
Vincent's angina	Borrelia Fusobacterium	Clindamycin 600 mg (IV) q8h x 2 weeks	Ceftizoxime 2 gm (IV) q8h x 2 weeks **or** Any beta-lactam (IV) x 2 weeks	Clindamycin 300 mg (PO) q8h x 2 weeks **or** Amoxicillin/ clavulanic acid 500/125 mg (PO) q8hx 2 weeks
Ludwig's angina	Group A streptococci	Clindamycin 600 mg (IV) q8h x 2 weeks	Ceftizoxime 2 gm (IV) q8h x 2 weeks **or** Any beta-lactam (IV) x 2 weeks	Clindamycin 300 mg (PO) q8h x 2 weeks **or** Amoxicillin/ clavulanic acid 500/125 mg (PO) q8h x 2 weeks
Stomatitis	Normal mouth flora	Not applicable	Not applicable	Not applicable
Herpangina	Coxsackie A virus	Not applicable	Not applicable	Not applicable
Herpes gingivo-stomatitis	HSV-1	Not applicable	PO Therapy Valacyclovir 500 mg (PO) q12h x 1 week **or** Famciclovir 500 mg (PO) q12h x 1 week **or** Acyclovir 400 mg (PO) 5x/day x 1 week	
Herpes labialis (cold sores/ fever blisters)	HSV-1 (recurrent)	Not applicable	PO Therapy Valacyclovir 2 gm (PO) q12h x 1 day (2 doses) started at onset of symptoms (tingling/burning) Topical Therapy Penciclovir 1% cream q2h while awake x 4 days **or** Acyclovir 5% cream 5x/d x 4 days	
Aphthous ulcers	Normal mouth flora	Not applicable	Not applicable	

Duration of therapy represents total time IV, PO, or IV + PO. Most patients on IV therapy able to take PO meds should be switched to PO therapy soon after clinical improvement (usually < 72 hours)

Clinical Presentation: Painful mouth ulcers/vesicles without fever

Vincent's Angina (Borrelia/Fusobacterium)

Diagnostic Considerations: Foul breath, poor dental hygiene/pyorrhea
Pitfalls: Do not attribute foul breath to poor dental hygiene without considering other serious causes (e.g., lung abscess, renal failure)
Therapeutic Considerations: After control of acute infection, refer to dentist
Prognosis: Excellent with early treatment

Ludwig's Angina (Group A streptococci)

Diagnostic Considerations: Fever with elevated floor of mouth is diagnostic. Massive neck swelling may be evident
Pitfalls: C_{1q} deficiency has perioral/tongue swelling, but no fever or floor of mouth elevation
Therapeutic Considerations: Surgical drainage is not necessary. May need airway emergently; have tracheotomy set at bedside
Prognosis: Early airway obstruction has adverse impact on prognosis

Stomatitis (normal mouth flora)

Diagnostic Considerations: Diagnosis based on clinical appearance
Pitfalls: Do not miss a systemic cause (e.g., acute leukemia)
Therapeutic Considerations: Painful; treat symptomatically.
Prognosis: Related to severity of underlying systemic disease

Herpangina (Coxsackie A virus)

Diagnostic Considerations: Ulcers located posteriorly in pharynx. No gum involvement or halitosis
Pitfalls: Do not confuse with anterior vesicular lesions of HSV
Therapeutic Considerations: No good treatment available. Usually resolves spontaneously in 2 weeks
Prognosis: Good, but may be recurrent

Herpes Gingivostomatitis (HSV-1)

Diagnostic Considerations: Anterior ulcers in pharynx. Associated with bleeding gums, not halitosis
Pitfalls: Do not miss a systemic disease associated with bleeding gums (e.g., acute myelogenous leukemia). Periodontal disease is not usually associated with oral ulcers
Therapeutic Considerations: Oral analgesic solutions may help in swallowing
Prognosis: Excellent with early treatment

Herpes Labialis (Cold Sores/Fever Blisters) (HSV-1)

Diagnostic Considerations: Caused by recurrrent HSV-1 infection, which appears as painful vesicular lesions on/near the vermillion border of lips. Attacks may be triggered by stress, sun exposure, mestruation, and often begin with pain or tingling before vesicles appear. Vesicles crust over and attacks usually resolve by 1 week. "Fever blisters" are not triggered by temperature elevations per se, but may accompany malaria, pneumococcal/meningococcal meningitis. Diagnosis is clinical
Pitfalls: Do not confuse with perioral impetigo; impetigo has crusts (not vesicles), is itchy (not painful), and does not involve the vermillion border of the lips
Therapeutic Considerations: Treatment is not always needed. If valacyclovir if used, it should be started when pain/tingling appear to decrease symptoms/vesicles/duration of attack. Valacyclovir is of no proven value once vesicles have appeared. Non-prescription topical products (docosanol 10%, tetracaine cream) may decrease pain/itching. Once-daily suppressive therapy may be considered for frequent recurrences or during times of increased risk (e.g., sun exposure). Sun screen may be helpful
Prognosis: Tends to be recurrent in normal hosts. May be severe in compromised hosts

Aphthous Ulcers (normal mouth flora)

Diagnostic Considerations: Usually an isolated finding. Ulcers are painful
Pitfalls: May be a clue to systemic disorder (e.g., Behcet's syndrome). Mouth ulcers in SLE are painless
Therapeutic Considerations: Usually refractory to all treatment and often recurrent. Steroid ointment (Kenalog in orabase) may be helpful. **Prognosis:** Good, but tends to recur

Deep Neck Infections, Lemierre's Syndrome, Severe Dental Infections

Subset	Usual Pathogens	Preferred IV Therapy	Alternate IV Therapy	IV-to-PO Switch
Deep neck infections (lateral pharyngeal, retropharyngeal, prevertebral space)	Oral anaerobes Oral streptococci	Meropenem 1 gm (IV) q8h x 2 weeks **or** Piperacillin/ tazobactam 4.5 gm (IV) q8h x 2 weeks **or** Ertapenem 1 gm (IV) q24h x 2 weeks	Clindamycin 600 mg (IV) q8h x 2 weeks **or** Ceftizoxime 2 gm (IV) q8h x 2 weeks **or** Imipenem 500 mg (IV) q6h x 2 weeks	Clindamycin 300 mg (PO) q8h x 2 weeks **or** Doxycycline 200 mg (PO) q12h x 3 days, then 100 mg (PO) q12h x 11 days*
Lemierre's Syndrome	Fusobacterium necrophorum	Treat as deep neck infection, above		
Severe dental infections	Oral anaerobes Oral streptococci	Clindamycin 600 mg (IV) q8h x 2 weeks **or** Piperacillin/ tazobactam 4.5 gm (IV) q8h x 2 weeks	Meropenem 1 gm (IV) q8h x 2 weeks **or** Imipenem 500 mg (IV) q6h x 2 weeks **or** Ertapenem 1 gm (IV) q24h x 2 weeks	Clindamycin 300 mg (PO) q8h x 2 weeks **or** Doxycycline 200 mg (PO) q12h x 3 days, then 100 mg (PO) q12h x 11 days*

Duration of therapy represents total time IV or IV + PO. Most patients on IV therapy able to take PO meds should be switched to PO therapy after clinical improvement
* Loading dose is not needed PO if given IV with the same drug

Clinical Presentation: Neck pain and fever
Diagnosis: Clinical presentation plus confirmatory CT/MRI scan

Deep Neck Infections
(lateral pharyngeal, retropharyngeal, prevertebral space)
Diagnostic Considerations: Patients are usually toxemic with unilateral posterior pharyngeal soft tissue mass on oral exam. Neck stiffness may be present with retropharyngeal space infection/abscess
Pitfalls: Retropharyngeal "danger space" infection may extend to mediastinum and present as mediastinitis
Therapeutic Considerations: Obtain ENT consult for surgical drainage
Prognosis: Poor without surgical drainage

Lemierre's Syndrome

Clinical Presentation: Jugular vein septic thrombophlebitis with fever, toxemic appearance, and tenderness over angle of jaw/jugular vein

Diagnostic Considerations: May present as multiple septic pulmonary emboli. Usually follows recent dental infection

Pitfalls: Suspect Lemierre's syndrome in patients with sore throat and shock

Therapeutic Considerations: If unresponsive to antibiotic therapy, may need venotomy

Prognosis: Poor with septic pulmonary emboli/shock

Severe Dental Infections

Diagnostic Considerations: Obtain CT/MRI of jaws to rule out osteomyelitis or abscess

Pitfalls: Chronic drainage in a patient with an implant is diagnostic of chronic osteomyelitis/abscess until proven otherwise

Therapeutic Considerations: Abscesses must be drained for cure

Prognosis: Poor prognosis and recurrent without adequate surgical drainage

Epiglottitis

Subset	Usual Pathogens	Preferred IV Therapy	Alternate IV Therapy	IV-to-PO Switch
Epiglottitis	S. pneumoniae H. influenzae Respiratory viruses	Ceftriaxone 1 gm (IV) q24h x 2 weeks **or** Ceftizoxime 2 gm (IV) q8h x 2 weeks	Meropenem 1 gm (IV) q8h x 2 weeks **or** Imipenem 500 mg (IV) q6h x 2 weeks **or** Gatifloxacin 400 mg (IV) q24h x 2 weeks **or** Levofloxacin 500 mg (IV) q24h x 2 weeks **or** Moxifloxacin 400 mg (IV) q24h x 2 weeks	Gatifloxacin 400 mg (PO) q24h x 2 weeks **or** Levofloxacin 500 mg (PO) q24h x 2 weeks **or** Moxifloxacin 400 mg (PO) q24h x 2 weeks **or** Cefprozil 500 mg (PO) q12h x 2 weeks

Duration of therapy represents total time IV or IV + PO. Most patients on IV therapy able to take PO meds should be switched to PO therapy after clinical improvement

Clinical Presentation: Stridor with upper respiratory infection

Diagnostic Considerations: Lateral film of neck shows epiglottic edema. Neck CT/MRI may help if neck films are non-diagnostic

Pitfalls: Do not attempt to culture the epiglottis (may precipitate acute upper airway obstruction)

Therapeutic Considerations: Treat empirically as soon as possible. Obtain ENT consult

Prognosis: Early airway obstruction is associated with an adverse prognosis

Empiric Therapy of Lower Respiratory Tract Infections

Acute Exacerbation of Chronic Bronchitis (AECB)

Subset	Pathogens	PO Therapy
AECB	S. pneumoniae H. influenzae M. catarrhalis	Quinolone* (PO) q24h x 5 days **or** Amoxicillin/clavulanic acid 500/125 mg (PO) q12h x 5 days **or** Telithromycin 800 mg (PO) q24h x 5 days **or** Clarithromycin XL 1 gm (PO) q24h x 5 days **or** Doxycycline 100 mg (PO) q12h x 5 days **or** Azithromycin 500 mg (PO) x 3 days

* Moxifloxacin 400 mg or levofloxacin 500 mg or gatifloxacin 400 mg or gemifloxacin 320 mg

Clinical Presentation: Productive cough and negative chest x-ray in a patient with chronic bronchitis
Diagnostic Considerations: Diagnosis by productive cough, purulent sputum, and chest x-ray negative for pneumonia. H. influenzae is relatively more common than other pathogens
Pitfalls: Do not obtain sputum cultures in chronic bronchitis; cultures usually reported as normal/mixed flora and should not be used to guide therapy
Therapeutic Considerations: Treated with same antibiotics as for community-acquired pneumonia, since pathogens are the same (even though H. influenzae is relatively more frequent). Respiratory viruses/C. pneumoniae may initiate AECB, but is usually followed by bacterial infection, which is responsible for symptoms and is the aim of therapy. Bronchodilators are helpful for bronchospasm
Prognosis: Related to underlying cardiopulmonary status

Mediastinitis

Subset	Usual Pathogens	Preferred IV Therapy	Alternate IV Therapy	IV-to-PO Switch
Following esophageal perforation or thoracic surgery	Oral anaerobes	Piperacillin/tazobactam 4.5 gm (IV) q8h x 2 weeks **or** Ampicillin/sulbactam 3 gm (IV) q6h x 2 weeks	Meropenem 1 gm (IV) q8h x 2 weeks **or** Imipenem 500 mg (IV) q6h x 2 weeks **or** Ertapenem 1 gm (IV) q24h x 2 wks	Amoxicillin/clavulanic acid 500/125 mg (PO) q8h x 2 weeks **or** Quinolone* (PO) q24h x 2 weeks

Duration of therapy represents total time IV or IV + PO. Most patients on IV therapy able to take PO meds should be switched to PO therapy after clinical improvement
* Moxifloxacin 400 mg or levofloxacin 500 mg or gatifloxacin 400 mg

Diagnostic Considerations: Chest x-ray usually shows perihilar infiltrate in mediastinitis. Pleural effusions from esophageal tears have elevated amylase levels
Pitfalls: Do not overlook esophageal tear in mediastinitis with pleural effusions
Therapeutic Considerations: Obtain surgical consult if esophageal perforation is suspected
Prognosis: Related to extent, location, and duration of esophageal tear/mediastinal infection

Community-Acquired Pneumonia (CAP)

Subset	Usual Pathogens*	IV Therapy		PO Therapy or IV-to-PO Switch

Pathogen unknown	S. pneumoniae
	H. influenzae
	M. catarrhalis
	Legionella sp.
	Mycoplasma
	  pneumoniae
	Chlamydia
	  pneumoniae
		Quinolone[†] (IV) q24h x 1-2 weeks
		or combination therapy with
		Ceftriaxone 1 gm (IV) q24h x 1-2 weeks
		or
		Ertapenem 1 gm (IV) q24h x 1-2 weeks
		plus either
		Azithromycin 500 mg (IV) q24h x 1-2 weeks (minimum 2 doses before switching to PO therapy)
		or
		Doxycycline[‡] (IV) x 1-2 weeks
				Quinolone[†] (PO) q24h x 1-2 weeks
				or
				Telithromycin 800 mg (PO) q24h x 1-2 weeks
				or
				Doxycycline[‡] (PO) x 1-2 weeks
				or
				Macrolide[††] (PO) q24h x 1-2 weeks

Typical bacterial pathogens *Adults*	S. pneumoniae H. influenzae M. catarrhalis	<u>Preferred IV</u> Quinolone[†] (IV) q24h x 1-2 weeks **or** Ertapenem 1 gm (IV) q24h x 1-2 weeks **or** Ceftriaxone 1 gm (IV) q24h x 1-2 weeks	<u>Alternate IV</u> Doxycycline[‡] (IV) x 1-2 weeks **or** Azithromycin 500 mg (IV) q24h x 1-2 weeks (minimum 2 doses before switching to PO therapy)	Quinolone[†] (PO) q24h x 1-2 weeks **or** Amoxicillin/clavulanic acid XR 2 tablets (PO) q12h x 7-10 days **or** Any of above (see pathogen unknown) **or** Cephalosporin** (PO) x 1-2 weeks
Children > 3 months	S. pneumoniae H. influenzae M. catarrhalis	<u>Hospitalized</u> Ceftriaxone 25 mg/kg (IV) q12h x 1-2 weeks **or** Azithromycin 5 mg/kg (IV) q12h x 1-2 weeks	<u>Ambulatory</u> Amoxicillin/clavulanic acid suspension 45 mg/kg (PO) q12h x 1-2 weeks **or** Cephalosporin[¶] (PO) x 1-2 weeks **or** Azithromycin 10 mg/kg (PO) x 1 dose followed by 5 mg/kg (PO) q24h x 4 days **or** Clarithromycin 7.5 mg/kg (PO) q12h x 1-2 weeks	
	B. pertussis B. parapertussis B. bronchio- septica	<u>IV Therapy:</u> Azithromycin 5 mg/kg q12h x 5 days **or** Erythromycin 10 mg/kg q6h x 2 weeks. <u>PO Therapy:</u> Azithromycin 10 mg/kg x 1 dose followed by 5 mg/kg q24h x 4 days **or** Clarithromycin 7.5 mg/kg q12h x 1 week **or** Erythromycin 10 mg/kg q6h x 2 weeks. <u>Macrolide-intolerant:</u> TMP-SMX 5 mg/kg (IV/PO) q6h x 2 weeks		

Duration of therapy represents total time IV or IV, PO, or IV + PO. Most patients on IV therapy able to take PO meds should be switched to PO therapy after clinical improvement

*   Compromised hosts may require longer courses of therapy
†   Moxifloxacin 400 mg or levofloxacin 500 mg or gatifloxacin 400 mg or gemifloxacin 320 mg. Levofloxacin 750 mg (PO) q24h x 5 days may be considered
†† Azithromycin 500 mg or clarithromycin XL 1 gm
‡   Doxycycline 200 mg (IV or PO) q12h x 3 days, then 100 mg (IV or PO) q12h x 4-11 days
** Adults: cefdinir 300 mg q12h or cefditoren 400 mg q12h or cefixime 400 mg q12h or cefpodoxime 200 mg q12h
¶   Children: cefprozil 15 mg/kg (PO) q12h or cefuroxime axetil 15 mg/kg (PO) q12h or cefdinir 7 mg/kg (PO) q12h or 14 mg/kg (PO) q24h or cefpodoxime 5 mg/kg (PO) q12h

Community-Acquired Pneumonia (CAP) (cont'd)

Subset	Usual Pathogens*	Preferred IV Therapy	Alternate IV Therapy	PO Therapy or IV-to-PO Switch
Atypical pathogens *Zoonotic*	Chlamydia psittaci (psittacosis) Coxiella burnetii (Q fever) Francisella tularensis (tularemia)	Doxycycline 200 mg (IV) q12h x 3 days, then 100 mg (IV) q12h x 2 weeks	Quinolone[†] (IV) q24h x 2 weeks	Doxycycline 200 mg (PO) q12h x 3 days, then 100 mg (PO) q12h x 11 days** **or** Quinolone[†] (PO) q24h x 2 weeks
SARS	SARS-associated coronavirus (SARS-CoV)	See therapeutic considerations, p. 50		
Non-zoonotic	Legionella sp.[‡] Mycoplasma pneumoniae[‡] Chlamydia pneumoniae[‡]	Moxifloxacin 400 mg (IV) q24h x 1-2 weeks **or** Levofloxacin 500 mg (IV) q24h x 1-2 weeks **or** Gatifloxacin 400 mg (IV) q24h x 1-2 weeks	Doxycycline 200 mg (IV) q12h x 3 days, then 100 mg (IV) q12h x 4-11 days **or** Azithromycin 500 mg (IV) q24h x 1-2 weeks (minimum of 2 doses before switching to PO therapy)	Quinolone[†] (PO) q24h x 1-2 weeks **or** Telithromycin 800 mg (PO) q24h x 1-2 weeks **or** Azithromycin 500 mg (PO) q24h x 1-2 weeks **or** Clarithromycin XL 1 gm (PO) q24h x 1-2 weeks **or** Doxycycline 200 mg (PO) q12h x 3 days, then 100 mg (PO) q12h x 4-11 days**
Influenza *Severe/ pneumonia*	Influenza virus, type A	Rimantadine 100 mg (PO) q12h x 7-10 days	Amantadine 200 mg (PO) q24h x 7-10 days	Start treatment as soon as possible after onset of symptoms, preferably within 2 days. Rimantidine/ amantadine miss Influenza type B, which is usually a milder illness
Mild/ moderate	Influenza virus, type A/B	Oseltamivir (Tamiflu) 75 mg (PO) q24h x 5 days	Zanamivir (Relenza) 10 mg (2 puffs via oral inhaler) q12h x 5 days	

Duration of therapy represents total time IV or IV, PO, or IV + PO
* *Compromised hosts may require longer courses of therapy*
** *Loading dose is not needed PO if given IV with the same drug*
† *Moxifloxacin 400 mg or levofloxacin 500 mg or gatifloxacin 400 mg or gemifloxacin 320 mg*
‡ *May require prolonged therapy: Legionella (4 weeks); Mycoplasma (2-3 weeks); Chlamydia (up to 6 weeks)*

Community-Acquired Pneumonia (CAP) (cont'd)

Subset	Usual Pathogens*	Preferred IV Therapy	Alternate IV Therapy	PO Therapy or IV-to-PO Switch
Aspiration	Oral anaerobes S. pneumoniae H. influenzae M. catarrhalis	Ceftriaxone 1 gm (IV) q24h x 2 weeks **or** Quinolone† (IV) q24h x 2 weeks	Doxycycline 200 mg (IV) q12h x 3 days, then 100 mg (IV) q12h x 11 days	Clarithromycin XL 1 gm (PO) q24h x 2 weeks **or** Doxycycline 200 mg (PO) q12h x 3 days, then 100 mg (PO) q12h x 4-11 days** **or** Quinolone† (PO) q24h x 2 weeks

Subset	Usual Pathogens	
Tuberculosis (TB)	M. tuberculosis	INH 300 mg (PO) q24h x 6-12 months **plus** Rifampin 600 mg (PO) q24h x 6-12 months <u>If multiresistant TB strain likely, also add:</u> EMB 15 mg/kg (PO) q24h x 6-12 months **plus** PZA 25 mg/kg (PO) q24h x 6-12 months
Atypical tuberculosis	Mycobacterium avium-intracellulare (MAI)	<u>Treat for 6 months after sputum negative for MAI:</u> Ethambutol 15 mg/kg (PO) q24h ***plus either*** Clarithromycin 500 mg (PO) q12h ***or*** Azithromycin 500 mg (PO) q24h <u>May also choose to add:</u> Ciprofloxacin 750 mg (PO) q12h **or** ofloxacin 400 mg (PO) q12h **or** levofloxacin 500 mg (PO) q24h
	M. kansasii	<u>Preferred therapy</u> Rifampin 600 mg (PO) q24h **plus** INH 300 mg (PO) q24h **plus** pyridoxine 50 mg (PO) q24h **plus** EMB 15 mg/kg (PO) q24h. Treat x 18 months with 12 months of negative sputum <u>Alternate therapy</u> Clarithromycin 500 mg (PO) q12h **plus** INH 900 mg (PO) q24h **plus** pyridoxine 50 mg (PO) q24h **plus** EMB 25 mg/kg (PO) q24h **plus** sulfamethoxazole 1 gm (PO) q8h. Treat x 18 months with 12 months of negative sputum <u>For severe cases,</u> add streptomycin 0.5-1 gm (IM) 3x/week during first 3 months of preferred/alternate therapy

Duration of therapy represents total time IV or IV, PO, or IV + PO
* *Compromised hosts are predisposed to organisms listed, but may be infected by usual pathogens in normal hosts*
** *Loading dose is not needed PO if given IV with the same drug*
† *Moxifloxacin 400 mg or levofloxacin 500 mg or gatifloxacin 400 mg*

Community-Acquired Pneumonia (CAP) (cont'd)

Subset	Usual Pathogens*	Preferred IV Therapy	Alternate IV Therapy	PO Therapy or IV-to-PO Switch
Chronic alcoholics	K. pneumoniae S. pneumoniae H. influenzae M. catarrhalis	Ceftriaxone 1 gm (IV) q24h x 2 weeks	Quinolone‡ (IV) q24h x 2 weeks	Quinolone‡ (PO) q24hx 2 weeks
Post-viral influenza	S. aureus S. pneumoniae H. influenzae	Quinolone‡ (IV) q24hx 2 weeks **plus either** Nafcillin 2 gm (IV) q4h x 2 weeks **or** Clindamycin 600 mg (IV) q8h x 2 weeks	Ceftriaxone 1 gm (IV) q24h x 2 weeks **plus either** Vancomycin 1 gm (IV) q12h x 2 weeks **or** Linezolid 600 mg (IV) q12h x 2 weeks **or** Clindamycin 600 mg (IV) q8h x 2 weeks	Quinolone‡ (PO) q24hx 2 weeks
Bronchiectasis, cystic fibrosis	P. aeruginosa	Treat as nosocomial pneumonia (p. 54)		
Nursing home-acquired pneumonia (NHAP)	H. influenzae S. pneumoniae M. catarrhalis C. pneumoniae	Cefepime 2 gm (IV) q12h x 2 weeks **or** Ceftriaxone 1 gm (IV or IM) q24h x 2 weeks	Quinolone‡ (IV) q24h x 2 weeks **or** Doxycycline 200 mg (IV) q12h x 3 days, then 100 mg (IV) q12h x 11 days	Quinolone‡ (PO) q24hx 2 weeks **or** Doxycycline 200 mg (PO) q12h x 3 days, then 100 mg (PO) q12h x 11 days**
Chronic steroid therapy† (If perihilar infiltrates/ hypoxemia, treat as PCP [next page] until lung biopsy)	Aspergillus	Itraconazole 200 mg (IV) q12h x 2 days, then 200 mg (IV) q24h until cured **or** Caspofungin 70 mg (IV) x 1 dose, then 50 mg (IV) q24h until cured	Amphotericin B deoxycholate 1 mg/kg (IV) q24h until 2-3 grams **or** Lipid-associated formulation of amphotericin B (p. 297) (IV) q24h x 4-6 weeks **or** Voriconazole 6 mg/kg (IV) q12h x 1 day, then 4 mg/kg IV q12h until cured	Itraconazole 200 mg (IV) q12h x 2 days, then 200 mg (PO) solution q12h until cured** **or** Voriconazole (see "usual dose," p. 400) until cured

Duration of therapy represents total time IV or IV, PO, or IV + PO. Most patients on IV therapy able to take PO meds should be switched to PO therapy soon after clinical improvement
*   *Compromised hosts are predisposed to organisms listed, but may be infected by usual pathogens in normal hosts*
** *Loading dose is not needed PO if given IV with the same drug*
†   *Treat only IV or IV-to-PO switch*
‡   *Moxifloxacin 400 mg or levofloxacin 500 mg or gatifloxacin 400 mg*

Community-Acquired Pneumonia (CAP) (cont'd)

Subset	Usual Pathogens*	Preferred IV Therapy	Alternate IV Therapy	IV-to-PO Switch
Chronic steroids† (cont'd)	P. carinii (PCP)	TMP-SMX 5 mg/kg (IV) q6h x 3 weeks	Pentamidine 4 mg/kg (IV) q24h x 3 weeks	TMP-SMX 5 mg/kg (PO) q6h x 3 weeks
Organ transplants†	CMV	Ganciclovir 5 mg/kg (IV) q12h until clinical improvement followed by valganciclovir 900 mg (PO) q12h until cured **plus** CMV immunoglobulin (CMV-IG) 500 mg/kg (IV) q48h x 2 weeks		
	P. carinii (PCP)	Same as for chronic steroid therapy, above		
Other pathogens	For Blastomyces, Histoplasma, Coccidioides, Paracoccidioides, Actinomyces, Nocardia, Pseudallescheria boydii, Sporothrix, Mucor, see pp. 198-199			

Duration of therapy represents total time IV or IV + PO. Most patients on IV therapy able to take PO meds should be switched to PO therapy soon after clinical improvement
* *Compromised hosts are predisposed to organisms listed, but may be infected by usual pathogens in normal hosts*
† *Treat only IV or IV-to-PO switch*

Clinical Presentation: Fever, cough, respiratory symptoms, chest x-ray consistent with pneumonia
Diagnosis: Identification of organism on sputum gram stain/culture. Same organism is found in blood if blood cultures are positive

Community-Acquired Pneumonia (Typical Bacterial Pathogens)
Diagnostic Considerations: Sputum is useful if a single organism predominates and is not contaminated by saliva. Purulent sputum, pleuritic chest pain, pleural effusion favor typical pathogens
Pitfalls: Obtain a chest x-ray to verify the diagnosis and rule out non-infectious mimics (e.g., heart failure). Treat COPD/chronic bronchitis patients empirically (sputum is unhelpful; usually shows "mixed/normal flora")
Therapeutic Considerations: Do not switch to narrow-spectrum antibiotic after organism is identified on gram stain/blood culture. Pathogen identification is important for prognostic and public health reasons, not for therapy. Severity of CAP is related to the degree of cardiopulmonary/immune dysfunction and impacts the length of hospital stay, not the therapeutic approach or antibiotic choice
Prognosis: Related to cardiopulmonary status and splenic function

Community-Acquired Pneumonia (Pertussis)
Clinical Presentation: Rhinorrhea over 1-2 weeks (catarrhal stage) progressing to paroxysms of cough (paroxysmal stage) lasting 2-4 weeks, often with a characteristic inspiratory whoop, followed by a convalescent stage lasting 1-2 weeks during which cough paroxysms decrease in frequency/severity. Fever is low grade or absent. In children < 6 months, whoop is frequently absent and apnea may occur. Older children/adults may present with persistent cough (without whoop) lasting 2-6 weeks
Diagnostic Considerations: A positive culture for Bordetella pertussis from a nasopharyngeal swab inoculated on fresh selective media is diagnostic
Pitfalls: Be sure to consider pertussis in older children and adults with prolonged coughing illness
Therapeutic Considerations: By the paroxysmal stage, antibiotics have minimal effect on the course of the illness but are indicated to decrease transmission
Prognosis: Good, despite the prolonged course

Community-Acquired Pneumonia (Atypical Pathogens)
Clinical Presentation: CAP with extra-pulmonary symptoms, signs, or laboratory abnormalities
Diagnosis: Confirm by specific serological tests

Zoonotic Infections (Psittacosis, Q fever, Tularemia)

Diagnostic Considerations: Zoonotic contact history is key to presumptive diagnosis: psittacosis (parrots and relatives); Q fever (sheep, parturient cats); tularemia (rabbit, deer, deer fly bite)
Pitfalls: Organisms are difficult/dangerous to grow. Do not culture. Use serological tests for diagnosis
Therapeutic Considerations: Q fever endocarditis requires prolonged therapy. Bioterrorist Q fever/tularemia pneumonia presents clinically and is treated the same as naturally-acquired infection
Prognosis: Good except for Q fever with complications (e.g., SBE)

Zoonotic Infections (Severe Acute Respiratory Syndrome; SARS)

Presentation: Influenza-like illness with fever, dry cough, and myalgias. Patients are short of breath/hypoxic. Auscultation of the lungs resembles viral influenza (i.e., quiet, no rales). Laboratory tests are non-specific but helpful in narrowing diagnostic possibilities. Chest x-ray shows bilateral interstitial (upper/lower lobe) infiltrates. Lower lobe infiltrates may be large/ovid. WBC and platelet counts are usually normal or slightly decreased. Relative lymphopenia is present early. Mild increases in SGOT/SGPT, LDH, CPK are common
Diagnostic Considerations: Diagnosis by viral isolation or specific SARS serology. Important to exclude influenza A, Legionnaires' disease and tularemic pneumonia serologically
Pitfalls: Most likely to be confused with viral influenza A—both present with fever, myalgias, hypoxia. Chest x-ray in SARS has discrete infiltrates (influenza does not unless superimposed on CAP) that are ovid and unlike most infiltrates in CAP. Legionella (L. micdadei) and tularemia can present with ovid infiltrates on chest x-ray, but hypoxemia is not prominent in Legionella or tularemic CAP. Mycoplasma is unlikely to be confused with SARS (i.e., hypoxemia is not prominent, patients are not critically ill, and WBC, platelet count, and LFT's are usually normal in mycoplasma CAP)
Therapeutic Considerations: Most patients are severely hypoxemic and require oxygen/ventilatory support. In a preliminary study, some patients benefitted from corticosteroids (pulse-dosed methylprednisolone 500 mg [IV] q24h x 3 days followed by taper/step down with prednisone [PO] to complete 20 days) plus Interferon alfacon-1 (9 mcg [SQ] q24h x at least 2 days, increased to 15 mcg/d if no response) x 8-13 days (JAMA 290;3222-28, 2003)
Prognosis: Related to underlying cardiopulmonary/immune status. Frequently fatal

Non-Zoonotic Infections (Legionella sp., M. pneumoniae, C. pneumoniae)

Diagnostic Considerations: Each atypical pathogen has a different and characteristic pattern of extra-pulmonary organ involvement. Legionnaire's disease is suggested by relative bradycardia, ↓ PO_4^-, ↑ SGOT, microscopic hematuria, abdominal pain, diarrhea
Pitfalls: Failure to respond to beta-lactams should suggest diagnosis of atypical CAP
Therapeutic Considerations: Treat Legionella x 4 weeks. Treat Mycoplasma or Chlamydia x 2 weeks
Prognosis: Related to severity of underlying cardiopulmonary disease

Influenza (Infuenza virus, type A/B)

Clinical Presentation: Acute onset of fever, headache, myalgias/arthralgias, sore throat, prostration. Severity ranges from mild flu to life-threatening pneumonia
Diagnositic Considerations: Mild cases with headache, sore throat, and rhinorrhea resemble the common cold/respiratory viruses (influenza-like illnesses) and can be caused by type A or B. Severe flu is usually due to type A. Influenza virus may be cultured from respiratory secretions and typed
Pitfalls: Influenza pneumonia has no auscultatory finding in the chest, and the chest x-ray is normal/near normal. Severe influenza pneumonia is accompanied by an oxygen diffusion defect (↑ A-a gradient), and patients are hypoxemic/cyanotic. Pleuritic chest pain indicates pleural irritation ± pleural effusion, which is characteristic of bacterial CAPs. Viral pneumonias are not associated with pleuritic chest pain, but Influenza virus can invade the intercostal muscles to mimic pleuritic chest pain. Chest x-ray in viral influenza is normal/near normal without focal/segmental infiltrates or pleural effusion. Infiltrates on chest x-ray with viral influenza indicate concurrent/subsequent bacterial pneumonia
Therapeutic Considerations: Mild/moderate influenza can be treated with neuraminidase inhibitors (Tamiflu/Relenza), which reduce symptoms by 1-2 days. Start treatment within 2 days of symptom

onset, if possible. Reduce the dose of Tamiflu to 75 mg (PO) q48h for CrCl 10-30 cc/min. Relenza is generally not recommended for patients with underlying COPD/asthma (increased risk of bronchospasm) and should be discontinued if bronchospasm or a decline in respiratory function occurs. For severe influenza/pneumonia, treat with rimantadine or amantadine, which have both antiviral effects and increase peripheral airway dilatation/oxygenation. Reduce the dose of rimantadine to 100 mg (PO) q24h in the elderly, severe liver dysfunction, or CrCl < 10 cc/min. Reduce the dose of amantadine to 100 mg (PO) q24h for age > 65 years. For renal dysfunction, give amantadine 200 mg (PO) load followed by 100 mg q24h (CrCl 30-50 cc/min), 100 mg q48h (CrCl 15-29 cc/min), or 200 mg weekly (CrCl < 15 cc/min). Flu complicated by bacterial pneumonia is often due to S. aureus (MRSA/MSSA); in these cases, treat as post-viral influenza CAP (p. 48)

Prognosis: Good for mild/moderate flu. Severe flu may be fatal due to pneumonia with profound hypoxemia. Prognosis is worse if complicated by bacterial pneumonia, particularly if due to S. aureus.

Aspiration Pneumonia
Diagnostic Considerations: Sputum not diagnostic. No need for transtracheal aspirate culture
Pitfalls: Lobar location varies with patient position during aspiration
Therapeutic Considerations: Oral anaerobes are sensitive to all beta-lactams and most antibiotics used to treat CAP. Additional anaerobic (B. fragilis) coverage is not needed
Prognosis: Related to severity of CNS/esophageal disease

Pneumonia in HIV
Pneumocystis carinii Pneumonia (PCP) (see p. 248)
Sputum Positive for AFB (TB/MAI) (see pp. 248, 251)
Sputum Negative for AFB
Clinical Presentation: CAP in HIV patient with focal infiltrate(s) and normal/slightly depressed CD$_4$
Diagnostic Considerations: Diagnosis by sputum gram stain/culture ± positive blood cultures (bacterial pathogens) or Legionella/Chlamydia serology (atypical pathogens). Blood cultures are most often positive for S. pneumoniae or H. influenzae. Only cover S. aureus in IV drug abusers with pre-terminal disease
Pitfalls: Atypical chest x-ray appearance is not uncommon. Treat syndrome of CAP, not chest x-ray. CAP in HIV does not resemble PCP, which presents with profound hypoxemia without focal infiltrates
Therapeutic Considerations: Treat the same as CAP in normal hosts
Prognosis: Clinically resolves the same as CAP in normal hosts

Tuberculous (TB) Pneumonia
Clinical Presentation: Community-acquired pneumonia with single/multiple infiltrates
Diagnostic Considerations: Diagnosis by sputum AFB smear/culture. Respiratory isolation important. Lower lobe effusion common in lower lobe primary TB. Reactivation TB is usually bilateral/apical ± old, healed Ghon complex; cavitation/fibrosis are common, but pleural effusion is absent
Pitfalls: Primary TB may present as CAP; reactivation TB presents as chronic pneumonia
Therapeutic Considerations: 1-2 weeks of therapy is usually required to eliminate AFBs from sputum
Prognosis: Related to underlying health status

Mycobacterium avium-intracellulare (MAI) Pneumonia
Clinical Presentation: Community-acquired pneumonia in normal hosts or immunosuppressed/HIV patient with focal single/multiple infiltrates indistinguishable from TB
Diagnostic Considerations: Diagnosis by AFB culture. In HIV, MAI may disseminate, resembling miliary TB. Diagnosis by culture of blood, liver, or bone marrow
Pitfalls: Must differentiate TB from MAI by AFB culture, as therapy for MAI differs from TB
Therapeutic Considerations: MAI in normal hosts is readily treatable, but MAI in HIV patients requires life-long suppressive therapy after initial treatment
Prognosis: Related to degree of immunosuppression/CD$_4$ count

Mycobacterium kansasii Pneumonia

Clinical Presentation: Subacute CAP resembling TB/MAI that can occur in clusters/outbreaks

Diagnostic Considerations: Chest x-ray infiltrates/lung disease plus M. kansasii in a single sputum specimen. M. kansasii can cause disseminated infection, like TB, and is diagnosed by culturing M. kansasii from the blood, liver, or bone marrow

Pitfalls: M. kansasii in sputum with a normal chest x-ray does not indicate infection

Therapeutic Considerations: M. kansasii is more readily treatable than TB. Use the alternate regimen for rifampin-resistant strains

Prognosis: Good in normal hosts. May be rapidly progressive/fatal without treatment in HIV patients

Pneumonia in Chronic Alcoholics

Diagnostic Considerations: Klebsiella pneumoniae usually occurs only in chronic alcoholics, and is characterized by blood-flecked "currant jelly" sputum and cavitation (typically in 3-5 days)

Pitfalls: Suspect Klebsiella in "pneumococcal" pneumonia that cavitates. Empyema is more common than pleural effusion

Therapeutic Considerations: Monotherapy with newer anti-Klebsiella agents is as effective or superior to "double-drug" therapy with older agents

Prognosis: Related to degree of hepatic/splenic dysfunction

Post-Viral Influenza Pneumonia

Diagnostic Considerations: S. aureus pneumonia usually only affects patients with viral influenza pneumonia, and is characterized by cyanosis and rapid cavitation on chest x-ray. Do not diagnose staphylococcal pneumonia without these signs

Pitfalls: Bacterial pneumonia may be superimposed or follow viral influenza pneumonia

Therapeutic Considerations: Usually no need to cover MRSA

Prognosis: Related to severity of influenza pneumonia and type of superinfection

Bronchiectasis/Cystic Fibrosis (P. aeruginosa)

Diagnostic Considerations: Cystic fibrosis/bronchiectasis is characterized by viscous secretions ± low grade fevers; less commonly may present as lung abscess. Onset of pneumonia/lung abscess heralded by cough/decrease in pulmonary function

Pitfalls: Sputum colonization is common (e.g., S. maltophilia, B. cepacia); may not reflect pathogens

Therapeutic Considerations: Important to select antibiotics with low resistance potential and good penetration into respiratory secretions (e.g., quinolones, meropenem). Treated the same as nosocomial pneumonia

Prognosis: Related to extent of underlying lung disease/severity of infection

Nursing Home-Acquired Pneumonia (NHAP)

Diagnostic Considerations: Difficult to obtain sputum in elderly/debilitated patients. H. influenzae is common; K. pneumoniae is uncommon in non-alcoholics, even in this population

Pitfalls: Resembles community-acquired pneumonia in terms of pathogens and length of hospital stay, not nosocomial pneumonia

Therapeutic Considerations: Treat as community-acquired pneumonia, not nosocomial pneumonia. No need to cover P. aeruginosa

Prognosis: Related to underlying cardiopulmonary status

Pneumonia in Chronic Steroid Therapy

If fungal infection is suspected, obtain lung biopsy to confirm diagnosis/identify causative organism. Non-responsiveness to appropriate antibiotics should suggest fungal infection. Avoid empirically treating fungi; due to the required duration of therapy, it is advantageous to confirm the diagnosis by lung biopsy first. Prognosis related to degree of immunosuppression

Acute Aspergillus Pneumonia

Clinical Presentation: Chest x-ray shows progressive necrotizing pneumonia unresponsive to antibiotic therapy. No characteristic appearance on chest x-ray. Usually seen only in compromised hosts
Diagnostic Considerations: Diagnosis by lung biopsy (not broncho-alveolar lavage) demonstrating hyphae invading lung parenchyma/blood vessels. Usually occurs only in patients receiving chronic steroids or cancer chemotherapy, organ transplants, leukopenic compromised hosts, or patients with chronic granulomatous disease
Pitfalls: Aspergillus pneumonia does not occur in normal hosts
Prognosis: Almost always fatal despite appropriate therapy

Pneumonia in Organ Transplants

Clinical Presentation: CAP with perihilar infiltrates and hypoxemia
Diagnostic Considerations: CMV is diagnosed by stain/culture of lung biopsy
Therapeutic Considerations: Treat as CMV pneumonia if CMV is predominant pathogen on lung biopsy. CMV may progress despite ganciclovir therapy
Prognosis: Related to degree of immunosuppression

Other Pneumonias (Blastomyces, Histoplasma, Coccidioides, Paracoccidioides, Actinomyces, Nocardia, Pseudallescheria boydii, Sporothrix, Mucor) (see pp. 198-199)

Lung Abscess/Empyema

Subset	Usual Pathogens	Preferred IV Therapy	Alternate IV Therapy	PO Therapy or IV-to-PO Switch
Lung abscess/ empyema	Oral anaerobes S. aureus S. pneumoniae	Clindamycin 600 mg (IV) q8h* **or** Meropenem 1 gm (IV) q8h* **or** Piperacillin/ tazobactam 4.5 gm (IV) q8h*	Imipenem 500 mg (IV) q6h* **or** Ertapenem 1 gm (IV) q24h*	Clindamycin 300 mg (PO) q8h* **or** Quinolone[†] (PO) q24h*
Bronchiectasis, cystic fibrosis	P. aeruginosa	Treat as nosocomial pneumonia (p. 54)		

* Treat until resolved. Duration of therapy represents total time IV, PO, or IV + PO. Most patients on IV therapy able to take PO meds should be switched to PO therapy soon after clinical improvement (usually < 72 hours)
† Moxifloxacin 400 mg or levofloxacin 500 mg or gatifloxacin 400 mg

Clinical Presentation: Lung abscess presents as single/multiple cavitary lung lesion(s) with fever. Empyema presents as persistent fever with pleural effusion that does not layer out on lateral decubitus chest x-ray
Diagnostic Considerations: In lung abscess, plain film/CT scan demonstrates cavitary lung lesions appearing > 1 week after pneumonia. Most CAPs are not associated with pleural effusion, and few develop empyema. In empyema, pleural fluid pH is ≤ 7.2; culture purulent exudate for pathogen
Pitfalls: Pleural effusions secondary to CAP usually resolve rapidly with treatment. Suspect empyema in patients with persistent pleural effusions with fever
Therapeutic Considerations: Chest tube/surgical drainage needed for empyema. Treat lung abscess until it resolves (usually 3-12 months)
Prognosis: Good if adequately drained

Nosocomial Pneumonia (NP) / Hospital-Acquired Pneumonia (HAP) / Ventilator-Associated Pneumonia (VAP)

Subset	Usual Pathogens	Preferred IV Therapy*	Alternate IV Therapy	IV-to-PO Switch
Empiric therapy	P. aeruginosa* E. coli K. pneumoniae S. marcescens	Meropenem 1 gm (IV) q8h x 2 weeks **or** Imipenem 500 mg (IV) q6h x 2 weeks† **or** Cefepime 2 gm (IV) q8h x 2 weeks **or** Piperacillin/tazobactam 4.5 gm (IV) q6h x 2 weeks **or** Combination therapy (see P. aeruginosa, below)		Ciprofloxacin 750 mg (PO) q12h x 2 weeks **or** Levofloxacin 750 mg (PO) q24h x 2 weeks
Specific therapy	P. aeruginosa	Any empiric monotherapy agent (above) **plus either** Ciprofloxacin 400 mg (IV) q8h x 2 weeks **or** Levofloxacin 750 mg (IV) q24h x 2 weeks **or** Aztreonam 2 gm (IV) q8h x 2 weeks **or** Amikacin 1 gm (IV) q24h x 2 weeks		Ciprofloxacin 750 mg (PO) q12h x 2 weeks **or** Levofloxacin 750 mg (PO) q24h x 2 weeks
	S. aureus‡ (MRSA)	Linezolid 600 mg (IV) q12h x 2 weeks **or** Vancomycin 1 gm (IV) q12h x 2 weeks	Quinupristin/ dalfopristin 7.5 mg/kg (IV) q8h x 2 weeks	Linezolid 600 mg (PO) q12h x 2 weeks **or** Minocycline 100 mg (PO) q12h x 2 weeks
	S. aureus‡ (MSSA)	Nafcillin 2 gm (IV) q4h x 2 weeks **or** Clindamycin 600 mg (IV) q8h x 2 weeks **or** Linezolid 600 mg (IV) q12h x 2 wks	Vancomycin 1 gm (IV) q12h x 2 weeks	Linezolid 600 mg (PO) q12h x 2 weeks **or** Clindamycin 300 mg (PO) q8h x 2 weeks **or** Cephalexin 1 gm (PO) q6h x 2 weeks

MSSA/MRSA = methicillin-sensitive/resistant S. aureus. Duration of therapy represents total time IV or IV + PO. Most patients on IV therapy able to take PO meds should be switched to PO therapy after clinical improvement
* For confirmed P. aeruginosa pneumonia, use combination IV therapy
† For moderately susceptible organisms (e.g., P. aeruginosa), use imipenem 1 gm (IV) q6-8h
‡ If lab report identifies gram-positive cocci in clusters, treat initially for MRSA. If later identified as MSSA, treat as MSSA or continue MRSA therapy

Clinical Presentation: Pulmonary infiltrate compatible with a bacterial pneumonia occurring ≥ 1 week in-hospital ± fever/leukocytosis

Diagnostic Considerations: Leukocytosis and fever are nonspecific/nondiagnostic of NP. Definitive diagnosis by culture of lung biopsy. P. aeruginosa and S. aureus are common colonizers in CCU-ventilated patients and manifest as necrotizing pneumonias with rapid cavitation (< 72 hours), microabscesses, and blood vessel invasion. S. aureus (MSSA/MRSA) rarely cause NP despite being cultured from 25% of ET tube respiratory secretions. Acinetobacter/Legionella NP occur usually in outbreak situations

Pitfalls: Do not cover non-pulmonary pathogens cultured from respiratory secretions in ventilated patients (Enterobacter, P. cepacia, P. maltophilia, Citrobacter, Flavobacterium, Enterococci); these organisms rarely if ever cause NP. S. aureus (MSSA/MRSA) cultured from BAL fluid is not diagnostic of S. aureus NP. Semi-quantitative BAL/protected brush specimens reflect airway colonization, not lung pathogens. Tissue (lung) culture is needed for definitive diagnosis of P. aeruginosa/S. aureus NP

Therapeutic Considerations: NP (HAP/VAP) is defined as pneumonia acquired > 7 hospital days. Except for MSSA/MRSA, there are no other NP gram-positive pathogens. So called "early" NP/HAP occuring < 3 days of hospitalization, which may be due to S. pneumoniae (including DRSP strains) or H. influenzae, actually represents CAP that manifests early after hospital admission. Empiric therapy recommendations (p. 54) cover "early" and "late" NP pathogens except MRSA. Monotherapy is as effective as combination therapy for non-P. aeruginosa NP, but 2-drug therapy is recommended for confirmed P. aeruginosa NP. After 2 weeks of appropriate antibiotic therapy, non-progressive/stable pulmonary infiltrates with fever and leukocytosis are usually due to a non-infectious cause, rather than persistent infection. Anaerobes are not pathogens in HAP/VAP

Prognosis: Related to underlying cardiopulmonary status

Empiric Therapy of Cardiovascular Infections

Subacute Bacterial Endocarditis (SBE)

Subset	Usual Pathogens	Preferred IV Therapy	Alternate IV Therapy	PO Therapy or IV-to-PO Switch
No obvious source	S. viridans Group B,C,G streptococci Nutritionally-variant streptococci	Ceftriaxone 2 gm (IV) q24h x 2 weeks **plus** Gentamicin 120 mg (IV) q24h x 2 weeks **or monotherapy with** Ceftriaxone 2 gm (IV) q24h x 2 weeks	Penicillin G 3 mu (IV) q4h x 2 weeks **plus** Gentamicin 180 mg (IV) q24h x 2 weeks **or monotherapy with** Vancomycin 1 gm (IV) q12h x 2 weeks **or** Linezolid 600 mg (IV) q12h x 2 weeks	Amoxicillin 1 gm (PO) q8h x 2 weeks **or** Linezolid 600 mg (PO) q12h x 2 weeks
GI/GU source likely (Treat initially for E. faecalis; if later identified as E. faecium, treat accordingly)	E. faecalis	Vancomycin 1 gm (IV) q12h x 4-6 wks **plus** Gentamicin 80 mg (IV) q8h x 4-6 weeks **or monotherapy with** Ampicillin 2 gm (IV) q4h x 4-6 weeks	Meropenem 1 gm (IV) q8h x 4-6 weeks **or** Imipenem 500 mg (IV) q6h x 4-6 weeks **or** Linezolid 600 mg (IV) q12h x 4-6 weeks	Amoxicillin 1 gm (PO) q8h x 4-6 weeks **or** Linezolid 600 mg (PO) q12h x 4-6 weeks

Subacute Bacterial Endocarditis (SBE) (cont'd)

Subset	Usual Pathogens	Preferred IV Therapy	Alternate IV Therapy	PO Therapy or IV-to-PO Switch
GI/GU source likely (cont'd)	E. faecium (VRE)	Linezolid 600 mg (IV) q12h x 4-6 weeks	Quinupristin/ dalfopristin 7.5 mg/kg (IV) q8h x 4-6 weeks	Linezolid 600 mg (PO) q12h x 4-6 weeks
	S. bovis	Treat the same as "no obvious source" subset (previous page)		
Apparent "culture negative" SBE*	Hemophilus sp. Actinobacillus actinomycetem-comitans Cardiobacterium hominis Eikenella corrodens Kingella kingae	Ceftriaxone 2 gm (IV) q24h x 4 wks **or** Any 3rd generation cephalosporin (IV) x 4 wks **or** Cefepime 2 gm (IV) q12h x 4 wks	Ampicillin 2 gm (IV) q4h x 4 wks **plus** Gentamicin 120 mg (IV) q24h x 4 wks **or monotherapy with** Quinolone† (IV) q24h x 4-6 weeks	Quinolone† (PO) q24h x 4-6 weeks
True "culture negative" SBE*	Legionella Coxiella burnetii (Q fever) Chlamydia psittaci Brucella	Quinolone† (IV) q24h x 4-6 weeks	Doxycycline 200 mg (IV) q12h x 3 days, then 100 mg (IV) q12h x 4-6 weeks	Quinolone† (PO) q24h x 4-6 weeks **or** Doxycycline 200 mg (PO) q12h x 3 days, then 100 mg (PO) q12h x 4-6 weeks**

VRE = vancomycin-resistant enterococci. Duration of therapy represents total time IV, PO, or IV + PO. Most patients on IV therapy able to take PO meds should be switched to PO therapy soon after clinical improvement
* Treat only IV or IV-to-PO switch
† Gatifloxacin 400 mg (IV or PO) or levofloxacin 500 mg (IV or PO) or moxifloxacin 400 mg (IV or PO)
** Loading dose is not needed PO if given IV with the same drug

Clinical Presentation: Subacute febrile illness ± localizing symptoms/signs in a patient with a heart murmur. Peripheral manifestations are commonly absent with early diagnosis/treatment
Diagnosis: Positive blood cultures plus vegetation on transthoracic/transesophageal echo

SBE (No Obvious Source)
Diagnostic Considerations: Most common pathogen is S. viridans. Source is usually from the mouth, although oral/dental infection is usually inapparent clinically
Pitfalls: Vegetations without positive blood cultures or peripheral manifestations of SBE are not diagnostic of endocarditis. SBE vegetations may persist after antibiotic therapy, but are sterile
Therapeutic Considerations: In penicillin-allergic (anaphylactic) patients, vancomycin may be used alone or in combination with gentamicin. Follow ESR weekly to monitor antibiotic response. No need to repeat blood cultures unless patient has persistent fever or is not responding clinically. Two-week treatment is acceptable for uncomplicated S. viridans SBE. Treat nutritionally-variant streptococci (B$_6$/pyridoxal deficient streptococci) the same as for S. viridans SBE
Prognosis: Related to extent of embolization/severity of heart failure

SBE (GI/GU Source Likely)

Diagnostic Considerations: Commonest pathogens from GI/GU source are Enterococci (especially E. faecalis). If S. bovis, look for GI polyp, tumor. Enterococcal SBE commonly follows GI/GU instrumentation

Therapeutic Considerations: E. faecalis SBE may be treated with ampicillin alone; gentamicin may be added if synergy testing is positive (e.g., isolate sensitive to < 500 mcg/mL of gentamicin). Do not add gentamicin if MIC > 500 mcg/mL. For penicillin-allergic patients, use vancomycin plus gentamicin; vancomycin alone is inadequate for enterococcal (E. faecalis) SBE. Treat enterococcal PVE the same as for native valve enterococcal SBE. Treat S. bovis SBE the same as S. viridans SBE. Non-enterococcal Group D streptococci (S. bovis) is penicillin sensitive, unlike Group D enterococci (E. faecalis)

Prognosis: Related to extent of embolization/severity of heart failure

Apparent "Culture Negative" SBE

Diagnostic Considerations: Culture of HACEK organisms requires enhanced CO_2/special media (Castaneda vented bottles) and prolonged incubation (2-4 weeks). True "culture negative" SBE is rare, and is characterized by peripheral signs of SBE with a murmur, vegetation, and negative blood cultures

Pitfalls: Most cases of "culture negative" SBE are not really culture negative, but due to fastidious organisms (HACEK group) requiring prolonged incubation with enhanced CO_2 atmosphere for growth. Sterile vegetations may persist after antibiotic therapy

Therapeutic Considerations: Follow clinical improvement with serial ESRs, which should return to pretreatment levels with therapy. Verification of cure by blood culture is not needed if patient is afebrile and clinically well

Prognosis: Related to extent of embolization/severity of heart failure

True "Culture Negative" SBE

Diagnostic Considerations: Diagnosis by specific serology. Large vessel emboli suggests culture negative SBE in patients with negative blood cultures but signs of SBE

Pitfalls: Do not diagnose culture negative SBE in patients with a heart murmur and negative blood cultures if peripheral SBE manifestations are absent

Therapeutic Considerations: Treatment is based on specific organism identified by diagnostic tests

Prognosis: Related to extent of embolization/severity of heart failure

Acute Bacterial Endocarditis (ABE)

Subset	Usual Pathogens	Preferred IV Therapy	Alternate IV Therapy	PO Therapy or IV-to-PO Switch
Normal hosts* (Treat initially for MSSA; if later identified as MRSA, treat accordingly)	S. aureus (MSSA)	Nafcillin 2 gm (IV) q4h x 4-6 weeks **or** Meropenem 1 gm (IV) q8h x 4-6 weeks **or** Imipenem 500 mg (IV) q6h x 4-6 weeks	Linezolid 600 mg (IV) q12h x 4-6 weeks **or** Vancomycin 1 gm (IV) q12h x 4-6 wks	Minocycline 100 mg (PO) q12h x 4-6 wks **or** Cephalexin 1 gm (PO) q6h x 4-6 weeks **or** Linezolid 600 mg (PO) q12h x 4-6 weeks
	S. aureus (MRSA)	*Treat (IV) x 4-6 weeks* with either linezolid 600 mg q12h **or** daptomycin 6 mg/kg q24h **or** quinupristin/dalfopristin 7.5 mg/kg q8h **or** vancomycin 1 gm q12h **or** minocycline 100 mg q12h		Linezolid 600 mg (PO) q12h x 4-6 wks **or** Minocycline 100 mg (PO) q12h x 4-6 wks

Acute Bacterial Endocarditis (ABE) (cont'd)

Subset	Usual Pathogens	Preferred IV Therapy	Alternate IV Therapy	PO Therapy or IV-to-PO Switch
IV drug abusers (Treat as MSSA before culture results; treat according to pathogen after culture results)	S. aureus (MSSA)	<u>Before culture results</u> Vancomycin 1 gm (IV) q12h **plus either** Gentamicin 120 mg (IV) q24h **or** Amikacin 500 mg (IV) q24h	<u>After culture results</u> Nafcillin 2 gm (IV) q4h x 4 weeks **or** Meropenem 1 gm (IV) q8h x 4 weeks **or** Linezolid 600 mg (IV) q12h x 4 weeks **or** Vancomycin 1 gm (IV) q12h x 4 weeks	<u>After culture results</u> Linezolid 600 mg (PO) q12h x 4 weeks **or** Minocycline 100 mg (PO) q12h x 4 weeks **or** Cephalexin 1 gm (PO) q6h x 4 weeks
	S. aureus (MRSA)	<u>Before culture results</u> Treat the same as MSSA	<u>After culture results</u> Linezolid 600 mg (IV) q12h x 4 weeks **or** Vancomycin 1 gm (IV) q12h x 4 weeks **or** Minocycline 100 mg (IV) q12h x 4 weeks	<u>After culture results</u> Linezolid 600 mg (PO) q12h x 4 weeks **or** Minocycline 100 mg (PO) q12h x 4 weeks
	P. aeruginosa*	<u>Before culture results</u> Treat the same as MSSA	<u>After culture results</u> **One "A" drug + one "B" drug** **"A" Drugs** Piperacillin/tazobactam 4.5 gm (IV) q8h x 4-6 wks **or** Cefepime 2 gm (IV) q8h x 4-6 weeks **or** Meropenem 1 gm (IV) q8h x 4-6 weeks **"B" Drugs** Amikacin 500 mg (IV) q24h x 4-6 weeks **or** Aztreonam 2 gm (IV) q8h x 4-6 weeks	<u>After culture results</u> Ciprofloxacin 750 mg (PO) q12h x 4-6 weeks

MSSA/MRSA = methicillin-sensitive/resistant S. aureus. Duration of therapy represents total time IV, PO, or IV + PO. Most patients on IV therapy able to take PO meds should be switched to PO therapy after clinical improvement
*   *Treat only IV or IV-to-PO switch*

Acute Bacterial Endocarditis

Diagnostic Considerations: Patients are critically ill and febrile (temperature ≥ 102°F). Vegetations are almost always present

Pitfalls: Obtain a baseline echocardiogram; watch for valve destruction, heart failure, ring/perivalvular abscess. Obtain cardiology consultation

Therapeutic Considerations: Treat for 4-6 weeks. Follow teichoic acid antibody levels weekly in S. aureus ABE, which fall (along with the ESR) with effective therapy

Prognosis: Related to extent of embolization/severity of heart failure

Acute Bacterial Endocarditis (IV Drug Abusers)

Diagnostic Considerations: IVDAs with S. aureus usually have mild ABE, permitting oral treatment

Pitfalls: IVDAs with new aortic or tricuspid regurgitation should be treated IV ± valve replacement

Therapeutic Considerations: After pathogen is isolated, may switch from IV to PO regimen to complete treatment course

Prognosis: Prognosis is better than for normal hosts (endocarditis usually milder) if not complicated by abscess, valve regurgitation, or heart failure

Prosthetic Valve Endocarditis (PVE)

Subset	Usual Pathogens	Before Culture Results	After Culture Results
Early PVE (< 60 days post-PVR)	S. aureus (MSSA/MRSA) Entero-bacteriaceae	Vancomycin 1 gm (IV) q12h **plus** Gentamicin 120 mg (IV) q24h	<u>MSSA/Enterobacteriaceae</u> Cefotaxime 3 gm (IV) q6h x 4-6 weeks **or** Ceftizoxime 4 gm (IV) q8h x 4-6 weeks **or** Cefepime 2 gm (IV) q8-12h x 4-6 weeks **or** Meropenem 1 gm (IV) q8h x 4-6 weeks <u>MRSA</u> Linezolid 600 mg (IV or PO) q12h x 4-6 weeks **or** Vancomycin 1 gm (IV) q12h x 4-6 weeks* **or** Minocycline 100 mg (IV or PO) q12h x 4-6 weeks
Late PVE (> 60 days post-PVR)	S. viridans S. epidermidis (MSSE/MRSE)	Linezolid 600 mg (IV or PO) q12h **or combination therapy with** Vancomycin 1 gm (IV) q12h **plus** Gentamicin 120 mg (IV) q24h	<u>S. viridans</u> Ceftriaxone 2 gm (IV) q24h x 4-6 weeks **or** Cefotaxime 3 gm (IV) q6h x 4-6 weeks **or** Ceftizoxime 4 gm (IV) q8h x 4-6 weeks <u>MSSE/MRSE</u> Linezolid 600 mg (IV or PO) q12h x 4-6 weeks **or** Vancomycin 1 gm (IV) q12h x 4-6 weeks*

MSSA/MRSA = methicillin-sensitive/resistant S. aureus; MSSE/MRSE = methicillin-sensitive/resistant S. epidermidis. Duration of therapy represents total time IV or IV + PO. Most patients on IV therapy able to take PO meds should be switched to PO therapy after clinical improvement

* ± Rifampin 300 mg (PO) q12h x 4-6 weeks

Clinical Presentation: Prolonged fevers and chills following prosthetic valve replacement (PVR)
Diagnosis: High-grade blood culture positivity (3/4 or 4/4) with endocarditis pathogen and no other source of infection

Early PVE (< 60 days post-PVR)
Diagnostic Considerations: Blood cultures persistently positive. Temperature usually ≤ 102°F
Pitfalls: Obtain baseline TTE/TEE. Premature closure of mitral leaflet is early sign of impending aortic valve regurgitation
Therapeutic Considerations: Patients improve clinically on treatment, but are not cured without valve replacement. Replace valve as soon as possible (no advantage in waiting)
Prognosis: Related to extent of embolization/severity of heart failure

Late PVE (> 60 days post-PVR)
Pitfalls: Culture of removed valve may be negative, but valve gram stain will be positive
Therapeutic Considerations: Late PVE resembles S. viridans SBE clinically. Valve removal for S. epidermidis PVE may be necessary for cure
Prognosis: Related to extent of embolization/severity of heart failure

Pericarditis/Myocarditis

Subset	Usual Pathogens	Preferred Therapy
Viral pericarditis/ myocarditis	Coxsackie virus	No treatment available
TB pericarditis	M. tuberculosis	Treat the same as pulmonary TB (p. 47)
Suppurative pericarditis	S. pneumoniae S. aureus	Treat the same as lung abscess/empyema (p. 53)

Clinical Presentation: Viral pericarditis presents with acute onset of fever/chest pain (made worse by sitting up) following a viral illness. Viral myocarditis presents with heart failure, arrhythmias ± emboli. TB pericarditis is indolent in presentation, with ↑ jugular venous distension (JVD), pericardial friction rub (40%), paradoxical pulse (25%), and chest x-ray with cardiomegaly ± left-sided pleural effusion. Suppurative pericarditis presents as acute pericarditis (patients are critically ill). Develops from contiguous (e.g., pneumonia) or hematogenous spread (e.g., S. aureus bacteremia)
Diagnostic Considerations: Pericarditis/effusion manifests cardiomegaly with decreased heart sounds ± tamponade. Diagnosis by culture/biopsy of pericardial fluid or pericardium for viruses, bacteria, or acid-fast bacilli (AFB). Diagnosis of myocarditis is clinical ± myocardial biopsy
Pitfalls: Consider other causes of pericardial effusion (malignancy, especially with bloody effusion, uremia, etc.). Rule out treatable non-viral causes of myocarditis (e.g., RMSF, Lyme disease, diphtheria)
Therapeutic Considerations: No specific treatment for viral myocarditis/pericarditis. TB pericarditis is treated the same as pulmonary TB ± pericardiectomy. Suppurative pericarditis is treated the same as lung abscess plus surgical drainage (pericardial window)
Prognosis: For viral pericarditis, the prognosis is good, but viral myocarditis may be fatal. For TB pericarditis, the prognosis is good if treated before constrictive pericarditis/adhesions develop. Suppurative pericarditis is often fatal without early pericardial window/antibiotic therapy

IV Line and Pacemaker Infections

Subset	Usual Pathogens	Preferred IV Therapy	Alternate IV Therapy	IV-to-PO Switch
Central IV line infection (temporary) *Bacterial* (Treat initially for MSSA; if later identified as MRSA, treat accordingly)	S. aureus (MSSA) Entero-bacteriaceae	Cefepime 2 gm (IV) q12h* **or** Meropenem 1 gm (IV) q8h* **or** Imipenem 500 mg (IV) q6h*	Ceftizoxime 2 gm (IV) q8h* **or** Cefotaxime 2 gm (IV) q6h*	Clindamycin 300 mg (PO) q8h* **plus** Quinolone‡ (PO) q24h*
	S. aureus (MRSA)	Linezolid 600 mg (IV) q12h* **or** Vancomycin 1 gm (IV) q12h*	Quinupristin/ dalfopristin 7.5 mg/kg (IV) q8h* **or** Minocycline 100 mg (IV) q12h*	Linezolid 600 mg (PO) q12h* **or** Minocycline 100 mg (PO) q12h*
Candida (Treat initially for C. albicans; if later identified as non-albicans Candida, treat accordingly. For candidemia not associated with IV lines, see pp. 120/122)	C. albicans	Itraconazole 200 mg (IV) q12h x 2 days, then 200 mg (IV) q24h*	Caspofungin 70 mg (IV) x 1 dose, then 50 mg (IV) q24h*	Itraconazole 200 mg (PO) solution q12h*†
	Non-albicans Candida	Itraconazole 200 mg (IV) q12h x 2 days, then 200 mg (IV) q24h* **or** Caspofungin 70 mg (IV) x 1 dose, then 50 mg (IV) q24h*	Fluconazole 800 mg (IV) x 1, then 400 mg (IV) q24h* **or** Amphotericin 1.5 mg/kg (IV) q24h*	Itraconazole 200 mg (PO) solution q12h*† **or** Fluconazole 800 mg (PO) x 1, then 400 mg (PO) q24h*†
Central IV line infection (semi-permanent); Hickman/ Broviac *Bacterial* (Treat initially for S. aureus; if later identified as S. epidermidis, treat accordingly)	S. aureus (MSSA/MRSA)	Linezolid 600 mg (IV) q12h* **or** Vancomycin 1 gm (IV) q12h*	Quinupristin/ dalfopristin 7.5 mg/kg (IV) q8h*	Linezolid 600 mg (PO) q12h* **or** Minocycline 100 mg (PO) q12h*
	S. epidermidis (MSSE/MRSE)	Linezolid 600 mg (IV) q12h* **or** Vancomycin 1 gm (IV) q12h*	Quinupristin/ dalfopristin 7.5 mg/kg (IV) q8h*	Linezolid 600 mg (PO) q12h*

* For S. aureus (MSSA/MRSA), treat x 2 weeks after line removal; for all other pathogens, treat x 1 week after line removal
† Loading dose is not needed PO if given IV with the same drug
‡ Gatifloxacin 400 mg or levofloxacin 500 mg or moxifloxacin 400 mg

IV Line and Pacemaker Infections (cont'd)

Subset	Usual Pathogens	Preferred IV Therapy	Alternate IV Therapy	IV-to-PO Switch
Pacemaker wire/generator infection (Treat initially for S. aureus; if later identified as S. epidermidis, treat accordingly)	S. aureus (MSSA/MRSA)	Linezolid 600 mg (IV) q12h*† **or** Vancomycin 1 gm (IV) q12h*†	Quinupristin/ dalfopristin 7.5 mg/kg (IV) q8h*†	Linezolid 600 mg (PO) q12h*† **or** Minocycline 100 mg (PO) q12h*†
	S. epidermidis (MSSE/MRSE)	Linezolid 600 mg (IV) q12h† **or** Vancomycin 1 gm (IV) q12h†	Quinupristin/ dalfopristin 7.5 mg/kg (IV) q8h†	Linezolid 600 mg (PO) q12h†
Septic thrombophlebitis (Treat initially for MSSA; if later identified as MRSA, treat accordingly)	S. aureus (MSSA)	Nafcillin 2 gm (IV) q4h x 2 weeks* **or** Meropenem 1 gm (IV) q8h x 2 weeks* **or** Imipenem 500 mg (IV) q6h x 2 weeks* **or** Linezolid 600 mg (IV) q12h x 2 weeks*	Ceftizoxime 2 gm (IV) q8h x 2 weeks* **or** Cefotaxime 2 gm (IV) q6h x 2 weeks*	Linezolid 600 mg (PO) q12h x 2 weeks* **or** Clindamycin 300 mg (PO) q8h x 2 weeks* **or** Cephalexin 1 gm (PO) q6h x 2 weeks*
	S. aureus (MRSA)	Linezolid 600 mg (IV) q12h x 2 weeks* **or** Vancomycin 1 gm (IV) q12h x 2 weeks*	Quinupristin/ dalfopristin 7.5 mg/kg (IV) q8h x 2 weeks*	Linezolid 600 mg (PO) q12h x 2 weeks* **or** Minocycline 100 mg (PO) q12h x 2 weeks*

MSSA/MRSA = methicillin-sensitive/resistant S. aureus; MSSE/MRSE = methicillin-sensitive/resistant S. epidermidis.
Duration of therapy represents total time IV or IV + PO. Most patients on IV therapy able to take PO meds should be switched to PO therapy after clinical improvement
*   Obtain teichoic acid antibody titers after 2 weeks. If titers are 1:4 or less, 2 weeks of therapy is sufficient. If titers are > 1:4, rule out endocarditis and complete 4-6 weeks of therapy
†   Treat x 2 weeks after wire/generator removal

Central IV Line Infection (Temporary)

Clinical Presentation: Temperature ≥ 102°F ± IV site erythema

Diagnostic Considerations: Diagnosis by semi-quantitative catheter tip culture with ≥ 15 colonies plus blood cultures with same pathogen. If no other explanation for fever and line has been in place ≥ 7 days, remove line and obtain semi-quantitative catheter tip culture. Suppurative thrombophlebitis presents with hectic/septic fevers and pus at IV site ± palpable venous cord

Pitfalls: Temperature ≥ 102° F with IV line infection, in contrast to phlebitis

Therapeutic Considerations: Line removal is usually curative, but antibiotic therapy is usually given for 1 week after IV line removal for gram-negative bacilli or 2 weeks after IV line removal for S. aureus (MSSA/MRSA). Antifungal therapy is usually given for 1 week after IV line removal for Candidemia

Prognosis: Good if line is removed before endocarditis/metastatic spread

Central IV Line Infection (Semi-Permanent) Hickman/Broviac

Clinical Presentation: Fever ± IV site erythema

Diagnostic Considerations: Positive blood cultures plus gallium scan pickup on catheter is diagnostic

Pitfalls: Antibiotics will lower temperature, but patient will usually not be afebrile without line removal

Therapeutic Considerations: Lines usually need to be removed for cure. Rifampin 600 mg (PO) q24h may be added to IV/PO regimen if pathogen is S. aureus

Prognosis: Good with organisms of low virulence

Pacemaker Wire/Generator Infection

Clinical Presentation: Persistently positive blood cultures without endocarditis in a pacemaker patient

Diagnostic Considerations: Positive blood cultures with gallium scan pickup on wire/pacemaker generator is diagnostic. Differentiate wire from pacemaker pocket infection by chest CT/MRI

Pitfalls: Positive blood cultures are more common in wire infections than pocket infections. Blood cultures may be negative in both, but more so with pocket infections

Therapeutic Considerations: Wire alone may be replaced if infection does not involve pacemaker generator. Replace pacemaker generator if involved; wire if uninvolved can usually be left in place

Prognosis: Good if pacemaker wire/generator replaced before septic complications develop

Septic Thrombophlebitis

Clinical Presentation: Temperature ≥ 102°F with local erythema and signs of sepsis

Diagnostic Considerations: Palpable venous cord and pus at IV site when IV line is removed

Pitfalls: Suspect diagnosis if persistent bacteremia and no other source of infection in a patient with a peripheral IV

Therapeutic Considerations: Remove IV catheter. Surgical venotomy is usually needed for cure

Prognosis: Good if removed early before septic complications develop

Vascular Graft Infections

Subset	Usual Pathogens	Preferred IV Therapy	Alternate IV Therapy	IV-to-PO Switch
AV graft/shunt infection (Treat initially for MSSA, etc.; if later identified as MRSA, treat accordingly)	S. aureus (MSSA) Enterococci Entero-bacteriaceae	Meropenem 1 gm (IV) x 1 dose*† **or** Imipenem 500 mg (IV) x 1 dose*† **or** Piperacillin/ tazobactam 4.5 gm (IV) x 1 dose*†	Vancomycin 1 gm (IV) x 1 dose*† **plus** Gentamicin 240 mg (IV) x 1 dose*†	Gatifloxacin 400 mg (IV or PO) x 1 dose*† **or** Levofloxacin 500 mg (IV or PO) x 1 dose*† **or** Moxifloxacin 400 mg (IV or PO) x 1 dose*†
	S. aureus (MRSA)	Linezolid 600 mg (IV) x 1 dose*†	Vancomycin 1 gm (IV) x 1 dose*†	Linezolid 600 mg (PO) x 1 dose*†
Aortic graft infection	S. aureus (MSSA) Entero-bacteriaceae P. aeruginosa	Cefepime 2 gm (IV) q12h† **or** Meropenem 1 gm (IV) q8h† **or** Piperacillin/ tazobactam 4.5 gm (IV) q8h†	Imipenem 500 mg (IV) q6h†	Gatifloxacin 400 mg (PO) q24h† **or** Levofloxacin 500 mg (PO) q24h† **or** Moxifloxacin 400 mg (PO) q24h†

MSSA/MRSA = methicillin-sensitive/resistant S. aureus. Duration of therapy represents total time IV or IV + PO. Most patients on IV therapy able to take PO meds should be switched to PO therapy after clinical improvement

*   Follow with maintenance dosing for renal failure (CrCl < 10 mL/min) and type of dialysis (see Chapter 7)

†   Treat until graft is removed/replaced

AV Graft Infection
Clinical Presentation: Persistent fever/bacteremia without endocarditis in a patient with an AV graft on hemodialysis
Diagnostic Considerations: Diagnosis by persistently positive blood cultures and gallium scan pickup over infected AV graft. Gallium scan will detect deep AV graft infection not apparent on exam
Pitfalls: Antibiotics will lower temperature, but patient will usually not become afebrile without AV graft replacement
Therapeutic Considerations: Graft usually must be removed for cure. MRSA is a rare cause of AV graft infection; if present, treat with linezolid 600 mg (IV or PO) q12h until graft is removed/replaced
Prognosis: Good if new graft does not become infected at same site

Aortic Graft Infection
Clinical Presentation: Persistently positive blood cultures without endocarditis in a patient with an aortic graft
Diagnostic Considerations: Diagnosis by positive blood cultures plus gallium scan pickup over infected aortic graft or abdominal CT/MRI scan
Pitfalls: Infection typically occurs at anastomotic sites

Therapeutic Considerations: Graft must be removed for cure. Operate as soon as diagnosis is confirmed (no value in waiting for surgery). MRSA is a rare cause of AV graft infection; if present, treat with linezolid 600 mg (IV or PO) q12h until graft is replaced

Prognosis: Good if infected graft is removed before septic complications develop

Empiric Therapy of GI Tract Infections

Esophagitis

Subset	Usual Pathogens	Preferred IV Therapy	Alternate IV Therapy	PO Therapy or IV-to-PO Switch
Fungal	Candida albicans	Fluconazole 200 mg (PO) x 1 dose, then 100 mg (PO) q24h x 3 weeks	Itraconazole 200 mg (IV) q12h x 2 days, then 200 mg (IV) q24h x 3 weeks **or** Amphotericin B deoxycholate 0.5 mg/kg (IV) q24h x 3 weeks **or** Caspofungin 50 mg (IV) q24h x 3 weeks	Itraconazole 200 mg (PO) solution q24h x 3 weeks **or** Fluconazole 200 mg (PO) x 1 dose, then 100 mg (PO) q24h x 3 weeks*
	Fluconazole-resistant C. albicans	Itraconazole 200 mg (PO) solution q24h or 100 mg (PO) solution q12h x 3 weeks		
	Non-albicans Candida	Itraconazole 200 mg (PO) solution q24h or 100 mg (PO) solution q12h x 3 weeks		
Viral	HSV-1	Acyclovir 5 mg/kg (IV) q8h x 3 weeks	Valacyclovir 500 mg (PO) q12h x 3 weeks **or** Famciclovir 500 mg (PO) q12h x 3 weeks	
	CMV	Ganciclovir 5 mg/kg (IV) q12h x 3 weeks	Valganciclovir 900 mg (PO) q12h x 3 weeks	

Duration of therapy represents total time IV, PO, or IV + PO. Most patients on IV therapy able to take PO meds should be switched to PO therapy soon after clinical improvement (usually < 72 hours)
* Loading dose is not needed PO if given IV with the same drug

Clinical Presentation: Pain on swallowing
Diagnosis: Stain/culture for fungi/HSV/CMV on biopsy specimen

Fungal (Candida) Esophagitis
Diagnostic Considerations: Rarely if ever in normal hosts. Often (but not always) associated with Candida in mouth. If patient is not alcoholic or diabetic and not receiving antibiotics, test for HIV
Pitfalls: Therapy as a diagnostic trial is apropapriate. Suspect CMV-related disease and proceed to endoscopy if a patient with a typical symptom complex fails to respond to antifungal therapy
Therapeutic Considerations: In normal hosts, treat for 1 week after clinical resolution. HIV patients respond more slowly than normal hosts and may need higher doses/treatment for 2-3 weeks after

clinical resolution (p. 250)
Prognosis: Related to degree of immunosuppression

Viral Esophagitis
Diagnostic Considerations: Rarely in normal hosts. May occur in non-HIV immunosuppressed patients
Pitfalls: Viral and non-viral esophageal ulcers look similar; need biopsy for specific viral diagnosis
Therapeutic Considerations: In normal hosts, treat for 2-3 weeks after clinical resolution. HIV patients respond more slowly and may need treatment for weeks after clinical resolution for cure
Prognosis: Related to degree of immunosuppression

Peptic Ulcer Disease

Subset	Usual Pathogens	Preferred Therapy
Peptic ulcer disease	Helicobacter pylori	Omeprazole 20 mg (PO) q12h x 2 weeks **plus** Clarithromycin 500 mg (PO) q12h x 2 weeks **plus** Amoxicillin 1 gm (PO) q8h x 2 weeks

Clinical Presentation: Periodic mid/upper abdominal pain relieved by meals. No fever
Diagnostic Considerations: Diagnosis by positive urea breath test
Pitfalls: Confirm diagnosis before starting therapy
Therapeutic Considerations: Regimens containing metronidazole or doxycycline are less effective
Prognosis: Excellent

Gastric Perforation

Subset	Usual Pathogens	Preferred IV Therapy	Alternate IV Therapy	IV-to-PO Switch
Gastric perforation	Oral anaerobes	Cefazolin 1 gm (IV) q8h x 2 weeks	Any β-lactam (IV) x 2 weeks	Amoxicillin 1 gm (PO) q8h x 2 weeks **or** Cephalexin 500 mg (PO) q6h x 2 weeks **or** Gatifloxacin 400 mg (PO) q24h x 2 weeks **or** Levofloxacin 500 mg (PO) q24h x 2 weeks **or** Moxifloxacin 400 mg (PO) q24h x 2 weeks

Duration of therapy represents total time IV or IV + PO. Most patients on IV therapy able to take PO meds should be switched to PO therapy after clinical improvement

Clinical Presentation: Presents acutely with fever and peritonitis
Diagnostic Considerations: Obtain CT/MRI of abdomen to determine site of perforation
Pitfalls: No need to cover B. fragilis with perforation of stomach/small intestine
Therapeutic Considerations: Obtain surgical consult for possible repair
Prognosis: Good if repaired

Infectious Diarrhea/Typhoid (Enteric) Fever

Subset	Usual Pathogens	Preferred Therapy	Alternate Therapy
Acute watery diarrhea	E. coli Campylobacter Yersinia Salmonella Vibrio sp.	Quinolone† (IV or PO) x 5 days	Doxycycline 100 mg (IV or PO) q12h x 5 days **or** TMP-SMX 1 DS tablet (PO) q12h x 5 days
Antibiotic-associated diarrhea/colitis (AAD/AAC)	Clostridium difficile	<u>AAD</u>: Vancomycin 125 mg (PO) q6h x 7-10 days <u>AAC</u>: Metronidazole 1 gm (IV) q24h or 500 mg (IV) q12h until cured	<u>AAD</u>: Metronidazole 250 mg (PO) q6h x 7-10 days <u>AAC</u>: Metronidazole 500 mg (PO) q12h until cured
Typhoid (enteric) fever	Salmonella typhi/non-typhi	Quinolone† (IV or PO) x 10-14 days **or** TMP-SMX 5 mg/kg (IV or PO) q6h x 10-14 days	Chloramphenicol 500 mg (IV or PO) q6h x 10-14 days **or** Any 3rd generation cephalosporin (IV or PO) x 10-14 days
Chronic watery diarrhea	Giardia lamblia*	Metronidazole 250 mg (PO) q8h x 5 days	Albendazole 400 mg (PO) q24h x 5 days **or** Quinacrine 100 mg (PO) q8h x 5 days
	Cryptosporidia*	No good treatment	Paromomycin 500-750 mg (PO) q8h until response **or** Azithromycin 600 mg (PO) q24h x 4 weeks
	Cyclospora*	TMP-SMX 1 DS tablet (PO) q12h x 2-4 weeks	
Acute dysentery	E. histolytica	Metronidazole 750 mg (PO) q8h x 10 days **followed by either** Iodoquinol 650 mg (PO) q8h x 20 days **or** Paromomycin 500 mg (PO) q8h x 7 days	Tinidazole 1 gm (PO) q12h x 3 days
	Shigella	Quinolone† (IV or PO) x 3 days	TMP-SMX 1 DS tablet (PO) q12h x 3 days **or** Azithromycin 500 mg (PO) q24h x 3 days

Duration of therapy represents total time IV, PO, or IV + PO. Most patients on IV therapy able to take PO meds should be switched to PO therapy soon after clinical improvement (usually < 72 hours)

* *May also present as acute watery diarrhea*

† *Ciprofloxacin 400 mg (IV) or 500 mg (PO) q12h or gatifloxacin 400 mg (IV or PO) q24h or levofloxacin 500 mg (IV or PO) q24h or moxifloxacin 400 mg (IV or PO) q24h*

Acute Watery Diarrhea

Clinical Presentation: Acute onset of watery diarrhea without blood/mucus

Diagnostic Considerations: Diagnosis by culture of organism from stool specimens

Pitfalls: Recommended antibiotics are active against most susceptible bacterial pathogens causing diarrhea, but not viruses/parasites. Concomitant transient lactase deficiency may prolong diarrhea if dairy products are taken during an infectious diarrhea

Therapeutic Considerations: Avoid norfloxacin and ciprofloxacin due to resistance potential. V. cholerae may be treated with a single dose of any oral quinolone or doxycycline

Prognosis: Excellent. Most recover with supportive treatment

Antibiotic-Associated Diarrhea/Colitis (Clostridium difficile)

Clinical Presentation: Watery diarrhea following exposure to patients with C. difficile diarrhea or recent cancer/antibiotic therapy. Clinically indistinguishable from other toxigenic community-acquired watery diarrheas. Most often associated with clindamycin or beta-lactams. Rarely due to quinolones, aminoglycosides, linezolid, doxycycline, TMP-SMX, carbapenems, vancomycin, piperacillin/tazobactam, cefoperazone, or cefepime

Diagnostic Considerations: Watery diarrhea with positive C. difficile toxin in stool specimen. Temperature is usually < 102°F. In patients receiving enteral feeds and antibiotics, diarrhea is much more likely due to enteral feeds than C. difficile

Pitfalls: In a patient with C. difficile diarrhea, C. difficile colitis is suggested by the presence of abdominal pain and temperature > 102° F; confirm diagnosis with CT/MRI of abdomen

Therapeutic Considerations: Oral vancomycin is more often effective than oral metronidazole. C. difficile diarrhea begins to improve and usually resolves by 5-7 days, although some patients require 10 days of therapy. Do not continue treating C. difficile toxin-negative diarrhea with vancomycin or metronidazole. For relapses/recurrences, treat with vancomycin 250 mg (PO) q6h x 10-14 days. For C. difficile colitis, treat until colitis resolves with metronidazole 1 gm (IV) q24h or 500 mg (IV) q12h or 500 mg (PO) q6-12h. IV vancomycin is *not* useful for C. difficile diarrhea/colitis

Pitfalls: C. difficile toxin may remain positive in stools for weeks following treatment; do not treat positive stool toxin unless patient has persistent diarrhea

Prognosis: Good with early treatment. Worse if treated late or patient has colitis. Prognosis with C. difficile colitis is related to severity of the colitis

Typhoid (Enteric) Fever (Salmonella typhi/non-typhi)

Clinical Presentation: High fevers (> 102°F) increasing in a stepwise fashion accompanied by relative bradycardia in a patient with watery diarrhea/constipation, headache, abdominal pain, cough/sore throat ± Rose spots

Diagnostic Considerations: Most community-acquired watery diarrheas are not accompanied by temperatures > 102°F and relative bradycardia. Diagnosis is confirmed by demonstrating Salmonella in blood, bone marrow, Rose spots, or stool cultures. Culture of bone marrow is the quickest/most reliable method of diagnosis. WBC count is usually low/low normal. Leukocytosis should suggest another diagnosis or bowel perforation, which may occur during 2nd week of typhoid fever

Pitfalls: Rose spots are few/difficult to see and not present in all cases. Typhoid fever usually presents with constipation, not diarrhea. Suspect another diagnosis in the absence of headache

Therapeutic Considerations: 2nd generation cephalosporins, aztreonam, and aminoglycosides are ineffective. Since Salmonella strains causing enteric fever are intracellular pathogens, treat for a full 2 weeks to maximize cure rates/minimize relapses. Treat relapses with the suggested antibiotics x 2-3 weeks. Salmonella excretion into feces usually persists < 3 months. Persistent excretion > 3 months suggests a carrier state—rule out hepatobiliary/urinary calculi

Prognosis: Good if treated early. Poor with late treatment/bowel perforation

Chronic Watery Diarrhea

Clinical Presentation: Watery diarrhea without blood/mucus lasting > 1 month

Diagnostic Considerations: Diagnosis by demonstrating organisms/cysts in stool specimens. Multiple fresh daily stool samples often needed for diagnosis
Pitfalls: Concomitant transient lactase deficiency may prolong diarrhea if dairy products are taken during an infectious diarrhea
Therapeutic Considerations: Cryptosporidia and Cyclospora are being recognized increasingly in acute/chronic diarrhea in normal hosts
Prognosis: Excellent in well-nourished patients. Untreated patients may develop malabsorption

Giardia lamblia
Clinical Presentation: Acute/subacute onset of diarrhea, abdominal cramps, bloating, flatulence. Incubation period 1-2 weeks. Malabsorption may occur in chronic cases. No eosinophilia
Diagnostic Considerations: Diagnosis by demonstrating trophozoites or cysts in stool/antigen detection assay. If stool exam and antigen test are negative and Giardiasis is suspected, perform "string test"/duodenal aspirate and biopsy
Pitfalls: Eggs intermittently excreted into stool. Usually need multiple stool samples for diagnosis. Often accompanied by transient lactose intolerance
Therapeutic Considerations: Diarrhea may be prolonged if milk (lactose-containing) products are ingested after treatment/cure
Prognosis: Related to severity of malabsorption and health of host

Cryptosporidia
Clinical Presentation: Acute/subacute onset of diarrhea. Usually occurs in HIV/AIDS patients with CD_4 counts < 200. Biliary cryptosporidiosis is seen only in HIV; may present as acalculous cholecystitis or sclerosing cholangitis with RUQ pain, fever, ↑ alkaline phosphatase, but bilirubin is normal
Diagnostic Considerations: Diagnosis by demonstrating organism in stool/intestinal biopsy specimen. Cholera-like illness in normal hosts. Chronic watery diarrhea in compromised hosts
Pitfalls: Smaller than Cyclospora. Oocyst walls are smooth (not wrinkled) on acid fast staining
Prognosis: Related to adequacy of fluid replacement/underlying health of host

Cyclospora
Clinical Presentation: Acute/subacute onset of diarrhea. Incubation period 1-14 days
Diagnostic Considerations: Diagnosis by demonstrating organism in stool/intestinal biopsy specimen. Clinically indistinguishable from cryptosporidial diarrhea (intermittent watery diarrhea without blood or mucus). Fatigue/weight loss common
Pitfalls: Oocysts only form seen in stool and are best identified with modified Kinyoun acid fast staining. Acid fast fat globules stain pink with acid fast staining. "Wrinkled wall" oocysts are characteristic of Cyclospora, not Cryptosporidia. Oocysts are twice the size of similar appearing Cryptosporidia (~ 10 µm vs. 5 µm)
Prognosis: Related to adequacy of fluid replacement/underlying health of host

Acute Dysentery
Entamoeba histolytica
Clinical Presentation: Acute/subacute onset of bloody diarrhea/mucus. Fecal WBC/RBCs due to mucosal invasion. E. histolytica may also cause chronic diarrhea. Colonic ulcers secondary to E. histolytica are round and may form "collar stud" abscesses
Diagnostic Considerations: Diagnosis by demonstrating organism/trophozoites in stool/intestinal biopsy specimen. Serology is negative in amebic dysentery, but positive with extra-intestinal forms. Test to separate E. histolytica from non-pathogenic E. dispar cyst passers. On sigmoidoscopy, ulcers due to E. histolytica are round with normal mucosa in between, and may form "collar stud" abscesses. In contrast, ulcers due to Shigella are linear and serpiginous without normal intervening mucosa. Bloody dysentery is more subacute with E. histolytica compared to Shigella
Pitfalls: Intestinal perforation/abscess may complicate amebic colitis. Rule out infectious causes of

bloody diarrhea with mucus before diagnosing/treating inflammatory bowel disease (IBD). Obtain multiple stool cultures for bacterial pathogens/parasites. Do not confuse E. histolytica in stool specimens with E. hartmanni, a non-pathogen protozoa similar in appearance but smaller in size
Therapeutic Considerations: E. histolytica cyst passers should be treated, but metronidazole is ineffective against cysts. Use paromomycin 500 mg (PO) q8h x 7 days for asymptomatic cysts. Recommended antibiotics treat both luminal and hepatic E. histolytica
Prognosis: Good if treated early. Related to severity of dysentery/ulcers/extra-intestinal amebiasis

Shigella
Clinical Presentation: Acute onset of bloody diarrhea/mucus
Diagnostic Considerations: Diagnosis by demonstrating organism in stool specimens. Shigella ulcers in colon are linear, serpiginous, and rarely lead to perforation
Therapeutic Considerations: Shigella dysentery is more acute/fulminating than amebic dysentery. Shigella has no carrier state, unlike Entamoeba
Prognosis: Good if treated early. Severity of illness related to Shigella species: S. dysenteriae (most severe) > S. flexneri > S. boydii/S. sonnei (mildest)

Cholecystitis

Subset	Usual Pathogens	Preferred IV Therapy	Alternate IV Therapy	PO Therapy or IV-to-PO Switch
Normal host	E. coli Klebsiella Enterococci	Quinolone[‡] (IV)* **or** Piperacillin/ tazobactam 4.5 gm (IV) q8h*	Cefazolin 1 gm (IV) q8h* **plus** Ampicillin 1 gm (IV) q4h*	Quinolone[‡] (PO)*
Emphy-sematous cholecystitis[†]	Clostridium perfringens	Meropenem 1 gm (IV) q8h x 1 week after cholecystectomy **or** Imipenem 500 mg (IV) q6h x 1 week after cholecystectomy **or** Ertapenem 1 gm (IV) q24h x 1 week after cholecystectomy	Piperacillin/ tazobactam 4.5 gm (IV) q8h x 1 week after cholecystectomy **or** Ticarcillin/clavulanate 3.1 gm (IV) q6h x 1 week after cholecystectomy	Clindamycin 300 mg (PO) q8h x 1 week after cholecystectomy

Duration of therapy represents total time IV, PO, or IV + PO. Most patients on IV therapy able to take PO meds should be switched to PO therapy after clinical improvement
† *Treat only IV or IV-to-PO switch*
‡ *Ciprofloxacin 400 mg (IV) or 500 mg (PO) q12h or gatifloxacin 400 mg (IV or PO) q24h or levofloxacin 500 mg (IV or PO) q24h or moxifloxacin 400 mg (IV or PO) q24h*
* *If no cholecystectomy, treat x 1-2 weeks. If cholecystectomy is peformed, treat x 1 week post-operatively*

Cholecystitis in Normal Hosts
Clinical Presentation: RUQ pain, fever usually ≤ 102°F, positive Murphy's sign, no percussion tenderness over right lower ribs
Diagnostic Considerations: Diagnosis by RUQ ultrasound/positive HIDA scan
Pitfalls: No need to cover B. fragilis
Therapeutic Considerations: Obtain surgical consult for possible cholecystectomy

Prognosis: Related to cardiopulmonary status

Emphysematous Cholecystitis

Clinical Presentation: Clinically presents as cholecystitis. Usually seen in diabetics
Diagnostic Considerations: RUQ/gallbladder gas on flat plate of abdomen
Pitfalls: Requires immediate cholecystectomy
Therapeutic Considerations: Usually a difficult/prolonged post-op course
Prognosis: Related to speed of gallbladder removal

Cholangitis

Subset	Usual Pathogens	Preferred IV Therapy	Alternate IV Therapy	IV-to-PO Switch
Normal host	E. coli Klebsiella Enterococci	Meropenem 1 gm (IV) q8h x 2 weeks **or** Piperacillin/ tazobactam 4.5 gm (IV) q8h x 2 weeks **or** Cefoperazone 2 gm (IV) q12h x 2 weeks	Ampicillin/sulbactam 3 gm (IV) q6h x 2 weeks **or** Imipenem 500 mg (IV) q6h x 2 weeks **or** Ticarcillin/clavulanate 3.1 gm (IV) q6h x 2 weeks	Ciprofloxacin 500 mg (PO) q12h x 2 weeks **or** Gatifloxacin 400 mg (PO) q24h x 2 weeks **or** Levofloxacin 500 mg (PO) q24h x 2 weeks **or** Moxifloxacin 400 mg (PO) q24h x 2 weeks

Duration of therapy represents total time IV or IV + PO. Most patients on IV therapy able to take PO meds should be switched to PO therapy after clinical improvement

Clinical Presentation: RUQ pain, fever > 102°F, positive Murphy's sign, percussion tenderness over right lower ribs
Diagnostic Considerations: Obstructed common bile duct on ultrasound/CT/MRI of abdomen
Pitfalls: Charcot's triad (fever, RUQ pain, jaundice) is present in only 50%
Therapeutic Considerations: Obtain surgical consult to relieve obstruction
Prognosis: Related to speed of surgical relief of obstruction

Gallbladder Wall Abscess/Perforation

Subset	Usual Pathogens	Preferred IV Therapy	Alternate IV Therapy	IV-to-PO Switch
Gallbladder wall abscess/ perforation	E. coli Klebsiella Enterococci	Meropenem 1 gm (IV) q8h x 2 weeks **or** Piperacillin/ tazobactam 4.5 gm (IV) q8h x 2 weeks **or** Cefoperazone 2 gm (IV) q12h x 2 weeks	Ampicillin/sulbactam 3 gm (IV) q6h x 2 weeks **or** Imipenem 500 mg (IV) q6h x 2 weeks **or** Ticarcillin/clavulanate 3.1 gm (IV) q6h x 2 weeks	Ciprofloxacin 500 mg (PO) q12h x 2 weeks **or** Gatifloxacin 400 mg (PO) q24h x 2 weeks **or** Levofloxacin 500 mg (PO) q24h x 2 weeks **or** Moxifloxacin 400 mg (PO) q24h x 2 weeks

Duration of therapy represents total time IV or IV + PO. Most patients on IV therapy able to take PO meds should be switched to PO therapy after clinical improvement

Clinical Presentation: RUQ pain, fever ≤ 102°F, positive Murphy's sign, no percussion tenderness over right lower ribs
Diagnostic Considerations: Diagnosis by CT/MRI of abdomen. Bile peritonitis is common
Pitfalls: Bacterial peritonitis may be present
Therapeutic Considerations: Obtain surgical consult for possible gallbladder removal. Usually a difficult and prolonged post-op course
Prognosis: Related to removal of gallbladder/repair of perforation

Acute Pancreatitis

Subset	Usual Pathogens	Preferred IV Therapy	Alternate IV Therapy	IV-to-PO Switch
Edematous pancreatitis	None	Not applicable	Not applicable	Not applicable
Hemorrhagic/ necrotizing pancreatitis	Entero- bacteriaceae B. fragilis	Meropenem 1 gm (IV) q8h x 2 weeks **or** Imipenem 500 mg (IV) q6h x 2 weeks **or** Ertapenem 1 gm (IV) q24h x 2 weeks	Piperacillin/ tazobactam 4.5 gm (IV) q8h x 2 weeks **or** Ampicillin/sulbactam 3 gm (IV) q6h x 2 weeks **or** Ticarcillin/clavulanate 3.1 gm (IV) q6h x 2 weeks	Clindamycin 300 mg (PO) q8h x 2 weeks **plus either** Ciprofloxacin 500 mg (PO) q12h x 2 weeks **or** Gatifloxacin 400 mg (PO) q24h x 2 weeks **or** Levofloxacin 500 mg (PO) q24h x 2 weeks **or monotherapy with** Moxifloxacin 400 mg (PO) q24h x 2 weeks

Duration of therapy represents total time IV or IV + PO. Most patients on IV therapy able to take PO meds should be switched to PO therapy after clinical improvement

Edematous Pancreatitis
Clinical Presentation: Sharp abdominal pain with fever ≤ 102°F ± hypotension
Diagnostic Considerations: Diagnosis by elevated serum amylase and lipase levels with normal methemalbumin levels. May be drug-induced (e.g., steroids)
Pitfalls: Amylase elevation alone is not diagnostic of acute pancreatitis
Therapeutic Considerations: NG tube is not needed. Aggressively replace fluids
Prognosis: Good with adequate fluid replacement

Hemorrhagic/Necrotizing Pancreatitis
Clinical Presentation: Sharp abdominal pain with fever ≤ 102° F ± hypotension. Grey-Turner/Cullen's sign present in some
Diagnostic Considerations: Mildly elevated serum amylase and lipase levels with high methemalbumin levels
Pitfalls: With elevated lipase, amylase level is inversely related to severity of disease

Therapeutic Considerations: Obtain surgical consult for possible peritoneal lavage as adjunct to antibiotics. Serum albumin/dextran are preferred volume expanders
Prognosis: Poor with hypocalcemia or shock

Pancreatic Abscess

Subset	Usual Pathogens	Preferred IV Therapy	Alternate IV Therapy	IV-to-PO Switch
Pancreatic abscess	Entero-bacteriaceae B. fragilis	Meropenem 1 gm (IV) q8h x 2 weeks **or** Piperacillin/ tazobactam 4.5 gm (IV) q8h x 2 weeks **or** Ertapenem 1 gm (IV) q24h x 2 weeks	Imipenem 500 mg (IV) q6h x 2 weeks **or** Ampicillin/sulbactam 3 gm (IV) q6h x 2 weeks **or** Ticarcillin/clavulanate 3.1 gm (IV) q6h x 2 weeks	Clindamycin 300 mg (PO) q8h x 2 weeks **plus** Quinolone[†] (PO) x 2 weeks **or monotherapy with** Moxifloxacin 400 mg (PO) q24h x 2 weeks

Duration of therapy represents total time IV or IV + PO. Most patients on IV therapy able to take PO meds should be switched to PO therapy after clinical improvement
† *Ciprofloxacin 500 mg q12h or gatifloxacin 400 mg q24h or levofloxacin 500 mg q24h*

Clinical Presentation: Follows acute pancreatitis or develops in a pancreatic pseudocyst. Fevers usually ≥ 102°F
Diagnostic Considerations: CT/MRI of abdomen demonstrates pancreatic abscess
Pitfalls: Peritoneal signs are typically absent
Prognosis: Related to size/extent of abscess and adequacy of drainage

Liver Abscess

Subset	Usual Pathogens	Preferred IV Therapy	Alternate IV Therapy	PO Therapy or IV-to-PO Switch
Liver abscess	Entero-bacteriaceae Enterococci B. fragilis	Meropenem 1 gm (IV) q8h* **or** Piperacillin/ tazobactam 4.5 gm (IV) q8h* **or** Imipenem 500 mg (IV) q6h*	Quinolone[†] (IV)* **plus either** Metronidazole 1 gm (IV) q24h* **or** Clindamycin 600 mg (IV) q8h* **or monotherapy with** Moxifloxacin 400 mg (IV) q24h*	Quinolone[†] (PO)* **plus either** Metronidazole 500 mg (PO) q12h* **or** Clindamycin 300 mg (PO) q8h* **or monotherapy with** Moxifloxacin 400 mg (PO) q24h*
	E. histolytica	See p. 203		

Duration of therapy represents total time IV, PO, or IV + PO. Most patients on IV therapy able to take PO meds should be switched to PO therapy after clinical improvement
* *Treat until abscess(es) are no longer present or stop decreasing in size on CT scan*
† *Ciprofloxacin 400 mg (IV) or 500 mg (PO) q12h or gatifloxacin 400 mg (IV or PO) q24h or levofloxacin 500 mg (IV or PO) q24h*

Clinical Presentation: Fever, RUQ tenderness, negative Murphy's sign, and negative right lower rib percussion tenderness

Diagnostic Considerations: Diagnosis by CT/MRI scan of liver and aspiration of abscess. CT shows multiple lesions in liver. Source is usually either the colon (diverticulitis or diverticular abscess with portal pyemia) or retrograde infection from the gallbladder (cholecystitis or gallbladder wall abscess)

Pitfalls: Bacterial abscesses are usually multiple and involve multiple lobes of liver; amebic abscesses are usually solitary and involve the right lobe of liver

Therapeutic Considerations: Liver laceration/trauma usually requires ~ 2 weeks of antibiotics

Prognosis: Good if treated early

Hepatosplenic Candidiasis

Subset	Usual Pathogens	Preferred IV Therapy	Alternate IV Therapy	IV-to-PO Switch
Hepato-splenic candidiasis	Candida albicans	Fluconazole 800 mg (IV) x 1 dose, then 400 mg (IV) q24h x 2-4 weeks **or** Caspofungin 70 mg (IV) x 1 dose, then 50 mg (IV) q24h x 2-4 weeks **or** Itraconazole 200 mg (IV) q12h x 2 days, then 200 mg (IV) q24h x 2-4 weeks	Amphotericin B deoxycholate 0.7 mg/kg (IV) q24h x 2-4 weeks **or** Lipid-associated formulation of amphotericin B (p. 297) (IV) q24h x 2-4 weeks	Fluconazole 800 mg (PO) x 1 dose, then 400 mg (PO) q24h x 2-4 weeks* **or** Itraconazole 200 mg (PO) solution q12h x 2-4 weeks

Duration of therapy represents total time IV or IV + PO. Most patients on IV therapy able to take PO meds should be switched to PO therapy after clinical improvement
* *Loading dose is not needed PO if given IV with the same drug*

Clinical Presentation: New high spiking fevers with RUQ/LUQ pain after 2 weeks in a patient with afebrile leukopenia

Diagnostic Considerations: Diagnosis by abdominal CT/MRI showing mass lesions in liver/spleen

Pitfalls: Do not overlook RUQ tenderness and elevated alkaline phosphatase in leukopenic cancer patients as a clue to the diagnosis

Therapeutic Considerations: Treat until liver/spleen lesions resolve. Should be viewed as a form of disseminated disease

Prognosis: Related to degree/duration of leukopenia

Granulomatous Hepatitis (BCG)

Subset	Pathogen	Preferred Therapy
BCG hepatitis	Bacille Calmette-Guérin (BCG)	INH 300 mg (PO) q24h x 6 months + rifampin 600 mg (PO) q24h x 6 months

Clinical Presentation: Fever, chills, anorexia, weight loss, hepatomegaly ± RUQ pain days to weeks after intravesicular BCG for bladder cancer

Diagnostic Considerations: ↑ alkaline phosphatase > ↑ SGOT/SGPT. Liver biopsy is negative for AFB/positive for granulomas

Pitfalls: Exclude other causes of hepatomegaly
Therapeutic Considerations: INH plus rifampin x 6 months is curative
Prognosis: Excellent with early treatment

Viral Hepatitis

Subset	Pathogens	PO/SQ Therapy
Acute	HAV, HBV, HCV, HDV, HEV, HFV, HGV, EBV, CMV: no acute therapy	
Chronic	HBV	Adefovir (Hepsera) 10 mg (PO) q24h x 52 weeks **or** lamivudine 100 mg (PO) q24h x 52 weeks
	HCV	Pegylated interferon (Pegasys) alfa-2a (40 KD) 180 mcg/week (SQ) x 48 weeks *plus* ribavirin 500-600 mg (PO) q12h x 48 weeks (see p. 372 for dosage adjustments) **or** Pegylated interferon (Peg-Intron) alfa-2b (12 KD) 1 mcg/kg/week (SQ) x 1 year (see Table 1, below, and p. 373 for dosing adjustments) **or** Pegylated interferon (Peg-Intron) alfa-2b (12 KD) 1.5 mcg/kg/week (SQ) x 1 year (see Table 2, below, and p. 373 for dosing adjustments) *plus* ribavirin 400 mg (PO) q12h x 1 year

Table 1. Recommended PEG-Intron Monotherapy Dosing

Weight (kg)	PEG Interferon alfa-2b		
	Vial Strength (mcg/0.5 mL)	Amount to Administer (mcg)	Volume to Administer (mL)
≤ 45	50	40	0.4
46-56		50	0.5
57-72	80	64	0.4
73-88		80	0.5
89-106	120	96	0.4
107-136		120	0.5
137-160	150	150	0.5

Table 2. Recommended PEG-Intron Combination Therapy Dosing

Weight (kg)	PEG Interferon alfa-2b		
	Vial Strength (mcg/0.5 mL)	Amount to Administer (mcg)	Volume to Administer (mL)
< 40	50	50	0.5
40-50	80	64	0.4
51-60		80	0.5
61-75	120	96	0.4
76-85		120	0.5
> 85	150	150	0.5

Acute Viral Hepatitis

Clinical Presentation: Anorexia, malaise, RUQ tenderness, temperature ≤ 102°F ± jaundice
Diagnostic Considerations: Diagnosis by elevated IgM serology with markedly elevated serum transaminases (SGOT ≥ 1000). Serum alkaline phosphatase is normal/mildly elevated. Percussion tenderness over right lower ribs distinguishes liver from gallbladder problem

Pitfalls: In patients without jaundice (anicteric hepatitis), rule out other hepatitic viruses (EBV, CMV)
Therapeutic Considerations: Patients feel better after temperature falls/jaundice appears
Prognosis: Excellent for hepatitis A (does not progress to chronic active hepatitis). Hepatitis B and C may progress to chronic hepatitis/cirrhosis. Serum transaminases are not a good predictor/indicator of liver injury in hepatitis C. HGV infection may moderate HIV infection

EBV/CMV Hepatitis
Clinical Presentation: Same as acute viral hepatitis plus bilateral posterior cervical adenopathy and fatigue
Diagnostic Considerations: EBV hepatitis occurs as part of infectious mononucleosis and may be the presenting sign in older adults. CMV hepatitis presents as a "mono-like" infection in normal hosts. Like EBV, CMV hepatitis in normal hosts is part of a systemic infection. In compromised hosts, particularly bone marrow/solid organ transplants (BMT/SOT), CMV hepatitis may be the primary manifestation of CMV infection. In the normal host, EBV and CMV infectious mono/hepatitis can be diagnosed by serology (positive mono spot test, ↑ EBV VCA IgM titer, ↑ CMV IgM titer). In BMT/SOT, CMV infection/hepatitis is diagnosed by liver biopsy, PCR, or semi-quantitative CMV antigenic assay
Pitfalls: In normal hosts and BMT/SOT patients with unexplained ↑ SGOT/SGPT, consider CMV hepatitis in the differential diagnosis and order appropriate diagnostic tests
Therapeutic Considerations: EBV/CMV hepatitis is not usually treated in normal hosts. However, for CMV in BMT/SOT, early treatment with valganciclovir or gangciclovir can be life saving
Prognosis: EBV/CMV hepatitis is usually self-limiting in normal hosts. The prognosis of CMV hepatitis in BMT/SOT is related to the degree of immunosuppression and rapidity of treatment

Chronic Viral Hepatitis
Clinical Presentation: Persistently elevated serum transaminases
Diagnostic Considerations: Liver biopsy is used to diagnose chronic viral hepatitis, and to differentiate chronic persistent hepatitis (CPH) from chronic active hepatitis (CAH). Hepatitis B is diagnosed by serum HBV DNA or PCR. Hepatitis C is diagnosed by serum HCV RNA levels
Pitfalls: Do not confuse viral hepatitis with lupoid/autoimmune hepatitis, which may present in similar fashion but with elevated ANAs. With HCV, rule out co-infection with HIV
Therapeutic Considerations: For chronic HBV and lamivudine faillures, use adefovir (Hepsera) until HBV DNA levels fall and ALT normalizes. There is no advantage for adefovir plus lamivudine. Adefovir is also effective in HIV/HBV coinfected patients (no side effects/drug interactions with anti-HIV medications). For chronic HCV with early viral response (EVR) (i.e., ≥ 2 log decrease in viral load during first 12 weeks) to pegylated interferon plus ribavirin, continue treatment for 48 weeks; if no EVR, discontinue treatment. Pegasys monotherapy results in a sustained viral response in 30%. Pegasys plus ribavirin results in a 56% response.
Prognosis: CPH has a good prognosis. CAH has a worse prognosis and may progress to cirrhosis

Intraabdominal or Pelvic Peritonitis/Abscess

Subset	Usual Pathogens	Preferred IV Therapy	Alternate IV Therapy	PO Therapy or IV-to-PO Switch
Mild or moderate peritonitis (e.g, appendicitis, diverticulitis, septic pelvic thrombo-phlebitis[†])	Entero-bacteriaceae B. fragilis	Ceftriaxone 1-2 gm (IV) q24h x 2 weeks **plus** Metronidazole 1 gm (IV) q24h x 2 weeks	Moxifloxacin 400 mg (IV) q24h x 2 weeks **or** Ampicillin/sulbactam 1.5 gm (IV) q6h x 2 weeks **or** Ceftizoxime 2 gm (IV) q8h x 2 weeks **or** Cefoxitin 2 gm (IV) q6h x 2 weeks	Moxifloxacin 400 mg (PO) q24h x 2 weeks **or combination therapy with** Clindamycin 300 mg (PO) q8h x 2 weeks **plus** Quinolone[¶] (PO) q24h x 2 weeks
Severe peritonitis[‡] (e.g, appendicitis, diverticulitis, septic pelvic thrombo-phlebitis[†])	Entero-bacteriaceae B. fragilis	Meropenem 1 gm (IV) q8h x 2 weeks **or** Piperacillin/tazobactam 4.5 gm (IV) q8h x 2 weeks **or** Ertapenem 1 gm (IV) q24h x 2 weeks **or** Imipenem 500 mg (IV) q6h x 2 weeks	Clindamycin 600 mg (IV) q8h x 2 weeks **or** Metronidazole 1 gm (IV) q24h x 2 weeks **plus either** Ceftriaxone 1 gm (IV) q24h **or** Quinolone** (IV) x 2 weeks	Moxifloxacin 400 mg (PO) q24h x 2 weeks **or** Amoxicillin/clavulanic acid 875/125 mg (PO) q12h x 2 weeks **or combination therapy with** Clindamycin 300 mg (PO) q8h x 2 weeks **plus** Quinolone[¶] (PO) q24h x 2 weeks
Spontaneous bacterial peritonitis (SBP)[‡]	Entero-bacteriaceae	Ceftriaxone 1 gm (IV) q24h x 2 weeks **or** Quinolone** (IV) x 2 weeks	Aztreonam 2 gm (IV) q8h x 2 weeks **or** Any aminoglycoside (IV) q24h x 2 weeks	Quinolone** (PO) x 2 weeks **or** Amoxicillin/clavulanic acid 875/125 mg (PO) q12h x 2 weeks
Chronic TB peritonitis	M. tuberculosis	Not applicable		Treat the same as pulmonary TB (p. 47)
CAPD-associated peritonitis[‡]	S. epidermidis S. aureus Entero-bacteriaceae Non-fermentative gram (-) aerobic bacilli	<u>Before culture results</u> Vancomycin 1 gm (IV) loading dose* **plus** Gentamicin 5 mg/kg or 240 mg (IV) loading dose*	<u>After culture results</u> _MSSA/Enterobacteriaceae_ Ceftriaxone 1 gm (IV)* _or_ cefepime 2 gm (IV)* _or_ aztreonam 2 gm (IV)* _MRSA_ Vancomycin (IV load given before culture results)* _or_ linezolid 600 mg (IV or PO)*	

MSSA/MRSA = methicillin-sensitive/resistant S. aureus. Duration of therapy represents total time IV, PO, or IV + PO
‡ Treat only IV or IV-to-PO switch
† In addition to antibiotics, give heparin to maintain PTT ~ 2 times control x 7-14 days
* Follow with maintenance dosing x 2 weeks after culture results are available. For maintenance dosing, use renal failure (CrCl < 10 mL/min) and post-peritoneal dialysis dosing (Chapter 7)
¶ Gatifloxacin 400 mg or levofloxacin 500 mg
** Ciprofloxacin 400 mg (IV) or 500 mg (PO) q12h or gatifloxacin 400 mg (IV or PO) q24h or levofloxacin 500 mg (IV or PO) q24h or moxifloxacin 400 mg (IV or PO) q24h

Intraabdominal or Pelvic Peritonitis/Abscess (Appendicitis/Diverticulitis/Septic Pelvic Thrombophlebitis)

Clinical Presentation: Spiking fevers with acute abdominal pain and peritoneal signs. In diverticulitis, the pain is localized over the involved segment of colon. Appendicitis ± perforation presents as RLQ pain/rebound tenderness or mass. Peri-diverticular abscess presents the same as intraabdominal/pelvic abscess, most commonly in the LLQ. Septic pelvic thrombophlebitis (SPT) presents as high spiking fevers unresponsive to antibiotic therapy following delivery/pelvic surgery

Diagnostic Considerations: Diagnosis by CT/MRI scan of abdomen/pelvis

Pitfalls: Tympany over liver suggests abdominal/visceral perforation. Pelvic peritonitis/abscess presents the same as intraabdominal abscess/peritonitis, but peritoneal signs are often absent

Therapeutic Considerations: Patients with ischemic/inflammatory colitis should be treated the same as peritonitis, depending on severity. Obtain surgical consult for repair/lavage or abscess drainage. In SPT, fever rapidly falls when heparin is added to antibiotics

Prognosis: Related to degree/duration of peritoneal spillage and rapidity/completeness of lavage. Prognosis for SPT is good if treated early and clots remain limited to pelvic veins

Spontaneous Bacterial Peritonitis (SBP)

Clinical Presentation: Acute or subacute onset of fever ± abdominal pain

Diagnostic Considerations: Diagnosis by positive blood cultures of SBP pathogens. For patients with abdominal pain, ascites, and a negative CT/MRI, paracentesis ascitic fluid with > 500 WBCs and > 100 PMNs predicts a positive ascitic fluid culture and is diagnostic of SBP. Some degree of splenic dysfunction usually exists, predisposing to infection with encapsulated organisms

Pitfalls: Do not overlook GI source of peritonitis (e.g, appendicitis, diverticulitis); obtain CT/MRI

Therapeutic Considerations: B. fragilis/anaerobes are not common pathogens in SBP, and B. fragilis coverage is unnecessary

Prognosis: Related to degree of hepatic/splenic dysfunction

Chronic Non-bacterial (TB) Peritonitis (Mycobacterium tuberculosis)

Clinical Presentation: Abdominal pain with fevers, weight loss, ascites over 1-3 months

Diagnostic Considerations: "Doughy consistency" on abdominal palpation. Diagnosis by AFB on peritoneal biopsy/culture

Pitfalls: Chest x-ray is normal in ~ 70%. Increased incidence in alcoholic cirrhosis

Therapeutic Considerations: Treated the same as pulmonary TB

Prognosis: Good if treated early

CAPD-Associated Peritonitis

Clinical Presentation: Abdominal pain ± fever in a CAPD patient

Diagnostic Considerations: Diagnosis by gram stain/culture and ↑ WBC count in peritoneal fluid

Pitfalls: Fever is often absent

Therapeutic Considerations: Treat with systemic antibiotics, not with antibiotics into dialysate

Prognosis: Good with early therapy and removal of peritoneal catheter

Empiric Therapy of Genitourinary Tract Infections

Dysuria-Pyuria Syndrome (Acute Urethral Syndrome)

Subset	Usual Pathogens	IV Therapy	PO Therapy
Acute urethral syndrome	S. saprophyticus C. trachomatis E. coli (low concentration)	Not applicable	Doxycycline 100 mg (PO) q12h x 10 days **or** Quinolone (PO)* x 7 days

* Ciprofloxacin 500 mg q12h or gatifloxacin 400 mg q24h or levofloxacin 500 mg q24h

Clinical Presentation: Dysuria, frequency, urgency, lower abdominal discomfort, fevers < 102°F
Diagnostic Considerations: Diagnosis by symptoms of cystitis with pyuria and no growth or low concentration of E. coli (≤ 10^3 colonies/mL) by urine culture. Clue to S. saprophyticus is alkaline urinary pH and RBCs in urine
Pitfalls: Resembles "culture negative" cystitis
Therapeutic Considerations: S. saprophyticus is susceptible to most antibiotics used to treat UTIs
Prognosis: Excellent

Cystitis

Subset	Usual Pathogens	Therapy
Bacterial	Enterobacteriaceae E. faecalis S. saprophyticus	Amoxicillin 500 mg (PO) x q12h x 3 days **or** TMP-SMX 1 SS tablet (PO) x q12h x 3 days **or** Quinolone (PO)* q24h x 3 days
Fungal	C. albicans	Fluconazole 200 mg (PO) x 1 dose, then 100 mg (PO) q24h x 4 days
	Fluconazole-resistant C. albicans Non-albicans Candida (C. krusei, lusitaniae, dublinensis, tropicalis, pseudotropicalis, glabrata, lipolytica, guilliermondii)	Amphotericin B deoxycholate 0.3 mg/kg (IV) x 1 dose

* Ciprofloxacin XR 500 mg or gatifloxacin 400 mg or levofloxacin 500 mg

Bacterial Cystitis
Clinical Presentation: Dysuria, frequency, urgency, lower abdominal discomfort, fevers < 102°F
Diagnostic Considerations: Pyuria plus bacteriuria
Pitfalls: Compromised hosts (chronic steroids, diabetes, SLE, cirrhosis, multiple myeloma) may require 3-5 days of therapy. A single dose of amoxicillin or TMP-SMX may be sufficient in acute uncomplicated cystitis in normal hosts
Therapeutic Considerations: Pyridium 200 mg (PO) q8h after meals x 24-48h is useful to decrease dysuria (inform patients urine will turn orange)

Prognosis: Excellent in normal hosts

Candidal Cystitis
Diagnostic Considerations: Marked pyuria, urine nitrate negative ± RBCs. Speciate if not C. albicans
Pitfalls: Lack of response suggests renal candidiasis or a "fungus ball" in the renal collecting system
Therapeutic Considerations: If fluconazole fails, use amphotericin. For chronic renal failure/dialysis patients with candiduria, use amphotericin B deoxycholate bladder irrigation (as for catheter-associated candiduria, below)
Prognosis: Patients with impaired host defenses, abnormal collecting systems, cysts, renal disease or stones are prone to recurrent UTIs/urosepsis

Catheter-Associated Bacteriuria/Candiduria

Subset	Usual Pathogens	Therapy
Catheter-associated bacteriuria	E. coli E. faecalis	Nitrofurantoin 100 mg (PO) q12h x 5 days **or** Amoxicillin 500 mg (PO) q12h x 5 days
	E. faecium (VRE)	Nitrofurantoin 100 mg (PO) q12h x 5 days
Catheter-associated candiduria	Candida species (usually C. albicans)	Fluconazole 200 mg (PO) x 1 dose, then 100 mg (PO) q24h x 4 days **or** Amphotericin B deoxycholate continuous bladder irrigation (50 mg/L) 1 L (sterile water) q24h x 1-2 days **or** Amphotericin B deoxycholate intermittent bladder irrigation (50 mg/L) 200-300 mL (sterile water) q6-8h x 1-2 days

Clinical Presentation: Indwelling urinary (Foley) catheter with bacteriuria and pyuria; no symptoms
Diagnostic Considerations: Pyuria plus bacteriuria/candiduria. Usually afebrile or temperature < 101°F
Pitfalls: Bacteriuria/candiduria often represent colonization, not infection. Persistent candiduria after amphotericin B deoxycholate bladder irrigation suggests renal candidiasis
Therapeutic Considerations: Compromised hosts (diabetes, SLE, chronic steroids, multiple myeloma, cirrhosis) may require therapy for duration of catheterization. If bacteriuria/candiduria does not clear with appropriate therapy, change the catheter. For chronic renal failure/dialysis patients with candiduria, use amphotericin B deoxycholate bladder irrigation. Efficacy of therapy of catheter-associated candiduria is limited and relapse is frequent unless the catheter can be replaced or (preferably) removed
Prognosis: Excellent in normal hosts. Untreated bacteriuria/candiduria in compromised hosts may result in ascending infection (e.g., pyelonephritis) or bacteremia/candidemia

Epididymitis

Subset	Usual Pathogens	Preferred IV Therapy	Alternate IV Therapy	PO Therapy or IV-to-PO Switch
Acute *Young males*	C. trachomatis	Doxycycline 200 mg (IV) q12h x 3 days, then 100 mg (IV) q12h x 4 days	Ciprofloxacin 400 mg (IV) q12h x 7 days **or** Gatifloxacin 400 mg (IV) q24h x 7 days **or** Levofloxacin 500 mg (IV) q24h x 7 days	Doxycycline 200 mg (PO) q12h x 3 days, then 100 mg (PO) q12h x 4 days* **or** Azithromycin 1 gm (PO) x 1 dose **or** Ciprofloxacin 500 mg (PO) q12h x 7 days **or** Gatifloxacin 400 mg (PO) q24h x 7 days **or** Levofloxacin 500 mg (PO) q24h x 7 days
Elderly males	P. aeruginosa	Cefepime 2 gm (IV) q8h x 10 days **or** Piperacillin/tazo-bactam 4 gm (IV) q8h x 10 days	Ciprofloxacin 400 mg (IV) q12h x 10 days	Ciprofloxacin 750 mg (PO) q12h x 10 days
Chronic	M. tuberculosis B. dermatidis	Treat the same as pulmonary TB (p. 47) or pulmonary blastomycosis (p. 198)		

Duration of therapy represents total time IV, PO, or IV + PO. Most patients on IV therapy able to take PO meds should be switched to PO therapy soon after clinical improvement (usually < 72 hours)
* *Loading dose is not needed PO if given IV with the same drug*

Acute Epididymitis (Chlamydia trachomatis/Pseudomonas aeruginosa)
Clinical Presentation: Acute unilateral testicular pain ± fever
Diagnostic Considerations: Ultrasound to rule out torsion or tumor
Pitfalls: Rule out torsion by absence of fever and ultrasound
Therapeutic Considerations: Young males respond to treatment slowly over 1 week. Elderly males respond to anti-Pseudomonal therapy within 72 hours
Prognosis: Excellent in young males. Related to health of host in elderly

Chronic Epididymitis (Mycobacterium tuberculosis/ Blastomyces dermatiditis)
Clinical Presentation: Chronic epididymoorchitis with epididymal nodules
Diagnostic Considerations: Diagnosis by AFB on biopsy/culture of epididymus. TB epididymitis is always associated with renal TB. Blastomyces epididymitis is a manifestation of systemic infection
Pitfalls: Vasculitis (e.g., polyarteritis nodosum) and lymphomas may present the same way
Therapeutic Considerations: Treated the same as pulmonary TB/blastomycosis
Prognosis: Good

Pyelonephritis/Renal TB

Subset	Usual Pathogens	Preferred IV Therapy	Alternate IV Therapy	PO Therapy or IV-to-PO Switch
Acute bacterial pyelonephritis (Treat initially based on urine gram stain; see therapeutic considerations, below)	Entero-bacteriaceae	Ceftriaxone 1 gm (IV) q24h x 1-2 weeks **or** Quinolone† (IV) x 1-2 weeks	Aztreonam 2 gm (IV) q8h x 1-2 wks **or** Gentamicin 240 mg (IV) q24h x 1-2 weeks	Quinolone† (PO) x 1-2 weeks **or** Amoxicillin 1 gm (PO) q8h x 1-2 weeks
	Enterococcus faecalis	Ampicillin 1 gm (IV) q4h x 1-2 weeks **or** Linezolid 600 mg (IV) q12h x 1-2 weeks	Quinolone† (IV) x 1-2 weeks	Amoxicillin 1 gm (PO) q8h x 1-2 weeks **or** Linezolid 600 mg (PO) q12h x 1-2 weeks **or** Quinolone†(PO) x 1-2 weeks
	Enterococcus faecium (VRE)	Linezolid 600 mg (IV) q12h x 1-2 weeks	Quinupristin/ dalfopristin 7.5 mg/kg (IV) q8h x 1-2 weeks **or** Doxycycline 200 mg (IV) q12h x 3 days, then 100 mg q12h x 1-2 weeks	Linezolid 600 mg (PO) q12h x 1-2 weeks **or** Doxycycline 200 mg (PO) q12h x 3 days, then 100 mg (PO) q12h x 1-2 weeks*
Chronic bacterial pyelonephritis	Entero-bacteriaceae	IV Therapy Not applicable	Quinolone† (PO) x 4-6 weeks **or** TMP-SMX 1 DS tab (PO) q12h x 4-6 weeks **or** Doxycycline 200 mg (PO) q12h x 3 days, then 100 mg (PO) q12h x 4-6 weeks total	
Renal TB	M. tuberculosis	IV Therapy Not applicable	Treated the same as pulmonary TB (p. 47)	

VRE = vancomycin-resistant enterococci. Duration of therapy represents total time IV, PO, or IV + PO. Most patients on IV therapy able to take PO meds should be switched to PO therapy after clinical improvement (usually < 72 hours)
* *Loading dose is not needed PO if given IV with the same drug*
† *Ciprofloxacin XR 1000 mg (PO) q24h or ciprofloxacin 400 mg (IV) q12h or levofloxacin 500 mg (IV or PO) q24h or gatifloxacin 400 mg (IV or PO) q24h*

Acute Bacterial Pyelonephritis (Enterobacteriaceae, E. faecalis/E. faecium)
Clinical Presentation: Unilateral CVA tenderness with fevers ≥ 102°F
Diagnostic Considerations: Bacteriuria plus pyuria with unilateral CVA tenderness and temperature ≥ 102°F. Bacteremia usually accompanies acute pyelonephritis; obtain blood and urine cultures
Pitfalls: Temperature decreases in 72 hours with or without antibiotic treatment. If temperature does not fall after 72 hours of antibiotic therapy, suspect renal/perinephric abscess
Therapeutic Considerations: Initial treatment is based on the urinary gram stain: If gram-negative bacilli, treat as Enterobacteriaceae. If gram-positive cocci in chains (enterococcus), treat as E. faecalis; if enterococcus is subsequently identified as E. faecium, treat accordingly. Acute pyelonephritis is

usually treated initially for 1-3 days IV, then switched to PO to complete 4 weeks of antibiotics to minimize progression to chronic pyelonephritis. Obtain a CT/MRI in persistently febrile patients after 72 hours of antibiotics to rule out renal calculi, obstruction, abscess, or xanthomatous pyelonephritis
Prognosis: Excellent if first episode is adequately treated with antibiotics for 4 weeks

Chronic Bacterial Pyelonephritis (Enterobacteriaceae)
Clinical Presentation: Previous history of acute pyelonephritis with same symptoms as acute pyelonephritis but less CVA tenderness/fever
Diagnostic Considerations: Diagnosis by CT/MRI showing changes of chronic pyelonephritis plus bacteriuria/pyuria. Urine cultures may be intermittently negative before treatment. Chronic pyelonephritis is bilateral pathologically, but unilateral clinically
Pitfalls: Urine culture may be intermittently positive after treatment; repeat weekly x 4 to confirm urine remains culture-negative
Therapeutic Considerations: Treat x 4-6 weeks. Impaired medullary vascular blood supply/renal anatomical distortion makes eradication of pathogen difficult
Prognosis: Related to extent of renal damage

Renal TB (Mycobacterium tuberculosis)
Clinical Presentation: Renal mass lesion with ureteral abnormalities (pipestem, corkscrew, or spiral ureters) and sterile pyuria. Painless unless complicated by ureteral obstruction
Diagnostic Considerations: Combined upper/lower urinary tract abnormalities ± microscopic hematuria/urinary pH $\leq$ 5.5. Diagnosis by culture of TB from urine
Pitfalls: Chest x-ray is normal in 30%, but patients are PPD–positive. Rule out other infectious/inflammatory causes of sterile pyuria (e.g., Trichomonas, interstitial nephritis)
Therapeutic Considerations: Treat the same as pulmonary TB
Prognosis: Good if treated before renal parenchymal destruction/ureteral obstruction occur

Renal Abscess (Intrarenal/Perinephric)

Subset	Usual Pathogens	Preferred IV Therapy	Alternate IV Therapy	PO Therapy or IV-to-PO Switch
Cortical (Treat initially for MSSA; if later identified as MRSA, treat accordingly)	S. aureus	MSSA Nafcillin 2 gm (IV) q4h* **or** Ceftriaxone 1 gm (IV) q24h* **or** Clindamycin 600 mg (IV) q8h* MRSA Linezolid 600 mg (IV) q12h* **or** Minocycline 100 mg (IV) q12h*	MSSA Meropenem 1 gm (IV) q8h* **or** Imipenem 500 mg (IV) q6h* **or** Ertapenem 1 gm (IV) q24h* MRSA Vancomycin 1 gm (IV) q12h*	MSSA Clindamycin 300 mg (PO) q8h* MRSA Linezolid 600 mg (PO) q12h* **or** Minocycline 100 mg (PO) q12h*
Medullary	Entero-bacteriaceae	Quinolone (IV)†*	TMP-SMX 2.5 mg/kg (IV) q6h*	Quinolone (PO)†*

MSSA/MRSA = methicillin-sensitive/resistant S. aureus. Duration of therapy represents total time IV, PO, or IV + PO. Most patients on IV therapy able to take PO meds should be switched to PO therapy soon after clinical improvement
* Treat until renal abscess resolves completely or is no longer decreasing in size on CT/MRI
† Ciprofloxacin XR 1000 mg (PO) q24h or ciprofloxacin 400 mg (IV) q12h or levofloxacin 500 mg (IV or PO) q24h or gatifloxacin 400 mg (IV or PO) q24h

Clinical Presentation: Similar to pyelonephritis but fever remains elevated after 72 hours of antibiotics
Diagnostic Considerations: Obtain CT/MRI to diagnose perinephric/intra-renal abscess and rule out mass lesion. Cortical abscesses are usually secondary to hematogenous/contiguous spread. Medullary abscesses are usually due to extension of intrarenal infection
Pitfalls: Urine cultures may be negative with cortical abscesses
Therapeutic Considerations: Most large abscesses need to be drained. Multiple small abscesses are managed medically. Obtain urology consult
Prognosis: Related to degree of baseline renal dysfunction

Prostatitis/Prostatic Abscess

Subset	Usual Pathogens	Preferred IV Therapy	Alternate IV Therapy	PO Therapy or IV-to-PO Switch
Acute prostatitis/ acute prostatic abscess	Entero-bacteriaceae	Quinolone* (IV) x 2 weeks **or** Ceftriaxone 1 gm (IV) q24h x 2 weeks	TMP-SMX 2.5 mg/kg (IV) q6h x 2 weeks **or** Aztreonam 2 gm (IV) q8h x 2 weeks	Quinolone* (PO) x 2 weeks **or** Doxycycline 200 mg (PO) q12h x 3 days, then 100 mg (PO) q24h x 11 days **or** TMP-SMX 1 SS tablet (PO) q12h x 2 weeks
Chronic prostatitis	Entero-bacteriaceae	IV therapy not applicable	Quinolone* (PO) x 1-3 months **or** Doxycycline 100 mg (PO) q24h x 1-3 months **or** TMP-SMX 1 DS tablet (PO) q12h x 1-3 months	

Duration of therapy represents total time IV, PO, or IV + PO. Most patients on IV therapy able to take PO meds should be switched to PO therapy soon after clinical improvement (usually < 72 hours)
* *Ciprofloxacin XR 1000 mg (PO) q24h or ciprofloxacin 400 mg (IV) q12h or levofloxacin 500 mg (IV or PO) q24h or gatifloxacin 400 mg (IV or PO) q24h*

Acute Prostatitis/Acute Prostatic Abscess (Enterobacteriaceae)
Clinical Presentation: Acute prostatitis presents as an acute febrile illness in males with dysuria and no CVA tenderness. Prostatic abscess presents with hectic/septic fevers without localizing signs
Diagnostic Considerations: Acute prostatitis is diagnosed by bacteriuria plus pyuria with exquisite prostate tenderness, and is seen primarily in young males. Positive urine culture is due to contamination of urine as it passes through infected prostate. Prostatic abscess is diagnosed by transrectal ultrasound or CT/MRI of prostate
Pitfalls: Do not overlook acute prostatitis in males with bacteriuria without localizing signs, or prostatic abscess in patients with a history of prostatitis
Therapeutic Considerations: Treat acute prostatitis for 2 full weeks to decrease progression to chronic prostatitis. Prostatic abscess is treated the same as acute prostatitis plus surgical drainage
Prognosis: Excellent if treated early with full course of antibiotics (plus drainage for prostatic abscess)

Chronic Prostatitis (Enterobacteriaceae)
Clinical Presentation: Vague urinary symptoms (mild dysuria ± low back pain), history of acute prostatitis, and little or no fever

Diagnostic Considerations: Diagnosis by bacteriuria plus pyuria with "boggy prostate" ± mild tenderness. Urine/prostate expressate is culture positive. Chronic prostatitis with prostatic calcifications (rectal ultrasound) will not clear with antibiotics; treat with transurethral resection of prostate (TURP)
Pitfalls: Commonest cause of treatment failure is inadequate duration of therapy
Therapeutic Considerations: In sulfa-allergic patients, TMP alone may be used in place of TMP-SMX
Prognosis: Excellent if treated x 1-3 months. Prostatic abscess is a rare but serious complication (may cause urosepsis)

Urosepsis

Subset	Usual Pathogens	Preferred IV Therapy	Alternate IV Therapy	IV-to-PO Switch
Community-acquired (Treat initially based on urine gram stain)	Entero-bacteriaceae	Ceftriaxone 1 gm (IV) q24h x 7 days **or** Quinolone[†] (IV) x 7 days	Gentamicin 240 mg (IV) q24h x 7 days **or** Aztreonam 2 gm (IV) q8h x 7 days	Quinolone[†] (PO) x 7 days **or** TMP-SMX 1 SS tablet (PO) q12h x 7 days
	Enterococci (E. faecalis) Group B streptococci	Ampicillin 2 gm (IV) q4h x 7 days	Meropenem 1 gm (IV) q8h x 7 days **or** Imipenem 500 mg (IV) q6h x 7 days	Amoxicillin 1 gm (PO) q8h x 7 days **or** Quinolone[†] (PO) x 7 days
Related to urological procedure (Treat initially for P. aeruginosa, etc; if later identified as non-aeruginosa Pseudomonas, treat accordingly)	P. aeruginosa Enterobacter Klebsiella Serratia	Ciprofloxacin 400 mg (IV) q12h x 7 days **or** Cefepime 2 gm (IV) q8h x 7 days **or** Meropenem 1 gm (IV) q8h x 7 days	Piperacillin/tazobactam 4.5 gm (IV) q8h x 7 days **or** Aztreonam 2 gm (IV) q8h x 7 days **or** Gentamicin 240 mg (IV) q24h x 7 days	Quinolone[†] (PO) x 7 days
	Non-aeruginosa Pseudomonas (B. cepacia, S. maltophilia)	TMP-SMX 2.5 mg/kg (IV) q6h x 7 days	Meropenem 1 gm (IV) q8h x 7 days **or** Imipenem 500 mg (IV) q6h x 7 days	TMP-SMX 1 SS tablet (PO) q12h x 7 days **or** Quinolone[†] (PO) x 7 days

Duration of therapy represents total time IV or IV + PO. Most patients on IV therapy able to take PO meds should be switched to PO therapy after clinical improvement
† *Ciprofloxacin XR 1000 mg (PO) q24h or ciprofloxacin 400 mg (IV) q12h or levofloxacin 500 mg (IV or PO) q24h or gatifloxacin 400 mg (IV or PO) q24h*

Community-Acquired Urosepsis
Clinical Presentation: Sepsis from urinary tract source
Diagnostic Considerations: Blood and urine cultures positive for same uropathogen. If patient does not have diabetes, SLE, cirrhosis, myeloma, steroids, pre-existing renal disease or obstruction, obtain CT/MRI of GU tract to rule out abscess/obstruction. Prostatic abscess is rarely a cause of urosepsis
Pitfalls: Mixed gram-positive/negative urine cultures suggest specimen contamination or enterovesicular fistula
Therapeutic Considerations: Empiric treatment is based on urine gram stain. If gram-positive cocci,

treat as Group B/D streptococci (not S. aureus/S. pneumoniae). If gram-negative bacilli, treat as Enterobacteriaceae (not P. aeruginosa/B. fragilis)
Prognosis: Related to severity of underlying condition causing urosepsis and health of host

Urosepsis Following Urological Procedures

Clinical Presentation: Sepsis within 24 hours after GU procedure
Diagnostic Considerations: Blood and urine cultures positive for same uropathogen. Use pre-procedural urine culture to identify uropathogen and guide therapy
Pitfalls: If non-aeruginosa Pseudomonas in urine/blood, switch to TMP-SMX until susceptibility test results are available
Therapeutic Considerations: Empiric P. aeruginosa monotherapy will cover most other uropathogens
Prognosis: Related to severity of underlying condition causing urosepsis and health of host

Pelvic Inflammatory Disease (PID), Salpingitis, Tuboovarian Abscess, Endometritis/Endomyometritis, Septic Abortion

Subset	Usual Pathogens	Preferred IV Therapy	Alternate IV Therapy	PO Therapy or IV-to-PO Switch
Hospitalized patients[†]	B. fragilis Entero-bacteriaceae N. gonorrhoeae C. trachomatis	Doxycycline 200 mg (IV) q12h x 3 days, then 100 mg (IV) q12h x 11 days **plus either** Cefoxitin 2 gm (IV) q6h x 2 wks **or** Cefotetan 2 gm (IV) q12h x 2 weeks **or** Ertapenem 1 gm (IV) q24h x 3-10 days **or monotherapy with** Moxifloxacin 400 mg (IV) q24h x 2 weeks	Doxycycline 200 mg (IV) q12h x 3 days, then 100 mg (IV) q12h x 11 days **plus** Ampicillin/sulbactam 3 gm (IV) q6h x 2 weeks ___2nd Alternate___ Quinolone[‡] (IV) q24h x 2 weeks **plus** Metronidazole 1 gm (IV) q24h x 2 weeks	Moxifloxacin 400 mg (PO) q24h x 2 weeks **or combination therapy with** Quinolone[‡] (PO) q24h x 2 weeks **plus either** Doxycycline 200 mg (PO) q12h x 3 days, then 100 mg (PO) q12h x 11 days* **or** Metronidazole 500 mg (PO) q12h x 2 weeks
Outpatients (mild PID only)	N. gonorrhoeae C. trachomatis B. fragilis Entero-bacteriaceae	Moxifloxacin 400 mg (PO) q24h x 2 weeks **or** Doxycycline 100 mg (PO) q12h x 2 weeks **or combination therapy with** Quinolone[‡] (PO) x 2 weeks **plus** Metronidazole 500 mg (PO) q12h x 2 weeks		

Duration of therapy represents total time IV, PO, or IV + PO. Most patients on IV therapy able to take PO meds should be switched to PO therapy after clinical improvement
† Treat only IV or IV-to-PO switch for salpingitis, tuboovarian abscess, endometritis, endomyometritis, septic abortion, or severe PID
* Loading dose is not needed PO if given IV with the same drug
‡ Ciprofloxacin 400 mg (IV) or 500 mg (PO) q12h or gatifloxacin 400 mg (IV or PO) q24h or levofloxacin 500 mg (IV or PO) q24h or moxifloxacin 400 mg (IV or PO) q24h or ofloxacin 400 mg (IV or PO) q12h

Clinical Presentation: PID/salpingitis presents with cervical motion/adnexal tenderness, lower quadrant abdominal pain, and fever. Endometritis/endomyometritis presents with uterine tenderness ± cervical discharge/fever. Endomyometritis is the most common post-partum infection

Diagnostic Considerations: Unilateral lower abdominal pain in a female without a non-pelvic cause suggests PID/salpingitis

Pitfalls: Obtain CT/MRI of abdomen/pelvis to confirm diagnosis and rule out other pathology or tubo-ovarian abscess

Therapeutic Considerations: Tuboovarian abscess usually requires drainage/removal ± TAH/BSO, plus antibiotics (p. 86) x 1-2 weeks after drainage/removal. Septic abortion is treated the same as endometritis/endomyometritis plus uterine evacuation

Prognosis: Related to promptness of treatment/adequacy of drainage if tuboovarian abscess. Late complications of PID/salpingitis include tubal scarring/infertility

Empiric Therapy of Sexually Transmitted Diseases

Urethritis/Cervicitis

Subset	Usual Pathogens	IM Therapy	PO Therapy
Gonococcal	N. gonorrhoeae	Ceftriaxone 125 mg (IM) x 1 dose Alternate 3rd gen. cephalo-sporin 250-500 mg (IM) x 1 dose	Azithromycin 2 gm (PO) x 1 dose **or** Quinolone* (PO) x 1 dose **or** Cefixime 400 mg (PO) x 1 dose
Non-gonococcal	C. trachomatis U. urealyticum M. genitalium	Not applicable	Doxycycline 100 mg (PO) q12h x 7 days **or** Azithromycin 1 gm (PO) x 1 dose **or** Quinolone* (PO) x 7 days **or** Erythromycin 500 mg (PO) q6h x 7 days
	Trichomonas vaginalis	Not applicable	Metronidazole 2 gm (PO) x 1 dose **or** Metronidazole 500 mg (PO) q12h x 7 days

* Ciprofloxacin 500 mg q12h or gatifloxacin 400 mg q24h or levofloxacin 500 mg q24h or moxifloxacin 400 mg q24h or ofloxacin 300 mg q12h

Gonococcal Urethritis/Cervicitis (Neisseria gonorrhoeae)

Clinical Presentation: Purulent penile/cervical discharge with burning/dysuria 3-5 days after contact

Diagnostic Considerations: Diagnosis in males by gram stain of urethral discharge showing gram-negative diplococci. In females, diagnosis requires culture of cervical discharge, not gram stain. Obtain throat/rectal culture for N. gonorrhoeae. Co-infections are common; obtain VDRL and HIV serologies

Pitfalls: Gram stain of cervical discharge showing gram-negative diplococci is not diagnostic of N. gonorrhoeae; must confirm by culture. N. gonorrhoeae infections are asymptomatic in 10%

Therapeutic Considerations: Failure to respond suggests re-infection or infection with another agent

(e.g., Trichomonas, Ureaplasma). Treat pharyngeal/rectal GC the same as GC urethritis
Prognosis: Increased risk of disseminated infection with pharyngeal/rectal GC

Non-Gonococcal Urethritis/Cervicitis (Chlamydia/Ureaplasma/Mycoplasma)

Clinical Presentation: Non-purulent penile/cervical discharge ± dysuria ~ 1 week after contact
Diagnostic Considerations: Diagnosis by positive chlamydial antigen test/Ureaplasma or Mycoplasma culture of urethral/cervical discharge. Culture urethral/cervical discharge to rule out N. gonorrhoeae. Co-infections are common; obtain VDRL and HIV serologies
Pitfalls: C. trachomatis infections are asymptomatic in 25%
Therapeutic Considerations: Failure to respond to anti-Chlamydia therapy suggests re-infection or Trichomonas/Ureaplasma/Mycoplasma infection. Quinolones are also active against N. gonorrhoeae
Prognosis: Tubal scarring/infertility in chronic infection

Trichomonas Urethritis/Cervicitis (Trichomonas vaginalis)

Clinical Presentation: Frothy, pruritic, vaginal discharge; not foul smelling
Diagnostic Considerations: Trichomonas by wet mount/culture on special media
Pitfalls: Classic "strawberry cervix" is infrequently seen
Therapeutic Considerations: Use week-long regimen if single dose fails
Prognosis: Excellent if partner is also treated

Vaginitis/Balanitis

Subset	Usual Pathogens	IV Therapy	PO Therapy
Bacterial vaginosis/ vaginitis	Gardnerella vaginalis Mobiluncus Prevotella Mycoplasma hominis	Not applicable	Metronidazole 2 gm (PO) x 1 dose **or** Metronidazole 500 mg (PO) q12h x 7 days **or** Clindamycin 300 mg (PO) q12h x 7 days **or** Moxifloxacin 400 mg (PO) q24h x 7 days
Candida vaginitis/ balanitis	Candida	Not applicable	Fluconazole 150 mg (PO) x 1 dose **or** Itraconazole 100 mg (PO) solution q24h x 7 days

Bacterial Vaginosis/Vaginitis

Clinical Presentation: Non-pruritic vaginal discharge with "fishy" odor
Diagnostic Considerations: Diagnosis by "clue cells" in vaginal fluid wet mount. Vaginal pH ≥ 4.5. "Fishy" odor emanates from smear of vaginal secretions when 10% KOH solution is added (positive "whiff test")
Pitfalls: Do not confuse "clue cells" with darkly staining bodies of H. ducreyi (chancroid)
Therapeutic Considerations: As an alternative to oral therapy, clindamycin cream 2% intravaginally qHS x 7 days or metronidazole gel 0.075% 1 application intravaginally q12h x 5 days can be used
Prognosis: Excellent

Candida Vaginitis/Balanitis

Clinical Presentation: Pruritic white plaques in vagina/glans penis
Diagnostic Considerations: Diagnosis by gram stain/culture of whitish plaques
Pitfalls: Rule out Trichomonas, which also presents with pruritus in females

Therapeutic Considerations: Treat both partners with oral anti-Candida therapy. If single-dose fluconazole therapy fails, treat with fluconazole 100 mg (PO) q24h x 7 days. Use itraconazole for non-albicans Candida

Prognosis: Good with systemic therapy. Diabetics/uncircumcised males may need prolonged therapy

Genital Vesicles

Subset	Usual Pathogens	IV Therapy	PO Therapy
Genital vesicles	HSV-2 (genital herpes)	Not applicable	Acyclovir 400 mg (PO) q8h x 7-10 days **or** Valacyclovir 1 gm (PO) q12h x 7-10 days **or** Famciclovir 250 mg (PO) q8h x 7-10 days

Clinical Presentation: Painful vesicles on genitals with painful bilateral regional adenopathy ± low-grade fever

Diagnostic Considerations: Diagnosis by clinical presentation/culture. "Satelliting" vesicles are characteristic of HSV-2

Pitfalls: Elevated IgG HSV-2 titer indicates past exposure, not acute infection

Therapeutic Considerations: If concomitant rectal herpes, increase acyclovir to 800 mg (PO) q8h x 7 days. For recurrent genital herpes, use acyclovir or valacyclovir (dose same as primary infection) for 7 days after each relapse. Recurrent episodes of HSV-2 are less painful than primary infection, and inguinal adenopathy is less prominent/painful

Prognosis: HSV-2 tends to recur, especially during the first year

Genital Ulcers

Subset	Usual Pathogens	IM Therapy	PO Therapy
Primary syphilis	Treponema pallidum	Benzathine penicillin 2.4 mu (IM) x 1 dose	Doxycycline 100 mg (PO) q12h x 2 weeks
Chancroid	Hemophilus ducreyi	Ceftriaxone 250 mg (IM) x 1 dose <u>Alternate</u> Any 3rd generation cephalosporin 250-500 mg (IM) x 1 dose	Azithromycin 1 gm (PO) x 1 dose **or** Quinolone* (PO) x 3 days **or** Erythromycin base 500 mg (PO) q6h x 7 days

* *Ciprofloxacin 500 mg q12h or gatifloxacin 400 mg or levofloxacin 500 mg or moxifloxacin 400 mg q24h*

Primary Syphilis (Treponema pallidum)

Clinical Presentation: Painless, indurated ulcers (chancres) with bilateral painless inguinal adenopathy. Syphilitic chancres are elevated, clean and raised, but not undermined

Diagnostic Considerations: Diagnosis by spirochetes on darkfield examination of ulcer exudate. Elevated VDRL titers after 1 week

Pitfalls: VDRL titers fall slowly within 1 year; failure to decline suggests treatment failure/HIV

Therapeutic Considerations: Parenteral penicillin is the preferred antibiotic for all stages of syphilis. If treatment fails/VDRL does not decline, obtain HIV serology

Prognosis: Good with early treatment

Chancroid (Hemophilus ducreyi)

Clinical Presentation: Ragged, undermined, painful ulcer(s) + painful unilateral inguinal adenopathy

Diagnostic Considerations: Diagnosis by streptobacilli in "school of fish" configuration on gram-stained smear of ulcer exudate/culture of H. ducreyi

Pitfalls: Co-infection is common; obtain VDRL and HIV serologies

Therapeutic Considerations: In HIV, multiple dose regimens or azithromycin is preferred. Resistance to erythromycin/ciprofloxacin has been reported

Prognosis: Good with early treatment

Suppurating Inguinal Adenopathy

Subset	Usual Pathogens	IV Therapy	PO Therapy
Lympho-granuloma venereum (LGV)	Chlamydia trachomatis (L_{1-3} serotypes)	Not applicable	Doxycycline 100 mg (PO) q12h x 3 weeks **or** Erythromycin 500 mg (PO) q6h x 3 weeks
Granuloma inguinale (Donovanosis)	Calymmato-bacterium granulomatosis	Not applicable	Doxycycline 100 mg (PO) q12h x 3 weeks **or** Erythromycin 500 mg (PO) q6h x 3 weeks **or** TMP-SMX 1 DS tablet (PO) q12h x 3 weeks **or** Ciprofloxacin 500 mg (PO) q12h x 3 weeks

Lymphogranuloma Venereum (Chlamydia trachomatis) LGV

Clinical Presentation: Unilateral inguinal adenopathy ± discharge/sinus tract

Diagnostic Consideration: Diagnosis by very high Chlamydia trachomatis L_{1-3} titers. Do not biopsy site (often does not heal and may form a fistula). May present as FUO

Pitfalls: Initial papule not visible at clinical presentation

Therapeutic Considerations: Rectal LGV may require additional courses of treatment

Prognosis: Fibrotic perirectal/pelvic damage does not reverse with therapy

Granuloma Inguinale (Calymmatobacterium granulomatosis) Donovanosis

Clinical Presentation: Accentuated inguinal groove ± discharge. Pseudolymphadenopathy ("groove sign") due to prominent soft tissue swelling

Diagnostic Consideration: Donovan bodies ("puffed-wheat" appearance) in tissue biopsy

Pitfalls: No true inguinal adenopathy, as opposed to LGV infection

Therapeutic Considerations: Doxycycline or erythromycin preferred

Prognosis: Good if treated early

Genital/Perianal Warts (Condylomata Acuminata)

Subset	Pathogens	Therapy
Genital/perianal warts	Human papilloma virus (HPV)	Podophyllin 10-25% in tincture of benzoin **or** surgical/laser removal/cryotherapy with liquid nitrogen **or** ciofovir gel (1%) QHS x 5 days every other week for 6 cycles **or** tricholoracetic acid (TCA)/bichloroacetic acid (BCA) **or** intralesional interferon

Clinical Presentation: Single/multiple verrucous genital lesions ± pigmentation usually without inguinal adenopathy

Diagnostic Considerations: Diagnosis by clinical appearance. Genital warts are usually caused by HPV types 11,16. Anogenital warts caused by HPV types 16,18,31,33,35 are associated with cervical neoplasia. Females with anogenital warts need serial cervical PAP smears to detect cervical dysplasia/neoplasia

Pitfalls: Most HPV infections are asymptomatic

Therapeutic Considerations: Cidofovir cures/halts HPV progression in 50% of cases

Prognosis: Related to HPV serotypes with malignant potential (HPV types 16,18,31,33,35)

Syphilis

Subset	Usual Pathogens	Preferred IV/IM Therapy	Alternate IV/IM Therapy	PO Therapy
Primary, secondary, or early latent (duration < 1 year) syphilis	Treponema pallidum	Benzathine penicillin 2.4 mu (IM) x 1 dose	Not applicable	Doxycycline 100 mg (PO) q12h x 2 weeks **or** Erythromycin 500 mg (PO) q6h x 2 weeks
Late latent (duration > 1 year) or tertiary syphilis	Treponema pallidum	Benzathine penicillin 2.4 mu (IM) weekly x 3 weeks	Not applicable	Doxycycline 100 mg (PO) q12h x 4 weeks
Neurosyphilis	Treponema pallidum	Penicillin G 3-4 mu (IV) q4h or continuous infusion x 10-14 days	Procaine penicillin 2.4 mu (IM) q24h x 10-14 days **plus** Probenecid 500 mg (PO) q6h x 10-14 days **or monotherapy with** Ceftriaxone 1 gm (IV) q24h x 10-14 days	Doxycycline 100 mg (PO) q12h x 10-14 days **or** Minocycline 100 mg (PO) q12h x 10-14 days

Duration of therapy represents total time IV, IM, or PO. All stages of syphilis in HIV/AIDS patients usually respond to therapeutic regimens recommended for normal hosts. Syphilis in pregnancy should be treated according to the stage of syphilis; penicillin-allergic pregnant patients should be desensitized and treated with penicillin

Primary Syphilis (Treponema pallidum)

Clinical Presentation: Painless, indurated ulcer(s) (chancre) with bilateral painless inguinal adenopathy

Diagnostic Considerations: Diagnosis by spirochetes on darkfield examination of ulcer exudate. Elevated VDRL titers after 1 week

Pitfalls: VDRL titers fall slowly within 1 year; failure to decline suggests treatment failure

Therapeutic Considerations: Parenteral penicillin is the preferred antibiotic for all stages of syphilis; if treatment fails/VDRL does not decline, obtain HIV serology

Prognosis: Good with early treatment

Secondary Syphilis (Treponema pallidum)

Clinical Presentation: Facial/truncal macular, papular, papulosquamous, non-pruritic, tender, symmetrical rash which may involve the palms/soles. Usually accompanied by generalized adenopathy. Typically appears 4-10 weeks after primary chancre, although stages may overlap. Alopecia aereata, condyloma lata, mucous patches, iritis/uveitis may be present. Renal involvement ranges from mild proteinuria to nephrotic syndrome. Without treatment, spontaneous resolution occurs after 3-12 weeks

Diagnostic Considerations: Diagnosis by clinical findings and VDRL in high titers ($\geq$ 1:256). After treatment, VDRL titers usually return to non-reactive within 2 years. Syphilitic hepatitis is characterized by elevated alkaline phosphatase > elevated SGOT

Pitfalls: Palmar/foot rashes are not due to 2° syphilis if VDRL is positive in low titer

Therapeutic Considerations: Parenteral penicillin is the preferred antibiotic for all stages of syphilis. VDRL titers that remain reactive after 2 years suggest reinfection and should be retreated

Prognosis: Excellent with early treatment

Latent Syphilis (Treponema pallidum)

Clinical Presentation: Patients are asymptomatic with elevated VDRL/FTA-ABS titers

Diagnostic Considerations: Diagnosis by positive serology ± prior history, but no signs/symptoms of syphilis. Asymptomatic syphilis < 1 year in duration is termed "early" latent syphilis; asymptomatic syphilis > 1 year/unknown duration is termed "late" latent syphilis. Secondary syphilis may relapse in up to 25% of patients with early latent syphilis, but relapse is rare in late latent syphilis. Evaluate patients for neurosyphilis

Pitfalls: FTA-ABS titers do not fall with treatment and may remain positive in low titer for life

Therapeutic Considerations: Parenteral penicillin is the preferred antibiotic for all stages of syphilis. Repeat VDRL titers at 6, 12, and 24 months; therapeutic response is defined as a 4-fold reduction in VDRL titers (2 tube dilutions).

Prognosis: Excellent even if treated late

Tertiary Syphilis (Treponema pallidum)

Clinical Presentation: May present with aortitis, neurosyphilis, iritis, or gummata 5-30 years after initial infection

Diagnostic Considerations: Diagnosis by history of syphilis plus positive VDRL/FTA-ABS with signs/symptoms of late syphilis

Pitfalls: Treat for signs of neurosyphilis on clinical exam or lumbar puncture, even if VDRL is non-reactive

Therapeutic Considerations: Parenteral penicillin is the preferred antibiotic for all stages of syphilis

Prognosis: Related to extent of end-organ damage

Neurosyphilis (Treponema pallidum)

Clinical Presentation: Patients are often asymptomatic, but may have ophthalmic/auditory symptoms, cranial nerve abnormalities, tabes dorsalis, paresis, psychosis, or signs of meningitis/dementia

Diagnostic Considerations: Diagnosis by elevated CSF VDRL titers; no need to obtain CSF FTA-ABS titers. CSF has pleocytosis, increased protein, and positive VDRL

Pitfalls: Persistent CSF abnormalities suggest treatment failure

Therapeutic Considerations: Parenteral penicillin is the preferred antibiotic for all stages of syphilis. CSF abnormalities should decrease in 6 months and return to normal after 2 years; repeat lumbar puncture 6 months after treatment. Failure rate with ceftriaxone is 20%

Prognosis: Related to extent of end-organ damage

Empiric Therapy of Bone and Joint Infections

Septic Arthritis/Bursitis

Subset	Usual Pathogens	Preferred IV Therapy	Alternate IV Therapy	PO Therapy or IV-to-PO Switch
Acute (Treat initially based on gram stain of synovial fluid. If gram positive cocci in clusters, treat initially for MSSA; if later identified as MRSA, treat accordingly)	S. aureus (MSSA)	Ceftriaxone 1 gm (IV) q24h x 3 weeks **or** Cefazolin 1 gm (IV) q8h x 3 weeks **or** Clindamycin 600 mg (IV) q8h x 3 weeks	Nafcillin 2 gm (IV) q4h x 3 weeks **or** Meropenem 1 gm (IV) q8h x 3 weeks **or** Imipenem 500 mg (IV) q6h x 3 weeks	Cephalexin 1 gm (PO) q6h x 3 weeks **or** Clindamycin 300 mg (PO) q8h x 3 weeks **or** Quinolone* (PO) q24h x 3 weeks
	S. aureus (MRSA)	Linezolid 600 mg (IV) q12h x 3 weeks **or** Vancomycin 1 gm (IV) q12h x 3 weeks	Quinupristin/ dalfopristin 7.5 mg/kg (IV) q8h x 3 weeks	Linezolid 600 mg (PO) q12h x 3 weeks **or** Minocycline 100 mg (PO) q12h x 3 weeks
	Group A,B,C,G streptococci	Ceftriaxone 1 gm (IV) q24h x 2 weeks **or** Clindamycin 600 mg (IV) q8h x 2 weeks	Cefazolin 1 gm (IV) q8h x 2 weeks **or** Ceftizoxime 2 gm (IV) q8h x 2 weeks	Clindamycin 300 mg (PO) q8h x 2 weeks **plus** Cephalexin 500 mg (PO) q6h x 2 weeks
	Entero-bacteriaceae	Ceftriaxone 1 gm (IV) q24h x 2 weeks **or** Cefepime 2 gm (IV) q12h x 2 weeks **or** Cefotaxime 2 gm (IV) q6h x 2 weeks **or** Ceftizoxime 2 gm (IV) q8h x 2 weeks	Aztreonam 2 gm (IV) q8h x 2 weeks **or** Ciprofloxacin 400 mg (IV) q12h x 2 weeks **or** Gatifloxacin 400 mg (IV) q24h x 2 weeks **or** Levofloxacin 750 mg (IV) q24h x 2 weeks **or** Moxifloxacin 400 mg (IV) q24h x 2 weeks	Ciprofloxacin 750 mg (PO) q12h x 2 weeks **or** Gatifloxacin 400 mg (PO) q24h x 2 weeks **or** Levofloxacin 750 mg (PO) q24h x 2 weeks **or** Moxifloxacin 400 mg (PO) q24h x 2 weeks

MSSA/MRSA = methicillin-sensitive/resistant S. aureus
* Gatifloxacin 400 mg or levofloxacin 500 mg or moxifloxacin 400 mg

Septic Arthritis/Bursitis (cont'd)

Subset	Usual Pathogens	Preferred IV Therapy	Alternate IV Therapy	PO Therapy or IV-to-PO Switch
Acute (cont'd)	P. aeruginosa	Meropenem 1 gm (IV) q8h x 3 weeks **or** Cefepime 2 gm (IV) q8h x 3 weeks	Aztreonam 2 gm (IV) q8h x 3 weeks **or** Piperacillin/ tazobactam 4.5 gm (IV) q8h x 3 weeks	Ciprofloxacin 750 mg (PO) q12h x 3 weeks
	N. gonorrhoeae	Ceftriaxone 1 gm (IV) q24h x 2 weeks **or** Ceftizoxime 2 gm (IV) q8h x 2 weeks	Ciprofloxacin 400 mg (IV) q24h x 2 weeks **or** Gatifloxacin 400 mg (IV) q24h x 2 weeks **or** Levofloxacin 500 mg (IV) q24h x 2 weeks **or** Moxifloxacin 400 mg (IV) q24h x 2 weeks	Ciprofloxacin 500 mg (PO) q24h x 2 weeks **or** Gatifloxacin 400 mg (PO) q24h x 2 weeks **or** Levofloxacin 500 mg (PO) q24h x 2 weeks **or** Moxifloxacin 400 mg (PO) q24h x 2 weeks
	Brucella	Streptomycin 1 gm (IM) q24h x 3 weeks **plus** Doxycycline 200 mg (IV) q12h x 3 days, then 100 mg (IV) q12h for 3-week total course	Gentamicin 5 mg/kg (IV) q24h x 3 weeks **plus** Doxycycline 200 mg (IV) q12h x 3 days, then 100 mg (IV) q12h for 3-week total course	Doxycycline 200 mg (PO) q12h x 3 days, then 100 mg (PO) q12h for 3-week total course[†] **plus** Rifampin 600 mg (PO) q24h x 3 weeks
	Salmonella	Ceftriaxone 2 gm (IV) q24h x 2-3 weeks **or** Quinolone* (IV) x 2-3 weeks	Aztreonam 2 gm (IV) q8h x 2-3 weeks **or** TMP-SMX 2.5 mg/kg (IV) q6h x 2-3 weeks	Quinolone* (PO) x 2-3 weeks **or** TMP-SMX 1 DS tablet (PO) q12h x 2-3 weeks

† Loading dose is not needed PO if given IV with the same drug
* Ciprofloxacin 400 mg (IV) or 500 mg (PO) q12h or gatifloxacin 400 mg (IV or PO) q24h or levofloxacin 500 mg (IV or PO) q24h or moxifloxacin 400 mg (IV or PO) q24h

Septic Arthritis/Bursitis (cont'd)

Subset	Usual Pathogens	Preferred IV Therapy	Alternate IV Therapy	PO Therapy or IV-to-PO Switch
Secondary to animal bite wound	P. multocida S. moniliformis E. corrodens	Piperacillin/ tazobactam 4.5 gm (IV) q8h x 2 weeks **or** Ampicillin/ sulbactam 3 gm (IV) q6h x 2 weeks **or** Ticarcillin/ clavulanate 3.1 gm (IV) q6h x 2 weeks	Meropenem 1 gm (IV) q8h x 2 weeks **or** Imipenem 500 mg (IV) q6h x 2 weeks **or** Ertapenem 1 gm (IV) q24h x 2 weeks **or** Doxycycline 200 mg (IV) q12h x 3 days, then 100 mg (IV) q12h x 11 days	Amoxicillin/ clavulanic acid 875/125 mg (PO) q12h x 2 weeks **or** Doxycycline 200 mg (PO) q12h x 3 days, then 100 mg (PO) q12h x 11 days[†] **or** Moxifloxacin 400 mg (PO) q24h x 2 weeks
Fungal arthritis	Coccidioides immitis	Not applicable	Itraconazole 200 mg (PO) solution q12h until cured **or** Fluconazole 800 mg (PO) q24h until cured	
	Sporothrix schenckii	Not applicable	Itraconazole 200 mg (PO) solution q12h until cured	
TB arthritis	M. tuberculosis	Not applicable	INH 300 mg (PO) q24h x 12 months **plus** Rifampin 600 mg (PO) q24h x 12 months If multiresistant TB strain likely, also add EMB 15 mg/kg (PO) q24h x 12 months **plus** PZA 25 mg/kg (PO) q24h x 12 months	

MSSA/MRSA = methicillin-sensitive/resistant S. aureus. Duration of therapy represents total time IV, PO, or IV + PO. Most patients on IV therapy able to take PO meds should be switched to PO therapy after clinical improvement
† Loading dose is not needed PO if given IV with the same drug

Acute Septic Arthritis/Bursitis

Clinical Presentation: Acute joint pain with fever. Septic joint unable to bear weight. Septic bursitis presents with pain on joint motion, but patient is able to bear weight

Diagnostic Considerations: Diagnosis by demonstrating organisms in synovial fluid by stain/culture. In septic bursitis (knee most common), there is pain on joint flexion (although the joint can bear weight), and synovial fluid findings are negative for septic arthritis. Except for N. gonorrhoeae, polyarthritis is not usually due to bacterial pathogens. Post-infectious polyarthritis is usually viral in origin, most commonly due to parvovirus B19, rubella, or HBV

Therapeutic Considerations: See specific pathogen, below. Treat septic bursitis as septic arthritis

Staphylococcus aureus

Diagnostic Considerations: Painful hot joint; unable to bear weight. Diagnosis by synovial fluid pleocytosis and positive culture for joint pathogen. Examine synovial fluid to rule out gout (doubly birefringent crystals) and pseudogout (calcium pyrophosphate crystals). May occur in setting of endocarditis with septic emboli to joints; other manifestations of endocarditis are usually evident

Pitfalls: Rule out causes of non-infectious arthritis (sarcoidosis, Whipple's disease, Ehlers-Danlos, etc.), which are less severe, but may mimic septic arthritis. In reactive arthritis following urethritis (C. trachomatis, Ureaplasma urealyticum, N. gonorrhoeae) or diarrhea (Shigella, Campylobacter, Yersinia, Salmonella), synovial fluid culture is negative, and synovial fluid WBCs counts are usually < 10,000/mm³ with normal synovial fluid lactic acid and glucose. Do not overlook infective endocarditis in mono/polyarticular arthritis without apparent cause

Therapeutic Considerations: For MRSA septic arthritis, vancomycin penetration into synovial fluid is unreliable; use linezolid instead. Most believe immobilization of infected joint during therapy is helpful. Local installation of antibiotics into synovial fluid has no advantage over IV/PO antibiotics

Prognosis: Treat as early as possible to minimize joint damage. Repeated aspiration/open drainage may be needed to preserve joint function

Group A, B, C, G Streptococci

Diagnostic Considerations: Usually monoarticular. Not usually due to septic emboli from endocarditis

Prognosis: Related to extent of joint damage and rapidity of antibiotic treatment

Enterobacteriaceae

Diagnostic Considerations: Diagnosis by isolation of gram-negative bacilli from synovial fluid

Pitfalls: Septic arthritis involving an unusual joint (e.g., sternoclavicular, sacral) should suggest IV drug abuse until proven otherwise

Therapeutic Considerations: Joint aspiration is essential in suspected septic arthritis of the hip and may be needed for other joints; obtain orthopedic surgery consult. Local installation of antibiotics into joint fluid is of no proven value

Prognosis: Related to extent of joint damage and rapidity of antibiotic treatment

Pseudomonas aeruginosa

Diagnostic Considerations P. aeruginosa septic arthritis/osteomyelitis may occur after water contaminated puncture wound (e.g., nail puncture of heel through shoes). Sternoclavicular/sacroiliac joint involvement is common in IV drug abusers (IVDAs)

Pitfalls: Suspect IVDA in P. aeruginosa septic arthritis without a history of trauma

Therapeutic Considerations: If ciprofloxacin is used, treat with 750 mg (not 500 mg) dose for P. aeruginosa septic arthritis/osteomyelitis

Prognosis: Related to extent of joint damage and rapidity of antibiotic treatment

Neisseria gonorrhoeae

Diagnostic Considerations: Gonococcal arthritis may present as a monoarticular arthritis, or multiple joints may be affected as part of gonococcal arthritis-dermatitis syndrome (disseminated gonococcal infection). Bacteremia with positive blood cultures occurs early during rash stage while synovial fluid cultures are negative. Joint involvement follows with typical findings of septic arthritis and synovial fluid cultures positive for N. gonorrhoeae; blood cultures are negative at this stage. Acute tenosynovitis is often a clue to gonococcal septic arthritis

Pitfalls: Spectinomycin is ineffective against pharyngeal gonorrhea

Therapeutic Considerations: Gonococcal arthritis-dermatitis syndrome is caused by very susceptible strains of N. gonorrhoeae. Cephalosporins also eliminate incubating syphilis

Prognosis: Excellent with arthritis-dermatitis syndrome; worse with only monoarticular arthritis

Brucella sp.
Diagnostic Considerations: Usually evidence of brucellosis elsewhere (meningitis, SBE, epididymoorchitis). Diagnosis by blood/joint cultures
Pitfalls: Brucella has predilection for bones/joints of spine
Therapeutic Considerations: Some patients may require 6 weeks of antibiotic therapy
Prognosis: Related to severity of infection and underlying health of host

Salmonella sp.
Diagnostic Considerations: Occurs in sickle cell disease and hemoglobinopathies. Diagnosis by blood/joint cultures
Pitfalls: S. aureus, not Salmonella, is the most common cause of septic arthritis in sickle cell disease
Prognosis: Related to severity of infection and underlying health of host

Septic Arthritis Secondary to Animal Bite Wound
Clinical Presentation: Penetrating bite wound into joint space
Diagnostic Considerations: Diagnosis by smear/culture of synovial fluid/blood cultures
Pitfalls: May develop metastatic infection from bacteremia
Therapeutic Considerations: Treat for at least 2 weeks of combined IV/PO therapy
Prognosis: Related to severity of infection and underlying health of host

Chronic Septic Arthritis
Clinical Presentation: Subacute/chronic joint pain with decreased range of motion and little or no fever. Able to bear weight on joint
Diagnostic Considerations: Diagnosis by smear/culture of synovial fluid/synovial biopsy

Coccidioides immitis
Diagnostic Considerations: Must grow organisms from synovium/synovial fluid for diagnosis
Pitfalls: Synovial fluid the same as in TB (lymphocytic pleocytosis, low glucose, increased protein)
Therapeutic Considerations: Oral therapy is preferred; same cure rates as amphotericin regimens. HIV/AIDS patients need life-long suppressive therapy
Prognosis: Related to severity of infection and underlying health of host

Sporothrix schenckii
Diagnostic Considerations: Usually a monoarticular infection secondary to direct inoculation/trauma
Pitfalls: Polyarticular arthritis suggests disseminated infection
Therapeutic Considerations: SSKI is useful for lymphocutaneous sporotrichosis, not bone/joint involvement
Prognosis: Excellent for localized disease (e.g., lymphocutaneous sporotrichosis). In disseminated disease, prognosis is related to host factors

Mycobacterium tuberculosis (TB)
Diagnostic Considerations: Clue is subacute/chronic tenosynovitis over involved joint. Unlike other forms of septic arthritis, which are usually due to hematogenous spread, TB arthritis is usually a complication of adjacent TB osteomyelitis. Synovial fluid findings include lymphocytic pleocytosis, low glucose, and increased protein
Pitfalls: Send synovial fluid for AFB smear/culture in unexplained chronic monoarticular arthritis
Therapeutic Considerations: TB arthritis is usually treated for 1 year
Prognosis: Related to severity of infection and underlying health of host

Lyme Disease/Lyme Arthritis

Subset	Usual Pathogens	Preferred IV Therapy	Alternate IV Therapy	PO Therapy or IV-to-PO Switch
Lyme disease/ arthritis	Borrelia burgdorferi	Ceftriaxone 1 gm (IV) q24h x 2 weeks	Ceftizoxime 2 gm (IV) q8h x 2 weeks	Amoxicillin 1 gm (PO) q8h x 2 weeks **or** Doxycycline 200 mg (PO) q12h x 3 days, then 100 mg (PO) q12h x 11 days

Duration of therapy represents total time IV, PO, or IV + PO. Most patients on IV therapy able to take PO meds should be switched to PO therapy after clinical improvement

Lyme Disease
Clinical Presentation: Can manifest acutely or chronically with local or disseminated disease following bite of tick infected with Borrelia spirochete. Erythema marginatum (expanding, erythematous, annular lesion with central clearing) occurs in ~ 75% within 2 weeks of tick bite and may be associated with fever, headache, arthralgias/myalgias, meningismus. Other possible acute manifestations include meningitis, encephalitis, Bell's palsy, peripheral neuropathy, mild hepatitis, myocarditis with heart block, or arthritis. Chronic disease may present with arthritis, peripheral neuropathy, meningoencephalitis, or acrodermatitis chronica atrophicans (usually > 10 years after infection)
Diagnostic Considerations: Diagnosis by clinical presentation plus elevated IgM Lyme titers (IFA/ELISA). If Lyme titer is borderline or suspected to be a false-positive, obtain an IgM Western blot to confirm the diagnosis. IgM titers may take 4-6 weeks to increase after tick bite. Ixodes ticks are the principal vector; small rodents are the primary reservoir. In the United States, most cases occur in the coastal Northeast, upper Midwest, California, and western Nevada
Pitfalls: Rash is not always seen, and tick bite is often painless and goes unnoticed (tick often spontaneously falls off after 1-2 days of feeding). Do not overlook Lyme disease in patients with unexplained heart block in areas where Ixodes ticks are endemic
Therapeutic Considerations: B. burgdorferi is highly susceptible to all beta-lactams. For Bell's palsy or neuroborreliosis, minocycline (100 mg PO q12h x 2 weeks) may be preferred to doxycycline
Prognosis: Excellent in normal hosts

Lyme Arthritis
Clinical Presentation: Acute Lyme arthritis presents with joint pain, decreased range of motion, ability to bear weight on joint, and little or no fever. Chronic Lyme arthritis resembles rheumatoid arthritis
Diagnostic Considerations: Usually affects children and large weight-bearing joints (e.g., knee). Acute Lyme arthritis is diagnosed by clinical presentation plus elevated IgM Lyme titer. Chronic Lyme arthritis is suggested by rheumatoid arthritis-like presentation with negative ANA and rheumatoid factor, and positive IgG Lyme titer and synovial fluid PCR
Pitfalls: Acute Lyme arthritis joint is red but not hot, in contrast to septic arthritis. In chronic Lyme arthritis, a negative IgG Lyme titer essentially rules out chronic Lyme arthritis, but an elevated IgG Lyme titer indicates only past exposure to B. burgdorferi and is not diagnostic of Lyme arthritis. Joint fluid in chronic Lyme disease is usually negative by culture, but positive by PCR; synovial fluid PCR, however, does not differentiate active from prior infection
Therapeutic Considerations: IgG Lyme titers remain elevated for life, and do not decrease with treatment. Joint symptoms often persist for months/years after effective antibiotic therapy due to autoimmune joint inflammation; treat with anti-inflammatory drugs, not repeat antibiotic courses. Oral

therapy as effective as IV therapy
Prognosis: Good in normal hosts. Chronic/refractory arthritis may develop in genetically predisposed patients with DRW 2/4 HLA types

Infected Joint Prosthesis

Subset	Usual Pathogens	Preferred IV Therapy	Alternate IV Therapy	IV-to-PO Switch
Staphylococcal (Treat initially for MSSA; if later identified as MRSA or S. epidermidis, treat accordingly)	S. epidermidis (MSSE/MRSE)	Linezolid 600 mg (IV) q12h* **or** Vancomycin 1 gm (IV) q12h*	Cefotaxime 2 gm (IV) q6h* **or** Ceftizoxime 2 gm (IV) q8h*	Linezolid 600 mg (PO) q12h*
	S. aureus (MSSA)	Ceftriaxone 1 gm (IV) q24h* **or** Clindamycin 600 mg (IV) q8h* **or** Cefazolin 1 gm (IV) q8h*	Nafcillin 2 gm (IV) q4h* **or** Meropenem 1 gm (IV) q8h* **or** Imipenem 500 mg (IV) q6h*	Clindamycin 300 mg (PO) q8h* **or** Linezolid 600 mg (PO) q12h* **or** Cephalexin 1 gm (PO) q6h*
	S. aureus (MRSA)	Linezolid 600 mg (IV) q12h* **or** Vancomycin 1 gm (IV) q12h*	Minocycline 100 mg (IV) q12h* **or** Quinupristin/ dalfopristin 7.5 mg/kg (IV) q8h*	Linezolid 600 mg (PO) q12h* **or** Minocycline 100 mg (PO) q12h*

MSSA/MRSA = methicillin-sensitive/resistant S. aureus; MSSE/MRSE = methicillin-sensitive/resistant S. epidermidis. Duration of therapy represents total time IV or IV + PO. Most patients on IV therapy able to take PO meds should be switched to PO therapy after clinical improvement
* Treat for 1 week after joint prosthesis is replaced

Clinical Presentation: Pain in area of prosthesis with joint loosening/instability ± low-grade fevers
Diagnostic Considerations: Infected prosthesis is suggested by prosthetic loosening/lucent areas adjacent to prosthesis on plain films ± positive blood cultures. Diagnosis confirmed by bone scan. Use joint aspiration to identify organism
Pitfalls: An elevated ESR with prosthetic loosening suggests prosthetic joint infection. Mechanical loosening without infection is comon many years after joint replacement, but ESR is normal
Therapeutic Considerations: Infected prosthetic joints usually must be removed for cure. Replacement prosthesis may be inserted anytime after infected prosthesis is removed. To prevent infection of new joint prosthesis, extensive debridement of old infected material is important. If replacement of infected joint prosthesis is not possible, chronic suppressive therapy may be used with oral antibiotics; adding rifampin 600 mg (PO) q24h may be helpful
Prognosis: Related to adequate debridement of infected material when prosthetic joint is removed

Osteomyelitis

Subset	Usual Pathogens	Preferred IV Therapy	Alternate IV Therapy	PO Therapy or IV-to-PO Switch
Acute (Treat initially for MSSA; if later identified as MRSA or Enterobacteriaceae, treat accordingly)	S. aureus (MSSA)	Ceftriaxone 1 gm (IV) q24h x 4-6 weeks **or** Meropenem 1 gm (IV) q8h x 4-6 weeks	Cefotaxime 2 gm (IV) q6h x 4-6 weeks **or** Ceftizoxime 2 gm (IV) q8h x 4-6 weeks	Clindamycin 300 mg (PO) q8h x 4-6 weeks **or** Cephalexin 1 gm (PO) q6h x 4-6 weeks **or** Quinolone‡ (PO) q24h x 4-6 weeks
	S. aureus (MRSA)	Linezolid 600 mg (IV) q12h x 4-6 weeks **or** Vancomycin 1 gm (IV) q12h x 4-6 weeks	Minocycline 100 mg (IV) q12h x 4-6 weeks **or** Quinupristin/ dalfopristin 7.5 mg/kg (IV) q8h x 4-6 weeks	Linezolid 600 mg (PO) q12h x 4-6 weeks **or** Minocycline 100 mg (PO) q12h x 4-6 weeks
	Enterobacteriaceae	Ceftriaxone 1 gm (IV) q24h x 4-6 wks **or** Quinolone† (IV) x 4-6 weeks	Cefotaxime 2 gm (IV) q6h x 4-6 wks **or** Ceftizoxime 2 gm (IV) q8h x 4-6 wks	Quinolone† (PO) x 4-6 weeks
Chronic *Diabetes mellitus*	Group A, B streptococci S. aureus (MSSA) E. coli P. mirabilis K. pneumoniae B. fragilis	Meropenem 1 gm (IV) q8h* **or** Piperacillin/ tazobactam 4.5 gm (IV) q8h* **or** Imipenem 500 mg (IV) q6h* **or** Ertapenem 1 gm (IV) q24h* **or combination therapy with** Ceftriaxone 1 gm (IV) q24h* **plus** Metronidazole 1 gm (IV) q24h*	Moxifloxacin 400 mg (IV) q24h* **or** Ceftizoxime 2 gm (IV) q8h* **or** Ampicillin/ sulbactam 3 gm (IV) q6h* **or combination therapy with** Clindamycin 600 mg (IV) q8h* **plus either** Ciprofloxacin 400 mg (IV) q12h* **or** Gatifloxacin 400 mg (IV) q24h* **or** Levofloxacin 500 mg (IV) q24h*	Clindamycin 300 mg (PO) q8h* **plus either** Ciprofloxacin 500 mg (PO) q12h* **or** Gatifloxacin 400 mg (PO) q24h* **or** Levofloxacin 500 (PO) q24h* **or monotherapy with** Moxifloxacin 400 mg (PO) q24h*

*   *Treat for 1 week after adequate debridement or amputation*
‡   *Gatifloxacin 400 mg or levofloxacin 500 mg or moxifloxacin 400 mg*
†   *Ciprofloxacin 400 mg (IV) or 500 mg (PO) q12h or gatifloxacin 400 mg (IV or PO) q24h or levofloxacin 500 mg (IV or PO) q24h or moxifloxacin 400 mg (IV or PO) q24h*

Osteomyelitis (cont'd)

Subset	Usual Pathogens	Preferred IV Therapy	Alternate IV Therapy	PO Therapy or IV-to-PO Switch
Chronic *Peripheral vascular disease (non-diabetics)*	S. aureus Group A, B streptococci Entero-bacteriaceae	Ceftriaxone 1 gm (IV) q24h x 2-4 weeks **or** Ceftizoxime 2 gm (IV) q8h x 2-4 weeks	Clindamycin 600 mg (IV) q8h x 2-4 weeks **plus** Quinolone* (IV) q24h x 2-4 weeks	Clindamycin 300 mg (PO) q8h x 2-4 weeks **plus** Quinolone* (PO) q24h x 2-4 weeks
TB osteomyelitis	M. tuberculosis	Not applicable		Treat the same as pulmonary TB (p. 47)

MSSA/MRSA = methicillin-sensitive/resistant S. aureus. Duration of therapy represents total time IV, PO, or IV + PO. Most patients on IV therapy able to take PO meds should be switched to PO therapy soon after clinical improvement
* *Gatifloxacin 400 mg or levofloxacin 500 mg or moxifloxacin 400 mg*

Acute Osteomyelitis
Clinical Presentation: Tenderness over infected bone. Fever and positive blood cultures common
Diagnostic Considerations: Diagnosis by elevated ESR with positive bone scan. Bone biopsy is not needed for diagnosis. Bone scan is positive for acute osteomyelitis in first 24 hours
Pitfalls: Earliest sign on plain films is soft tissue swelling; bony changes evident after 2 weeks
Therapeutic Considerations: Treat 4-6 weeks with antibiotics. Debridement is not necessary for cure
Prognosis: Related to adequacy/promptness of treatment

Chronic Osteomyelitis
Diabetes Mellitus
Clinical Presentation: Afebrile or low-grade fever with normal WBC counts and deep penetrating ulcers ± draining sinus tracts
Diagnostic Considerations: Diagnosis by elevated ESR and bone changes on plain films. Bone scan is not needed for diagnosis. Bone biopsy is preferred method of demonstrating organisms, since blood cultures are usually negative and cultures from ulcers/sinus tracts are unreliable
Pitfalls: P. aeruginosa is a common colonizer and frequently cultured from deep ulcers/sinus tracts, but is not a pathogen in chronic osteomyelitis in diabetics
Therapeutic Considerations: Surgical debridement is needed for cure; antibiotics alone are ineffective. Revascularization procedures usually do not help, since diabetes is a microvascular disease. Do not culture penetrating foot ulcers/draining sinus tracts; culture results reflect superficial flora. Bone biopsy during debridement is the best way to identify pathogen; if biopsy not possible, treat empirically
Prognosis: Related to adequacy of blood supply/surgical debridement

Non-Diabetics with Peripheral Vascular Disease (PVD)
Clinical Presentation: Absent or low-grade fever with normal WBC counts ± wet/dry digital gangrene
Diagnostic Considerations: Diagnosis by clinical appearance of dusky/cold foot ± wet/dry gangrene. Chronic osteomyelitis secondary to PVD/open fracture is often polymicrobial
Pitfalls: Wet gangrene usually requires surgical debridement/antibiotic therapy; dry gangrene may not
Therapeutic Considerations: Surgical debridement needed for cure. Antibiotics alone are ineffective. Revascularization procedure may help treat infection by improving local blood supply
Prognosis: Related to degree of vascular compromise

TB Osteomyelitis (Mycobacterium tuberculosis)
Clinical Presentation: Presents similar to chronic bacterial osteomyelitis. Vertebral TB (Pott's disease) affects disk spaces early and presents with chronic back/neck pain ± inguinal/paraspinal mass
Diagnostic Considerations: Diagnosis by AFB on biopsy/culture of infected bone. PPD–positive

Pitfalls: Chest x-ray is normal in 50%. May be confused with cancer or chronic bacterial osteomyelitis
Therapeutic Considerations: Treated the same as TB arthritis
Prognosis: Good for non-vertebral TB/vertebral (if treated before paraparesis/paraplegia)

Empiric Therapy of Skin and Soft Tissue Infections

Cellulitis (Erysipelas/Impetigo)/Lymphangitis/ Soft Tissue Infections

Subset	Usual Pathogens	Preferred IV Therapy	Alternate IV Therapy	PO Therapy or IV-to-PO Switch
Above-the-waist (including mastitis) (Treat initially for Gp. A strep, MSSA; if later identified as MRSA, treat accordingly)	Group A streptococci S. aureus (MSSA)	Ceftriaxone 1-2 gm (IV) q24h x 2 weeks **or** Cefazolin 1 gm (IV) q8h x 2 weeks	Nafcillin 2 gm (IV) q4h x 2 weeks **or** Clindamycin 600 mg (IV) q8h x 2 weeks	Cephalexin 500 mg (PO) q6h x 2 weeks **or** Clindamycin 300 mg (PO) q6h x 2 weeks
	S. aureus (MRSA)	Linezolid 600 mg (IV) q12h x 2 weeks Daptomycin 4 mg/kg (IV) q24h x 2 weeks **or** Quinupristin/dalfopristin 7.5 mg/kg (IV) q12h x 2 weeks **or** Vancomycin 1 gm (IV) q12h x 2 weeks **or** Minocycline 100 mg (IV) q12h x 2 weeks		Linezolid 600 mg (PO) q12h x 2 weeks **or** Minocycline 100 mg (PO) q12h x 2 weeks
Below-the-waist (Treat initially for Gp. A,B strep, etc.; if later identified as MRSA, treat accordingly)	Group A, B streptococci E. coli P. mirabilis K. pneumoniae S. aureus (MSSA)	Ceftriaxone 1-2 gm (IV) q24h x 2 weeks **or** Piperacillin/ tazobactam 4.5 gm (IV) q8h x 2 weeks	Quinolone* (IV) q24h x 2 weeks **or** Ampicillin/sulbactam 3 gm (IV) q6h x 2 weeks **or** Ticarcillin/clavulanate 3.1 gm (IV) q6h x 2 weeks	Cephalexin 500 mg (PO) q6h x 2 weeks **or combination therapy with** Clindamycin 300 mg (PO) q6h x 2 weeks **plus** Quinolone* (PO) q24h x 2 weeks
	S. aureus (MRSA)	Treat the same as for above-the-waist cellulitis (MRSA), above		Linezolid 600 mg (PO) q12h x 2 weeks **or** Minocycline 100 mg (PO) q12h x 2 weeks

MSSA/MRSA = methicillin-sensitive/resistant S. aureus. Duration of therapy represents total time IV, PO, or IV + PO.
Most patients on IV therapy able to take PO meds should be switched to PO therapy soon after clinical improvement
* Gatifloxacin 400 mg or levofloxacin 750 mg or moxifloxacin 400 mg

Clinical Presentation: Cellulitis presents as warm, painful, non-pruritic skin erythema without discharge. Impetigo is characterized by vesiculopustular lesions, most commonly on the face/extremities. Erysipelas resembles cellulitis, but is raised and sharply demarcated. Mastitis presents as cellulitis/abscess of the breast, and is treated the same as cellulitis above the waist

Diagnostic Considerations: Diagnosis by clinical appearance ± culture of pathogen from aspirated skin lesion(s). Group B streptococci are important pathogens in diabetics. Lower extremity cellulitis tends to recur. Chronic edema of an extremity predisposes to recurrent/persistent cellulitis

Pitfalls: Streptococcal and staphylococcal cellulitis may be indistinguishable clinically, but regional adenopathy/lymphangitis favors Streptococci, and bullae favor S. aureus

Therapeutic Considerations: Lower extremity cellulitis requires ~ 1 week of antibiotics to improve. Patients with peripheral vascular disease, chronic venous stasis, alcoholic cirrhosis, and diabetes take 1-2 weeks longer to improve and often require 3-4 weeks of treatment. Treat mastitis as cellulitis above-the-waist, and drain surgically if an abscess is present

Prognosis: Related to degree of vascular insufficiency

Complicated Soft Tissue Infections

Subset	Usual Pathogens	Preferred IV Therapy	Alternate IV Therapy	IV-to-PO Switch
Mixed aerobic-anaerobic deep soft tissue infection	Entero-bacteriaceae Group A streptococci S. aureus Anaerobic streptococci Fusobacterium	Meropenem 1 gm (IV) q8h x 2 weeks **or** Piperacillin/ tazobactam 4.5 gm (IV) q8h x 2 weeks **or** Ertapenem 1 gm (IV) q24h x 2 weeks	Moxifloxacin 400 mg (IV) q24h x 2 weeks **or** Imipenem 500 mg (IV) q6h x 2 weeks **or** Cefoxitin 2 gm (IV) q6h x 2 weeks **or combination therapy with** Clindamycin 600 mg (IV) q8h x 2 weeks **plus** Quinolone[†] (IV) x 2 weeks	Moxifloxacin 400 mg (PO) q24h x 2 weeks **or combination therapy with** Clindamycin 300 mg (PO) q8h x 2 weeks **plus** Quinolone[†] (PO) x 2 weeks
Clostridial myonecrosis (gas gangrene)	Clostridia sp.	Penicillin G 10 mu (IV) q4h x 2 weeks **or** Clindamycin 600 mg (IV) q8h x 2 weeks **or** Piperacillin/ tazobactam 4.5 gm (IV) q8h x 2 weeks	Meropenem 1 gm (IV) q8h x 2 weeks **or** Imipenem 500 mg (IV) q6h x 2 weeks **or** Ertapenem 1 gm (IV) q24h x 2 weeks	Not applicable

Duration of therapy represents total time IV or IV + PO. Most patients on IV therapy able to take PO meds should be switched to PO therapy after clinical improvement
† *Ciprofloxacin 400 mg (IV) or 500 mg (PO) q12h or gatifloxacin 400 mg (IV or PO) q24h or levofloxacin 750 mg (IV or PO) q24h*

Complicated Soft Tissue Infections (cont'd)

Subset	Usual Pathogens	Preferred IV Therapy	Alternate IV Therapy	IV-to-PO Switch
Necrotizing fasciitis/ synergistic gangrene	Group A streptococci Entero-bacteriaceae Anaerobic streptococci S. aureus (MSSA)	Meropenem 1 gm (IV) q8h x 2 weeks **or** Piperacillin/ tazobactam 4.5 gm (IV) q8h x 2 weeks **or** Ertapenem 1 gm (IV) q24h x 2 weeks **or** Imipenem 500 mg (IV) q6h x 2 weeks	Clindamycin 600 mg (IV) q8h x 2 weeks **plus either** Ciprofloxacin 400 mg (IV) q12h x 2 weeks **or** Gatifloxacin 400 mg (IV) q24h x 2 weeks **or** Levofloxacin 750 mg (IV) q24h x 2 weeks **or** Moxifloxacin 400 mg (IV) q24h x 2 weeks	Clindamycin 300 mg (PO) q8h x 2 weeks **plus either** Ciprofloxacin 500 mg (PO) q12h x 2 weeks **or** Gatifloxacin 400 mg (PO) q24h x 2 weeks **or** Levofloxacin 750 mg (PO) q24h x 2 weeks **or** Moxifloxacin 400 mg (PO) q24h x 2 weeks

Duration of therapy represents total time IV or IV + PO. Most patients on IV therapy able to take PO meds should be switched to PO therapy after clinical improvement

Mixed Aerobic/Anaerobic Deep Soft Tissue Infection

Clinical Presentation: Acutely ill patient with gross gas deep in soft tissues and usually high fevers
Diagnostic Considerations: Diagnosis by gram stain/culture of aspirated fluid. Patients usually have high fevers. Wound discharge is foul when present
Pitfalls: Gross crepitance/prominent gas in soft tissues on x-ray suggests a mixed aerobic/anaerobic necrotizing infection, not gas gangrene
Therapeutic Considerations: Prompt surgical debridement may be lifesaving. Control/cure of infection requires surgical debridement and antibiotics
Prognosis: Related to severity of infection, adequacy of debridement, and underlying health of host

Gas Gangrene (Clostridial Myonecrosis)

Clinical Presentation: Fulminant infection of muscle with little or no fever. Infected area is extremely painful, indurated, and discolored with or without bullae
Diagnostic Considerations: Diagnosis is clinical. Aspiration of infected muscle shows few PMNs and gram-positive bacilli without spores. Gas gangrene is not accompanied by high fever. Patients are often apprehensive with relative bradycardia ± diarrhea. Wound discharge, if present, is sweetish and not foul. Rapidly progressive hemolytic anemia is characteristic
Pitfalls: Gas gangrene (clostridial myonecrosis) has little visible gas on plain film x-rays; abundant gas should suggest a mixed aerobic/anaerobic infection, not gas gangrene
Therapeutic Considerations: Surgical debridement is life saving and the only way to control infection
Prognosis: Related to speed/extent of surgical debridement. Rapid progression/death may occur within hours

Necrotizing Fasciitis/Synergistic Gangrene

Clinical Presentation: Acutely ill patient with high fevers and extreme local pain without gas in tissues

Diagnostic Considerations: Diagnosis by CT/MRI of involved extremity showing infection confined to one or more muscle compartments/fascial planes. Patients are febrile and ill. Gas is not present on exam or x-rays. May be polymicrobial or due to a single organism. Foul smelling exudate from infected soft tissues indicates anaerobes are present

Pitfalls: Extreme pain in patients with deep soft tissue infections should suggest a compartment syndrome/necrotizing fasciitis. No hemolytic anemia, diarrhea, or bullae as with gas gangrene

Therapeutic Considerations: Control/cure of infection requires surgical decompression of infected compartment, debridement of dead tissue in necrotizing fasciitis, and antimicrobial therapy

Prognosis: Related to rapidity/extent of surgical debridement

Skin Ulcers

Subset	Usual Pathogens	Preferred IV Therapy	Alternate IV Therapy	PO Therapy or IV-to-PO Switch
Decubitus ulcers *Above the waist*	Group A streptococci E. coli P. mirabilis K. pneumoniae S. aureus (MSSA)	Cefazolin 1 gm (IV) q8h* **or** Ceftriaxone 1 gm (IV) q24h*	Cefotaxime 2 gm (IV) q6h* **or** Ceftizoxime 2 gm (IV) q8h*	Cephalexin 500 mg (PO) q6h*
Below the waist	Group A streptococci E. coli P. mirabilis K. pneumoniae B. fragilis S. aureus (MSSA)	Meropenem 1 gm (IV) q8h* **or** Piperacillin/ tazobactam 4.5 gm (IV) q8h* **or** Imipenem 500 mg (IV) q6h* **or** Ertapenem 1 gm (IV) q24h*	Moxifloxacin 400 mg (IV) q24h* **or combination therapy with** Clindamycin 600 mg (IV) q6h* **plus either** Ciprofloxacin 400 mg (IV) q12h* **or** Gatifloxacin 400 mg (IV) q24h* **or** Levofloxacin 500 mg (IV) q24h*	Moxifloxacin 400 mg (PO) q24h* **or combination therapy with** Clindamycin 300 mg (PO) q8h* **plus either** Ciprofloxacin 500 mg (PO) q12h* **or** Gatifloxacin 400 mg (PO) q24h* **or** Levofloxacin 500 mg (PO) q24h*

Duration of therapy represents total time IV, PO, or IV + PO. Most patients on IV therapy able to take PO meds should be switched to PO therapy soon after clinical improvement

* *Treat Stages I/II (superficial) decubitus ulcers with local care. Treat Stages III/IV (deep) decubitus ulcers with antibiotics for 1-2 weeks after adequate debridement*

Skin Ulcers (cont'd)

Subset	Usual Pathogens	Preferred IV Therapy	Alternate IV Therapy	PO Therapy or IV-to-PO Switch
Diabetic foot ulcers (chronic osteomyelitis)	Group A, B streptococci S. aureus (MSSA) E. coli P. mirabilis K. pneumoniae B. fragilis	Meropenem 1 gm (IV) q8h[†] **or** Piperacillin/ tazobactam 4.5 gm (IV) q8h[†] **or** Imipenem 500 mg (IV) q6h[†] **or** Ertapenem 1 gm (IV) q24h[†] **or combination therapy with** Ceftriaxone 1 gm (IV) q24h[†] **plus** Metronidazole 1 mg (IV) q24h[†]	Ceftizoxime 2 gm (IV) q8h[†] **or** Ampicillin/sulbactam 3 gm (IV) q6h[†] **or** Moxifloxacin 400 mg (IV) q24h[†] **or combination therapy with** Clindamycin 600 mg (IV) q8h[†] **plus either** Ciprofloxacin 400 mg (IV) q12h[†] **or** Gatifloxacin 400 mg (IV) q24h[†] **or** Levofloxacin 500 mg (IV) q24h[†]	Moxifloxacin 400 mg (PO) q24h[†] **or combination therapy with** Clindamycin 300 mg (PO) q8h[†] **plus either** Ciprofloxacin 500 mg (PO) q12h[†] **or** Gatifloxacin 400 mg (PO) q24h[†] **or** Levofloxacin 500 mg (PO) q24h[†]
Ischemic foot ulcers	Group A streptococci E. coli S. aureus (MSSA)	Ceftriaxone 1 gm (IV) q24h x 2 weeks **or** Piperacillin/ tazobactam 4.5 gm (IV) q8h x 2 weeks **or** Ceftizoxime 2 gm (IV) q8h x 2 weeks	Clindamycin 600 mg (IV) q8h x 2 weeks **plus either** Gatifloxacin 400 mg (IV) q24h x 2 weeks **or** Levofloxacin 750 mg (IV) q24h x 2 weeks **or** Moxifloxacin 400 mg (IV) q24h x 2 weeks	Gatifloxacin 400 mg (PO) q24h x 2 weeks **or** Levofloxacin 750 mg (PO) q24h x 2 weeks **or** Moxifloxacin 400 mg (PO) q24h x 2 weeks

MSSA = methicillin-sensitive S. aureus. Duration of therapy represents total time IV, PO, or IV + PO. Most patients on IV therapy able to take PO meds should be switched to PO therapy soon after clinical improvement
† *Treat for 1 week after adequate debridement or amputation*

Decubitus Ulcers

Clinical Presentation: Painless ulcers with variable depth and infectious exudate ± fevers ≤ 102°F

Diagnostic Considerations: Diagnosis by clinical appearance. Obtain ESR/bone scan to rule out underlying osteomyelitis with deep (Stage III/IV) decubitus ulcers

Pitfalls: Superficial decubitus ulcers do not require systemic antibiotics

Therapeutic Considerations: Deep decubitus ulcers require antibiotics and debridement, superficial ulcers do not. Coverage for B. fragilis is needed for deep perianal decubitus ulcers. Good nursing care is important in preventing/limiting extension of decubitus ulcers

Prognosis: Related to fecal contamination of ulcer and bone involvement (e.g., osteomyelitis)

Diabetic Foot Ulcers/Chronic Osteomyelitis

Clinical Presentation: Ulcers/sinus tracts on bottom of foot/between toes; usually painless. Fevers ≤ 102°F and a foul smelling exudate are common

Diagnostic Considerations: In diabetics, deep, penetrating, chronic foot ulcers/draining sinus tracts are diagnostic of chronic osteomyelitis. ESR ≥ 100 mm/hr in a diabetic with a foot ulcer/sinus tract is diagnostic of chronic osteomyelitis. Foot films confirm chronic osteomyelitis. Bone scan is needed only in acute osteomyelitis

Pitfalls: Do not rely on culture results of deep ulcers/sinus tracts to choose antibiotic coverage, since cultures reflect skin colonization, not bone pathogens. Treat empirically

Therapeutic Considerations: B. fragilis coverage is required in deep penetrating diabetic foot ulcers/fetid foot infection. P. aeruginosa is often cultured from diabetic foot ulcers/sinus tracts, but represents colonization, not infection. P. aeruginosa is a "water" organism that colonizes feet from moist socks/dressings, irrigant solutions, or whirlpool baths. Surgical debridement is essential for cure of chronic osteomyelitis in diabetics. Treat superficial diabetic foot ulcers the same as cellulitis in non-diabetics (p. 102)

Prognosis: Related to adequacy of debridement of infected bone

Ischemic Foot Ulcers

Clinical Presentation: Ulcers often clean/dry ± digital gangrene. No fevers/exudate

Diagnostic Considerations: Diagnosis by clinical appearance/location in a patient with peripheral vascular disease. Ischemic foot ulcers most commonly affect the toes, medial malleoli, dorsum of foot, or lower leg

Pitfalls: In contrast to ulcers in diabetics, ischemic ulcers due to peripheral vascular disease usually do not involve the plantar surface of the foot

Therapeutic Considerations: Dry gangrene should not be treated with antibiotics unless accompanied by signs of systemic infection. Wet gangrene should be treated as a mixed aerobic/anaerobic infection. Both dry/wet gangrene may require debridement for cure/control. Do not rely on ulcer cultures to guide treatment; treat empirically if necessary. Evaluate for revascularization

Prognosis: Related to degree of vascular insufficiency

Skin Abscesses/Infected Cysts
(Skin Pustules, Skin Boils, Furunculosis)

Subset	Usual Pathogens	Preferred IV Therapy	Alternate IV Therapy	PO Therapy or IV-to-PO Switch
Skin abscesses (Treat initially for MSSA; if later identified as MRSA, treat accordingly)	S. aureus (MSSA)	Clindamycin 600 mg (IV) q8h x 2 wks **or** Ceftriaxone 1 gm (IV) q24h x 2 weeks	Cefazolin 1 gm (IV) q8h x 2 weeks **or** Nafcillin 2 gm (IV) q4h x 2 weeks	Cephalexin 500 mg (PO) q6h x 2 weeks **or** Clindamycin 300 mg (PO) q8h x 2 weeks
	S. aureus (MRSA)	Linezolid 600 mg (IV) q12h x 2 weeks **or** Daptomycin 4 mg/kg (IV) q24h x 2 weeks **or** Vancomycin 1 gm (IV) q12h x 2 weeks **or** Minocycline 100 mg (IV) q12h x 2 weeks		Linezolid 600 mg (PO) q12h x 2 weeks **or** Minocycline 100 mg (PO) q12h x 2 weeks
Infected pilonidal cysts	Group A streptococci E. coli P. mirabilis K. pneumoniae S. aureus (MSSA)	Ceftriaxone 1 gm (IV) q24h x 2 weeks **or** Ceftizoxime 2 gm (IV) q8h x 2 weeks **or** Cefoxitin 2 gm (IV) q6h x 2 weeks	Gatifloxacin 400 mg (IV) q24h x 2 weeks **or** Levofloxacin 500 mg (IV) q24h x 2 weeks **or** Moxifloxacin 400 mg (IV) q24h x 2 weeks	Gatifloxacin 400 mg (PO) q24h x 2 weeks **or** Levofloxacin 500 mg (PO) q24h x 2 weeks **or** Moxifloxacin 400 mg (PO) q24h x 2 weeks
Hydradenitis suppurativa	S. aureus (MSSA)	Not applicable	TMP-SMX 1 SS tablet (PO) q12h x 2-4 weeks **or** Clindamycin 300 mg (PO) q8h x 2-4 weeks **or** Minocycline 100 mg (PO) q12h x 2-4 weeks	

MSSA/MRSA = methicillin-sensitive/resistant S. aureus. Duration of therapy represents total time IV, PO, or IV + PO. Most patients on IV therapy able to take PO meds should be switched to PO therapy soon after clinical improvement (usually < 72 hours)

Skin Abscesses

Clinical Presentation: Warm painful nodules ± bullae, low-grade fever ± systemic symptoms, no lymphangitis. Skin boils/furunculosis present as acute, chronic, or recurrent skin pustules, and remain localized without lymphangitis

Diagnostic Considerations: Specific pathogen diagnosed by gram stain of abscess. Recurring S. aureus abscesses are not uncommon and should be drained. Blood cultures are rarely positive. Suspect Job's syndrome if recurring abscesses with peripheral eosinophilia. Skin boils/furunculosis are diagnosed by clinical appearance (skin pustules)

Pitfalls: Recurring S. aureus skin infections may occur on an immune basis, but immunologic studies are usually negative

Therapeutic Considerations: Repeated aspiration of abscesses may be necessary. Surgical drainage is required if antibiotics fail. Treat boils/furunculosis as in hydradenitis suppurativa

Prognosis: Excellent if treated early

Infected Pilonidal Cysts
Clinical Presentation: Chronic drainage from pilonidal cysts
Diagnostic Considerations: Diagnosis by clinical appearance. Deep/systemic infection is rare
Pitfalls: Culture of exudate is usually unhelpful
Therapeutic Considerations: Surgical debridement is often necessary
Prognosis: Good with adequate excision

Hydradenitis Suppurativa
Clinical Presentation: Chronic, indurated, painful, raised axillary/groin lesions ± drainage/sinus tracts
Diagnostic Considerations: Diagnosis by clinical appearance/location of lesions. Infections are often bilateral and tend to recur
Pitfalls: Surgical debridement is usually not necessary unless deep/extensive infection
Therapeutic Considerations: Most anti-S. aureus antibiotics have poor penetration and usually fail
Prognosis: Good with recommended antibiotics. Surgery, if necessary, is curative

Skin Vesicles (non-genital)

Subset	Usual Pathogens	IV Therapy	PO Therapy
Herpes simplex	Herpes simplex virus (HSV)	Not applicable	Acyclovir 400 mg (PO) q8h x 10 days **or** Valacyclovir 1 gm (PO) q12h x 10 days **or** Famciclovir 250 mg (PO) q8h x 10 days
Herpes zoster, dermatomal	Varicella zoster virus (VZV)	Not applicable	Acyclovir 800 mg (PO) 5x/day x 7 days **or** Famciclovir 500 mg (PO) q8h x 7 days **or** Valacyclovir 1 gm (PO) q8h x 7 days
Herpes whitlow	HSV-1	Not applicable	Acyclovir 400 mg (PO) q8h x 1-2 weeks **or** Valacyclovir 1 gm (PO) q12h x 1-2 weeks **or** Famciclovir 250 mg (PO) q8h x 1-2 weeks

Herpes Simplex (HSV)
Clinical Presentation: Painful, sometimes pruritic vesicles that form pustules or painful erythematous ulcers. Associated with fever, myalgias
Diagnostic Considerations: Diagnosis by clinical appearance and demonstration of HSV by culture of vesicle fluid/vesicle base. May be severe in HIV/AIDS
Pitfalls: Painful vesicular lesions surrounded by prominent induration distinguishes HSV from insect bites (pruritic) and cellulitis (no induration)
Therapeutic Considerations: Topical acyclovir ointment may be useful early when vesicles erupt, but is ineffective after vesicles stop erupting. For severe/refractory cases, use acyclovir 5 mg/kg (IV) q8h x 2-7 days, then if improvement, switch to acyclovir 400 mg (PO) q8h to complete 10-day course
Prognosis: Related to extent of tissue involvement/degree of cellular immunity dysfunction

Herpes Zoster (VZV)
Clinical Presentation: Painful, vesicular eruption in dermatomal distribution. Pain may be difficult to diagnose
Diagnostic Considerations: Diagnosis by appearance/positive Tzanck test of vesicle base scrapings
Pitfalls: Begin therapy within 2 days of vesicle eruption
Therapeutic Considerations: Higher doses of acyclovir are required for VZV than HSV. See p. 252 for disseminated VZV, ophthalmic nerve/visceral involvement, or acyclovir-resistant strains
Prognosis: Good if treated early. Some patients develop painful post-herpetic neuralgia of involved dermatomes

Herpes Whitlow
Clinical Presentation: Multiple vesicopustular lesions on fingers and hands. Lymphangitis, adenopathy, fever/chills are usually present, suggesting a bacterial infection
Diagnostic Considerations: Common in healthcare workers giving patients oral care/suctioning
Pitfalls: No need for antibiotics even though lesions appear infected with "pus"
Therapeutic Considerations: Never incise/drain herpes whitlow; surgical incision will flare/prolong the infection
Prognosis: Excellent, unless incision/drainage has been performed

Wound Infections (for rabies, see pp. 276, 284)

Subset	Usual Pathogens	Preferred IV Therapy	Alternate IV Therapy	PO Therapy or IV-to-PO Switch
Animal bite wounds	Group A streptococci P. multocida Capnocytophaga (DF2) S. aureus (MSSA)	Piperacillin/ tazobactam 4.5 gm (IV) q8h x 2 weeks **or** Ampicillin/ sulbactam 3 gm (IV) q6h x 2 weeks	Meropenem 1 gm (IV) q8h x 2 weeks **or** Imipenem 500 mg (IV) q6h x 2 weeks **or** Ertapenem 1 gm (IV) q24h x 2 weeks	Amoxicillin/ clavulanic acid 500/125 mg (PO) q8h or 875/125 mg (PO) q12h x 2 weeks **or** Doxycycline 200 mg (PO) q12h x 3 days, then 100 mg (PO) q12h x 11 days
Human bite wounds	Oral anaerobes Group A streptococci E. corrodens S. aureus (MSSA)	Piperacillin/ tazobactam 4.5 gm (IV) q8h x 2 weeks **or** Ampicillin/ sulbactam 3 gm (IV) q6h x 2 weeks	Meropenem 1 gm (IV) q8h x 2 weeks **or** Imipenem 500 mg (IV) q6h x 2 weeks **or** Ertapenem 1 gm (IV) q24h x 2 weeks	Amoxicillin/ clavulanic acid 500/125 mg (PO) q8h or 875/125 mg (PO) q12h x 2 weeks **or** Doxycycline 200 mg (PO) q12h x 3 days, then 100 mg (PO) q12h x 11 days

MSSA = methicillin-sensitive S. aureus. Duration of therapy represents total time IV, PO, or IV + PO. Most patients on IV therapy able to take PO meds should be switched to PO therapy soon after clinical improvement

Wound Infections (cont'd) (for rabies, see pp. 276, 284)

Subset	Usual Pathogens	Preferred IV Therapy	Alternate IV Therapy	PO Therapy or IV-to-PO Switch
Cat scratch fever	Bartonella henselae	Doxycycline 200 mg (IV) q12h x 3 days, then 100 mg (IV) q12h x 4-8 weeks **or** Azithromycin 500 mg (IV) q24h x 4-8 weeks	Chloramphenicol 500 mg (IV) q6h x 4-8 weeks **or** Erythromycin 500 mg (IV) q6h x 4-8 weeks	Doxycycline 200 mg (PO) q12h x 3 days, then 100 mg (PO) q12h x 4-8 weeks* **or** Azithromycin 250 mg (PO) q24h x 4-8 weeks **or** Quinolone[‡] (PO) x 4-8 weeks
Burn wounds (severe)[†]	Group A streptococci Enterobacter P. aeruginosa	Cefepime 2 gm (IV) q8h x 2 weeks **or** Meropenem 1 gm (IV) q8h x 2 weeks	Piperacillin/ tazobactam 4.5 gm (IV) q8h x 2 weeks	Not applicable
Freshwater-exposed wounds	Aeromonas hydrophilia	Quinolone[‡] (IV) x 2 weeks **or** TMP-SMX 2.5 mg/kg (IV) q6h x 2 weeks	Ceftriaxone 1 gm (IV) q24h x 2 weeks **or** Aztreonam 2 gm (IV) q8h x 2 weeks **or** Gentamicin 240 mg (IV) q24h x 2 weeks	Quinolone[‡] (PO) x 2 weeks **or** TMP-SMX 1 SS tablet (PO) q12h x 2 weeks
Saltwater-exposed wounds	Vibrio vulnificus	Doxycycline 200 mg (IV) q12h x 3 days, then 100 mg (IV) q12h x 11 days **or** Quinolone[‡] (IV) x 2 weeks	Ceftriaxone 2 gm (IV) q12h x 2 weeks **or** Chloramphenicol 500 mg (IV) q6h x 2 weeks	Doxycycline 200 mg (PO) q12h x 3 days, then 100 mg (PO) q12h x 11 days* **or** Quinolone[‡] (PO) x 2 weeks

MSSA = methicillin-sensitive S. aureus. Duration of therapy represents total time IV, PO, or IV + PO. Most patients on IV therapy able to take PO meds should be switched to PO therapy soon after clinical improvement

†   Treat only IV or IV-to-PO switch

*   Loading dose is not needed PO if given IV with the same drug

‡   Ciprofloxacin 400 mg (IV) or 500 mg (PO) q12h or gatifloxacin 400 mg (IV or PO) q24h or levofloxacin 500 mg (IV or PO) q24h or moxifloxacin 400 mg (IV or PO) q24h

Animal Bite Wounds (for rabies, see p. 276)
Clinical Presentation: Cellulitis surrounding bite wound
Diagnostic Considerations: Diagnosis by culture of bite wound exudate. Deep bites may also cause tendinitis/osteomyelitis, and severe bites may result in systemic infection with bacteremia
Pitfalls: Avoid erythromycin in penicillin-allergic patients (ineffective against P. multocida)
Therapeutic Considerations: For facial/hand bites, consult a plastic surgeon
Prognosis: Related to adequacy of debridement and early antibiotic therapy

Human Bite Wounds
Clinical Presentation: Cellulitis surrounding bite wound
Diagnostic Considerations: Diagnosis by culture of bite wound exudate. Infection often extends to involve tendon/bone
Pitfalls: Compared to animal bites, human bites are more likely to contain anaerobes, S. aureus, and Group A streptococci
Therapeutic Considerations: Avoid primary closure of human bite wounds
Prognosis: Related to adequacy of debridement and early antibiotic therapy

Cat Scratch Fever/Disease (Bartonella henselae)
Clinical Presentation: Subacute presentation of obscure febrile illness associated with cat bite/contact. Usually accompanied by adenopathy
Diagnostic Considerations: Diagnosis by wound culture/serology for Bartonella. Cat scratch fever/disease may follow a cat scratch, but a lick from a kitten contaminating an inapparent micro-laceration is more common. May present as an FUO. Culture of exudate/node is unlikely to be positive, but silver stain of biopsy material shows organisms
Pitfalls: Rule out lymphoma, which may present in similar fashion
Therapeutic Considerations: Prolonged oral antibiotic therapy may be necessary. Treat until symptoms/signs resolve. Bartonella are sensitive in-vitro to cephalosporins and TMP-SMX, but these antibiotics are ineffective in-vivo
Prognosis: Related to health of host

Burn Wounds
Clinical Presentation: Severe (3rd/4th degree) burns ± drainage
Diagnostic Considerations: Semi-quantitative bacterial counts help differentiate colonization (low counts) from infection (high counts). Burn wounds quickly become colonized
Pitfalls: Treat only infected 3rd/4th degree burn wounds with systemic antibiotics
Therapeutic Considerations: Meticulous local care/eschar removal/surgical debridement is key in preventing and controlling infection
Prognosis: Related to severity of burns and adequacy of eschar debridement

Freshwater-Exposed Wounds (Aeromonas hydrophilia)
Clinical Presentation: Fulminant wound infection with fever and diarrhea
Diagnostic Considerations: Diagnosis by stool/wound/blood culture
Pitfalls: Suspect A. hydrophilia in wound infection with fresh water exposure followed by diarrhea
Therapeutic Considerations: Surgical debridement of devitalized tissue may be necessary
Prognosis: Related to severity of infection and health of host

Saltwater-Exposed Wounds (Vibrio vulnificus)
Clinical Presentation: Fulminant wound infection with fever, painful hemorrhagic bullae, diarrhea
Diagnostic Considerations: Diagnosis by stool/wound/blood culture. Vibrio vulnificus is a fulminant, life-threatening infection that may be accompanied by hypotension
Pitfalls: Suspect V. vulnificus in acutely ill patients with fever, diarrhea, and bullous lesions after salt-

water exposure

Therapeutic Considerations: Surgical debridement of devitalized tissue may be necessary

Prognosis: Related to extent of infection and health of host

Superficial Fungal Infections of Skin and Nails

Subset	Usual Pathogens	Topical Therapy	PO Therapy
Cutaneous (local/non-disseminated) candidiasis	C. albicans	<u>Interdigital, other local</u> Clotrimazole 1% cream twice daily x 2-4 weeks	<u>Onychomycosis (nail infection)</u> Itraconazole 200 mg (PO) solution q12h x 1 week per month for 2 months <u>Cutaneous (local/non-disseminated) candidiasis</u> Fluconazole 400 mg (PO) x 1 dose, then 200 mg (PO) q24h x 2 weeks
Tinea corporis (body ringworm)	Trichophyton rubrum Epidermophyton floccosum Microsporum canis Trichophyton mentagrophytes	Clotrimazole 1% cream twice daily x 4-8 weeks **or** Miconazole 2% cream twice daily x 2 weeks **or** Econazole 1% cream twice daily x 2 weeks	Terbinafine 250 mg (PO) q24h x 4 weeks **or** Ketoconazole 200 mg (PO) q24h x 4 weeks **or** Fluconazole 200 mg (PO) weekly x 4 weeks
Tinea capitis (scalp ringworm)	Same as Tinea corporis, above	Selenium sulfide shampoo daily x 2-4 weeks	Same as Tinea corporis, above
Tinea cruris (jock itch)	T. cruris	Same as Tinea corporis, above	Same as Tinea corporis, above
Tinea pedis (athlete's foot)	Same as Tinea corporis, above	Same as Tinea corporis, above	Terbinafine 250 mg (PO) q24h x 2 weeks **or** Ketoconazole 200 mg (PO) q24h x 4 weeks **or** Itraconazole 200 mg (PO) solution q24h x 4 weeks
Tinea versicolor (pityriasis)	M. furfur (Pityrosporum orbiculare)	Clotrimazole cream (1%) or miconazole cream (2%) or ketoconazole cream (2%) daily x 7 days	Ketoconazole 200 mg (PO) q24h x 7 days **or** Itraconazole 200 mg (PO) solution q24h x 7 days **or** Fluconazole 400 mg (PO) x 1 dose

Superficial Fungal Infections of Skin and Nails (cont'd)

Subset	Usual Pathogens	Topical Therapy	PO Therapy
Tinea unguium (onycho-mycosis)	Epidermophyton floccosum Trichophyton mentagrophytes Trichophyton rubrum	Not applicable	Terbinafine 250 mg (PO) q24h x 6 weeks (fingernail infection) or 12 weeks (toenail infection) **or** Itraconazole 200 mg (PO) solution q24h 1 week per month x 2 months (fingernail infection) or 3 months (toenail infection) **or** Fluconazole 200 mg (PO) q24h 1 week per month x 3 months (fingernail infection) or 6 months (toenail infection)

Cutaneous (Local/Non-disseminated) Candidiasis
Clinical Presentation: Primary cutaneous findings include an erythematous rash with satellite lesions, which may be papular, pustular, or ulcerated. Lesions can be limited or widespread over parts of body. Chronic mucocutaneous candidiasis manifests as recurrent candidal infections of skin, nails, or mucous membranes
Diagnostic Considerations: Diagnosis by demonstrating organism by stain/culture in tissue specimen. In HIV/AIDS, Candida is very common on skin/mucous membranes
Pitfalls: Do not confuse with the isolated, multinodular lesions of disseminated disease, which may resemble ecthyma gangrenosa or purpura fulminans
Therapeutic Considerations: Diabetics and other compromised hosts may require prolonged therapy. In contrast to local disease, nodular cutaneous candidiasis represents disseminated disease (p. 217)
Prognosis: Related to extent of disease/host defense status

Tinea Corporis (Body Ringworm)
Clinical Presentation: Annular pruritic lesions on trunk/face with central clearing
Diagnostic Considerations: Diagnosis by clinical appearance/skin scraping
Pitfalls: Do not confuse with erythema migrans, which is not pruritic
Therapeutic Considerations: If topical therapy fails, treat with oral antifungals
Prognosis: Excellent

Tinea Capitis (Scalp Ringworm)
Clinical Presentation: Itchy, annular scalp lesions
Diagnostic Considerations: Scalp lesions fluoresce with ultraviolet light. Culture hair shafts
Pitfalls: T. capitis is associated with localized areas of alopecia
Therapeutic Considerations: Selenium sulfide shampoo may be used first for 2-4 weeks. Treat shampoo failures with oral ketoconazole, terbinafine, or fluconazole
Prognosis: Excellent

Tinea Cruris (Jock Itch)
Clinical Presentation: Groin, inguinal, perineal, or buttock lesions that are pruritic and serpiginous with scaling borders/central clearing
Diagnostic Considerations: Diagnosis by clinical appearance/culture
Pitfalls: Usually spares penis/scrotum, unlike Candida

Therapeutic Considerations: In addition to therapy, it is important to keep area dry
Prognosis: Excellent

Tinea Pedis (Athlete's Foot)
Clinical Presentation: Painful cracks/fissures between toes
Diagnostic Considerations: Diagnosis by clinical appearance/skin scraping
Pitfalls: Must keep feet dry or infection will recur
Therapeutic Considerations: In addition to therapy, it is important to keep area dry
Prognosis: Excellent

Tinea Versicolor (Pityriasis)
Clinical Presentation: Oval hypo- or hyperpigmented scaly lesions that coalesce into large confluent areas typically on upper trunk; chronic/relapsing
Diagnostic Considerations: Diagnosis by clinical appearance and culture of affected skin lesions
Pitfalls: M. furfur also causes seborrheic dermatitis, but seborrheic lesions are typically on the face/scalp
Therapeutic Considerations: If topical therapy fails, treat with oral antifungals. Treat non-scalp seborrheic dermatitis with ketoconazole cream (2%) daily until cured
Prognosis: Excellent

Dermatophyte Nail Infections
Clinical Presentation: Chronically thickened, discolored nails
Diagnostic Considerations: Diagnosis by culture of nail clippings
Pitfalls: Nail clipping cultures often contaminated by bacterial/fungal colonizers. Green nail discoloration suggests P. aeruginosa, not a fungal nail infection; treat with ciprofloxacin 500 mg (PO) q12h x 2-3 weeks
Therapeutic Considerations: Lengthy therapy is required. However, terbinafine and itraconazole remain bound to nail tissue for months following dosing and thus therapy with these compounds is not continued until clearance of the nail bed
Prognosis: Excellent if infection is totally eradicated from nail bed. New nail growth takes months

Skin Infestations

Subset	Usual Pathogens	Topical Therapy
Scabies	Sarcoptes scabiei	Treat whole body with Permethrin cream 5% (Elimite); leave on for 8-10 hours
Head lice	Pediculus humanus var. capitis	Shampoo with Permethrin 5% (Elimite) or 1% (NIX) cream x 10 minutes
Body lice	Pediculus humanus var. corporis	Body lice removed by shower. Removed clothes should be washed in hot water or sealed in bags for 1 month, or treated with DDT powder 10% or malathion powder 1%
Pubic lice (crabs)	Phthirus pubis	Permethrin 5% (Elimite) or 1% (NIX) cream x 10 minutes to affected areas

Scabies (Sarcoptes scabiei)
Clinical Presentation: Punctate, serpiginous, intensely pruritic black spots in webbed spaces of hands/feet and creases of elbows/knees
Diagnostic Considerations: Diagnosis by visualization of skin tracts/burrows. Incubation period up

to 6 weeks after contact. Spread by scratching from one part of body to another
Pitfalls: Mites are not visible, only their skin tracks
Therapeutic Considerations: Permethrin cream is usually effective. If itching persists after treatment, do not retreat (itching is secondary to hypersensitivity reaction of eggs in skin burrows). Treat close contacts. Vacuum bedding/furniture
Prognosis: Norwegian scabies is very difficult to eradicate

Head Lice (Pediculus humanus var. capitis)
Clinical Presentation: White spots may be seen on hair shafts of head/neck, but not eyebrows
Diagnostic Considerations: Nits on hair are unhatched lice eggs, seen as white dots attached to hair shaft. May survive away from body x 2 days
Pitfalls: May need to retreat in 7 days to kill any lice that hatched from surviving nits
Therapeutic Considerations: Shampoo with Permethrin 5% (Elimite) or 1% (NIX) cream kills lice/nits. Clothes and non-washables should be tied off in plastic bags x 2 weeks to kill lice. Alternately, wash and dry clothes/bed linens; heat from dryer/iron kills lice
Prognosis: Related to thoroughness of therapy

Body Lice (Pediculus humanus var. corporis)
Clinical Presentation: Intense generalized pruritus
Diagnostic Considerations: Smaller than head lice and more difficult to see. May survive away from body x 1 week
Pitfalls: Body lice live in clothes; leave only for a blood meal, then return to clothing
Therapeutic Considerations: Can survive in seams of clothing x 1 week
Prognosis: Good if clothes are also treated

Pubic Lice (Phthirus pubis) Crabs
Clinical Presentation: Genital pruritus
Diagnostic Considerations: Seen on groin, eyelashes, axilla. May survive away from body x 1 day
Pitfalls: Smaller than head lice, but easily seen
Therapeutic Considerations: Treat partners. Wash, dry, and iron clothes; heat from dryer/iron kills lice. Non-washables may be placed in a sealed bag x 7 days
Prognosis: Good if clothes are also treated

Ischiorectal/Perirectal Abscess

Subset	Pathogens	Preferred Therapy
Ischiorectal/ perirectal abscess	Enterobacteriaceae B. fragilis	Treat the same as mild/severe peritonitis (p. 77) ± surgical drainage depending on abscess size/severity

Clinical Presentation: Presents in normal hosts with perirectal pain, pain on defecation, leukocytosis, erythema/tenderness over abscess ± fever/chills. In febrile neutropenia, there is only tenderness
Diagnostic Considerations: Diagnosis by erythema/tenderness over abscess or by CT/MRI
Pitfalls: Do not confuse with perirectal regional enteritis (Crohn's disease) in normal hosts, or with ecthyma gangrenosum in febrile neutropenics
Therapeutic Considerations: Antibiotic therapy may be adequate for mild cases. Large abscesses require drainage plus antibiotics x 1-2 weeks post-drainage. With febrile neutropenia, use an antibiotic that is active against both P. aeruginosa and B. fragilis (e.g., meropenem, piperacillin/tazobactam)
Prognosis: Good with early drainage/therapy

Sepsis, Septic Shock, Febrile Neutropenia

Sepsis/Septic Shock

Subset	Usual Pathogens	Preferred IV Therapy	Alternate IV Therapy	IV-to-PO Switch
Unknown source	Entero-bacteriaceae B. fragilis	Meropenem 1 gm (IV) q8h x 2 weeks **or** Piperacillin/ tazobactam 4.5 gm (IV) q8h x 2 weeks **or** Imipenem 500 mg (IV) q6h x 2 weeks **or** Ertapenem 1 gm (IV) q24h x 2 weeks **or combination therapy with** Ceftriaxone 1 gm (IV) q24h x 2 weeks **plus** Metronidazole 1 gm (IV) q24h x 2 weeks	Quinolone* (IV) x 2 weeks **plus either** Metronidazole 1 gm (IV) q24h x 2 weeks **or** Clindamycin 600 mg (IV) q8h x 2 weeks	Moxifloxacin 400 mg (PO) q24h x 2 weeks **or combination therapy with** Clindamycin 300 mg (PO) q8h x 2 weeks **plus either** Ciprofloxacin 500 mg (PO) q12h x 2 weeks **or** Gatifloxacin 400 mg (PO) q24h x 2 weeks **or** Levofloxacin 500 mg (PO) q24h x 2 weeks
	Group D streptococci[†] E. faecalis	Meropenem 1 gm (IV) q8h x 2 weeks **or** Piperacillin/ tazobactam 4.5 gm (IV) q8h x 2 weeks	Ampicillin/sulbactam 3 gm (IV) q6h x 2 weeks **or** Quinolone[‡] (IV) x 2 weeks	Quinolone[‡] (PO) x 2 weeks
	E. faecium (VRE)	Linezolid 600 mg (IV) q12h x 2 weeks	Chloramphenicol 500 mg (IV) q6h x 2 weeks **or** Doxycycline 200 mg (IV) q12h x 3 days, then 100 mg (IV) q12h x 11 days	Linezolid 600 mg (PO) q12h x 2 weeks **or** Doxycycline 100 mg (PO) q12h x 2 weeks

Duration of therapy represents total time IV or IV + PO
* *Ciprofloxacin 400 mg (IV) or 500 mg (PO) q12h or gatifloxacin 400 mg (IV or PO) q24h or levofloxacin 500 mg (IV or PO) q24h*
† *Treat initially for E. faecalis; if later identified as E. faecium (VRE), treat accordingly*
‡ *Ciprofloxacin 400 mg (IV) or 500 mg (PO) q12h or gatifloxacin 400 mg (IV or PO) q24h or levofloxacin 500 mg (IV or PO) q24h or moxifloxacin 400 mg (IV or PO) q24h*

Sepsis/Septic Shock (cont'd)

Subset	Usual Pathogens	Preferred IV Therapy	Alternate IV Therapy	IV-to-PO Switch
Lung source	S. pneumoniae H. influenzae K. pneumoniae	Ceftriaxone 1 gm (IV) q24h x 2 weeks **or** Cefepime 2 gm (IV) q12h x 2 weeks	Quinolone[‡] (IV) q24h x 2 weeks **or** Any 2nd generation cephalosporin (IV) x 2 weeks	Quinolone[‡] (PO) q24h x 2 weeks **or** Doxycycline 200 mg (PO) q12h x 3 days, then 100 mg (PO) q12h x 11 days
IV line sepsis *Bacterial* (Treat initially for MSSA; if later identified as MRSA, treat accordingly)	S. epidermidis S. aureus (MSSA) Klebsiella Enterobacter Serratia	Meropenem 1 gm (IV) q8h x 2 weeks **or** Cefepime 2 gm (IV) q12h x 2 weeks	Ceftriaxone 1 gm (IV) q24h x 2 wks **or** Quinolone* (IV) q24h x 2 weeks	Quinolone* (PO) q24h x 2 weeks **or** Cephalexin 500 mg (PO) q6h x 2 weeks
	S. aureus (MRSA)	Vancomycin 1 gm (IV) q12h x 2 weeks **or** Linezolid 600 mg (IV) q12h x 2 wks	Quinupristin/ dalfopristin 7.5 mg/kg (IV) q8h x 2 weeks	Linezolid 600 mg (PO) q12h x 2 wks **or** minocycline 100 mg (PO) q12h x 2 weeks
Fungal (Treat initially for non-albicans Candida; if later identified as C. albicans, treat accordingly)	Candida albicans	Preferred IV Therapy Fluconazole 800 mg (IV) x 1, then 400 mg (IV) q24h x 2 weeks Alternate IV Therapy Caspofungin 70 mg (IV) x 1 dose, then 50 mg (IV) q24h x 2 weeks **or** Lipid-associated formulation of amphotericin B (p. 297) (IV) q24h x 2 wks **or** Amphotericin B deoxycholate 0.7 mg/kg (IV) q24h x 2 weeks **or** Itraconazole 200 mg (IV) q12h x 2 days, then 200 mg (IV) q24h x 2 weeks		Fluconazole 400 mg (PO) q24h x 2 weeks **or** Itraconazole 200 mg (PO) solution q12h x 2 weeks
	Non-albicans Candida[¶]	Caspofungin **or** lipid amphotericin B **or** amphotericin B deoxycholate (see C. albicans, above) x 2 weeks	Fluconazole **or** itraconazole (see C. albicans, above) **or** voriconazole (see "usual dose," p. 400) x 2 weeks[¶]	Fluconazole (see C. albicans, above) **or** itraconazole 200 mg (PO) solution q24h **or** voriconazole (see "usual dose," p. 400) x 2 weeks[¶]

Duration of therapy represents total time IV or IV + PO

‡ *Ciprofloxacin 400 mg (IV) or 500 mg (PO) q12h or gatifloxacin 400 mg (IV or PO) q24h or levofloxacin 500 mg (IV or PO) q24h or moxifloxacin 400 mg (IV or PO) q24h*

* *Gatifloxacin 400 mg or levofloxacin 500 mg or moxifloxacin 400 mg*

¶ *Best agent depends on infecting species. Fluconazole-susceptibility varies predictably by species. C. glabrata (usually) and C. krusei (almost always) are resistant to fluconazole. C. lusitaniae is often resistant to amphotericin B (deoxycholate and lipid-associated formulations). Others are generally susceptible to all agents*

Sepsis/Septic Shock (cont'd)

Subset	Usual Pathogens	Preferred IV Therapy	Alternate IV Therapy	IV-to-PO Switch
IV line sepsis *Fungal* (cont'd)	Aspergillus	Voriconazole (see "usual dose, p. 400) x 2 weeks **or** Caspofungin 70 mg (IV) x 1 dose, then 50 mg (IV) q24h x 2 weeks **or** Itraconazole 200 mg (IV) q12h x 2 days, then 200 mg (IV) q24h x 2 weeks	Lipid-associated formulation of amphotericin B (p. 297) (IV) q24h x 2 weeks **or** Amphotericin B deoxycholate 1-1.5 mg/kg (IV) q24h x 2 weeks	Voriconazole (see "usual dose," p. 400) x 2 weeks **or** Itraconazole 200 mg (PO) solution q12h x 2 days, then 200 mg (PO) solution q24h x 2 weeks
Intra-abdominal/ pelvic source	Entero-bacteriaceae B. fragilis	Meropenem 1 gm (IV) q8h x 2 weeks **or** Piperacillin/ tazobactam 4.5 gm (IV) q8h x 2 weeks **or** Imipenem 500 mg (IV) q6h x 2 weeks **or** Ertapenem 1 gm (IV) q24h x 2 weeks **or combination therapy with** Ceftriaxone 1 gm (IV) q24h x 2 weeks **plus** Metronidazole 1 gm (IV) q24h x 2 weeks	Quinolone* (IV) x 2 weeks **plus either** Metronidazole 1 gm (IV) q24h x 2 weeks **or** Clindamycin 600 mg (IV) q8h x 2 weeks	Moxifloxacin 400 mg (PO) q24h x 2 weeks **or combination therapy with** Clindamycin 300 mg (PO) q8h x 2 weeks **plus either** Ciprofloxacin 500 mg (PO) q12h x 2 weeks **or** Gatifloxacin 400 mg (PO) q24h x 2 weeks **or** Levofloxacin 500 mg (PO) q24h x 2 weeks
Urosepsis *Gram (–) bacilli*	Entero-bacteriaceae	Ceftriaxone 1 gm (IV) q24h x 1-2 weeks **or** Quinolone (IV)* x 1-2 weeks	Aztreonam 2 gm (IV) q8h x 1-2 weeks **or** Any aminoglycoside (IV) x 1-2 weeks	Quinolone (PO)* x 1-2 weeks
Gram (+) streptococci (Treat initially for E. faecalis; if later identified as VRE, treat accordingly)	Gp. B streptococci E. faecalis	Quinolone (IV)* x 1-2 weeks	Ampicillin 1-2 gm (IV) q4h x 1-2 weeks **or** Vancomycin 1 gm (IV) q12h x 1-2 wks	Amoxicillin 1 gm (PO) q8h x 1-2 weeks **or** Quinolone (PO)* x 1-2 weeks

* Ciprofloxacin 400 mg (IV) or 500 mg (PO) q12h or gatifloxacin 400 mg (IV or PO) q24h or levofloxacin 500 mg (IV or PO) q24h † Loading dose not needed PO if given IV with the same drug

Sepsis/Septic Shock (cont'd)

Subset	Usual Pathogens	Preferred IV Therapy	Alternate IV Therapy	IV-to-PO Switch
Urosepsis *Gram (+) streptococci (cont'd)* (Treat initially for E. faecalis; if later identified as VRE, treat accordingly)	E. faecium (VRE)	Linezolid 600 mg (IV) q12h x 1-2 weeks	Quinupristin/ dalfopristin 7.5 mg/kg (IV) q8h x 1-2 weeks	Linezolid 600 mg (PO) q12h x 1-2 weeks **or** Doxycycline 200 mg (PO) q12h x 3 days, then 100 mg (PO) q12h x 4-11 days
Organism not known	Entero-bacteriaceae Gp. B, D streptococci	Quinolone (IV)* x 2 weeks	Piperacillin/ tazobactam 4.5 gm (IV) q8h x 1-2 weeks	Quinolone (PO)* x 1-2 weeks
Asplenia or hyposplenia	S. pneumoniae H. influenzae N. meningitidis	Ceftriaxone 2 gm (IV) q24h x 2 weeks **or** Quinolone† (IV) q24h x 2 weeks	Cefepime 2 gm (IV) q12h x 2 weeks **or** Cefotaxime 2 gm (IV) q6h x 2 weeks	Quinolone† (PO) q24h x 2 weeks **or** Amoxicillin 1 gm (PO) q8h x 2 weeks
Steroids (high chronic dose)	Candida Aspergillus	Treat the same as for fungal infection (pp. 118-119)		
Miliary TB	M. tuberculosis	Treat the same as pulmonary TB (p. 47) plus steroids x 1-2 wks		
Miliary BCG (disseminated)	Bacille Calmette-Guérin (BCG)	Treat with 4 anti-TB drugs (INH, rifampin, ethambutol, cycloserine) q24h x 6-12 months plus steroids (e.g., prednisolone 40 mg q24h) x 1-2 weeks		
Severe sepsis	Gram-negative or gram-positive bacteria	Appropriate antimicrobial therapy plus surgical decompression/drainage if needed **plus** drotrecogin alpha (Xigris) 24 mcg/kg/hr (IV) x 96 hours		

MSSA/MRSA = methicillin-sensitive/resistant S. aureus. Duration of therapy represents total time IV or IV + PO. Most patients on IV therapy able to take PO meds should be switched to PO therapy after clinical improvement
* Ciprofloxacin 400 mg (IV) or 500 mg (PO) q12h or gatifloxacin 400 mg (IV or PO) q24h or levofloxacin 500 mg (IV or PO) q24h
† Gatifloxacin 400 mg or levofloxacin 500 mg or moxifloxacin 400 mg

Sepsis, Unknown Source

Clinical Presentation: Abrupt onset of high spiking fevers, rigors ± hypotension

Diagnostic Considerations: Diagnosis suggested by high-grade bacteremia (2/4 - 4/4 positive blood cultures) with unexplained hypotension. Rule out pseudosepsis (GI bleed, myocardial infarction, pulmonary embolism, acute pancreatitis, adrenal insufficiency, etc.). Sepsis usually occurs from a GI, GU, or IV source, so coverage is directed against GI and GU pathogens if IV line infection is unlikely

Pitfalls: Most cases of fever/hypotension are *not* due to sepsis. Before the label of "sepsis" is applied to febrile/hypotensive patients, first consider treatable/reversible mimics (see above)

Therapeutic Considerations: Resuscitate shock patients initially with rapid volume replacement, followed by pressors, if needed. Do not give pressors before volume replacement or hypotension may continue/worsen. Use normal saline, plasma expanders, or blood for volume replacement, not D$_5$W. If patient is persistently hypotensive despite volume replacement, consider relative adrenal insufficiency: Obtain a serum cortisol level, then give cortisone 100 mg (IV) q6h x 24-72h; blood pressure will rise promptly if relative adrenal insufficiency is the cause of volume-unresponsive hypotension. Do not add/change antibiotics if patient is persistently hypotensive/febrile; look for GI bleed, myocardial infarction, pulmonary embolism, pancreatitis, undrained abscess, adrenal insufficiency, or IV line infection. Drain abscesses as soon as possible. Remove IV lines if the entry site is red or a central line has been in place for ≥ 7 days and there is no other explanation for fever/hypotension. In addition to antibiotic therapy/surgical drainage, selected patients with severe sepsis may benefit from activated protein C (Xigris); bleeding is the most serious side effect; avoid in patients with active bleeding, drugs/disorders associated with coagulopathies, or thrombocytopenia (platelets < 60,000/mm³)

Prognosis: Related to severity of septic process and underlying cardiopulmonary/immune status

Sepsis, Lung Source

Clinical Presentation: Normal hosts with community-acquired pneumonia (CAP) do not present with sepsis. CAP with sepsis suggests the presence of impaired immunity/hyposplenic function (see "sepsis in hyposplenia/asplenia," below)

Diagnostic Considerations: Impaired splenic function may be inferred by finding Howell-Jolly bodies (small, round, pinkish or bluish inclusion bodies in red blood cells) in the peripheral blood smear. The number of Howell-Jolly bodies is proportional to the degree of splenic dysfunction

Pitfalls: CAP with hypotension/sepsis should suggest hyposplenic function, impaired immunity, or an alternate diagnosis that can mimic CAP/shock. Be sure to exclude acute MI, acute heart failure/COPD, PE/infarction, overzealous diuretic therapy, concomitant GI bleed, and acute pancreatitis

Therapeutic Considerations: Patients with malignancies, myeloma, or SLE are predisposed to CAP, which is not usually severe or associated with shock. Be sure patients with CAP receiving steroids at less than "stress doses" do not have hypotension/shock from relative adrenal insufficiency. In patients with SLE, try to distinguish between lupus pneumonitis and CAP; lupus pneumonitis usually occurs as part of a lupus flare, CAP usually does not

Prognosis: Related to underlying cardiopulmonary/immune status. Early treatment is important

IV Line Sepsis

Clinical Presentation: Temperature ≥ 102°F ± IV site erythema

Diagnostic Considerations: Diagnosis by semi-quantitative catheter tip culture with ≥ 15 colonies plus blood cultures with same pathogen. If no other explanation for fever and line has been in place ≥ 7 days, remove line and obtain semi-quantitative catheter tip culture. Suppurative thrombophlebitis presents with hectic/septic fevers and pus at IV site ± palpable venous cord

Pitfalls: Temperature ≥ 102°F with IV line infection, in contrast to phlebitis

Therapeutic Considerations: Line removal is usually curative, but antibiotic therapy is usually given for 1 week after IV line removal for gram-negative bacilli or 2 weeks after IV line removal for S. aureus (MSSA/MRSA). Antifungal therapy is also usually given for 2 weeks after IV line removal for candidemia. Dilated ophthalmoscopy by an ophthalmologist is important to exclude candidal endophthalmitis following candidemia

Prognosis: Good if line is removed before endocarditis/metastatic spread

Sepsis, Intra-abdominal/Pelvic Source

Clinical Presentation: Fever, peritonitis ± hypotension. Usually a history of an intra-abdominal disorder that predisposes to sepsis (e.g., diverticulosis, gallbladder disease, recent intra-abdominal/pelvic surgery). Signs and symptoms are referable to the abdomen/pelvis

Diagnostic Considerations: Clinical presentation plus imaging studies (e.g., abdominal/pelvic CT or MRI to demonstrate pathology) are diagnostic

Pitfalls: Elderly patients may have little/no fever and may not have rebound tenderness. Be sure to exclude intra-abdominal mimics of sepsis (e.g., GI bleed, pancreatitis)

Therapeutic Considerations: Empiric coverage should be directed against aerobic gram-negative bacilli plus B. fragilis. Anti-enterococcal coverage is not essential. Antibiotic therapy is ineffective unless ruptured viscus is repaired, obstruction is relieved, abscesses are drained
Prognosis: Related to rapidity/adequacy of abscess drainage and repair/lavage of ruptured organs. The preoperative health of the host is also important

Urosepsis
Clinical Presentation: Fever/hypotension in a patient with diabetes mellitus, SLE, myeloma, pre-existing renal disease, stone disease, or partial/total urinary tract obstruction
Diagnostic Considerations: Urine gram stain determines initial empiric coverage. Pyuria is also present. Diagnosis confirmed by culturing the same isolate from urine and blood
Pitfalls: Pyuria without bacteriuria and bacteremia due to same pathogens is not diagnostic of urosepsis. Urosepsis does not occur in normal hosts; look for host defect (e.g., diabetes, renal disease)
Therapeutic Considerations: If stones/obstruction are not present, urosepsis resolves rapidly with appropriate therapy. Delayed/no response suggests infected/obstructed stent, stone, partial/total urinary tract obstruction, or renal abscess
Prognosis: Good if stone/stent removed, obstruction relieved, abscess drained

Sepsis in Hyposplenia/Asplenia
Clinical Presentation: Presents as overwhelming septicemia/shock with petechiae
Diagnostic Considerations: Diagnosis by gram stain of buffy coat of blood or by blood cultures. Organism may be stained/cultured from aspirated petechiae. Howell-Jolly bodies in the peripheral smear are a clue to decreased splenic function. Conditions associated with hyposplenism include sickle cell trait/disease, cirrhosis, rheumatoid arthritis, SLE, systemic necrotizing vasculitis, amyloidosis, celiac disease, chronic active hepatitis, Fanconi's syndrome, IgA deficiency, intestinal lymphangiectasia, intravenous gamma-globulin therapy, myeloproliferative disorders, non-Hodgkin's lymphoma, regional enteritis, ulcerative colitis, Sezary syndrome, splenic infarcts/malignancies, steroid therapy, systemic mastocytosis, thyroiditis, infiltrative diseases of spleen, mechanical compression of splenic artery/spleen, Waldenstrom's macroglobulinemia, hyposplenism of old age, congenital absence of spleen
Pitfalls: Suspect hyposplenia/asplenia in unexplained overwhelming infection
Therapeutic Considerations: In spite of early aggressive antibiotic therapy and supportive care, patients often die within hours from overwhelming infection, especially due to S. pneumoniae
Prognosis: Related to degree of splenic dysfunction

Sepsis in Patients on Chronic High-Dose Steroids (Candida, Aspergillus)
Clinical Presentation: Subacute onset of fever with disseminated infection in multiple organs
Diagnostic Considerations: Diagnosis by positive blood cultures for fungi or demonstration of invasive fungal infection from tissue biopsy specimens. Sepsis is most commonly due to fungemia
Pitfalls: Obtain blood cultures to diagnose fungemias and rule out bacteremias (uncommon)
Therapeutic Considerations: Use itraconazole, caspofungin, amphotericin B deoxycholate, fluconazole, or voriconazole for Candida or Aspergillus
Prognosis: Related to degree of immunosuppression

Miliary (Disseminated) TB (Mycobacterium tuberculosis)
Clinical Presentation: Unexplained, prolonged fevers without localizing signs
Diagnostic Considerations: Diagnosis by AFB on biopsy/culture of liver or bone marrow
Pitfalls: Chest x-ray is negative early in 1/3. Subtle miliary (2 mm) infiltrates on chest x-ray (1-4 weeks)
Therapeutic Considerations: Treated the same as pulmonary TB
Prognosis: Death within weeks without treatment

Miliary (Disseminated) BCG (Bacille Calmette-Guérin)
Clinical Presentation: Fever, circulatory collapse, DIC days to weeks after intravesicular BCG
Diagnostic Considerations: Usually occurs in compromised hosts (e.g., transplants, active TB,

congenital/acquired immunodeficiencies [e.g., HIV], leukemias/lymphomas). Rare in normal hosts
Pitfalls: Avoid intravesicular BCG immediately after traumatic catheterization, bladder biopsy, TURP
Therapeutic Considerations: Treat with 4 anti-TB drugs plus steroids. Do not repeat BCG therapy
Prognosis: Good with early treatment

Febrile Neutropenia

Subset	Usual Pathogens	Preferred IV Therapy	Alternate IV Therapy	IV-to-PO Switch
Febrile leukopenia < 7 days	P. aeruginosa Entero-bacteriaceae S. aureus (MSSA)	Cefepime 2 gm (IV) q8h* **or** Meropenem 1 gm (IV) q8h* **or** Piperacillin/ tazobactam 4.5 gm (IV) q8h*	Amikacin 1 gm (IV) q24h* **plus either** Aztreonam 2 gm (IV) q8h* **or** Quinolone† (IV)*	Ciprofloxacin 750 mg (PO) q12h* **or** Levofloxacin 750 mg (PO) q24h*
> 7 days	Candida Aspergillus	Caspofungin 70 mg (IV) x 1 dose, then 50 mg (IV) q24h* **or** Itraconazole 200 mg (IV) q12h x 2 days, then 200 mg (IV) q24h* **or** If Aspergillus deemed unlikely, Fluconazole 800 mg (IV) x 1, then 400 mg (IV) q24h*	Amphotericin B deoxycholate 1.5 mg/kg (IV) q24h until 1-2 gm given **or** Lipid-associated formulation of amphotericin B (IV) (p. 297) q24h* **or** Voriconazole 6 mg/kg (IV) q12h x 1 day, then 4 mg/kg (IV) q12h*	Itraconazole 200 mg (PO) solution q12h* **or** Voriconazole (see "usual dose," p. 400)* **or** If Aspergillus deemed unlikely, Fluconazole 800 mg (PO) x 1, then 400 mg (PO) q24h*‡

MSSA = methicillin-sensitive S. aureus. Duration of therapy represents total time IV or IV + PO. Most patients on IV therapy able to take PO meds should be switched to PO therapy after clinical improvement
† *Ciprofloxacin 400 mg q12h or gatifloxacin 400 mg q24h or levofloxacin 500 mg q24h or moxifloxacin 400 mg q24h* * *Treat until neutropenia resolves* ‡ *Loading dose is not needed PO if given IV with the same drug*

Clinical Presentation: Incidence of infection rises as PMN counts fall below 1000/mm³
Diagnostic Considerations: Febrile neutropenia < 7 days ± positive blood cultures. After blood cultures are drawn, anti-P. aeruginosa coverage should be initiated. Do not overlook ischiorectal or perirectal abscess as sources of fever
Pitfalls: Suspect fungemia if abrupt rise in temperature occurs after 7 days of appropriate anti-P. aeruginosa antibiotic therapy. Fungemias usually do not occur in first 7 days of neutropenia
Therapeutic Considerations: If a patient is neutropenic for > 2 weeks and develops RUQ/LUQ pain/increased alkaline phosphatase, suspect hepatosplenic candidiasis; confirm diagnosis with abdominal CT/MRI showing mass lesions in liver/spleen and treat as systemic/invasive candidiasis (p. 74). S. aureus is not a common pathogen in neutropenic compromised hosts without central IV lines, and B. fragilis/anaerobes are not usual pathogens in febrile neutropenia. If IV line infection/perirectal abscess are ruled out, consider tumor fever or drug fever before changing antibiotic therapy. If febrile neutropenia persists after 1 week of antibiotic therapy, treat empirically for Aspergillus with amphotericin B deoxycholate, caspofungin, voriconazole, or itraconazole
Prognosis: Related to degree and duration of neutropenia

Infections in Organ Transplants

Infections in Organ Transplants

Subset	Usual Pathogens	Preferred IV Therapy	Alternate IV Therapy	PO Therapy or IV-to-PO Switch
FEVER, SOURCE UNKNOWN				
Bacteremia *Bone marrow transplant (BMT)* *(leukopenic pre-engraftment)* *< 7 days*	P. aeruginosa Entero- bacteriaceae S. aureus (MSSA)	Cefepime 2 gm (IV) q8h* **or** Meropenem 1 gm (IV) q8h* **or** Piperacillin/ tazobactam 4.5 gm (IV) q8h*	Quinolone† (IV) q24h* **plus either** Aztreonam 2 gm (IV) q8h* **or** Amikacin 1 gm (IV) q24h*	Quinolone† (PO) q24h* **or** Ciprofloxacin 750 mg (PO) q12h*
> 7 days	Candida Aspergillus	Caspofungin 70 mg (IV) x 1 dose, then 50 mg (IV) q24h* **or** Itraconazole 200 mg (IV) q12h x 2 days, then 200 mg (IV) q24h*¶ **or** If Aspergillus deemed unlikely, Fluconazole 800 mg (IV) x 1, then 400 mg (IV) q24h*	Lipid-associated formulation of amphotericin B (p. 297) (IV) q24h* **or** Voriconazole 6 mg/kg (IV) q12h x 1 day, then 4 mg/kg (IV) q12h*¶ **or** Amphotericin B deoxycholate 1.5 mg/kg (IV) q24h until 1-2 gm given	Itraconazole 200 mg (PO) solution q12h*¶ **or** Voriconazole (see "usual dose," p. 400)*¶ **or** If Aspergillus deemed unlikely, Fluconazole 800 mg (PO) x 1, then 400 mg (PO) q24h*‡
Solid organ transplant (SOT) (Treat initially for MSSA; if later identified as MRSA, treat accordingly)	S. aureus (MSSA) Entero- bacteriaceae	Meropenem 1 gm (IV) q8h x 2 weeks **or** Ceftriaxone 1 gm (IV) q24h x 2 weeks	Quinolone† (IV) q24h x 2 weeks **or** Cefepime 2 gm (IV) q12h x 2 weeks	Quinolone† (PO) q24h x 2 weeks **or** Cephalexin 500 mg (PO) q6h x 2 weeks
	S. aureus (MRSA)	Linezolid 600 mg (IV) q12h x 2 weeks **or** Vancomycin 1 gm (IV) q12h x 2 weeks	Quinupristin/ dalfopristin 7.5 mg/kg (IV) q8h x 2 weeks	Linezolid 600 mg (PO) q12h x 2 weeks **or** Minocycline 100 mg (PO) q12h x 2 weeks

BMT/SOT = bone marrow/solid organ transplant, MSSA/MRSA = methicillin-sensitive/resistant S. aureus
† *Gatifloxacin 400 mg or levofloxacin 500 mg or moxifloxacin 400 mg*
* *Treat until neutropenia resolves*
‡ *Loading dose is not needed PO if given IV with the same drug*
¶ *Significant drug interactions are possible with usual immunosuppressive agents (e.g., tacrolimus). Review all concomitant medications for potential interactions*

Infections in Organ Transplants (cont'd)

Subset	Usual Pathogens	Preferred IV Therapy	Alternate IV Therapy	PO Therapy or IV-to-PO Switch
Fungemia	C. albicans	Same as for IV line sepsis (p. 118), except use higher dose of fluconazole: 1600 mg (IV) x 1, then 800 mg (IV) q24h x 2 weeks ¶	Same as for IV line sepsis (p. 118) x 2 weeks¶	Same as for IV line sepsis (p. 118), except use higher dose of fluconazole: 1600 mg (PO) x 1, then 800 mg (PO) q24h x 2 weeks‡
	Non-albicans Candida*	Same as for IV line sepsis (p. 118)¶	Same as for IV line sepsis (p. 118), except use higher dose of fluconazole: 1600 mg (IV) x 1, then 800 mg (IV) q24h x 2 weeks¶	Same as for IV line sepsis (p. 118), except use higher dose of fluconazole: 1600 mg (PO) x 1, then 800 mg (PO) q24h x 2 weeks‡¶
	Aspergillus	Voriconazole (see "usual dose, p. 400) x 2 weeks¶ **or** Caspofungin 70 mg (IV) x 1 dose, then 50 mg (IV) q24h x 2 weeks **or** Itraconazole 200 mg (IV) q12h x 2 days, then 200 mg (IV) q24h x 2 weeks¶	Lipid-associated formulation of amphotericin B (p. 297) (IV) q24h x 2 weeks **or** Amphotericin B deoxycholate 1-1.5 mg/kg (IV) q24h x 2 weeks	Voriconazole (see "usual dose," p. 400) x 2 weeks¶ **or** Itraconazole 200 mg (PO) solution q12h x 2 days, then 200 mg (PO) solution q24h x 2 weeks‡¶
CNS SOURCE				
Encephalitis/ meningitis	CMV	<u>Induction therapy</u> Ganciclovir 5 mg/kg (IV) q12h x 2 weeks **plus** CMV immunoglobulin (CMV-IG) 500 mg/kg (IV) q48h x 2 weeks For ganciclovir-induced neutropenia, foscarnet 60 mg/kg (IV) q8h can be substituted for ganciclovir until WBC ↑ to 2500-5000 WBC/mm³. GM-CSF 1-8 mcg/kg (IV) q24h can be given if neutropenia is prolonged/severe <u>Maintenance therapy (following induction therapy)</u> Valganciclovir 900 mg (PO) q24h x 3 months **plus** CMV-IG 100 mg/kg (IV) q48h x 3 months		

‡ *Loading dose is not needed PO if given IV with the same drug*
* *Best agent depends on infecting species. Fluconazole-susceptibility varies predictably by species. C. glabrata (usually) and C. krusei (almost always) are resistant to fluconazole. C. lusitaniae is often resistant to amphotericin B (deoxycholate and lipid-associated formulations). Others are generally susceptible to all agents*
¶ *Significant drug interactions are possible when voriconazole or itraconazole is administered with usual immunosuppressive agents (e.g., tacrolimus). Review all concomitant medications for potential interactions*

Infections in Organ Transplants (cont'd)

Subset	Usual Pathogens	Preferred IV Therapy	Alternate IV Therapy	PO Therapy or IV-to-PO Switch
Encephalitis/ meningitis (cont'd)	CMV, ganciclovir-resistant CMV MIC ≥ 3 mcg/mL (12 mcM)	<u>Induction Therapy:</u> Ganciclovir 5 mg/kg (IV) q24h x 2 weeks **plus** foscarnet 60 mg/kg (IV) q8h x 2 weeks **plus** CMV immunoglobulin (CMV-IG) 500 mg/kg (IV) q48h x 2 weeks <u>Maintenance Therapy (following induction therapy):</u> Ganciclovir 5 mg/kg (IV) q48h x 2 weeks **plus** foscarnet 60 mg/kg (IV) q48h x 2 weeks **with or without** CMV immunoglobulin (CMV-IG) 100 mg/kg (IV) q48h x 3 months		
	Listeria, HSV, C. neoformans, M. tuberculosis treated the same as in normal hosts (pp. 24-25)			
Brain abscess/ mass lesion	Aspergillus	Voriconazole 6 mg/kg (IV) q12h x 1 day, then 4 mg/kg (IV) q12h until cured¶	Lipid-associated formulation of amphotericin B (p. 297) (IV) q24h until cured **or** Caspofungin 70 mg (IV) x 1 dose, then 50 mg (IV) q24h until cured **or** Amphotericin B deoxycholate 1.5 mg/kg (IV) q24h until cured	Voriconazole (see "usual dose," p. 400) until cured¶
	Nocardia	TMP-SMX 5 mg/kg (IV) q6h until clinical improvement, then (PO) until cured	Minocycline 200 mg (IV) q12h until clinical improvement, then (PO) until cured	TMP-SMX 1 DS (PO) q6h **or** minocycline 200 mg (PO) q12h until cured
	T. gondii	<u>Preferred Therapy</u> Sulfadiazine 1.5-2 gm (PO) q6h + pyrimethamine 200 mg (PO) x 1 dose then 50 mg (PO) q6h + folinic acid 10 mg (PO) q24h x 6-8 weeks until CT/MRI clinical response. Follow with sulfadiazine 1 gm (PO) q12h + pyrimethamine 50 mg (PO) q24h + folinic acid 10 mg (PO) q24h until cured <u>Alternate Therapy</u> Clindamycin 600 mg (IV or PO) q6h + pyrimethamine 200 mg (PO) x 1 dose then 50 mg (PO) q6h + folinic acid 10 mg (PO) q24h x 6-8 weeks until CT/MRI clinical response. Follow with sulfadiazine 1 gm (PO) q12h + pyrimethamine 50 mg (PO) q24h + folinic acid 10 mg (PO) q24h until cured		
	C. neoformans	Treat the same as in chronic meningitis (p. 22)		

¶ *Significant drug interactions are possible when voriconazole or itraconazole is administered with usual immunosuppressive agents (e.g., tacrolimus). Review all concomitant medications for potential interactions*

Infections in Organ Transplants (cont'd)

Subset	Usual Pathogens	Preferred IV Therapy	Alternate IV Therapy	PO Therapy or IV-to-PO Switch
		LUNG SOURCE		
Focal/ segmental infiltrates *Acute*	S. pneumoniae Legionella	Treat the same as in normal hosts (pp. 45-46)		
Subacute	Aspergillus	<u>Preferred Therapy</u> Voriconazole 6 mg/kg (IV) q12h x 1 day, then 4 mg/kg (IV) q12h x 1-2 weeks, then 200 mg (PO) q12h until cured*¶ **or** Itraconazole 200 mg (IV) q12h x 2 days, then 200 mg (IV) q24h x 1-2 weeks, then 200 mg (PO) solution q12h until cured¶ **or** Caspofungin 70 mg (IV) x 1 dose, then 50 mg (IV) q24h x 1-2 weeks, then itraconazole 200 mg (PO) solution q12h until cured <u>Alternate Therapy</u> Lipid-associated amphotericin B (p. 297) (IV) q24h until cured **or** Amphotericin B deoxycholate 1 mg/kg (IV) q24h until 2-3 grams		
	M. tuberculosis C. neoformans	For TB, see p. 47. For C. neoformans, see p. 199		
Diffuse infiltrates	S. stercoralis (hyperinfection syndrome)	<u>Preferred Therapy</u> Thiabendazole 25-50 mg/kg (PO) q12h (max. 3 gm/day) until cured <u>Alternate Therapy</u> Ivermectin 200 mcg/kg (PO) q24h until cured		
	P. carinii (PCP) RSV	Treat the same as in other compromised hosts (p. 248)		
	CMV	Treat the same as CMV pneumonia (p. 49)		
		HEPATIC SOURCE		
Viral hepatitis	CMV	Treat the same as for CMV pneumonia (p. 49)		
	HBV, HCV	Treat the same as in normal hosts (p. 75)		

*Duration of therapy represents total time PO, IV, or IV + PO. Most patients on IV therapy able to take PO meds should be switched to PO therapy after clinical improvement * If < 40 kg, use 100 mg (PO) maintenance dose*
¶ Significant drug interactions are possible when voriconazole or itraconazole is administered with usual immunosuppressive agents (e.g., tacrolimus). Review all concomitant medications for potential interactions

Bacteremia
Clinical Presentation: Fever and shaking chills ± localizing signs. If localizing signs are present, the organ involved indicates the origin of the bacteremia (e.g., urinary tract findings suggest urosepsis)
Diagnostic Considerations: Diagnosis is clinical and is confirmed by positive blood cultures
Pitfalls: 3/4 or 4/4 positive blood cultures indicates bacteremia. Even 1/4 positive blood cultures of

an unusual pathogen may be clinically significant in BMT/SOT. The significance of 1/4 blood cultures with coagulase-negative staphylococci is less clear. S. epidermidis bacteremia is usually IV-line related, but in some compromised hosts, it may be pathogenic without an IV line focus

Therapeutic Considerations: In SOT, coverage should be directed against S. aureus (MSSA) and Enterobacteriaceae. Anti-P. aeruginosa coverage is not needed since these patients are not neutropenic. If the source of infection is a central IV line, the line should be removed. In pre-engraftment BMT, coverage should be directed against P. aeruginosa until leukopenia resolves. Continued fever after 1 week of appropriate antibiotic therapy suggests the presence of fungemia

Prognosis: Good with early antibiotic therapy and, if appropriate, IV line removal

Fungemia

Clinical Presentation: Fever and shaking chills ± localizing signs. If localizing signs are present, the organ involved indicates the origin of the fungemia (e.g, reddened central IV line site suggests IV line-related fungemia)

Diagnostic Considerations: Candida and Aspergillus are the commonest fungi associated with fungemia in BMT/SOT. Non-albicans Candida are more commonly cultured from the blood than C. albicans or Aspergillus

Pitfalls: Do not assume that all Candida are C. albicans. Non-albicans Candida are more common in SOT patients. Empiric therapy should be directed against non-albicans Candida pending speciation, which will also cover C. albicans (including fluconazole-resistant strains) and Aspergillus. Because mortality/morbidity associated with fungemia exceeds that of bacteremia, empiric therapy should be started as soon as fungemia is suspected

Prognosis: Related to underlying immune status and promptness of empiric antifungal therapy

Encephalitis/Meningitis

Clinical Presentation: Typical encephalitis/meningitis presentation (fever, headache, stiff neck, change in mental status)

Diagnostic Considerations: CSF usually reveals a lymphocytic predominance with a normal or ↑ CSF lactic acid and low glucose. The diagnosis of HSV/CMV encephalitis can be made by CSF PCR

Pitfalls: Patients with Listeria encephalitis often have a negative CSF Gram stain, but Listeria nearly always grow on CSF culture. HSV/Listeria encephalitis typically have RBCs in the CSF. Head CT/MRI rules out CNS mass lesions and is negative in encephalitis/meningitis

Therapeutic Considerations: CMV encephalitis is rare but treatable, resulting in clinical/radiological improvement. However, neurological deficits usually remain. CMV retinitis, common in HIV (p. 253), is unusual in BMT/SOT

Prognosis: Related to underlying immune status and promptness of therapy

Brain Abscess/Mass Lesions

Clinical Presentation: BMT/SOT patients with brain abscesses/mass lesions present with seizures/cranial nerve abnormalities. Mental status is clear, in contrast to patients with encephalitis, and nuchal rigidity is absent, in contrast to patients with meningitis

Diagnostic Considerations: Head CT/MRI is the preferred diagnostic modality, and brain biopsy is the definitive diagnostic method. CSF analysis is not usually helpful in mass lesions, with the exception of infection due to M. tuberculosis or C. neoformans. With C. neoformans, the CSF cryptococcal antigen test is positive, and the CSF India ink preparation may be positive. With M. tuberculosis, acid fast testing of the CSF is sometimes positive, but culture has a higher yield and PCR is the preferred diagnostic modality

Pitfalls: Patients with brain abscesses/mass lesions should have a head CT/MRI before lumbar puncture. To avoid herniation during lumbar puncture when a mass lesion is present, lumbar puncture should be performed by an experienced operator, and a minimal amount of CSF should be withdrawn

Therapeutic Considerations: M. tuberculosis and C. neoformans are readily treatable. Be sure to use antimicrobial therapy that penetrates into CSF/brain

Prognosis: Related to underlying immune status and promptness of therapy

Lung Focus, Focal or Segmental Pulmonary Infiltrates

Clinical Presentation: Acute or subacute community-acquired pneumonia (CAP) with respiratory symptoms and fever

Diagnostic Considerations: BMT/SOT patients with focal/segmental infiltrates are most commonly infected with the usual CAP pathogens affecting normal hosts (e.g., S. pneumoniae, H. influenzae, Legionella). The clinical presentation of CAP in organ transplants is indistinguishable from that in normal hosts. However, BMT/SOT patients presenting subacutely with focal/segmental infiltrates are usually infected with pulmonary pathogens with a slower clinical onset (e.g., Nocardia, Aspergillus). Empiric therapy will not cover all possible pathogens; tissue biopsy is necessary for definitive diagnosis and specific therapy. Preferred diagnostic modalities include transbronchial lung biopsy, percutaneous thin needle biopsy, or open lung biopsy, not BAL

Pitfalls: Patients presenting with subacute onset of CAP have a different pathogen distribution than those presenting with acute CAP. PCP/CMV does not present with focal/segmental infiltrates

Therapeutic Considerations: BMT/SOT patients with acute onset of CAP are treated with the same antibiotics used to treat CAP in normal hosts. Empiric coverage is directed against both typical and atypical bacterial pathogens. If no improvement in clinical status after 72 hours, proceed to lung biopsy to identify non-bacterial pathogens (e.g., Nocardia, Aspergillus)

Prognosis: Best with acute focal/segmental infiltrates. Not as good with subacute or chronic focal/segmental infiltrates

Lung Focus, Diffuse Pulmonary Infiltrates

Clinical Presentation: Insidious onset of interstitial pneumonia usually accompanied by low-grade fevers. Focal/segmental infiltrates are absent

Diagnostic Considerations: Bilateral diffuse infiltrates, which can be minimal or extensive, fall into two clinical categories: those with and without hypoxemia/↑ A-a gradient. Diffuse pulmonary infiltrates without hypoxemia suggest a noninfectious etiology (e.g., CHF, pulmonary drug reaction, pulmonary hemorrhage). The differential diagnosis of diffuse pulmonary infiltrates with hypoxemia includes PCP, CMV, HSV, RSV, others. For interstitial infiltrates with hypoxemia, the chest x-ray may be only minimally abnormal, but gallium/indium scans reveal intense bilateral, diffuse lung uptake, explaining the apparent discrepancy between clinical status and chest x-ray findings. RSV/HSV may be detected by specific monoclonal antibody tests of respiratory secretions. CMV/PCP require tissue biopsy for definitive diagnosis. A highly elevated LDH suggests the possibility of PCP. Transbronchial biopsy is preferable, but BAL may be used. The incidence of CMV pneumonia is highest in lung transplants. CMV has a predilection for infecting the transplanted organ. (T. gondii myocarditis is the most common opportunistic infection in the transplanted heart)

Pitfalls: Because infections in BMT/SOT are sequential, the majority of patients with PCP pneumonia may have underlying CMV as well. In BMT, CMV found alone on lung biopsy suggests it is the primary pathogen. Serological tests are unhelpful for CMV; a semiquantitative CMV antigenemic assay is preferred. Candida pneumonia does not exist as a separate entity but only as part of disseminated/invasive candidiasis

Therapeutic Considerations: Nocardia and Aspergillus should be treated aggressively until lesions resolve. Among the subacute diffuse pneumonias, PCP is readily treatable. Initiate treatment for CMV pneumonia with ganciclovir IV; after clinical improvement, complete therapy with valganciclovir (PO) until cured. If after treatment, there is an ↑ in CMV antigen levels, treat pre-emptively to prevent CMV pneumonia with valganciclovir 900 mg (PO) q24h until CMV antigen levels return to previous levels. Specific therapy exists for HSV and RSV but not adenovirus or HHV-6/7

Prognosis: Related to underlying immune status, promptness of therapy, and general health of host

Viral Hepatitis

Clinical Presentation: Fever < 102°F with ↑ SGOT/SGPT ± RUQ pain

Diagnostic Considerations: Because CMV is of such critical importance in BMT/SOT, CMV testing should always be done in organ transplants with ↑ SGOT/SGPT. The best test for CMV is semiquantitative CMV antigenemia assay (better than shell vial culture assay). Most patients undergoing organ transplant are immunized for HBV pre-transplant. HCV serology and EBV IgM VCA titers should be ordered. ↑ incidence of HCV in HIV patients. Viral hepatitis is usually accompanied by some degree of leukopenia. A few atypical lymphocytes may be present, and serum transaminases can be mildly or markedly elevated. CMV infectious mono is the commonest manifestation of CMV infection in BMT/SOT patients. CMV has a predilection for infecting the organ transplanted, and CMV hepatitis is particularly common in liver transplants. Anicteric hepatitis is more common than icteric hepatitis.

Pitfalls: The diagnosis of active CMV hepatitis in organ transplant patients is critical because it is an immunomodulating virus, adding to the net immunosuppressive effect of immunosuppressive therapy. Do not rely on CMV IgM/IgG titers for the diagnosis

Therapeutic Considerations: CMV and HCV should be treated aggressively to minimize their potentiating immunoregulatory defects, which may predispose to nonviral opportunistic pathogens. CMV antigen levels increase before CMV infection; therefore, when CMV antigen levels increase, begin early pre-emptive therapy with valganciclovir 900 mg (PO) q24h until CMV antigen levels return to previous levels. There is no treatment for EBV or HDV

Prognosis: Treated early, CMV responds well to therapy. HCV is more difficult to treat. Preserved functional capacity of the liver and early treatment are good prognostic factors. The incidence of hepatoma is increased with HCV (and markedly increased with HCV in HIV patients). Prognosis of HCV is worse with hepatoma

Toxin-Mediated Infectious Diseases

Toxin-Mediated Infectious Diseases

Subset	Usual Pathogens	IV Therapy	PO/IM Therapy or IV-to-PO Switch
Toxic shock syndrome (TSS)* (Treat initially for MSSA; if later identified as MRSA , treat accordingly)	S. aureus (MSSA)	<u>Preferred IV Therapy</u> Cefazolin 1 gm (IV) q8h x 2 weeks <u>Alternate IV Therapy</u> Nafcillin 2 gm (IV) q4h x 2 weeks **or** Clindamycin 600 mg (IV) q8h x 2 weeks	Cephalexin 500 mg (PO) q6h x 2 weeks **or** Clindamycin 300 mg (PO) q6h x 2 weeks
	S. aureus (MRSA)	<u>Preferred IV Therapy</u> Vancomycin 1 gm (IV) q12h x 2 weeks **or** Linezolid 600 mg (IV) q12h x 2 weeks <u>Alternate IV Therapy</u> Minocycline 100 mg (IV) q12h x 2 weeks **or** Quinupristin/dalfopristin 7.5 mg/kg (IV) q8h x 2 weeks	Linezolid 600 mg (PO) q12h x 2 weeks **or** Minocycline 100 mg (PO) q12h x 2 weeks

MSSA/MRSA = methicillin-sensitive/resistant S. aureus. Duration of therapy represents total time IV, PO, or IV + PO. Most patients on IV therapy able to take PO meds should be switched to PO therapy after clinical improvement
*   Treat only IV or IV-to-PO switch

Toxin-Mediated Infectious Diseases (cont'd)

Subset	Usual Pathogens	IV Therapy	PO/IM Therapy or IV-to-PO Switch
Botulism (food, infant, wound)	Clostridium botulinum	<u>Preferred Therapy</u> 2 vials of type-specific trivalent (types A,B,E) or polyvalent (types A,B,C,D,E) antitoxin (IV)	<u>Alternate Therapy</u> Amoxicillin 1 gm (PO) q8h x 7 days (wound botulism only)
Tetanus	Clostridium tetani	<u>Preferred Therapy</u> Tetanus immune globulin (TIG) antitoxin 3000-10,000 units (IM) (50% into deltoid, 50% into wound site) **plus either** Penicillin G 4 mu (IV) q4h x 10 days **or** Doxycycline 200 mg (IV or PO) q12h x 3 days, then 100 mg (IV or PO) x 7 days	<u>Alternate Therapy</u> Tetanus immune globulin (TIG) antitoxin 3000-10,000 units (IM) (50% into deltoid, 50% into wound site) **plus** Metronidazole 1 gm (IV) q12h x 10 days
Diphtheria (pharyngeal, nasal, wound)	Coryne-bacterium diphtheriae	Diphtheria antitoxin (IV) over 1 hour (pharyngeal diphtheria = 40,000 units; nasopharyngeal diphtheria = 60,000 units; systemic diphtheria or diphtheria > 3 days duration = 100,000 units) **plus either** Penicillin G 1 mu (IV) q4h x 14 days **or** Erythromycin 500 mg (IV) q6h x 14 days	Diphtheria antitoxin (IV) over 1 hour (pharyngeal diphtheria = 40,000 units; nasopharyngeal diphtheria = 60,000 units; systemic diphtheria or diphtheria > 3 days duration = 100,000 units) **plus** Procaine penicillin 600,000 units (IM) q24h x 14 days

Duration of therapy represents total time IV, PO, or IV + PO. Most patients on IV therapy able to take PO meds should be switched to PO therapy after clinical improvement

Toxic Shock Syndrome (S. aureus)

Clinical Presentation: Scarlatiniform rash ± hypotension. Spectrum ranges from minimal infection to multiorgan system failure/shock. ↑ CPK common

Diagnostic Considerations: Diagnosis by clinical presentation with mucous membrane, renal, liver, and skin involvement/culture of TSS-1 toxin-producing strain of S. aureus from mouth, nares, vagina, or wound

Pitfalls: Toxic shock syndrome wound discharge is clear, not purulent

Therapeutic Considerations: Remove source of toxin production if possible (e.g., remove tampon, drain collections). Support organ dysfunction until recovery

Prognosis: Good in early/mild form. Poor in late/multisystem disease form

Botulism (Clostridium botulinum)

Clinical Presentation: Descending symmetrical paralysis beginning with cranial nerve involvement, induced by botulinum toxin. Onset begins with blurry vision, followed rapidly by ocular muscle paralysis, difficulty speaking, and inability to swallow. Respiratory paralysis may occur in severe cases. Mental status is unaffected. Usual incubation period is 10-12 hours. Incubation is shortest for Type E strain (hours), longest for Type A strain (up to 10 days), and is inversely proportional to the quantity of toxin consumed (food botulism). Wound botulism (Types A or B) may follow C. botulinum entry into IV drug abuser injection site, surgical or traumatic wounds. Infant (< 1 year) botulism (most commonly Type A or B) is acquired from C. botulinum containing honey. Patients with botulism are afebrile, and have profuse vomiting without diarrhea

Diagnostic Considerations: Detection of botulinum toxin from stool, serum, or food (especially home canned foods with neutral or near neutral pH [~ 7] or smoked fish [Type E]) is diagnostic of food botulism. Wound botulism is diagnosed by culturing C. botulinum from the wound or by detecting botulinum toxin in the serum

Pitfalls: Clinical diagnosis based on descending paralysis with cranial nerve involvement in an afebrile patient must be differentiated from Guillain-Barre (fever, ascending paralysis, sensory component) and polio (fever, pure ascending motor paralysis). Do not diagnose botulism in the absence of ocular/pharyngeal paralysis

Therapeutic Considerations: Antitoxin neutralizes only unbound toxin, and does not reverse toxin-induced paralysis. Botulism is a toxin-mediated infection and antibiotic therapy (wound botulism) is adjunctive. Guanidine has been used with variable effect. Ventilator support is needed for respiratory paralysis. Bioterrorist botulism presents clinically and is treated the same as naturally-acquired botulism

Prognosis: Good if treated early, before respiratory paralysis

Tetanus (Clostridium tetani)

Clinical Presentation: Begins with jaw stiffness/difficulty chewing induced by C. tetani toxin (tetanospasmin). Trismus rapidly follows with masseter muscle spasm, followed by spasm of the abdominal/back muscles. Rigidity and convulsions may occur. Patients are afebrile unless there is hypothalamic involvement (central fever), in which case fevers may exceed 106°F. Usual incubation period is 3-21 days

Diagnostic Considerations: Diagnosis suggested by muscle spasms/rigidity in a patient with trismus

Pitfalls: In rabies, muscle spasms are localized and usually involve the face/neck, rather than primary involvement of the extremities, as in tetanus

Therapeutic Considerations: Tetanus is self-limited with intensive supportive care. Sedation is important, and avoidance of all stimuli is mandatory to reduce the risk of convulsions. Avoid unnecessary handling/movement of patient. Antitoxin is effective only in neutralizing unbound toxin. Tracheostomy/respiratory support can be lifesaving in severe cases

Prognosis: Good if not complicated by spinal fractures, aspiration pneumonia, or CNS involvement (hyperpyrexia, hyper/hypotension)

Diphtheria (Corynebacterium diphtheriae)

Clinical Presentation: Within 1 week following insidious onset of sore throat without fever, pharyngeal patches coalesce to form a gray diphtheric membrane (surrounded by a red border), which is adherent/bleeds easily when removed. Membrane begins unilaterally; may extend to the soft palate, uvula and contralateral posterior pharynx; are accompanied by prominent bilateral anterior adenopathy; become necrotic (green/black); and have a foul odor (fetor oris). Submandibular edema ("bull neck") and hoarseness (laryngeal stridor) precede respiratory obstruction/death. Cutaneous diphtheria may follow C. diphtheriae contaminated wounds (traumatic, surgical) or insect/human bites, and is characterized by a leathery eschar (cutaneous membrane) covering a deep punched out ulcer. Serosanguineous discharge is typical of nasal diphtheria (membrane in nares). Diphtheric myocarditis may complicate any form of diphtheria (most commonly follows pharyngeal form), and usually occurs in the second week, but may occur up to 8 weeks after infection begins. Diphtheric polyneuritis is a common complication. Cardiac/neurologic complications are due to elaboration of a potent toxin

Diagnostic Considerations: Diagnosis is suggested by unilateral membranous pharyngitis/palatal paralysis, absence of fever, and relative tachycardia. Diagnosis is confirmed by culture of C. diphtheriae from nares, membrane, or wound

Pitfalls: Differentiated from Arcanobacterium (Corynebacterium) haemolyticum (which also forms a pharyngeal membrane) by culture and absence of scarletiniform rash with C. diphtheriae

Therapeutic Considerations: Antibiotic therapy treats the infection and stops additional toxin production. Antitoxin is effective against unbound toxin, but will not reverse toxin-mediated myocarditis/neuropathy. Serum sickness is common 2 weeks after antitoxin. Respiratory/cardiac support may be lifesaving

Prognosis: Poor with airway obstruction or myocarditis. Myocarditis may occur despite early treatment

Bioterrorist Agents

Bioterrorist Agents in Adults¶

Subset	Pathogen	IV/IM Therapy	IV-to-PO Switch
Anthrax *Inhalation*	Bacillus anthracis	Doxycycline 200 mg (IV) q12h x 3 days, then 100 mg (IV) q12h x 11 days‡ **or** Penicillin G 4 MU (IV) q4h x 2 weeks **or** Quinolone* (IV) x 2 weeks	Doxycycline 100 mg (PO) q12h x 2 weeks **or** Amoxicillin 1 gm (PO) q8h x 2 weeks **or** Quinolone* (PO) x 2 weeks
Cutaneous		Not applicable	Treat using the same (PO) antibiotics as for inhalation anthrax x 1 week
Tularemia pneumonia	Francisella tularensis	Streptomycin 1 gm (IM) q12h x 2 weeks **or** Gentamicin 5 mg/kg (IM or IV) q24h x 2 weeks **or** Doxycycline 200 mg (IV) q12h x 3 days, then 100 mg (IV) q12h x 7 days‡ **or** Chloramphenicol 500 mg (IV) q6h x 10 days **or** Quinolone* (IV) x 2 weeks	Doxycycline 100 mg (PO) q12h x 10 days **or** Chloramphenicol 500 mg (PO) q6h x 10 days **or** Quinolone* (PO) x 2 weeks

Duration of therapy represents total treatment time. Most patients on IV therapy able to take PO meds should be switched to PO therapy after clinical improvement

‡ *Patients who remain critically ill after doxycycline 200 mg (IV) q12h x 3 days should continue receiving 200 mg (IV) q12h for the full course of therapy. For patients who have improved after 3 days, the dose may be decreased to 100 mg (IV or PO) q12h to complete the course of therapy*

* *Ciprofloxacin 400 mg (IV) q12h or 500 mg (PO) q12h or levofloxacin 500 mg (IV or PO) q24h or gatifloxacin 400 mg (IV or PO) q24h*

¶ *Additional information can be obtained at www.bt.cdc.gov. For post-exposure prophylaxis, see p. 277*

Bioterrorist Agents in Adults (cont'd)¶

Subset	Pathogen	IV/IM Therapy
Pneumonic plague	Yersinia pestis	Treat the same as tularemic pneumonia
Botulism	Clostridium botulinum	2 vials of type-specific trivalent (types A,B,E) or polyvalent (types A,B,C,D,E) antitoxin (IV). Antibiotics do not neutralize toxin
Smallpox	Variola virus	Smallpox vaccine ≤ 4 days after exposure
Ebola	Ebola virus	No specific therapy. Supportive therapy can be life saving

¶ Additional information can be obtained at www.bt.cdc.gov. For post-exposure prophylaxis, see p. 277

Anthrax (B. anthracis)

Clinical Presentation: Bioterrorist anthrax usually presents as cutaneous or inhalational anthrax. Cutaneous anthrax has the same clinical presentation as naturally-acquired anthrax: Lesions begin as painless, sometimes mildly pruritic papules, usually on the upper extremities, neck, or face, and evolve into a vesicular lesion which may be surrounded by satellite lesions. A "gelatinous halo" surrounds the vesicle as it evolves into an ulcer, and a black eschar eventually develops over the ulcer. Inhalational anthrax is a biphasic illness. Initially, there is a viral illness-like prodrome with fever, chills, and myalgias with chest discomfort 3-5 days after inhaling anthrax spores. Bacteremia is common. Patients often improve somewhat over the next 1-2 days, only to rapidly deteriorate and become critically ill with high fevers, dyspnea, cyanosis, crushing substernal chest pain, and shock

Diagnostic Considerations: Cutaneous anthrax is a clinical diagnosis suggested by the lack of pain relative to the size of the lesion. A presumptive microbiologic diagnosis is made by finding gram-positive bacilli in the fluid from the gelatinous halo surrounding the ulcer or from under the eschar. Blood cultures may reveal B. anthracis. Definitive diagnosis depends on identifying B. anthracis from culture of the skin lesions or blood cultures. Inhalation anthrax is suspected in patients with fevers, chest pain, and mediastinal widening accompanied by bilateral pleural effusions on chest x-ray. If chest x-ray findings are equivocal, then a chest CT/MRI is recommended to demonstrate mediastinal lymph node enlargement. Inhalational anthrax presents as a hemorrhagic mediastinitis, not community-acquired pneumonia. The diagnosis is clinical but supported by Gram stain of hemorrhagic pleural fluid demonstrating gram-positive bacilli. Patients with inhalation anthrax often have positive blood cultures and may have associated anthrax meningitis. If meningitis is present, the CSF is hemorrhagic and CSF Gram stain shows gram-positive bacilli, which, when cultured, is B. anthracis

Pitfalls: Cutaneous anthrax is most often initially confused with ringworm or a brown recluse spider bite. Subacute/chronic lesions may initially resemble ringworm, but the skin lesion in ringworm has an annular configuration, is painless, and is accompanied by prominent pruritis, particularly at the edges of the lesion. Patients with ringworm have no fever or systemic symptoms. Brown recluse spider bites produce extremely painful lesions with irregular edges, which eventually develop a necrotic center followed by eschar formation. The lesions of the brown recluse spider bite are irregular, not accompanied by fever, and intensely painful. In contrast, cutaneous anthrax lesions are painless, round, and are not primarily pruritic in nature. Be alert to the possibility of smallpox following outbreaks of other bioterrorist agents such as anthrax, as the genome of smallpox is easily modified and can be incorporated into bacteria

Therapeutic Considerations: B. anthracis is highly susceptible to nearly all antibiotics; in the U.S. bioterrorist experience, no strains were resistant to antibiotics. Traditionally, penicillin has been used to treat natural anthrax, but because of concern for resistant bioterrorist strains, doxycycline or quinolones are preferred. There is no need for double therapy or synergy for susceptible strains. However, clindamycin, which by itself is active against B. anthracis, has been used in combination with other agents because of its potential anti-exotoxin activity. Although the 2001 inhalational anthrax experience was limited to a few patients, some patients seemed to respond somewhat better when clindamycin 600 mg (IV) q8h or 300 mg (PO) q8h plus rifampin 300 mg (PO) q12h was added to either a quinolone or doxycycline

Prognosis: Prognosis of cutaneous anthrax is uniformly good. With inhalational anthrax, prognosis is related to the inhaled dose of the organism, underlying host status, and rapidity of initiating antimicrobial therapy. Inhalational anthrax remains a highly lethal infectious disease, but with early intervention/supportive care, some patients survive. Patients with associated anthrax meningitis have a poor prognosis

Tularemic Pneumonia (F. tularensis)

Clinical Presentation: Fever, chills, myalgias, headache, dyspnea and a nonproductive cough may occur, but encephalopathy is absent. Chest x-ray resembles other causes of community-acquired pneumonia, but tularemic pneumonia is usually accompanied by hilar adenopathy and pleural effusion, which is serosanguineous or frankly bloody. Cavitation sometimes occurs. Relative bradycardia is not present and serum transaminases are not elevated

Diagnostic Considerations: Tularemic pneumonia can resemble other atypical pneumonias, but in a patient presenting with community-acquired pneumonia, the presence of hilar adenopathy with pleural effusions should suggest the diagnosis. F. tularensis may be seen in the Gram stain of the sputum or bloody pleural effusion fluid as a small, bipolar staining, gram-negative bacillus. Diagnosis is confirmed serologically or by culture of the organism from respiratory fluid/blood

Pitfalls: Gram-negative bacilli in the sputum may resemble Y. pestis but are not bipolar staining. Chest x-ray may resemble inhalational anthrax (hilar adenopathy/mediastinal widening). Both tularemic pneumonia and inhalational anthrax may be accompanied by bloody pleural effusions. In contrast to inhalational anthrax (which may be accompanied by anthrax meningitis), CNS involvement is not a feature of tularemic pneumonia

Therapeutic Considerations: Streptomycin is the antibiotic traditionally used to treat tularemia. Gentamicin may be substituted for streptomycin if it is not available. Doxycycline, chloramphenicol, or a quinolone are also effective

Prognosis: Depends on inoculum size and health of host. Mortality rates for severe untreated infection can be as high as 30%, although early treatment is associated with mortality rates < 1%

Pneumonic Plague (Y. pestis)

Clinical Presentation: Bioterrorist plague presents as pneumonic plague and has the potential for person-to-person spread. After an incubation period of 1-4 days, the patient presents with acute onset of fever, chills, headache, myalgias and dizziness, followed by pulmonary manifestations including cough, chest pain, dyspnea. Hemoptysis may occur, and increasing respiratory distress and circulatory collapse are common. Compared to community-acquired pneumonia, patients presenting with plague pneumonia are critically ill. Sputum is pink and frothy and contains abundant bipolar staining gram-negative bacilli. Chest x-ray is not diagnostic

Diagnostic Considerations: Yersinia pestis may be demonstrated in sputum Gram stain (bipolar staining gram-negative bacilli) and may be recovered from blood cultures. Laboratory confirmation requires isolation of Y. pestis from body fluid or tissue culture. Consider the diagnosis in any critically ill patient with pneumonia and bipolar staining gram-negative bacilli in the sputum

Pitfalls: Plague pneumonia can resemble tularemic pneumonia, but there are several distinguishing features. Unlike plague, tularemic pneumonia is usually associated with hilar enlargement and pleural effusion. Although gram-negative bacilli may be present in the sputum of patients with tularemia, the organisms are not bipolar staining

Therapeutic Considerations: Streptomycin is the preferred drug for pneumonic plague. Doxycycline or a quinolone is also effective

Prognosis: Depends on inoculum size, health of the host, and the rapidity of treatment. Left untreated, mortality rates exceed 50%. ARDS, DIC, and other manifestations of gram-negative sepsis are more common when treatment is delayed

Botulism (C. botulinum) (see p. 131)

Smallpox

Clinical Presentation: After an incubation period of 1-12 days, typical smallpox is heralded by high fever, headache, and gastrointestinal complaints (vomiting, colicky pain). No rash is present at this time. After 1-2 days, the fever decreases to near normal level, and macules begin to appear on the head, usually at the hairline. Macules progress to papules, then vesicles, then finally pustules. The rash begins on the face/head and rapidly spreads to the extremities with relative sparing of the trunk. The mucous membranes of the oropharynx and upper/lower airways are also affected early. Lesions initially are umbilicated, then later lose their umbilication. The fully formed smallpox pustule is located deep in the dermis. The appearance of the pustules is accompanied by recrudescence of fever. Hemorrhagic smallpox is a fulminant form of smallpox that begins with petechial lesions in a "swimming trunk" distribution and results in widespread hemorrhage into the skin and mucous membranes. Patients look toxemic and have high fevers with no other signs of smallpox; death from toxemia often occurs before the typical rash appears

Diagnostic Considerations: Smallpox is most likely to be confused with chickenpox or drug eruptions. Patients with chickenpox are less toxemic and the lesion distribution is different from smallpox. Chickenpox lesions occur in crops for the first 72 hours, then stop. The lesions of chickenpox are superficial, not deep in the dermis like smallpox, and chickenpox vesicles are predominantly centripetal rather than centrifugal. The chickenpox vesicle has been described as a "dewdrop on a rose petal" because of its fragility and superficial location on the skin. If there is any doubt, a Tzanck test should be performed by unroofing the vesicle, scraping cells from the base of the vesicle, and staining the cells. A positive Tzanck test indicates chickenpox, not smallpox. Alternatively, a monoclonal VZV test can be performed on vesicle base cells. Drug eruptions are not accompanied by toxemia and are usually accompanied by relative bradycardia if fever is present

Pitfalls: Smallpox is easily missed before the rash and is difficult to diagnose. Look for the combination of high fever/headache with gastrointestinal symptoms (e.g., abdominal pain) that precedes the rash. GI complaints may be confused with appendicitis. A petechial rash in a swimming trunk distribution does not occur with any other infectious disease and should immediately suggest smallpox

Therapeutic Considerations: Smallpox vaccination should be initiated as soon as the diagnosis is suspected. Smallpox vaccine may be given at full strength or in a 1:5 dilution, which is also protective. In the future, chemoprophylaxis with oral HDP cidofovir may prove useful

Prognosis: Variable in typical smallpox, with deep, permanent scarring, especially on the face. Hemorrhagic smallpox is highly lethal

Ebola Virus

Clinical Presentation: After an incubation period of 3-9 days, there is abrupt onset of high fevers, severe headache/myalgias followed by diarrhea, extreme malaise, decreased sensorium, and a nonpruritic maculopapular rash on the face and neck that spreads to the extremities. Hemorrhagic phenomenon–GI, renal, vaginal, conjunctival bleeding–occur at 5-7 days. Patients rapidly become critically ill. Fever is usually accompanied by relative bradycardia, and patients usually have leukopenia, thrombocytopenia, and hepatic/renal dysfunction. Conjunctival suffusion is also an early finding in half the cases. If a patient is not a traveler from an endemic area (e.g., Africa), suspect bioterrorist Ebola

Diagnostic Considerations: Ebola is a hemorrhagic fever clinically indistinguishable from Yellow fever and other African hemorrhagic fevers (e.g., Lassa fever, Marburg virus disease). Presumptive diagnosis is clinical; definitive diagnosis is confirmed by specific virologic/serologic studies

Pitfalls: Patients with Ebola may complain initially of a sore throat and dry cough, with or without chest pain. Diarrhea/abdominal pain is not uncommon. The rash is maculopapular before it becomes hemorrhagic. Failure to consider the diagnosis may occur early when sore throat/GI symptoms are prominent (i.e., before hemorrhagic manifestations appear)

Therapeutic Considerations: There is no specific therapy available for Ebola infection. Supportive therapy can be life saving

Prognosis: Varies with severity of infection and health of the host

REFERENCES AND SUGGESTED READINGS

Adimora AA. Treatment of uncomplicated genital chlamydia trachomatis infections in adults. Clin Infect Dis 35 (Suppl 2):S183-6, 2002.

Allos BM. Campylobacter jejuni Infections: update on emerging issues and trends. Clin Infect Dis 32:1201-6, 2001.

Arathoon EG, Gotuzzo E, Noriega LM, et al. Randomized, double-blind, multicenter study of caspofungin versus amphotericin B for treatment of oropharyngeal and esophageal candidiases. Antimicrob Agents Chemother 46:451-7, 2002.

Arikan S, Lozano-Chiu M, Paetznick V, et al. In vitro synergy of caspofungin and amphotericin B against Aspergillus and Fusarium spp. Antimicrob Agents Chemother 46:245-7, 2002.

Ascioglu S, Rex JH, DePauw B, Bennett JE, et al. Defending opportunistic invasive fungal infections in immunocompromised patients with cancer: An international consensus. Clin Infect Dis 34:7-14, 2002.

Aubry A, Chosidow O, Caumes E, et al. Sixty-three cases of Mycobacterium marinum infection: clinical features, treatment, and antibiotic susceptibility of causative isolates. Arch Intern Med 162:1746-52, 2002.

Augenbraun MH. Treatment of syphilis 2002: nonpregnant adults. Clin Infect Dis 35 (Suppl 2):187-90, 2002.

Baddour LM, Bettmann MA, Bolger AF, et al. Nonvascular cardiovascular device-related infections. Circulation 108:2015-2031, 2003.

Bartlett JG. Antibiotic-associated diarrhea. N Engl J Med 346:334-339, 2002.

Bartlett JG, Inglesby TV Jr, Borio L. Management of anthrax. Clin Infect Dis 35:851-858, 2002.

Bisno AL. Acute pharyngitis. N Engl J Med 344:205-212, 2001.

Breman JG, Henderson DA. Diagnosis and management of smallpox. N Engl J Med 346:1300-1308, 2002.

Bryskier A. Bacillus anthracis and antibacterial agents. Clin Microbiol Infect 8:467-478, 2002.

Castiglioni B, Sutton DA, Rinaldi MG, et al. Pseudallescheria boydii (Anamorph Scedosporium apiospermum). Infection in solid organ transplant recipients in a tertiary medical center and review of the literature. Medicine (Baltimore). 81:333-48, 2002.

Cavusoglu C, Cicek-Saydam C, Darasu Z, et al. Mycobacterium tuberculosis infection and laboratory diagnosis in solid-organ transplant recipients. Clin Transplant 16:88, 2002.

Chastre J, Wolff M, Fagon JY, et al. Comparison of 8 vs 15 days of antibiotic therapy for ventilator-associated pneumonia in adults. JAMA 290:2588-2598, 2003.

Chen XM, Leithly JS, Paya CV, et al. Cryptosporidiosis. N Engl J Med 346:1723-1731, 2002.

Chocarro Martinez A, Gonzalez A, Garcia I. Caspofungin versus amphotericin B for the treatment of Candidal esophagitis. Clin Infect Dis 35:107-108, 2002.

Conti DJ, Rubin RH. Infections of the central nervous system in organ transplant recipients. Neurol Clin North Am 6:241-260, 1988.

Croft SL, Yardley V. Chemotherapy of leishmaniasis. Curr Pharm Des. 8:319-42, 2002.

Cunha BA. The use of meropenem in critical care. Antibiotics for Clinicians 4:59-66, 2000.

Cunha BA. Central nervous system infections in the compromised host. A diagnostic approach. Infect Dis Clin 15:67-590, 2001.

Cunha BA. Pulmonary infection in the compromised host. Infect Dis Clin 16:591-612, 2001.

Cunha BA. Effective antibiotic resistance and control strategies. Lancet 357:1307-1308, 2001.

Cunha BA. Nosocomial pneumonia: Diagnostic and therapeutic considerations. Medical Clinics of North America 85:79-114, 2001.

Cunha BA. Community acquired pneumonia: diagnostic and therapeutic considerations. Medical Clinics of North America 85:43-77, 2001.

Cunha BA. Antimicrobial selection in the penicillin allergic patient. Drugs for Today 37:337-383, 2001

Cunha BA. Clinical relevance of penicillin-resistant Streptococcus pneumoniae. Semin Respir Infect 17:204-14, 2002.

Cunha BA. Strategies to control antibiotic resistance. Semin Respir Infect 17:250-8, 2002.

Cunha BA. Bioterrorist anthrax: a clinician's perspective (part II). Infectious Disease Practice 26:81-85, 2002.

Cunha BA. Smallpox: An Oslerian primer. Infectious Disease Practice 26:141-148, 2002.

Cunha BA. Strategies to control the emergence of resistant organisms. Semin Respir Infect 17:250-258, 2002.

Cunha BA. Osteomyelitis in the elderly. Clin Infect Dis 35:287-273, 2002.

Cunha BA. Community-acquired pneumonias re-revisited. Am J Med 108:436-437, 2000.

Cunha BA. Pseudomonas aeruginosa: Resistance and therapy. Semin Respir Infect 17:231-9, 2002.

Cunha BA. Pneumonias in the comprised host. Infect Dis Clin 15:591-612, 2001.

Cunha BA. Bioterrorism in the emergency room: Anthrax, tularemia, plague, ebola and smallpox. Clinical Microbiology & Infection 8:489-503, 2002.

Darling RG, Catlett CL, Huebner KD, et al. Threats in bioterrorism. I. CDC category A agents. Emerg Med Clin North Am 20:273-309, 2002.

Davis GL. Combination treatment with interferon and ribavirin for chronic hepatitis C. Clin Liver Dis 1:811-26, 1999.

Demirturk N, Usluer G, Ozgunes I, et al. Comparison of different treatment combinations for chronic hepatitis B infection. J Chemother 14:285-9, 2002.

DiBisceglie AM. Combination therapy for hepatitis B. Gut 50:443-5, 2002.

Dill SR, Cobbs CG, McDonald CK. Subdural empyema: analysis of 32 cases and review. Clin Infect Dis 20:372-86, 1995.

Duff P. Antibiotic selection in obstetrics: making cost-effective choices. Clin Obstet Gynecol 45:59-72, 2002.

Emery VC. Human herpes virus 6 and 7 in solid organ transplant recipients. Clin Infect Dis 32:1357-1360, 2001.

Fihn SD. Acute uncomplicated urinary tract infection in women. N Engl J Med 349:259-66, 2003.

File TM Jr. Community-acquired pneumonia. Lancet 362:1991-2001, 2003.

Frieden TR, Sterling TR, Munsiff SS, et al. Tuberculosis. Lancet 362:887-99, 2003.

Frothingham R. Lipid formulations of amphotericin B for empirical treatment of fever and neutropenia. Clin Infect Dis 35:896-7, 2002.

Gerding DN, Johnson S, Peterson LR, et al. Clostridium difficile-associated diarrhea and colitis. Infect Control Hosp Epidemiol 16:459-77, 1995.

Gnann JW, Whitley ARJ. Herpes zoster. N Engl J Med 347:340-346, 2002.

Goh KL. Update on the management of Helicobacter pylori infection, including drug-resistant organisms. J Gastroenterol Hepatol 17:482-7, 2002.

Graninger W, Assadian O, Lagler H, et al. The role of glycopeptides in the treatment of intravascular catheter-related infections. Clin Microbiol Infect 8:310-5, 2002.

Grunow R, Finke EJ. A procedure for differentiating between the intentional release of biological warfare agents and natural outbreaks of disease: its use in analyzing the tularemia outbreak in Kosovo in 1999 and 2000. Clin Microbiol Infect 8:510-521, 2002.

Hall WA, Mattinez AJ, Dummer JS, et al. Central nervous system infections in heart and heart-lung transplant recipients. Arch Neurol 46:173-177, 1989.

Hanekom WA, Yogev R. Cerebrospinal fluid shunt infections. Adv Pediatr Infect Dis 11:29-54, 1996.

Heldman AW, Hartert TV, Ray SC, et al. Oral antibiotic treatment of right-sided staphylococcal endocarditis in injection drug users: prospective randomized comparison with parenteral therapy. Am J Med 101:68-76, 1996.

Heffelfinger JD, Dowell SF, Jorgensen JH, et al. Management of community-acquired pneumonia in the era of pneumococcal resistance: a report from the Drug-Resistant Streptococcus pneumoniae Therapeutic Working Group. Arch Intern Med 160:1399-408, 2000.

Hemsel DL, Ledger WJ, Martens M, et al. Concerns regarding the Centers for Disease Control's published guidelines for pelvic inflammatory disease. Clin Infect Dis 32:103-7, 2001.

Hemsel DL, Little BB, Faro S, et al. Comparison of three regimens recommended by the Centers for Disease Control and Prevention for the treatment of women hospitalized with acute pelvic inflammatory disease. Clin Infect Dis 19:720-7, 1994.

Hooper DC, Pruitt AA, Rubin RH. Central nervous system infections in the chronically immunosuppressed. Medicine (Baltimore) 61:166-188, 1982.

Hotchkiss RS, Karl IE. The pathophysiology and treatment of sepsis. N Engl J Med 348:138-50, 2003.

Inglesby TV, Henderson DA, Bartlett JG, et al. Anthrax as a biological weapon: medical and public health management. Working Group on Civilian Biodefense. JAMA 281:1735-45, 1999.

Johnson DH, Cunha BA. Infections in alcoholic cirrhosis. Infectious Disease Clinics 15:1-32, 2001.

Joseph SM, Peiris MD, D. Phil et al. The severe acute respiratory syndrome. N Engl J Med 349:2431-41, 2003.

Kaplan EL, Gooch III UM, Notano GF, Craft JC. Macrolide therapy of group A streptococcal pharyngitis: 10 days of macrolide therapy (clarithromycin) is more effective in streptococcal eradication than 5 days (azithromycin). Clin Infect Dis 32:1798-802, 2001.

Kauffman CA. Endemic mycoses in patients with hematologic malignancies. Semin Respir Infect 17:106-12, 2002.

Klein NC, Cunha BA. New uses for older antibiotics. Med Clin North America 85:125-132, 2001

Klein NC, Go J, Cunha BA. Infectious in patients on steroids. Infect Dis Clin 16:423-421, 2001

Kovacs JA, Gill VJ, Meshnick S, et al. New insights into transmission, diagnosis, and drug treatment of Pneumocystis carinii pneumonia. JAMA 286:2450-60, 2001.

Krause PJ. Babesiosis. Med Clin North Am 86:361-73, 2002.

Kremery V, Barnes AJ. Non-albicans Candida spp. causing fungaemia: pathogenicity and antifungal resistance. J Hosp Infect 50:243-60, 2002.

Kuti JL, Caron MF. Drotrecogin alfa (activated) (Xigris). Antibiotics for Clinicians 6:113-119, 2002

Lai CL, Ratziu V, Yuen MF, et al. Viral hepatitis B. Lancet 362:2089-94, 2003.

Lau CY, Qureshi AK. Azithromycin versus doxycycline for genital chlamydial infections: a metaanalysis of randomized clinical trials. Sex Transm Dis 29:497-502, 2002.

Lauder MG, Walker BD. Hepatitis C virus infection. N Engl J Med 345:41-52, 2001.

Leather HL, Wingard JR. Infections following hematopoietic stem cell transplantation. Infect Dis Clin North Am 15:483-520, 2001.

Limaye AP. Ganciclovir-resistant cytomegalovirus in organ transplant recipients. Clin Infect Dis 1;35:866-72, 2002.

Linden PK. Treatment options for vancomycin-resistant enterococcal infections. Drugs 62:425-41, 2002.

Loddenkemper R, Sagebiel D, Brendel A. Strategies against multidrug-resistant tuberculosis. Eur Respir J Suppl 36:66s-77s, 2002.

Lok AS. Chronic hepatitis B. N Engl J Med 346:1682-3, 2002.

Lonks JR, Garau J, Gomez L, et al. Failure of macrolide antibiotic treatment in patients with bacteremia due to erythromycin-resistant Streptococcus pneumoniae. Clin Infect Dis 35:556-64, 2002.

Mandell LA, Bartlett JG, Dowell SF. Update of practice guidelines for the management of community-acquired pneumonia in immunocompetent adults. Clin Infect Dis 37:1405-33, 2003.

Marr KA. Empirical antifungal therapy–new options, new tradeoffs. N Engl J Med 346:278-80, 2002.

Martin DF, Sierra-Madero J, Walmsley S, et al. A controlled trial of valganciclovir as induction therapy for cytomegalovirus retinitis. N Engl J Med 346:1119-26, 2002.

Meduri GU, Mauldin GL, Wunderink RG, et al. Causes of fever and pulmonary densities in patients with clinical manifestations of ventilator-associated pneumonia. Chest. 106:221-35, 1994.

Minnaganti V, Cunha BA. Infections associated with uremia and dialysis. Infect Dis Clin 16:385-406, 2001.

Montoya JG, Giraldo LF, Efron B, et al. Infectious complications among 620 consecutive heart transplant patients at Stanford University Medical Center. Clin Infect Dis 33:629-640, 2001.

Mylonakis E, Calderwood SB. Infective endocarditis in adults. N Engl J Med 345:1318, 2001.

Naber KG, Weidner W. Chronic prostatitis-an infectious disease? J Antimicrob Chemother 46:157-61, 2000.

Nicholson KG, Wood JM, Zambon M. Influenza. Lancet 362:1733-45, 2003.

Nicolle LE. Urinary tract infection: traditional pharmacologic therapies. Am J Med 113 (Suppl 1A):35S-44S, 2002.

Nulens E, Voss A. Laboratory diagnosis and biosafety issues of biological warfare agents. Clin Microbiol Infect 8:455-466, 2002.

Ortiz-Ruiz G, Caballero-Lopez J, Friedland IR, et al. A study evaluating the efficacy, safety, and tolerability of ertapenem versus ceftriaxone for the treatment of community-acquired pneumonia in adults. Clin Infect Dis 34:1076-83, 2002.

Owens RC, Jr. Antimicrobial associated QTc prolongation. Antibiotics for Clinicians 6:125-134, 2002.

Pappas PG, Rex JH. Therapeutic approaches to candida sepsis. In: Mandell GL and Tunkel A (eds), Current Infectious Diseases Reports, 1:245-252, 2000.

Parry CM, Hien TT, Dougan G, et al. Typhoid fever. N Engl J Med 347:1770-82, 2002.

Paya CV. Prevention of cytomegalovirus disease in recipients of solid-organ transplants. Clin Infect Dis 15:596-603, 2001.

Peacock JE, Herrington DA, Wade JC, et al. Ciprofloxacin plus piperacillin compared with tobramycin plus piperacillin as empirical therapy in febrile neutropenic patients. A randomized, double-blind trial. Ann Intern Med 137:77-87, 2002.

Peipert JF. Genital Chlamydial Infections. N Engl J Med 349:2424-30, 2003.

Perea S, Patterson TF. Invasive Aspergillus infections in hematological malignancy patients. Semin Respir Infect 17:99-105, 2002.

Pevsdos G, Cunha BA. Methicillin-resistant Staphylococcus aureus septic arthritis of the knee secondary to steroid/anesthetic injection. Infectious Disease in Clinical Practice 10:49-51, 2002.

Puri J, Mishra B, Mal A, et al. Catheter associated urinary tract infections in neurology and neurosurgical units. J Infect 44:171-5, 2002.

Quagliarello VJ, Scheld WM. Treatment of bacterial meningitis. N Engl J Med 336:708-16, 1997.

Ramsey PG, Rubin RH, Tolkoff-Rubin NE, et al. The renal transplant patient with fever and pulmonary infiltrates: etiology, clinical manifestations, and management. Medicine (Baltimore) 59:206-22, 1980

Rao N, White GJ. Successful treatment of Enterococcus faecalis prosthetic valve endocarditis with linezolid. Clin Infect Dis 35:902-4, 2002.

Rex JH. Approach to the treatment of systemic fungal infectious. In: Kelley WN (ed), Kelley's Textbook of Internal Medicine, 4th ed., 2279-2281, 2000.

Rex JH, Anaissie EF, Boutati E, et al. Systemic antifungal prophylaxis reduces invasive fungal infections in acute myelogenous leukemia: a retrospective review of 833 episodes of neutropenia in 322 adults. Leukemia 16:1197-1199, 2002.

Rex JH, Rinaldi MG, Pfaller MA. Resistance of Candida species to fluconazole. Antimicrob Agents Chemother 39:1-8, 1995.

Richard GA, Mathew CP, Kirstein JM, et al. Single-dose fluoroquinolone therapy of acute uncomplicated urinary tract infection in women: results from a randomized, double-blind, multicenter trial comparing single-dose to 3-day fluoroquinolone regimens. Urology 59:334-9, 2002.

Rijnders BJ, Vandecasteele SJ, Van Wijngaerden E. Use of semiautomatic treatment advice to improve compliance with Infectious Diseases Society of America guidelines for treatment of intravascular catheter-related infection: a before-after study. Clin Infect Dis 37:980-3, 2003.

Rissing JP. Antimicrobial therapy for chronic osteomyelitis in adults: role of the quinolones. Clin Infect Dis 25:1327-33, 1997.

Rivkina A, Rybalov S. Chronic hepatitis B: current and future treatment options. Pharmacotherapy 22:721-37, 2002.

Rodriguez LJ, Rex JH, Galgiani JN. Susceptibility testing of fungi: Current status of the correlation of in vitro data with clinical outcome. J Clin Microbiol 34:489-495, 1996.

Rodriguez-Bano J. Selection of empiric therapy in patients with catheter-related infections. Clin Microbiol Infect 8:275-81, 2002.

Ross AGP, Bartley PB, Sleigh AC, et al. Schistosomiasis. N Engl J Med 346:1212-1220, 2002.

Rubin MA, Carroll KC, Cahill BC. Caspofungin in combination with itraconazole for the treatment of invasive aspergillosis in humans. Clin Infect Dis 34:1160-1, 2002.

Rubin RH, Hooper DC. Central nervous system infection in the compromised host. Med Clin North Am 69:281-296, 1985.

Ryan ET, Wilson ME, Lain KC. Illness after international travel. N Engl J Med 347:505-516, 2002.

Safdar A, Bryan CS, Stinfon S, et al. Prosthetic valve endocarditis due to vancomycin-resistant Enterococcus faecium: treatment with chloramphenicol plus minocycline. Clin Infect Dis 34:61-3, 2002.

Sanz MA, Lopez J, Lahureta JJ, et al. Cefepime plus amikacin versus piperacillin-tazobactam plus amikacin for initial antibiotic therapy in hematology patients with febrile neutropenia: results of an open, randomized, multicentre trial. J Antimicrob Chemother 50:79-88, 2002.

Schaad UB, Kaplan SL, McCracken GH Jr. Dill SR, Cobbs CG, McDonald CK. Steroid therapy for bacterial meningitis. Clin Infect Dis 20:685-90, 1995.

Scowden EB, Schaffner W, Stone WJ. Overwhelming strongyloidiasis: An unappreciated opportunistic infection. Medicine (Baltimore) 57:527-44, 1978.

Sejvar JJ, Haddad MB, Tierney BC. Neurologic manifestations and outcome of west nile virus infection. Jama 290:511-515, 2003.

Sharkey PK, Kauffman CA, Graybill JR, et al. Itraconazole treatment of sporotrichosis. Am J Med 95:279-285, 1993.

Sher LD, McAdoo MA, Bettis RB, et al. A multicenter, randomized, investigator-blinded study of 5- and 10-day gatifloxacin versus 10-day amoxicillin/clavulanate in patients with acute bacterial sinusitis. Clin Ther 24:269-81, 2002.

Simon DM, Levin S. Infectious complications of solid organ transplantations. Infect Dis Clin North Am 15:521-49, 2001.

Small PM, Fujiwara PI. Management of tuberculosis in the United States. N Engl J Med 345:189-200, 2001.

Snydman DR, Jacobus NV, McDermott LA, et al. National survey on the susceptibility of Bacteroides fragilis: report and analysis of trends for 1997-2000. Clin Infect Dis 35(Suppl 1):S126-34, 2002.

Solomkin JS, Mazuski JE, Baron EJ. Guidelines for the selection of anti-infective agents for complicated intra-abdominal infections. Clin Infect Dis 37:997-1005, 2003.

Stanek G, Strle F. Lyme borreliosis. Lancet 362:1639-47, 2003.

Talan DA, Stamm WE, Hooton TM, et al. Comparison of ciprofloxacin (7 days) and trimethoprim-sulfamethoxazole (14 days) for acute uncomplicated pyelonephritis in women: a randomized trial. JAMA 283:1583-90, 2000.

Tegnell A, Wahren B, Elgh G. Smallpox – eradicated, but a growing terror threat. Clin Microbiol Infect 8:504-509, 2002.

Thielman NM, Guerrant RL. Acute infectious diarrhea. N Engl J Med 350:38-47, 2004.

Thompson WW, Shay DK, Weintraub E et al. Mortality associated with influenza and respiratory syncytial virus in the United States. Jama 289:179-186, 2003.

Tolkoff-Rubin NE, Rubin RH. Recent advances in the diagnosis and management of infection in the organ transplant recipient. Semin Nephrol 20:148-163, 2000.

Tomioka H, Sato K, Shimizu T, et al. Anti-mycobacterium tuberculosis activities of new fluoroquinolones in combination with other antituberculous drugs. J Infect 44:160-5, 2002.

Voitl P, Scheibenpflug C, Weber T, et al. Combined antifungal treatment of visceral mucormycosis with caspofungin and liposomal amphotericin B. Eur J Clin Microbiol Infect Dis 21:632-4, 2002.

Walsh TJ, Rex JH. All catheter-related candidemia is not the same: assessment of the balance between the risks and benefits of removal of vascular catheters. Clin Infect Dis 34:600-602, 2002.

Wendel Jr GD, Sheffield JS, Hollier LM, et al. Treatment of syphilis in pregnancy and prevention of congenital syphilis. Clin Infect Dis 35 (Suppl 2):S200-9, 2002.

Whitley RJ, Roizman B. Herpes simplex virus infections. Lancet 357:1513-18, 2001.

Wilson WR, Karchmer AW, Dajani AS, et al. Antibiotic treatment of adults with infective endocarditis due to streptococci, enterococci, staphylococci, and HACEK microorganisms. American Heart Association. JAMA 274:1706-13, 1995.

Winstanley PA, Ward SA, Snow RW. Clinical status and implications of antimalarial drug resistance. Microbes Infect 4:157-64, 2002.

Winston DJ, Gale RP, Meyer DV, et al. Infectious complications of human bone marrow transplantation. Medicine (Baltimore) 58:1-31, 1979.

Winston DJ, Busuttil RW. Randomized controlled trial of oral itraconazole solution versus intravenous/oral fluconazole for prevention of fungal infections in liver transplant recipients. Transplantation 74:688-95, 2002.

Yuen KY, Woo PC. Tuberculosis in blood and marrow transplant recipients. Hematol Oncol 20:51-62, 2002.

GUIDELINES

Bartlett JG, Dowell SF, Mandell LA, File Jr TM, Musher DM, Fine MJ. Practice guidelines for the management of community-acquired pneumonia in adults. Infectious Diseases Society of America. Clin Infect Dis 31:347-82, 2000 .

Bisno AL, Gerber MA, Gwaltney JM Jr, Kaplan EL, Schwartz RH. Practice guidelines for the diagnosis and management of group A streptococcal pharyngitis. Infectious Diseases Society of America. Clin Infect Dis 35:113-25, 2002.

Chapman SW, Bradsher RW Jr, Cambell CD Jr, et al. Practice guidelines for the management of patients with blastomycosis. Infectious Diseases Society of America. Clin Infect Dis 30:679-83, 2000.

Clarke SM, Mulcahy FM, Tjia J, Reynolds HE, Gibbons SE, Barry MG. Pharmacokinetic interactions of nevirapine and methadone and guidelines for use of nevirapine to treat injection drug users. Clin Infect Dis 34:730-51, 2002.

Dykewicz CA. Summary of the guidelines for preventing opportunistic infectious among hematopoietic stem cell transplant recipients. Clin Infect Dis 33:139-44, 2001.

Galgiani JN, Ampel NM, Catanzaro A. et al. Practice guidelines for the treatment of coccidioidomycosis. Infectious Diseases Society of America. Clin Infect Dis 30:658-61, 2000.

Gardner P, Pickering LK, Orenstein WA, Gershon AA, Nichol KL. Guidelines for quality standards for immunization. Clin Infect Dis 35:503-11, 2002.

Goodman EL. Practice guidelines for evaluating new fever in critically ill adult patients. Clin Infect Dis 30:234, 2000.

Gross PA, Asch S, Kitahata NM, Freedberg KA, et al. Performance measures for guidelines on preventing opportunistic infections in patients infected with human immunodeficiency virus. Clin Infect Dis 30(Suppl 1):S85-93, 2000.

Guerrant RL, Van Gilder T, Sterner TS, Thielman NM, Slutsker L, et al. Practice guidelines for the management of infectious diarrhea. Clin Infect Dis 15:321-4, 2001.

Horsburgh CR Jr, Feldman S, Ridzon R. Practice guidelines for the treatment of tuberculosis. Clin Infect Dis 31:633-9, 2000.

Hughes WT, Armstrong D, Bodey GP, Bow EJ, Brown AE, Calandra T. 2002 guidelines for the use of antimicrobial agents in neutropenic patients with cancer. Clin Infect Dis 34:730-51, 2002.

Kaplan JE, Masur H, Holmes KK, Freedberg KA, et al. An overview of the 1999 US Public Service Infectious Diseases Society of America Guidelines for preventing opportunistic infections in human immunodeficiency virus-infectious persons. Clin Infect Dis 30 (Suppl 1):S15-28, 2000.

Kauffman CA, Hajjeh R, Chapman SW. Practice guidelines for the management of patients with sporotrichosis. For the mycoses study group, Infectious Diseases Society of America. Clin Infect Dis 30:684-7, 2000.

Mandell LA. Guidelines for community-acquired pneumonia: a tale of 3 countries. Clin Infect Dis 31:422-5, 2000.

Marr K, Boeckh M. Practice guidelines for fungal infections: a risk-guided approach. Clin Infect Dis 32:331-51, 2001.

Mermel LA, Farr BM, Sheretz RJ, Raad II, O'Grady N, Harris JS, Craven GE. Guidelines for the management of intravascular catheter-related infections. Clin Infect Dis 32:1249-82, 2001.

Nathwani D, Rubinstein E, Barlow G, Davey P. Do guidelines for community-acquired pneumonia improve the cost-effectiveness of hospital care? Clin Infect Dis 32:728-41, 2001.

Rex JH, Walsh TJ, Sobel JD, Filler SG, et al. Practice guidelines for the treatment of candidiasis. Infectious Diseases Society of America. Clin Infect Dis 30:679-83, 2000.

Saag MS, Graybill RJ, Larsen RA, Pappas PG, et al. Practice guidelines for the management of cryptococcal disease. Infectious Diseases Society of America. Clin Infect Dis 30:710-8, 2000.

Shales DM, Gerding DN, John JF Jr, Craig WA, et al. Society for Healthcare Epidemiology of America Joint Committee on the Prevention of Antimicrobial Resistance: guidelines for the prevention of antimicrobial resistance in hospitals. Clin Infect Dis 25:584-99, 1997.

Sobel JD. Practice guidelines for the treatment of fungal infections. For the Mycoses Study Group. Infectious Diseases Society of America. Clin Infect Dis 30:652, 2000.

Stevens DA, Dan VL, Judson MA, Morrison VA, et al. Practice guidelines for diseases caused by Aspergillus. Infectious Diseases Society of America. Clin Infect Dis 30:696-709, 2000.

Talmor M, Li P, Barie PS. Acute paranasal sinusitis in critically ill patients: guidelines for prevention, diagnosis, and treatment. Clin Infect Dis 25:1441-6, 1997.

Walder CK, Workowski KA, Washington AE, Soper D, Sweet RL. Anaerobes in pelvic inflammatory disease: implications for the Centers for Disease Control and Prevention's guidelines for sexually transmitted diseases. Clin Infect Dis 28 (Suppl 1):S29-36, 1999.

Warren JW, Abrutyn E, Hebel JR, Johnson JR, et al. Guidelines for antimicrobial treatment of uncomplicated acute bacterial cystitis and acute pyelonephritis in women. Infectious Diseases Society of America. Clin Infect Dis 29:745-58, 1999.

Wheat J, Sarosi G, McKinsey D, Hammil R, et al. Practice guidelines for the management of patients with histoplasmosis. Infectious Diseases Society of America. Clin Infect Dis 30:688-95, 2000.

Workowski KA, Berman SM. CDC sexually transmitted diseases treatment guidelines. Clin Infect Dis 35 (Suppl 2):S135-7, 2002.

Wormser GP, Nadelman RB, Battwyler RJ, et al. Practice guidelines for the treatment of Lyme disease. Infectious Disease Society of America. Clin infect Dis 31 (Suppl 1):1-14, 2000.

TEXTBOOKS

Andriole VT, Bodey GP (eds). Systemic Antifungal Therapy. Scientific Therapeutic Information, Springfield, NJ, 1994.

Arikan S and Rex JH (eds). Antifungal Drugs in Manual of Clinical Microbiology, 8th edition, 2003.

Balows A, Hausler WJ, Jr., Ohashi M, Turano A (eds). Laboratory Diagnosis of Infectious Diseases. Principles and Practice (vol 1). New York, Springer-Verlag, 1988.

Bodey GP, Fainstein V (eds). Candidiasis. New York, Raven Press, 1985.

Brandstetter R, Cunha BA, Karetsky M (eds). The Pneumonias. Mosby, Philadelphia, 1999.

Calderone RA (ed). Candida and Candidiasis. ASM Press, Washington DC, 2002.

Cimolai N (ed). Laboratory Diagnosis of Bacterial Infections. New York, Marcel Dekker, 2001.

Cohen DM, Rex JH. Antifungal Therapy. In: Scholssberg DM (ed). Current therapy of infectious diseases, 1996.

Cook GC (ed). Manson's Tropical Diseases, 20th edition. W.B. Saunders Company Ltd., London, 1996.

Cunha BA (ed). Tick-Borne Infectious Diseases. Marcel Dekker, New York, 2000.

Cunha BA (ed). Infectious Disease in Critical Care Medicine. Marcel Dekker, New York, 1998.

Cunha BA (ed). Infectious Disease in the Elderly. John Wright & Co., London, 1988.

Emmons CW, Binford CH, Utz JP, Kwon-Chung KJ (eds). Medical mycology, 3rd edition. Philadelphia, Lea & Febiger, 1977.

Faro S, Soper DE (eds). Infectious Diseases in Women. WB Saunders Company, Philadelphia, 2001.

Frey D, Oldfield RJ, Bridger RC (eds). Color Atlas of Pathogenic Fungi. Year Book Medical Publishers, Chicago, 1979.

Gorbach SL, Bartlett JG, Blacklow NR (eds). Infectious Diseases, 2nd Edition. W.B. Saunders Company, Philadelphia, 1999.

Guerrant RL, Walker DH, Weller PF (eds). Tropical Infectious Disease: Principles, Pathogens & Practice. Churchill Livingstone, Philadelphia, 1999.

Howard DH. Pathogenic Fungi in Humans and Animals, 2nd Edition. Marcel Dekker, New York, 2003.

Mandell GL, Bennett JE, Dolin R (eds). Mandell, Douglas and Bennett's Principles and Practice of Infectious Disease, 5th Edition. Churchill Livingstone, Philadelphia, 2000

Martins MD, Rex JH. Antifungal Therapy. In: Parillo JE (ed). Current therapy in Critical Care Medicine, 3rd Edition. 1997.

Merck & Co. Introduction to Medical Mycology. North Whales Press, North Whales, 2001.

Pastorek III JG (ed). Obstetric and Gynecologic Infectious Diseases. Raven Press, New York, 1994.

Plotkin SA, Orenstein WA (eds). Vaccines, 3rd edition. W. B. Saunders, Philadelphia, 1999.

Rex JH, Sobel JD, Powderly WB. Candida Infections. In: Yu VL, Jr., Merigan TC, Jr., and Barriere SL (eds.). Antimicrobial Therapy & Vaccines. Williams & Wilkins, Baltimore, MD, 1998.

Rex JH, Pappas PG. Hematogenously Disseminated Fungal Infections. In: Anaissie EJ, Pfaller MA, McGinnis M (eds.), Clinical Mycology, Churchill-Livingstone, Edinburgh, 2002.

Rippon JW (ed). Medical Mycology, 3rd ed. W. B. Saunders, Philadelphia, 1988.

Ristuccia AM, Cunha BA (eds). Antimicrobial Therapy. Raven Press, New York,1984.

Rubin RH, Young LS, (eds). Clinical Approach to Infection in the Compromised Host, 3rd edition, Plenum Medical Book Co., New York, 1994.

Root RK (ed). Clinical Infectious Disease: A Practical Approach. Oxford University Press, New York, 1999.

Sarosi GA, Davies SF (eds). Fungal Diseases of the Lung. Grune & Stratton, New York, 1986.

Schlossberg D (ed). Current Therapy of Infectious Disease 2nd Edition. Mosby-Yearbook, St. Louis, 2001.

Singh N, Aguado JM (eds). Infectious Complications in Transplant Patients. Kluwer Academic Publishers, Boston, 2000.

Strickland GT (ed). Hunter's Tropical Medicine and Emerging Infectious Diseases, 8th Edition. W.B. Saunders Company, Philadelphia, 2000.

Sweet RL, Gibbs RS (eds). Infectious Diseases on the Female Genital Tract, 2nd Edition. Williams & Wilkins, Baltimore, 1990.

Yoshikawa TT, Norman DC (eds). Antimicrobial Therapy in the Elderly. Marcel Dekker, New York, 1994.xx

Chapter 3

Initial Therapy of Isolates Pending Susceptibility Testing

Burke A. Cunha, MD
Paul E. Schoch, PhD
John H. Rex, MD

Introduction

When bacteria are isolated from a body site and reported, the clinical significance of the organism should be determined before deciding on potential antibiotic treatment.

The tables in this chapter serve as a guide to the clinical significance of bacterial and fungal isolates recovered from various body sites, including CSF, blood, sputum, urine, stool, and wound. In general, isolates listed as pathogens (P) should be treated with antibiotics, while those listed as non-pathogens (NP), colonizers (C), or skin contaminants (C*) ordinarily should not. The antibiotics recommended in this section should be effective initial therapy pending susceptibility testing.

Isolates by Gram Stain, Arrangement, Oxygen Requirements

AEROBIC ISOLATES

*   *Enterobacteriaceae (oxidase negative, catalase positive)*
**   *Oxidase negative*

CAPNOPHILIC ISOLATES[+]

+   *Capnophilic organisms grow best under increased CO_2 tension*

ANAEROBIC ISOLATES[++]

++ *Microaerophilic organisms. Grow best under decreased O_2 concentration*

YEASTS/FUNGI

Alphabetical Index of Isolates

Table 1. Clinical Significance of AEROBIC Isolates Pending Susceptibility Testing

GRAM-POSITIVE COCCI (CLUSTERS)

Isolate	Isolate Significance	Preferred Therapy	Alternate Therapy	Comments
Staphylococcus aureus (MSSA/MRSA)	• CSF = C*, P (CNS shunts) • Blood = C*, P (from soft tissue/bone infection, abscess, IV line infection, ABE, PVE) • Sputum = C, P (S. aureus pneumonia is rare; usually only after viral influenza) • Urine = C, P (S. aureus in urine is usually due to skin contamination or rarely overwhelming S. aureus bacteremia) • Stool = C, P (enterocolitis) • Wound = C, P (cellulitis, abscess)	<u>MSSA</u> Nafcillin (IV) Cefazolin (IV) Clindamycin (IV/PO) <u>MRSA</u> Linezolid (IV/PO) Daptomycin (IV) Quinupristin/dalfopristin (IV) Vancomycin (IV) Minocycline (IV/PO)	<u>MSSA</u> Any 2nd, 3rd generation cephalosporin (IV) (except ceftazidime, ceftriaxone) Meropenem (IV) Imipenem (IV) Ertapenem (IV) Linezolid (IV/PO)	For oral treatment, 1st generation cephalosporins are better tolerated and have more reliable blood levels than oral anti-staphylococcal penicillins (e.g., dicloxacillin). MRSA in-vitro susceptibility testing is unreliable; treat infection empirically with one of agents listed. Do not treat MRSA colonization. Cannot substitute doxycycline for minocycline for MRSA. Some antibiotics are associated with an increase in MRSA (e.g., ceftazidime)
Staphylococcus epidermidis (MSSE/MRSE) or coagulase-negative staphylococci	• CSF = C*, P (CNS shunts) • Blood = C*, P (from IV lines, infected implants, PVE, rarely native valve SBE) • Sputum = C • Urine = C (may be reported as S. saprophyticus; request novobiocin sensitivity to differentiate from other coagulase-negative staph) • Stool = NP • Wound = C, P (infected foreign body drainage)	<u>MSSE</u> Linezolid (IV/PO) Vancomycin (IV) Meropenem (IV) Ertapenem (IV) <u>MRSE</u> Linezolid (IV/PO) Vancomycin (IV) ± rifampin (PO)	<u>MSSE</u> Clindamycin (IV/PO) Gatifloxacin (IV/PO) Levofloxacin (IV/PO) Moxifloxacin (IV/PO) Imipenem (IV) <u>MRSE</u> Quinupristin/dalfopristin (IV)	Usually non-pathogenic in absence of prosthetic/implant materials. Common cause of PVE; rare cause of native valve SBE. Treat foreign body-related infection until foreign body is removed

C = colonizer; C* = skin contaminant; NP = non-pathogen at site; P = pathogen at site; (IV/PO) = IV or PO. See p. 1 for all other abbreviations

Table 1. Clinical Significance of AEROBIC Isolates Pending Susceptibility Testing (cont'd)

Isolate	Isolate Significance	Preferred Therapy	Alternate Therapy	Comments
GRAM-POSITIVE COCCI (CLUSTERS)				
Staphylococcus saprophyticus (coagulase-negative staphylococci)	• CSF = NP • Blood = NP • Sputum = NP • Urine = P (cystitis, pyelo) • Stool = NP • Wound = NP	Amoxicillin (PO) TMP-SMX (PO) Nitrofurantoin (PO)	Any quinolone (PO) Any 1st generation cephalosporin (PO)	S. saprophyticus UTI is associated with a urinary "fishy odor," alkaline urine pH, and microscopic hematuria. Novobiocin sensitivity differentiates coagulase-negative staphylococci (sensitive) from S. saprophyticus (resistant)
GRAM-POSITIVE COCCI (CHAINS)				
Enterococcus faecalis	• CSF = NP (except from S. stercoralis hyperinfection or V-P shunt infection) • Blood = C*, P (from GI/GU source, SBE) • Sputum = NP • Urine = C, P (cystitis, pyelonephritis) • Stool = NP • Wound = C, P (cellulitis)	Non-SBE Ampicillin (IV) Amoxicillin (PO) Meropenem (IV) Piperacillin/tazobactam Linezolid (IV/PO) Daptomycin (IV) SBE Gentamicin (IV) plus either ampicillin (IV) or vancomycin (IV) Meropenem (IV) Piperacillin/tazobactam Linezolid (IV/PO) Daptomycin (IV)	Non-SBE Cefoperazone (IV) Chloramphenicol (IV) Any quinolone (IV/PO) Nitrofurantoin (PO) (UTIs only) SBE Any quinolone (IV/PO) Cefoperazone (IV) Imipenem (IV)	Sensitive to ampicillin, not penicillin. Cause of intermediate (in-between ABE and SBE) endocarditis, hepatobiliary infections, and UTIs. Enterococci (E. faecalis, E. faecium) are the only cause of SBE from GI/GU sources. Permissive pathogen (i.e., usually does not cause infection alone) in the abdomen/pelvis. Cefoperazone is the only cephalosporin with anti-E. faecalis activity (MIC ~ 32 mcg/mL). Quinupristin/dalfopristin is not active against E. faecalis
Enterococcus faecium (VRE)	• CSF = NP (except from S. stercoralis hyperinfection or V-P shunt infection) • Blood = C*, P (from GI/GU source, SBE) • Sputum = C • Urine = C, P (cystitis, pyelo) • Stool = NP • Wound = C, P (cellulitis)	Non-SBE Linezolid (IV/PO), quinupristin/dalfopristin (IV), doxycycline (IV/PO), chloramphenicol (IV), nitrofurantoin (PO) (UTIs only) SBE Linezolid (IV/PO) Quinupristin/dalfopristin (IV)		Same spectrum of infection as E. faecalis. Colonization is more common than infection. Fecal carriage is intermittent but prolonged. In-vitro antibiotic sensitivity predicts in-vivo efficacy. Increased prevalence of E. faecalis (VRE) infections related to IV vancomycin use, not PO vancomycin

C = colonizer; C* = skin contaminant; NP = non-pathogen at site; P = pathogen at site; (IV/PO) = IV or PO. See p. 1 for all other abbreviations

Table 1. Clinical Significance of AEROBIC Isolates Pending Susceptibility Testing (cont'd)

		GRAM-POSITIVE COCCI (CHAINS)		
Isolate	Isolate Significance	Preferred Therapy	Alternate Therapy	Comments
Group A streptococci	• CSF = C*, P (rare cause of meningitis) • Blood = P (from skin/soft tissue infection) • Sputum = P (rare cause of CAP) • Urine = NP • Stool = NP • Wound = C, P (cellulitis) • Throat = C, P (pharynx is colonized with Group A streptococci in ~ 30% of patients with EBV mono)	Amoxicillin (PO) Clindamycin (IV/PO) Any β-lactam (IV/PO)	Penicillin (PO) Clarithromycin XL (PO) Azithromycin (PO)	For Group A streptococcal pharyngitis, amoxicillin is preferred over penicillin. Clindamycin is best for elimination of carrier states, and for penicillin-allergic patients with streptococcal pharyngitis. Any β-lactam is equally effective against Group A streptococci. Nafcillin is the most active anti-staphylococcal penicillin against Group A streptococcus. Erythromycin is no longer reliable against Group A streptococcus due to increasing resistance. Doxycycline has little/no activity against Group A streptococci
Group B streptococci (S. agalactiae)	• CSF = P (ABM) • Blood = P (from IV line/urine source, SBE) • Sputum = NP • Urine = P (CAB, UTIs, especially in diabetics, elderly) • Stool = NP • Wound = C, P (diabetic foot infections)	Non-SBE, non-CNS Clindamycin (IV/PO) Any 1st, 2nd, 3rd generation cephalosporin (IV/PO) SBE Ceftriaxone (IV) Penicillin (IV) Vancomycin (IV) CNS Ceftriaxone (IV) Penicillin (IV)	Non-SBE, non-CNS Vancomycin (IV) Amoxicillin (PO) SBE Imipenem (IV) Meropenem (IV) Ertapenem (IV) Linezolid (IV/PO) CNS Chloramphenicol (IV) Linezolid (IV/PO)	Cause of UTIs and IV line infections in diabetics and the elderly. Cause of neonatal meningitis. Infection is uncommon in the general population. Rarely a cause of SBE in non-pregnant adults. Aminoglycosides are ineffective

C = colonizer; C* = skin contaminant; NP = non-pathogen at site; P = pathogen at site; (IV/PO) = IV or PO. See p. 1 for all other abbreviations

Table 1. Clinical Significance of AEROBIC Isolates Pending Susceptibility Testing (cont'd)

		GRAM-POSITIVE COCCI (CHAINS)		
Isolate	Isolate Significance	Preferred Therapy	Alternate Therapy	Comments
Group C, F, G streptococci	• CSF = P (meningitis) • Blood = P (from skin/soft tissue infection, SBE) • Sputum = P (rare cause of CAP) • Throat = C (especially with viral pharyngitis), P (pharyngitis in medical personnel) • Urine = NP • Stool = NP • Wound = P (cellulitis)	Ceftriaxone (IV) Penicillin (IV) Ampicillin (IV) Clindamycin (IV/PO)	Vancomycin (IV) Amoxicillin (PO) Any 1st,2nd,3rd generation cephalosporin (IV) Imipenem (IV) Meropenem (IV) Ertapenem (IV)	Group C, G streptococci may cause pharyngitis, wound infections, and rarely SBE. Common pharyngeal colonizers in medical personnel
Streptococcus bovis	• CSF = NP • Blood = P (SBE from GI source) • Sputum = NP • Urine = NP • Stool = NP • Wound = NP	Ceftriaxone (IV) Ampicillin (IV) Clindamycin (IV/PO)	Vancomycin (IV) Amoxicillin (PO) Any 1st,2nd,3rd generation cephalosporin (IV)	Associated with GI malignancies. Non-enterococcal Group D streptococci (e.g., S. bovis) are sensitive to penicillin
Streptococcus viridans group (S. mitior, milleri, mitis, mutans, oralis, sanguis, parasanguis, salivarius)	• CSF = NP • Blood = C*, P (1° bacteremia, SBE) • Sputum = NP • Urine = NP • Stool = NP • Wound = NP	Ceftriaxone (IV) Penicillin (IV)	Amoxicillin (PO) Any 1st,2nd,3rd generation cephalosporin (IV/PO) Meropenem (IV) Ertapenem (IV) Vancomycin (IV)	S. viridans is commonly isolated from blood cultures. Low-grade blood culture positivity (1/4) indicates contamination during venipuncture. High-grade blood culture positivity (3/4 or 4/4) indicates SBE until proven otherwise. S. milleri is associated with metastatic abscesses

C = colonizer; C* = skin contaminant; NP = non-pathogen at site; P = pathogen at site; (IV/PO) = IV or PO. See p. 1 for all other abbreviations

Table 1. Clinical Significance of AEROBIC Isolates Pending Susceptibility Testing (cont'd)

GRAM-POSITIVE COCCI (PAIRS)

Isolate	Isolate Significance	Preferred Therapy	Alternate Therapy	Comments
Leuconostoc	• CSF = NP • Blood = P (PVE) • Sputum = NP • Urine = P (UTIs) • Stool = NP • Wound = NP	Penicillin (IV) Ampicillin (IV) Clindamycin (IV/PO)	Amoxicillin (PO) Erythromycin (IV) Minocycline (IV/PO) Clarithromycin XL (PO)	Coccobacillary forms resemble streptococci/enterococci. Cause of infection in compromised hosts. Rare cause of IV line infection. Vancomycin resistant
Streptococcus pneumoniae	• CSF = P (ABM) • Blood = P (from respiratory tract source) • Sputum = C, P • Urine = NP • Stool = NP • Wound = P (cellulitis only in SLE)	**PCN-resistant** Amoxicillin/clavulanic acid (XR, ES-600) (PO); ceftriaxone (IV); any respiratory quinolone (IV/PO); telithromycin (PO); imipenem (IV); ertapenem (IV); meropenem (IV); cefepime (IV); linezolid (IV/PO); vancomycin (IV) **Sensitive or relatively PCN-resistant** Doxycycline (IV/PO); any cephalosporin (IV/PO); clindamycin (IV/PO)		Penicillin-resistant S. pneumoniae are still sensitive to full-dose/high-dose β-lactams

GRAM-NEGATIVE COCCI (PAIRS)

Isolate	Isolate Significance	Preferred Therapy	Alternate Therapy	Comments
Neisseria gonorrhoeae (GC)	• CSF = NP • Blood = P (from pharyngitis, proctitis, ABE) • Sputum = NP • Urine = P (urethritis) • Stool = NP • Wound = NP • Rectal discharge = P (GC proctitis)	**Penicillin-sensitive N. gonorrhoeae** Ceftriaxone (IV/IM) Any quinolone (IV/PO) **PPNG** Ceftriaxone (IV/IM)	**Penicillin-sensitive N. gonorrhoeae** Penicillin (IV/IM) Amoxicillin (PO) Doxycycline (IV/PO) **PPNG** Spectinomycin (IM) Any quinolone (PO) Any 1st, 2nd, 3rd gen. cephalosporin (IV/IM)	Cause of "culture negative" right-sided ABE. May be cultured from synovial fluid/blood in disseminated GC infection (arthritis-dermatitis syndrome). Treat possible Chlamydia trachomatis co-infection and sexual partners. Spectinomycin is ineffective against pharyngeal GC/ incubating syphilis. PPNG are tetracycline-resistant (TRNG). GC strains from Hawaii/California have increased quinolone resistance; use ceftriaxone for such strains

C = colonizer; C* = skin contaminant; NP = non-pathogen at site; P = pathogen at site; (IV/PO) = IV or PO. See p. 1 for all other abbreviations

Table 1. Clinical Significance of AEROBIC Isolates Pending Susceptibility Testing (cont'd)

GRAM-NEGATIVE COCCI (PAIRS)

Isolate	Isolate Significance	Preferred Therapy	Alternate Therapy	Comments
Neisseria meningitidis	• CSF = P (ABM) • Blood = P (acute/chronic meningococcemia) • Sputum = C, P (only in closed populations, e.g., military recruits) • Urine C, P (urethritis rarely) • Stool = NP • Wound = NP	Penicillin (IV) Ampicillin (IV) Any 3rd generation cephalosporin (IV)	Chloramphenicol (IV) Cefepime (IV) Meropenem (IV)	In ABM, do not decrease meningeal dose of β-lactam antibiotics as patient improves, since CSF penetration/concentration decreases as meningeal inflammation decreases. Chloramphenicol is an excellent choice for penicillin-allergic patients. Preferred meningococcal prophylaxis is an oral quinolone (single dose)

GRAM-POSITIVE BACILLI

Isolate	Isolate Significance	Preferred Therapy	Alternate Therapy	Comments
Arcanobacterium (Corynebacterium) haemolyticum	• CSF = NP • Blood = NP • Sputum = P (oropharyngeal secretions) • Urine = NP • Stool/Wound = NP	Doxycycline (PO)	Erythromycin (PO) Azithromycin (PO) Any 1st, 2nd, 3rd generation cephalosporin (PO) Clarithromycin XL (PO)	Causes membranous pharyngitis with scarlet fever-like rash. Differentiate from C. diphtheriae by culture. Penicillin and ampicillin are less effective than erythromycin or doxycycline
Bacillus anthracis	• CSF = P (ABM) • Blood = P (septicemia; isolation required; dangerous) • Sputum = P (mediastinitis; anthrax pneumonia rare) • Urine = NP • Stool = NP • Wound = P (ulcer; isolation required; dangerous)	Penicillin (IV) Doxycycline (IV/PO) Any quinolone (IV/PO)	Amoxicillin (PO) Ampicillin (IV)	Doxycycline may be used for therapy/outbreak prophylaxis. Streptobacillary configuration in blood. Causes hemorrhagic meningitis, wound infections, and bacteremia. Quinolones are effective, but experience is limited. Alert microbiology laboratory of potentially biohazardous specimens. Do not culture. Bioterrorist and naturally-acquired anthrax are treated the same

C = colonizer; C* = skin contaminant; NP = non-pathogen at site; P = pathogen at site; (IV/PO) = IV or PO. See p. 1 for all other abbreviations

Table 1. Clinical Significance of AEROBIC Isolates Pending Susceptibility Testing (cont'd)

| | GRAM-POSITIVE BACILLI | | | |
Isolate	Isolate Significance	Preferred Therapy	Alternate Therapy	Comments
Bacillus cereus, subtilis, megaterium	• CSF = NP • Blood = C*, P (leukopenic compromised hosts) • Sputum = NP • Urine = NP • Stool = NP • Wound = NP	Vancomycin (IV) Clindamycin (IV/PO)	Imipenem (IV) Meropenem (IV/PO) Any quinolone (IV/PO)	Soil organisms not commonly pathogenic for humans. Suspect pseudoinfection if isolated from clinical specimens. Look for soil/dust contamination of blood culture tube top/apparatus. Rare pathogen in leukopenic compromised hosts
Corynebacterium diphtheriae	• CSF = NP • Blood = NP • Sputum = P (oropharyngeal secretions) • Urine = NP • Stool = NP • Wound = P (wound diphtheria)	Penicillin (IV) Erythromycin (IV) Clindamycin (IV/PO)	Doxycycline (IV/PO) Clarithromycin XL (PO) Rifampin (PO)	Administer diphtheria antitoxin as soon as possible (p. 131). Antibiotic therapy is adjunctive, since diphtheria is a toxin-mediated disease. Patients may die unexpectedly from toxin-induced myocarditis during recovery
Corynebacterium jeikeium (CDC group JK)	• CSF = C*, P (CSF shunts) • Blood = C*, P (from IV lines) • Sputum = NP • Urine/Stool = NP • Wound = C	Vancomycin (IV) Linezolid (IV/PO)	Quinupristin/ dalfopristin (IV)	Cause of IV line/foreign body infections. In-vitro testing is not always reliable. Highly resistant to most anti-gram positive antibiotics
Erysipelothrix rhusiopathiae	• CSF = NP • Blood = P (from SBE) • Sputum = NP • Urine = NP • Stool = NP • Wound = P (chronic erysipelas-like skin lesions)	Penicillin (IV) Ampicillin (IV)	Any 3rd generation cephalosporin (IV) Any quinolone (IV/PO)	Cause of "culture-negative" SBE. One of the HACEK organisms. Resistant to clindamycin and metronidazole

C = colonizer; C* = skin contaminant; NP = non-pathogen at site; P = pathogen at site; (IV/PO) = IV or PO. See p. 1 for all other abbreviations

Table 1. Clinical Significance of AEROBIC Isolates Pending Susceptibility Testing (cont'd)

GRAM-POSITIVE BACILLI

Isolate	Isolate Significance	Preferred Therapy	Alternate Therapy	Comments
Listeria monocytogenes	• CSF = P (ABM) • Blood = P (1° bacteremia, SBE) • Sputum = NP • Urine = NP • Stool = NP • Wound = NP	Ampicillin (IV) Amoxicillin (PO) Chloramphenicol (IV) **CNS** Ampicillin (IV) TMP-SMX (IV/PO) Chloramphenicol (IV) **SBE** Ampicillin (IV)	Doxycycline (IV/PO) Erythromycin (IV)	Listeria ABM is common in T-cell deficiencies (e.g., lymphoma, steroids, HIV). Causes SBE in normal hosts, and is the commonest cause of bacteremia in non-neutropenic cancer patients. 3rd generation cephalosporins are ineffective against Listeria
Nocardia asteroides, brasiliensis	• CSF = P (brain abscess) • Blood = P (from lung/soft tissue source) • Sputum = P (pneumonia, lung abscess) • Urine/Stool = NP • Wound = P (skin lesions from direct inoculation or dissemination)	TMP-SMX (IV/PO) Minocycline (IV/PO)	Imipenem (IV) plus either amikacin (IV) or any 3rd generation cephalosporin (IV)	Branched, filamentous, beady hyphae are typical, but coccobacillary and bacillary forms are also common. Nocardia are gram-positive, aerobic, and acid fast. Quinolones and macrolides are usually ineffective
Rhodococcus equi	• CSF = NP • Blood = P (from pneumonia, lung abscess) • Sputum = P (pneumonia with abscess/cavitation) • Urine = NP • Stool = NP • Wound = NP	Any quinolone (IV/PO) Vancomycin (IV)	Erythromycin (IV) Imipenem (IV) Meropenem (IV) Doxycycline (IV/PO) TMP-SMX (IV/PO)	Causes TB-like community-acquired pneumonia in AIDS patients. Filamentous bacteria break into bacilli/cocci. Aminoglycosides and β-lactams are relatively ineffective

C = colonizer; C* = skin contaminant; P = pathogen at site; NP = non-pathogen at site; (IV/PO) = IV or PO. See p. 1 for all other abbreviations

Table 1. Clinical Significance of AEROBIC Isolates Pending Susceptibility Testing (cont'd)

GRAM-NEGATIVE BACILLI

Isolate	Isolate Significance	Preferred Therapy	Alternate Therapy	Comments
Acinetobacter baumannii, lwoffi, calcoaceticus, haemolyticus	• CSF = C*, P (ABM) • Blood = P (from IV line, lung, or urine source) • Sputum = C, P (VAP) • Urine = C, P (CAB) • Stool = NP • Wound = C (common), P (rare)	Ampicillin/sulbactam (IV) Piperacillin/tazobactam (IV) Imipenem (IV) Meropenem (IV)	Any 3rd generation cephalosporin (IV) (except ceftazidime) Cefepime (IV)	Usually associated with respiratory support equipment. Occurs in outbreaks of ventilator-associated pneumonia. Ertapenem is inactive
Actinobacillus actinomycetem-comitans	• CSF = NP • Blood = P (from abscess, SBE) • Sputum = NP • Urine/Stool = NP • Wound = P (from abscess, draining fistulous tract)	Any quinolone (IV/PO) Any 3rd generation cephalosporin (IV/PO)	Penicillin (IV) + gentamicin (IV) TMP-SMX (IV/PO)	Cause of "culture-negative" SBE. One of the HACEK organisms. Found with Actinomyces in abscesses. Resistant to erythromycin and clindamycin
Aeromonas hydrophila	• CSF = NP • Blood = P (from wound, urine, or GI source) • Sputum = NP • Urine = C, P (CAB) • Stool = P (diarrhea) • Wound = P (cellulitis)	Gentamicin (IV) TMP-SMX (IV/PO) Any quinolone (IV/PO)	Doxycycline (IV/PO) Any 3rd generation cephalosporin (IV/PO) Imipenem (IV) Meropenem (IV) Aztreonam (IV)	Cause of wound infection, septic arthritis, diarrhea, and necrotizing soft tissue infection resembling gas gangrene
Alcaligenes (Achromobacter) xylosoxidans	• CSF = P (rarely ABM) • Blood = P (from urine) • Sputum = NP • Urine = P (CAB) • Stool = NP • Wound = P (cellulitis rare)	Imipenem (IV) Meropenem (IV) Any 3rd generation cephalosporin (IV/PO) Piperacillin/tazobactam (IV)	Any quinolone (IV/PO) Cefepime (IV) Aztreonam (IV) Ticarcillin/clavulanic acid (IV/PO)	Water-borne pathogen resembling Acinetobacter microbiologically. Resistant to aminoglycosides and 1st, 2nd generation cephalosporins

C = colonizer; C* = skin contaminant; NP = non-pathogen at site; P = pathogen at site; (IV/PO) = IV or PO. See p. 1 for all other abbreviations

Table 1. Clinical Significance of AEROBIC Isolates Pending Susceptibility Testing (cont'd)

GRAM-NEGATIVE BACILLI

Isolate	Isolate Significance	Preferred Therapy	Alternate Therapy	Comments
Bartonella henselae, quintana, bacilliformis	• CSF = NP • Blood = P (from skin source, SBE) • Sputum = NP • Urine = NP • Stool = NP • Wound = P (skin lesions)	Doxycycline (IV/PO), Azithromycin (PO)	Clarithromycin XL (PO) Any quinolone (IV/PO) Any aminoglycoside (IV)	Causes bacillary angiomatosis or verruga peruana in AIDS patients. Also the cause of Cat Scratch disease and Aroya fever. May present as FUO. TMP-SMX and cephalosporins are ineffective
Bordetella pertussis, parapertussis	• CSF = NP • Blood = P (from respiratory tract source) • Sputum = C, P (pertussis) • Urine = NP • Stool = NP • Wound = NP	Erythromycin (IV) Clarithromycin XL (PO) Azithromycin (IV/PO)	Any quinolone (IV/PO) TMP-SMX (IV/PO)	Causes pertussis in children and incompletely/non-immunized adults. Macrolides remain the preferred therapy. Resistant to penicillins, cephalosporins, and aminoglycosides
Brucella abortus, canis, suis, melitensis	• CSF = P (meningitis) • Blood = P (from abscess, SBE) • Sputum = NP • Urine = P (pyelonephritis) • Stool/Wound = NP	Doxycycline (IV/PO) + gentamicin (IV) Doxycycline + streptomycin (IM)	TMP-SMX (IV/PO) + gentamicin (IV) Doxycycline (IV/PO) + rifampin (PO) Any quinolone (IV/PO) + rifampin (PO)	Causes prolonged relapsing infection. Zoonotic cause of brucellosis/Malta fever. Resistant to penicillins
Burkholderia (Pseudomonas) cepacia	• CSF = NP • Blood = P (usually from IV line/urinary tract infection) • Sputum = C (not a cause of VAP) • Urine = C • Stool = NP • Wound = NP	TMP-SMX (IV/PO)	Chloramphenicol (IV) Minocycline (IV/PO) Any quinolone (IV/PO) Meropenem (IV) Cefepime (IV) Piperacillin/ tazobactam (IV)	Rare cause of urosepsis following urologic instrumentation. Common water-borne colonizer in intensive care units. Opportunistic pathogen in cystic fibrosis/bronchiectasis. Resistant to aminoglycosides

C = colonizer; C* = skin contaminant; NP = non-pathogen at site; P = pathogen at site; (IV/PO) = IV or PO. See p. 1 for all other abbreviations

Table 1. Clinical Significance of AEROBIC Isolates Pending Susceptibility Testing (cont'd)

		GRAM-NEGATIVE BACILLI		
Isolate	Isolate Significance	Preferred Therapy	Alternate Therapy	Comments
Burkholderia (Pseudomonas) pseudomallei	• CSF = NP • Blood = P (from septicemic melioidosis) • Sputum = P (chronic cavitary pneumonia) • Urine = NP • Stool = NP • Wound = NP	TMP-SMX (IV/PO) Ceftazidime (IV)	Imipenem (IV) Meropenem (IV) Chloramphenicol (IV)	Causes melioidosis, which resembles chronic fibrocaseating TB, but in lower lobe distribution. Resistant to aminoglycosides
Campylobacter fetus	• CSF = P (ABM) • Blood = P (from vascular source) • Sputum = NP • Urine = NP • Stool = NP • Wound = NP	Gentamicin (IV) Imipenem (IV) Meropenem (IV)	Chloramphenicol (IV) Ampicillin (IV) Any 3rd generation cephalosporin (IV)	Causes invasive infection with spread to CNS. CNS infection may be treated with meningeal doses of chloramphenicol, ampicillin, or a 3rd generation cephalosporin. Resistant to erythromycin
Campylobacter jejuni	• CSF = NP • Blood = P (from GI source) • Sputum = NP • Urine = NP • Stool = P (diarrhea) • Wound = NP	Any quinolone (IV/PO) Erythromycin (PO) Doxycycline (IV/PO)	Azithromycin (PO) Clarithromycin XL (PO)	Commonest cause of acute bacterial diarrhea. Resistant to TMP-SMX
Cardiobacterium hominis	• CSF = NP • Blood = P (from SBE) • Sputum = NP • Urine = NP • Stool = NP • Wound = NP	Penicillin (IV) + gentamicin (IV) Ampicillin (IV) + gentamicin (IV)	Any 3rd generation cephalosporin (IV) + gentamicin (IV)	Pleomorphic bacillus with bulbous ends. Often appears in clusters resembling rosettes. Cause of "culture-negative" SBE (one of the HACEK organisms). Rare cause of abdominal abscess. Grows best with CO_2 enhancement. Resistant to macrolides and clindamycin

C = colonizer; C* = skin contaminant; NP = non-pathogen at site; P = pathogen at site; (IV/PO) = IV or PO. See p. 1 for all other abbreviations

Table 1. Clinical Significance of AEROBIC Isolates Pending Susceptibility Testing (cont'd)

GRAM-NEGATIVE BACILLI

Isolate	Isolate Significance	Preferred Therapy	Alternate Therapy	Comments
Chromobacterium violaceum	• CSF = NP • Blood = P (from wound infection) • Sputum = NP • Urine = NP • Stool = NP • Wound = P (drainage from deep soft tissue infection)	Gentamicin (IV) Doxycycline (IV/PO)	Chloramphenicol (IV)	Cause of cutaneous lesions primarily in tropical/subtropical climates. Often mistaken for Vibrio or Alcaligenes. Resistant to β-lactams
Chryseobacterium (Flavobacterium) meningosepticum	• CSF = P (ABM) • Blood = P (from IV line infection, PVE) • Sputum = NP • Urine = C, P (from urologic instrumentation) • Stool = NP • Wound = C, P (cellulitis)	CNS TMP-SMX (IV/PO) Non-CNS Vancomycin (IV) + rifampin (PO) Any quinolone (IV/PO)	CNS Chloramphenicol (IV) Non-CNS Clarithromycin XL (PO) + rifampin (PO) Clindamycin (IV/PO)	Rare cause of ABM in newborns and PVE in adults. Only unencapsulated Flavobacterium species. Clindamycin, clarithromycin, and vancomycin are useful only in non-CNS infections. Resistant to aztreonam and carbapenems
Citrobacter diversus, freundii, koseri	• CSF = C*, P (from NS procedure) • Blood = C*, P (from IV line/ urinary tract infection) • Sputum = C (not pneumonia) • Urine = C, P (from urologic instrumentation) • Stool = NP • Wound = C, P (rarely in compromised hosts)	Any quinolone (IV/PO) Meropenem (IV) Imipenem (IV) Ertapenem (IV) Cefepime (IV)	Aztreonam (IV) Piperacillin/tazobactam (IV) Any 3rd generation cephalosporin (IV)	Common wound/urine colonizer. Rare pathogen in normal hosts. Often aminoglycoside resistant (C. freundii is usually more resistant than C. koseri)

C = colonizer; C* = skin contaminant; NP = non-pathogen at site; P = pathogen at site; (IV/PO) = IV or PO. See p. 1 for all other abbreviations

Table 1. Clinical Significance of AEROBIC Isolates Pending Susceptibility Testing (cont'd)

GRAM-NEGATIVE BACILLI

Isolate	Isolate Significance	Preferred Therapy	Alternate Therapy	Comments
Edwardsiella tarda	• CSF = NP • Blood = P (from liver abscess) • Sputum/Urine = NP • Stool = P • Wound C, P (wound infection)	Ampicillin (IV) Amoxicillin (PO) Any quinolone (IV/PO)	Doxycycline (IV/PO) Any 3rd generation cephalosporin (IV/PO)	Cause of bacteremia, usually from liver abscess or wound source
Enterobacter agglomerans, aerogenes, cloacae	• CSF = C*, P (from NS procedure) • Blood = C*, P (from IV line/ urinary tract infection) • Sputum = C (not a cause of pneumonia) • Urine = C, P (post-urologic instrumentation) • Stool = NP • Wound = C, P (rarely in compromised hosts)	Cefepime (IV) Any quinolone (IV/PO) Aztreonam (IV)	Piperacillin/tazobactam (IV) Meropenem (IV) Ertapenem (IV)	Not a cause of community-acquired or nosocomial pneumonia. Common colonizer of respiratory secretions and wound/urine specimens. Treatment of Enterobacter colonizers with ceftazidime or ciprofloxacin may cause multi-drug resistance
Escherichia coli	• CSF = P (ABM) • Blood = P (from GI/ GU source) • Sputum = P (rarely CAP from urinary source, VAP) • Urine = C, P (CAB, cystitis, pyelonephritis) • Stool = C, P (diarrhea) • Wound = P (cellulitis)	Ceftriaxone (IV) Amoxicillin (PO) TMP-SMX (IV/PO) Any quinolone (IV/PO)	Any 1st, 2nd, 3rd generation cephalosporin (IV/PO) Aztreonam (IV) Gentamicin (IV) Nitrofurantoin (PO) (UTIs only)	Common pathogen, usually from GI/ GU source. Many strains are resistant to ampicillin and some to 1st generation cephalosporins. ESBL-producing E. coli may be treated with ampicillin/sulbactam, cefepime, imipenem, meropenem ± amikacin

C = colonizer; C* = skin contaminant; NP = non-pathogen at site; P = pathogen at site; (IV/PO) = IV or PO. See p. 1 for all other abbreviations

Table 1. Clinical Significance of AEROBIC Isolates Pending Susceptibility Testing (cont'd)

GRAM-NEGATIVE BACILLI

Isolate	Isolate Significance	Preferred Therapy	Alternate Therapy	Comments
Francisella tularensis	• CSF = NP • Blood = P (isolation required; dangerous) • Sputum = P (tularemic pneumonia; isolation required; dangerous) • Urine/Stool = NP • Wound = P (isolation required; dangerous)	Doxycycline (IV/PO) Gentamicin (IV/IM) Streptomycin (IM)	Chloramphenicol (IV/PO) Any quinolone (IV/PO)	Six clinical tularemia syndromes. Alert microbiology laboratory of potentially biohazardous specimens. Do not culture. Resistant to penicillins and cephalosporins. Bioterrorist tularemia is treated the same as naturally-acquired tularemia
Hafnia alvei	• CSF = C, P (from NS procedure) • Blood = C*, P (from IV line/ urinary tract infection) • Sputum = C (not pneumonia) • Urine = C, P (post-urologic instrumentation) • Stool = NP • Wound = C, P (rarely in compromised hosts)	Cefepime (IV) Any quinolone (IV/PO)/ Aztreonam (IV)	Piperacillin/tazobactam (IV) Imipenem (IV) Meropenem (IV)	Formerly Enterobacter hafniae. Uncommon nosocomial pathogen. Rarely pathogenic in normal hosts. Cause of UTIs in compromised hosts
Helicobacter (Campylobacter) pylori	• CSF = NP • Blood = NP • Sputum = NP • Urine = NP • Stool = P (from upper GI tract biopsy specimens, not stool) • Wound = NP	Omeprazole (PO) + clarithromycin XL (PO) Omeprazole (PO) + amoxicillin (PO) Metronidazole (PO) + amoxicillin (PO) + bismuth subsalicylate (PO)	Doxycycline (PO) + metronidazole (PO) + bismuth subsalicylate (PO)	Do not treat H. pylori gastritis, only peptic ulcer disease and MALT lymphomas. Optimal therapy awaits definition. Treat until cured. Some strains of clarithromycin-resistant H. pylori may respond to re-treatment with higher clarithromycin doses. TMP-SMX is ineffective

C = colonizer; C* = skin contaminant; NP = non-pathogen at site; P = pathogen at site; (IV/PO) = IV or PO. See p. 1 for all other abbreviations

Table 1. Clinical Significance of AEROBIC Isolates Pending Susceptibility Testing (cont'd)

GRAM-NEGATIVE BACILLI

Isolate	Isolate Significance	Preferred Therapy	Alternate Therapy	Comments
Hemophilus influenzae, parainfluenzae, aphrophilus, paraphrophilus	• CSF = P (ABM) • Blood = P (from respiratory tract or cardiac source) • Sputum = C, P (CAP) • Urine = NP • Stool = NP • Wound = NP	**Ampicillin-sensitive H. influenzae** Any 2nd,3rd generation cephalosporin (IV/PO) Any quinolone (IV/PO) Telithromycin (PO) Doxycycline (IV/PO) **Ampicillin-resistant H. influenzae** Any 2nd,3rd generation cephalosporin (IV/PO) Any quinolone (IV/PO) Telithromycin (PO) Doxycycline (IV/PO)	**For all Hemophilus species** Chloramphenicol (IV) TMP-SMX (IV/PO) Azithromycin (PO) Aztreonam (IV) **Ampicillin-resistant H. influenzae** Meropenem (IV) Imipenem (IV) Ertapenem (IV) Aztreonam (IV) Cefepime (IV)	1st generation cephalosporins, erythromycin, and clarithromycin have limited anti-H. influenzae activity; doxycycline and azithromycin are better. Hemophilus species are common colonizers of the respiratory tract. Rarely a cause of "culture-negative" SBE (H. parainfluenzae/aphrophilus are HACEK organisms). Growth enhanced with CO_2. Penicillin has little anti-H. influenzae activity
Kingella (Moraxella) kingae	• CSF = NP • Blood = P (from skeletal or cardiac source) • Sputum = C • Urine = NP • Stool/wound = NP	Ampicillin (IV) + any aminoglycoside (IV)	Any 3rd generation (IV) cephalosporin + any aminoglycoside (IV) Imipenem (IV) Meropenem (IV) Any quinolone (IV/PO)	Common colonizer of respiratory tract, but rarely a respiratory pathogen. Causes septic arthritis/osteomyelitis in children and endocarditis in adults (one of HACEK organisms). Oxidase positive. Growth enhanced with CO_2
Klebsiella pneumoniae, oxytoca	• CSF = P (ABM) • Blood = P (from respiratory, GI, GU source) • Sputum = C, P (CAP/VAP), P • Urine = C (CAB), P • Stool = NP • Wound = C, P (cellulitis)	Ceftriaxone (IV) Cefepime (IV) Meropenem (IV) Ertapenem (IV) Any quinolone (IV/PO)	Piperacillin/tazobactam (IV) Any 3rd generation cephalosporin (IV,PO) Aztreonam (IV)	TMP-SMX may be ineffective in systemic infection, but is acceptable for UTIs. Anti-pseudomonal penicillins have limited anti-Klebsiella activity. ESBL-producing Klebsiella may be treated with ampicillin/sulbactam, cefepime, imipenem, meropenem ± amikacin

C = colonizer; C* = skin contaminant; NP = non-pathogen at site; P = pathogen at site; (IV/PO) = IV or PO. See p. 1 for all other abbreviations

Table 1. Clinical Significance of AEROBIC Isolates Pending Susceptibility Testing (cont'd)

GRAM-NEGATIVE BACILLI

Isolate	Isolate Significance	Preferred Therapy	Alternate Therapy	Comments
Klebsiella ozaenae, rhinoscleromatis	• CSF = NP • Blood = NP • Sputum = NP • Urine = NP • Stool = NP • Wound = P (rhinoscleromatis lesions)	Any quinolone (PO)	TMP-SMX (PO) + rifampin (PO)	Skin infection usually requires prolonged treatment for cure (weeks-to-months)
Legionella sp.	• CSF = NP • Blood = NP • Sputum = P (CAP or VAP) • Urine = NP • Stool = NP • Wound = NP	Any quinolone (IV/PO) Doxycycline (IV/PO) Telithromycin (PO) Azithromycin (IV/PO)	Clarithromycin XL (PO) Erythromycin (IV)	Anti-Legionella activity: respiratory quinolones > doxycycline > erythromycin. Erythromycin failures are not uncommon. In compromised hosts (e.g., organ transplants), optimal treatment is a quinolone plus azithromycin. Rarely a cause of culture-negative SBE/PVE
Leptospira interrogans	• CSF = P (ABM) • Blood = P (1° bacteremia) • Sputum = NP • Urine = P (excreted in urine) • Stool = NP • Wound = NP	Doxycycline (IV/PO) Penicillin G (IV)	Amoxicillin (PO)	Blood/urine cultures may be positive during initial/bacteremic phase, but are negative during immune phase. Relapse is common. Resistant to chloramphenicol
Moraxella (Branhamella) catarrhalis	• CSF = NP • Blood = P (rarely from CAP) • Sputum = C, P (CAP) • Urine = NP • Stool = NP • Wound = NP	Any 2nd, 3rd generation cephalosporin (IV/PO) Any quinolone (IV/PO) Telithromycin (PO) Doxycycline (IV/PO)	Azithromycin (PO) Clarithromycin XL (PO) TMP-SMX (IV/PO)	Almost all strains are β-lactamase positive and resistant to penicillin/ampicillin. β-lactamase-resistant β-lactams are effective

C = colonizer; C* = skin contaminant; NP = non-pathogen at site; P = pathogen at site; (IV/PO) = IV or PO. See p. 1 for all other abbreviations

Table 1. Clinical Significance of AEROBIC Isolates Pending Susceptibility Testing (cont'd)

GRAM-NEGATIVE BACILLI

Isolate	Isolate Significance	Preferred Therapy	Alternate Therapy	Comments
Morganella morganii	• CSF = NP • Blood = P (from GU source) • Sputum = NP • Urine = P (CAB, cystitis, pyelonephritis) • Stool = NP • Wound = P (cellulitis rare)	Any quinolone (IV/PO) Any 3rd generation cephalosporin (IV) Cefepime (IV) Meropenem (IV) Ertapenem (IV)	Any aminoglycoside (IV) Aztreonam (IV) Imipenem (IV)	Common uropathogen. Causes bacteremia with urosepsis. Rare cause of wound infections
Ochrobactrum anthropi (CDC group Vd)	• CSF = NP • Blood = P (from IV line infections) • Sputum = C • Urine = C • Stool/Wound = C	Any quinolone (IV/PO) TMP-SMX (IV/PO)	Any aminoglycoside (IV) Imipenem (IV) Meropenem (IV)	Pathogen in compromised hosts. Oxidase and catalase positive. Resistant to β-lactams
Pasteurella multocida	• CSF = P (ABM) • Blood = P (from respiratory source, bite wound/abscess) • Sputum = C, P (CAP) • Urine = C, P (pyelonephritis) • Stool = NP • Wound = P (human/animal bites)	Amoxicillin (PO) Doxycycline (IV/PO) Penicillin G (IV)	Ampicillin/sulbactam (IV) Piperacillin/tazobactam (IV) Any quinolone (IV/PO)	Common cause of infection following dog/cat bites. Many antibiotics are effective, but erythromycin is ineffective
Plesiomonas shigelloides	• CSF = NP • Blood = P (from GU source) • Sputum = NP • Urine = NP • Stool = P (diarrhea) • Wound = NP	Any quinolone (PO) TMP-SMX (PO)	Doxycycline (PO) Aztreonam (PO)	Infrequent cause of diarrhea, less commonly dysentery. Oxidase positive. β-lactamase strains are increasing. Resistant to penicillins

C = colonizer; C* = skin contaminant; NP = non-pathogen at site; P = pathogen at site; (IV/PO) = IV or PO. See p. 1 for all other abbreviations

Table 1. Clinical Significance of AEROBIC Isolates Pending Susceptibility Testing (cont'd)

GRAM-NEGATIVE BACILLI

Isolate	Isolate Significance	Preferred Therapy	Alternate Therapy	Comments
Proteus mirabilis, vulgaris	• CSF = NP • Blood = P (from urinary source) • Sputum = C • Urine = C, P (from urologic instrumentation) • Stool = NP • Wound = C, P (wound infection)	<u>P. mirabilis, indole (−)</u> Ampicillin (IV) Any 1st, 2nd, 3rd gen. cephalosporin (IV/PO) <u>P. vulgaris, indole (+)</u> Any 3rd generation cephalosporin (IV/PO) Cefepime (IV) Any quinolone (IV/PO)	<u>P. mirabilis, indole (−)</u> TMP-SMX (IV/PO) Amoxicillin (PO) <u>P. vulgaris, indole (+)</u> Aztreonam (IV) Imipenem (IV) Meropenem (IV) Ertapenem (IV) Any aminoglycoside (IV)	Usually a uropathogen. Most antibiotics are effective against P. mirabilis (indole-negative), but indole-positive Proteus require potent antibiotics to treat non-UTIs
Providencia alcalifaciens, rettgeri, stuartii	• CSF = NP • Blood = C*, P (from GU source) • Sputum/Stool = NP • Urine = C, P • Wound = C, P (rare)	Any quinolone (IV/PO) Any 3rd generation cephalosporin (IV/PO) Cefepime (IV) Meropenem (IV) Ertapenem (IV)	Any aminoglycoside (IV) Aztreonam (IV) Piperacillin/tazobactam (IV) Imipenem (IV)	Almost always a uropathogen. Formerly classified as indole-positive Proteus
Pseudomonas aeruginosa	• CSF = NP • Blood = P (from respiratory, GU source) • Sputum = C (usually), P (rarely indicates VAP) • Urine = C, P (from urologic instrumentation) • Stool = NP • Wound = C (almost always)	<u>Monotherapy</u> Meropenem (IV) Cefepime (IV) Piperacillin/ tazobactam (IV) <u>Combination therapy</u> Meropenem (IV) or cefepime (IV) or piperacillin/tazo-bactam (IV) plus either ciprofloxacin (IV) or gatifloxacin (IV) or levofloxacin (IV)	<u>Monotherapy</u> Amikacin (IV) Aztreonam (IV) Polymyxin B (IV) <u>Combination therapy</u> Piperacillin/ tazobactam (IV) plus either amikacin (IV) or cefepime (IV)	For serious P. aeruginosa infection, double-drug therapy is preferred. All double anti-P. aeruginosa regimens are equally effective. Individual differences in activity (MICs) are unimportant if combination therapy is used

C = colonizer; C* = skin contaminant; NP = non-pathogen at site; P = pathogen at site; (IV/PO) = IV or PO. See p. 1 for all other abbreviations

Table 1. Clinical Significance of AEROBIC Isolates Pending Susceptibility Testing (cont'd)

			GRAM-NEGATIVE BACILLI		
Isolate	Isolate Significance	Preferred Therapy	Alternate Therapy	Comments	
Pseudomonas (Chryseomonas) luteola (CDC group Ve-1)	• CSF = NP • Blood = P (from IV line infection) • Sputum = NP • Urine = NP • Stool = NP • Wound = NP	Imipenem (IV) Meropenem (IV) Cefepime (IV)	Piperacillin/tazobactam (IV) Aztreonam (IV)	Opportunistic pathogen primarily in compromised hosts	
Pseudomonas (Flavimonas) oryzihabitans (CDC group Ve-2)	• CSF = P (NS procedures) • Blood = P (from IV line infection) • Sputum = NP • Urine = NP • Stool = NP • Wound = P (rare)	Imipenem (IV) Meropenem (IV) Cefepime (IV)	Any 3rd generation cephalosporin (IV) Piperacillin/tazobactam (IV) Aztreonam (IV)	Rare cause of central IV line infections in compromised hosts (usually in febrile neutropenics). Rare cause of peritonitis in CAPD patients. Oxidase negative, unlike other Pseudomonas species	
Salmonella typhi, non-typhi	• CSF = NP • Blood = P (from GI source) • Sputum = NP • Urine = P (only with enteric fever) • Stool = C (carrier), P (gastroenteritis, enteric fever) • Wound = NP	Any quinolone (IV/PO) Any 3rd generation cephalosporin (IV)	Chloramphenicol (IV) TMP-SMX (IV/PO) Doxycycline (IV/PO)	Carrier state is best eliminated by a quinolone or TMP-SMX. If drug therapy fails to eliminate carrier state, look for hepatic/bladder calculi for persistent focus. Many strains are resistant to ampicillin/amoxicillin	

C = colonizer; C* = skin contaminant; NP = non-pathogen; P = pathogen at site; (IV/PO) = IV or PO. See p. 1 for all other abbreviations

Table 1. Clinical Significance of AEROBIC Isolates Pending Susceptibility Testing (cont'd)

Isolate	Isolate Significance	Preferred Therapy	Alternate Therapy	Comments
		GRAM-NEGATIVE BACILLI		
Serratia marcescens	• CSF = P (from NS procedures) • Blood = P (from IV line or urinary source) • Sputum = C, P (rarely in VAP) • Urine = C, P (post-urologic instrumentation) • Stool = NP • Wound = C, P (rare)	Any 3rd generation cephalosporin (IV/PO) (except ceftazidime) Any quinolone (IV/PO) Cefepime (IV)	Imipenem (IV) Meropenem (IV) Ertapenem (IV) Gentamicin (IV) Aztreonam (IV) Piperacillin/tazobactam (IV)	Enterobacteriaceae. Associated with water sources. Common colonizer of respiratory secretions/urine in ICU. Serratia nosocomial pneumonia and PVE are rare. Cause of septic arthritis, osteomyelitis, and SBE (IV drug abusers). Among aminoglycosides, gentamicin has the greatest anti-Serratia activity
Shigella boydii, sonnei, flexneri, dysenteriae	• CSF = NP • Blood = P (from GI source) • Sputum = NP • Urine = NP • Stool = P (Shigella dysentery) • Wound = NP	Any quinolone (IV/PO)	TMP-SMX (IV/PO) Azithromycin (IV/PO)	No carrier state. Severity of dysentery varies with the species: S. dysenteriae (most severe) > S. flexneri > S. sonnei/boydii (least severe)
Stenotrophomonas (Xanthomonas, Pseudomonas) maltophilia	• CSF = C, P (from NS procedures) • Blood = C*, P (from IV line infection, GU source) • Sputum = C (not VAP) • Urine = C, P (from urologic instrumentation) • Stool = NP • Wound = C, P (rarely in compromised hosts)	TMP-SMX (IV/PO) Ticarcillin/clavulanic acid (IV)	Minocycline (IV/PO) Aztreonam (IV) Ceftazidime (IV)	Not a cause of community-acquired or nosocomial pneumonia. Potential pulmonary pathogen only in bronchiectasis/cystic fibrosis. Resistant to aminoglycosides

C = colonizer; C* = skin contaminant; NP = non-pathogen at site; P = pathogen at site; (IV/PO) = IV or PO. See p. 1 for all other abbreviations

Table 1. Clinical Significance of AEROBIC Isolates Pending Susceptibility Testing (cont'd)

GRAM-NEGATIVE BACILLI

Isolate	Isolate Significance	Preferred Therapy	Alternate Therapy	Comments
Streptobacillus moniliformis	• CSF = P (brain abscess) • Blood = P (from wound) • Sputum = P (lung abscess) • Urine = NP • Stool = NP • Wound = P (from rat bite)	Penicillin (IV) Ampicillin (IV) Amoxicillin (PO)	Doxycycline (IV/PO) Erythromycin (IV) Clindamycin (IV/PO)	Cause of Haverhill fever and rat-bite fever, with abrupt onset of severe headache/arthralgias after bite wound has healed. Morbilliform/petechial rash. Arthritis in 50%. May cause SBE
Vibrio cholerae	• CSF = NP • Blood = P (from GI source) • Sputum = NP • Urine = NP • Stool = P (cholera) • Wound = NP	Doxycycline (IV/PO) Any quinolone (IV/PO)	TMP-SMX (IV/PO)	No carrier state. Treat for 3 days. Single-dose therapy is often effective. Resistant to ampicillin
Vibrio parahaemolyticus	• CSF = NP • Blood = P (from GI source) • Sputum = NP • Urine = NP • Stool = P (diarrhea) • Wound = P	Doxycycline (IV/PO)	Any quinolone (IV/PO)	Most cases of gastroenteritis caused by V. parahaemolyticus are self-limited and require no treatment
Vibrio vulnificus, alginolyticus	• CSF = NP • Blood = P (from GI/wound source) • Sputum = NP • Urine = NP • Stool = P (diarrhea) • Wound = P (water-contaminated wound)	Doxycycline (IV/PO) Any quinolone (IV/PO)	Piperacillin/tazobactam (IV) Ampicillin/sulbactam (IV)	Causes necrotizing soft tissue infection resembling gas gangrene. Patients are critically ill with fever, bullous lesions, diarrhea, and hypotension. Treat wound infection, bacteremia. Aminoglycoside susceptibilities are unpredictable

C = colonizer; C* = skin contaminant; NP = non-pathogen at site; P = pathogen at site; (IV/PO) = IV or PO. See p. 1 for all other abbreviations

Table 1. Clinical Significance of AEROBIC Isolates Pending Susceptibility Testing (cont'd)

GRAM-NEGATIVE BACILLI

Isolate	Isolate Significance	Preferred Therapy	Alternate Therapy	Comments
Yersinia enterocolitica	• CSF = NP • Blood = P (from GI source) • Sputum = NP • Urine = NP • Stool = P (diarrhea) • Wound = NP	Any quinolone (IV/PO) Gentamicin (IV) Doxycycline (IV/PO)	TMP-SMX (IV/PO) Any 3rd generation cephalosporin (IV/PO)	Cause of diarrhea with abdominal pain. If pain in is right lower quadrant, may be mistaken for acute appendicitis
Yersinia pestis	• CSF = NP • Blood = P (septicemic plague; isolation required; dangerous) • Sputum = P (pneumonic plague; isolation required; dangerous) • Urine = NP • Stool = NP • Wound = P (lymph nodes, lymph node drainage; bubonic plague; isolation required; dangerous)	Doxycycline (IV/PO) Streptomycin (IM)	Chloramphenicol (IV) Gentamicin (IV)	Cause of bubonic, septicemic, and pneumonic plagues. Doxycycline may be used for prophylaxis. Alert microbiology laboratory of potentially biohazardous specimens. Do not culture. Bioterrorist plague is treated the same as naturally-acquired plague

C = colonizer; C* = skin contaminant; NP = non-pathogen at site; P = pathogen at site; (IV/PO) = IV or PO. See p. 1 for all other abbreviations

Table 1. Clinical Significance of AEROBIC Isolates Pending Susceptibility Testing (cont'd)

SPIROCHETES

Isolate	Isolate Significance	Preferred Therapy	Alternate Therapy	Comments
Borrelia burgdorferi	• CSF = P (neuroborreliosis) • Blood = P (rarely isolated; requires special media) • Sputum = NP • Urine = NP • Stool = NP • Wound = P (rarely isolated from erythema migrans lesions)	Doxycycline (PO) Amoxicillin (PO)	Any cephalosporin (PO) Azithromycin (PO) Erythromycin (PO)	Cause of Lyme disease. β-lactams and doxycycline are effective. Erythromycin least effective for erythema migrans. Minocycline may be better than doxycycline for CNS Lyme disease
Borrelia recurrentis	• CSF = P (ABM) • Blood = P (1° bacteremia) • Sputum = NP • Urine = NP • Stool = NP • Wound = NP	Doxycycline (IV/PO) Azithromycin (IV/PO)	Erythromycin (IV) Penicillin (IV) Ampicillin (IV) Any 1st,2nd,3rd generation cephalosporin (IV/PO)	Cause of relapsing fever. May be recovered from septic metastatic foci. Septic emboli may cause sacroilitis, SBE, myositis, orchitis, or osteomyelitis.
Spirillum minus	• CSF = NP • Blood = P (from wound source, SBE) • Sputum = NP • Urine = NP • Stool = NP • Wound = P (from rat bite)	Penicillin (IV) Amoxicillin (PO)	Doxycycline (IV/PO) Any quinolone (IV/PO)	Cause of rat-bite fever. Bite wound heals promptly, but 1-4 weeks later becomes painful, purple and swollen, and progresses to ulceration and eschar formation. Painful regional adenopathy. Central maculopapular rash is common (rarely urticarial). Arthralgias/arthritis is rare compared to rat-bite fever from Streptobacillus moniliformis. Rarely causes SBE

C = colonizer; C* = skin contaminant; NP = non-pathogen at site; P = pathogen at site; (IV/PO) = IV or PO. See p. 1 for all other abbreviations

Table 2. Clinical Significance of CAPNOPHILIC Isolates Pending Susceptibility Testing

		GRAM-NEGATIVE BACILLI		
Isolate	Isolate Significance	Preferred Therapy	Alternate Therapy	Comments
Capnocytophaga canimorsus (CDC group DF-2)	• CSF = NP • Blood = P (from GI source, bite wound) • Sputum = NP • Urine = NP • Stool = NP • Wound = P (from dog/cat bite)	Ampicillin/sulbactam (IV) Piperacillin/tazobactam (IV) Imipenem (IV) Meropenem (IV) Ertapenem (IV)	Clindamycin (IV/PO) Any quinolone (IV/PO) Doxycycline (IV/PO)	Associated with animal bites or cancer. May cause fatal septicemia in cirrhotics/asplenics. Resistant to aminoglycosides, metronidazole, TMP-SMX, and aztreonam
Capnocytophaga ochraceus (CDC group DF-1)	• CSF = NP • Blood = P (from GI, wound, abscess source) • Sputum = NP • Urine = NP • Stool = NP • Wound = P	Ampicillin/sulbactam (IV) Piperacillin/tazobactam (IV) Imipenem (IV) Meropenem (IV) Ertapenem (IV)	Clindamycin (IV/PO) Any quinolone (IV/PO) Doxycycline (IV/PO)	Thin, spindle-shaped bacilli resemble Fusobacteria morphologically. "Gliding motility" seen in hanging drop preparations. Cause of septicemia, abscesses, and wound infections. Resistant to aminoglycosides, metronidazole, TMP-SMX, and aztreonam
Eikenella corrodens	• CSF = NP • Blood = P (SBE in IV drug abusers) • Sputum = NP • Urine = NP • Stool = NP • Wound = P (IV drug abusers)	Penicillin (IV) Ampicillin (IV) Imipenem (IV) Meropenem (IV) Ertapenem (IV)	Piperacillin/tazobactam (IV) Ampicillin/sulbactam (IV) Doxycycline (IV/PO) Amoxicillin (PO)	Cause of "culture-negative" SBE (one of the HACEK organisms). Resistant to clindamycin and metronidazole

C = colonizer; C* = skin contaminant; P = pathogen at site; P = pathogen at site; NP = non-pathogen at site; (IV/PO) = IV or PO. See p. 1 for all other abbreviations

Table 3. Clinical Significance of ANAEROBIC Isolates Pending Susceptibility Testing

GRAM-POSITIVE COCCI (CHAINS)

Isolate	Isolate Significance	Preferred Therapy	Alternate Therapy	Comments
Peptococcus	• CSF = P (brain abscess) • Blood = P (from GI/pelvic source) • Sputum = C, P (aspiration pneumonia, lung abscess) • Urine/Stool = NP • Wound = P (rarely a sole pathogen)	Penicillin (IV) Ampicillin (IV) Amoxicillin (PO) Clindamycin (IV/PO)	Chloramphenicol (IV) Erythromycin (IV) Imipenem (IV) Meropenem (IV) Ertapenem (IV) Moxifloxacin (IV/PO)	Normal flora of mouth, GI tract, and pelvis. Associated with mixed aerobic/anaerobic dental, abdominal, and pelvic infections, especially abscesses
Pepto-streptococcus	• CSF = P (brain abscess) • Blood = P (GI/pelvic source) • Sputum = C, P (aspiration pneumonia, lung abscess) • Urine/Stool = NP • Wound = P (rarely a sole pathogen)	Penicillin (IV) Ampicillin (IV) Amoxicillin (PO) Clindamycin (IV/PO)	Chloramphenicol (IV) Erythromycin (IV) Imipenem (IV) Meropenem (IV) Ertapenem (IV) Moxifloxacin (IV/PO)	Normal flora of mouth, GI tract, and pelvis. Associated with mixed aerobic/anaerobic dental, abdominal, and pelvic infections, especially abscesses

GRAM-POSITIVE BACILLI

Isolate	Isolate Significance	Preferred Therapy	Alternate Therapy	Comments
Actinomyces israelii, odontolyticus	• CSF = P (brain abscess) • Blood = NP • Sputum = C, P (lung abscess) • Urine = NP • Stool = NP • Wound = P (fistulas/ underlying abscess)	Amoxicillin (PO) Doxycycline (PO)	Erythromycin (PO) Clindamycin (PO)	Anaerobic and non-acid fast. Usually presents as cervical, facial, thoracic, or abdominal masses/fistulas. Prolonged (6-12 month) treatment is needed for cure. Unlike Nocardia, Actinomyces rarely causes CNS infections. May be cultured from polymicrobial brain abscess of pulmonary origin. Quinolones, aminoglycosides, metronidazole, and TMP-SMX have little activity

C = colonizer; C* = skin contaminant; NP = non-pathogen at site; P = pathogen at site; (IV/PO) = IV or PO. See p. 1 for all other abbreviations

Table 3. Clinical Significance of ANAEROBIC Isolates Pending Susceptibility Testing (cont'd)

GRAM–POSITIVE BACILLI

Isolate	Isolate Significance	Preferred Therapy	Alternate Therapy	Comments
Arachnia propionica	• CSF = P (brain abscess) • Blood = P (from dental, GI, lung source) • Sputum = C, P (lung abscess) • Urine = NP • Stool = NP • Wound = NP	Clindamycin (IV/PO) Ampicillin (IV) + gentamicin (IV)	Erythromycin (IV)	Polymicrobial pathogen in dental, lung, and brain abscesses
Bifidobacterium sp.	• CSF = P (brain abscess) • Blood = NP • Sputum = C, P (lung abscess) • Urine/Stool = NP • Wound = NP	Clindamycin (IV/PO) Ampicillin (IV) + gentamicin (IV)	Erythromycin (IV)	Usually part of polymicrobial infection
Clostridium botulinum	• CSF = NP • Blood = NP • Sputum = NP • Urine/Stool = NP • Wound = P (wound botulism)	Penicillin (IV)	Clindamycin (IV/PO) Imipenem (IV) Meropenem (IV)	Give trivalent equine antitoxin (p. 131) as soon as possible. Antibiotic therapy is adjunctive
Clostridium difficile	• CSF = NP • Blood = P (rarely from GI source) • Sputum = NP • Urine = NP • Stool = C (normal fecal flora), P (antibiotic-associated diarrhea/colitis) • Wound = NP	Antibiotic-associated diarrhea (AAD) Vancomycin (PO) Antibiotic-associated colitis (AAC) Metronidazole (IV)	Antibiotic-associated diarrhea (AAD) Metronidazole (PO) Antibiotic-associated colitis (AAC) Metronidazole (PO)	For C. difficile diarrhea, PO vancomycin is more consistently effective than PO metronidazole. For C. difficile colitis, use IV or PO metronidazole (IV/PO vancomycin is ineffective). Diagnose AAD by stool C. difficile toxin assay, not stool culture

C = colonizer; C* = skin contaminant; NP = non-pathogen at site; P = pathogen at site; (IV/PO) = IV or PO. See p. 1 for all other abbreviations

Table 3. Clinical Significance of ANAEROBIC Isolates Pending Susceptibility Testing (cont'd)

GRAM-POSITIVE BACILLI

Isolate	Isolate Significance	Preferred Therapy	Alternate Therapy	Comments
Clostridium perfringens, septicum, novyi	• CSF = NP • Blood = P (from GI source/malignancy) • Sputum = NP • Urine = NP • Stool = NP • Wound = P (gas gangrene)	Penicillin (IV) Piperacillin/tazobactam (IV) Meropenem (IV) Ertapenem (IV)	Clindamycin (IV) Chloramphenicol (IV) Imipenem (IV)	Usual cause of myonecrosis (gas gangrene). Surgical debridement is crucial; antibiotic therapy is adjunctive. Also causes emphysematous cholecystitis/cystitis
Clostridium tetani	• CSF = NP • Blood = NP • Sputum = NP • Urine/Stool = NP • Wound = P (wound tetanus)	Penicillin (IV) Clindamycin (IV)	Imipenem (IV) Meropenem (IV)	Prompt administration of tetanus immune globulin is crucial (p. 131). Antibiotic therapy is adjunctive
Eubacterium sp.	• CSF = P (brain abscess) • Blood = P (from dental, GI, GU, lung source) • Sputum = P (lung abscess) • Urine/Stool = NP • Wound = NP	Clindamycin (IV/PO) Ampicillin (IV) + gentamicin (IV)	Erythromycin (IV)	Pathogen in lung/pelvic/brain abscesses, and chronic periodontal disease. Eubacterium bacteremias are associated with malignancies
Lactobacillus sp.	• CSF = P (ABM) • Blood = P (1° bacteremia, SBE, or from endometritis) • Sputum = NP • Urine = P (rare) • Stool = NP • Wound = NP	Ampicillin (IV) + gentamicin (IV) Clindamycin (IV/PO)	Erythromycin (IV)	Uncommon pathogen in normal/compromised hosts. Rare cause of SBE. Variably resistant to cephalosporins and quinolones. Some clindamycin-resistant strains. Resistant to metronidazole and vancomycin

C = colonizer; C* = skin contaminant; NP = non-pathogen at site; P = pathogen at site; (IV/PO) = IV or PO. See p. 1 for all other abbreviations

Table 3. Clinical Significance of ANAEROBIC Isolates Pending Susceptibility Testing (cont'd)

GRAM–POSITIVE BACILLI

Isolate	Isolate Significance	Preferred Therapy	Alternate Therapy	Comments
Propionibacterium acnes	• CSF = C*, P (meningitis from NS shunts) • Blood = C*, P (from IV line infection), SBE) • Sputum = NP • Urine = NP • Stool = NP • Wound = C (acne)	Penicillin (IV) Clindamycin (IV/PO)	Doxycycline (IV/PO)	Common skin colonizer/blood culture contaminant. Rarely causes prosthetic joint infection, endocarditis, or CNS shunt infection

GRAM–NEGATIVE BACILLI

Isolate	Isolate Significance	Preferred Therapy	Alternate Therapy	Comments
Bacteroides fragilis group (B. distasonis, ovatus, thetaiotao-micron, vulgatus)	• CSF = P (meningitis from Strongyloides hyperinfection) • Blood = P (from GI/pelvic source) • Sputum = NP • Urine = NP, P (only from colonic fistula) • Stool = NP • Wound = NP	Meropenem (IV) Piperacillin/tazobactam (IV) Ertapenem (IV)	Imipenem (IV) Clindamycin (IV/PO) or metronidazole (IV/PO) plus either ciprofloxacin (IV/PO) or gatifloxacin (IV/PO) or levofloxacin (IV/PO) Moxifloxacin (IV/PO) Ampicillin/sulbactam (IV)	Major anaerobe below the diaphragm. Usually part of polymicrobial lower intra-abdominal and pelvic infections. Cefotetan is less effective against B. fragilis DOT strains (B. distasonis, B. ovatus, B. thetaiotaomicron). Resistant to penicillin
Fusobacterium nucleatum	• CSF = P (brain abscess) • Blood = P (from lung, GI source) • Sputum = P (aspiration pneumonia, lung abscess) • Urine = NP • Stool = NP • Wound = P (rarely)	Clindamycin (IV/PO) Piperacillin/tazobactam (IV) Ampicillin/sulbactam (IV)	Chloramphenicol (IV) Metronidazole (IV/PO)	Mouth flora associated with dental infections and anaerobic lung infections. F. nucleatum is associated with jugular vein septic phlebitis and GI cancer

C = colonizer; C* = skin contaminant; P = pathogen at site; NP = non-pathogen at site; (IV/PO) = IV or PO. See p. 1 for all other abbreviations

Table 3. Clinical Significance of ANAEROBIC Isolates Pending Susceptibility Testing (cont'd)

Isolate	Isolate Significance	Preferred Therapy	Alternate Therapy	Comments
Prevotella (Bacteroides) bivia	• CSF = NP • Blood = P (from dental, lung, pelvic source) • Sputum = P (lung abscess) • Urine = NP • Stool = NP • Wound = NP	Penicillin (IV/PO) Any β-lactam (IV/PO)	Any quinolone (IV/PO) Doxycycline (IV/PO) Clindamycin (IV/PO)	Cause of dental, oropharyngeal, and female genital tract infections
Prevotella (Bacteroides) melaninogenicus, intermedius	• CSF = P (brain abscess) • Blood = P (from oral/pulmonary source) • Sputum = P (from aspiration pneumonia, lung abscess) • Urine = NP • Stool = NP • Wound = NP	_Aspiration pneumonia/ lung abscess_ Any β-lactam (IV/PO) Any quinolone (IV/PO) _Brain abscess_ Penicillin (IV)	_Aspiration pneumonia/ lung abscess_ Doxycycline (IV/PO) _Brain abscess_ Chloramphenicol (IV)	Predominant anaerobic flora of mouth. Known as "oral pigmented" Bacteroides (e.g., B. melanogenicus). Antibiotics used to treat community-acquired pneumonia are effective against oral anaerobes (e.g., Prevotella) in aspiration pneumonia; does not require anti-B. fragilis coverage with clindamycin, metronidazole, or moxifloxacin

C = colonizer; C* = skin contaminant; NP = non-pathogen at site; P = pathogen at site; (IV/PO) = IV or PO. See p. 1 for all other abbreviations

GRAM-NEGATIVE BACILLI

Table 4. Clinical Significance of YEAST/FUNGI Pending Susceptibility Testing

Isolate	Isolate Significance	Preferred Therapy	Alternate Therapy	Comments
		YEAST/FUNGI		
Aspergillus species	• CSF = P (only from disseminated infection) • Blood = C, P (1° fungemia or from pulmonary source) • Sputum = C, P (pneumonia) • Urine = NP • Stool = NP • Wound = NP	Voriconazole (IV/PO) Caspofungin (IV/PO) Itraconazole (IV/PO)	Amphotericin B deoxycholate (IV) Amphotericin B lipid formulation (IV)	A. fumigatus is the usual cause of invasive aspergillosis. Growth of Aspergillus sp. from a specimen can represent airborne contamination, but repeated growth or growth from a significantly immunocompromised patient with a consistent syndrome should be considered as evidence of possible infection. Aspergillus pneumonia and disseminated aspergillosis are common in patients receiving chronic steroids or immunosuppressive therapy (esp. organ transplants). Recovery of Aspergillus from respiratory tract is not diagnostic of Aspergillus pneumonia; tissue biopsy is required for diagnosis
Candida non-albicans group	• CSF = P (only from disseminated infection) • Blood = P (1° candidemia or from IV line infection) • Sputum = NP • Urine = C (indwelling catheters), P (from cystitis, pyelonephritis) • Stool = C (source of candiduria) • Wound = NP	Caspofungin (IV) Voriconazole (IV/PO) Itraconazole (IV/PO)	Fluconazole (IV/PO) Amphotericin B deoxycholate (IV/PO) Amphotericin B lipid formulation (IV)	Non-albicans Candida cause the same spectrum of invasive disease as C. albicans. Fluconazole-susceptibility varies predictably by species. C. glabrata (usually) and C. krusei (almost always) are resistant to fluconazole. C. lusitaniae is often resistant to amphotericin B (deoxycholate and lipid-associated formulations). Other species are generally susceptible to all agents

C = colonizer; C* = skin contaminant; NP = non-pathogen at site; P = pathogen at site; (IV/PO) = IV or PO. See p. 1 for all other abbreviations

Table 4. Clinical Significance of YEAST/FUNGI Pending Susceptibility Testing (cont'd)

YEAST/FUNGI

Isolate	Isolate Significance	Preferred Therapy	Alternate Therapy	Comments
Candida albicans	• CSF = P (only from disseminated infection) • Blood = P (1° candidemia or from IV line infection) • Sputum = C, P (only from disseminated infection) • Urine = C, P (from cystitis, pyelonephritis) • Stool = C (source of candiduria) • Wound = NP	Fluconazole (IV/PO) Caspofungin (IV) Itraconazole (IV/PO)	Amphotericin B deoxycholate (IV/PO) Amphotericin B lipid formulation (IV)	Common colonizer of GI/GU tracts. Colonization is common in diabetics, alcoholics, and patients receiving steroids/antibiotics. Commonest cause of fungemia in hospitalized patients. Candidemia secondary to central IV lines does not prove disseminated candidiasis, but repeated blood cultures and careful follow-up (including ophthalmoscopy) should be undertaken to exclude possibile occult dissemination following even a single positive blood culture. Primary candidal pneumonia is rare
Cryptococcus neoformans	• CSF = P (meningitis, brain abscess) • Blood = P (from pulmonary source) • Sputum = P (pneumonia) • Urine = NP • Stool = NP • Wound = NP	CNS Amphotericin B deoxycholate (IV) ± flucytosine (PO) Non-CNS Amphotericin B deoxycholate (IV) Amphotericin B lipid formulation (IV)	CNS Fluconazole (IV/PO) Non-CNS Itraconazole (IV/PO) Fluconazole (IV/PO)	C. neoformans meningitis may occur with or without dissemination. Cryptococcal pneumonia frequently disseminates to CNS. C. neoformans in blood cultures occurs in compromised hosts (e.g., HIV/AIDS) and indicates disseminated infection

C = colonizer; C* = skin contaminant; NP = non-pathogen at site; P = pathogen at site; (IV/PO) = IV or PO. See p. 1 for all other abbreviations

Table 4. Clinical Significance of YEAST/FUNGI Pending Susceptibility Testing (cont'd)

YEAST/FUNGI

Isolate	Isolate Significance	Preferred Therapy	Alternate Therapy	Comments
Histoplasma capsulatum	• CSF = P (from disseminated infection, pneumonia) • Blood = P (1° fungemia, rarely SBE) • Sputum = P (pneumonia, mediastinitis) • Urine = P • Stool = P • Wound = P	Itraconazole (IV/PO) Amphotericin B deoxycholate (IV)	Fluconazole (IV/PO) Amphotericin B lipid formulation (IV)	Histoplasma recovered from CSF/blood cultures indicates dissemination. Disseminated (reactivated latent) histoplasmosis is most common in compromised hosts (e.g., HIV/AIDS). Itraconazole is ineffective for meningeal histoplasmosis, but is preferred for chronic suppressive therapy
Malassezia furfur	• CSF = NP • Blood = P (from IV line infection) • Sputum = NP • Urine = NP • Stool = NP • Wound = P (eosinophilic folliculitis)	Itraconazole (IV/PO) Ketoconazole (PO)	Fluconazole (IV/PO)	M. furfur IV line infections are associated with IV lipid hyperalimentation emulsions. Fungemia usually resolves with IV line removal. Morphology in blood is blunt buds on a broad base yeast. M. furfur requires long chain fatty acids for growth (overlay agar with thin layer of olive oil, Tween 80, or oleic acid)
Penicillium marneffei	• CSF = NP • Blood = P (usually from dissemination) • Sputum = P (pneumonia) • Urine = NP • Stool = NP • Wound = NP	Amphotericin B deoxycholate (IV) Itraconazole (IV/PO)	Amphotericin B lipid formulation (IV)	Histoplasma-like yeast forms seen in lymph nodes, liver, skin, bone marrow, blood. Characteristic red pigment diffuses into agar. Causes granulomatous tissue reaction ± necrosis. Skin lesions indicate dissemination. Rash may be papular, or resembles molluscum contagiosum with central umbilication. Hepatosplenomegaly is common. Dissemination is common in HIV

C = colonizer; C* = skin contaminant; NP = non-pathogen at site; P = pathogen at site; (IV/PO) = IV or PO. See p. 1 for all other abbreviations

Table 5. Technique for Gram Stain and Giemsa Stain

GRAM STAIN

Clinical applications: CSF, sputum, urine

Technique:
1. Place specimen on slide
2. Heat fix smear on slide by passing it quickly over a flame
3. Place crystal violet solution on slide for 20 seconds
4. Wash gently with water
5. Apply Gram iodine solution to slide for 20 seconds
6. Decolorize the slide quickly in solution of acetone/ethanol
7. Wash slide gently with water
8. Counterstain slide with safranin for 10 seconds
9. Wash gently with water; air dry or blot dry with bibulous paper

Interpretation: Gram-negative organisms stain red; gram-positive organisms stain blue. B fragilis stains weakly pink. Fungi stain deep blue. See Tables 2-5 for interpretation of Gram stain findings in CSF, urine, sputum, and feces, respectively

GIEMSA STAIN

Clinical applications: Blood, buffy coat, bone marrow

Technique:
1. Place specimen on slide
2. Fix smear by placing slide in 100% methanol for 1 minute
3. Drain methanol off slide
4. Flood slide with Giemsa stain (freshly diluted 1:10 with distilled water) for 5 minutes
5. Wash slide gently with water; air dry

Interpretation: Fungi/parasites stain light/dark blue

Table 6. Clinical Use of CSF Gram Stain, WBC Type, Glucose

Gram Stain	Organism/Condition	
Gram-positive bacilli	Pseudomeningitis (Bacillus, Corynebacteria)	Listeria
Gram-negative bacilli	H. influenzae (small, encapsulated, pleomorphic)	Non-enteric/enteric aerobic bacilli (larger, unencapsulated)
Gram-positive cocci	Gp A, B, D, streptococci (pairs/chains) S. pneumoniae (pairs)	S. aureus (pairs/clusters) S. epidermidis (pairs/clusters)
Gram-negative cocci	Neisseria meningitidis	
Mixed organisms (polymicrobial)	Pseudomeningitis Anaerobic organisms (brain abscess with meningeal leak) Iatrogenic infection	Neonatal meningitis Meningitis 2° to penetrating head trauma

WBC Type/Glucose	Organism/Condition	
Purulent CSF, no organisms	Neisseria meningitidis	S. pneumoniae
Clear CSF, no organisms	Viral meningitis TB/fungal meningitis Sarcoidosis meningitis Meningeal carcinomatosis Brain abscess Parameningeal infection Septic emboli 2° to endocarditis Lupus cerebritis Lyme's disease Rocky Mountain Spotted Fever	Lymphocytic choriomeningitis Viral encephalitis Listeria HIV Syphilis Leptospirosis Bacterial meningitis (very early/partially-treated) Meningitis in leukopenic host
Cloudy CSF, no WBCs	S. pneumoniae	
Predominantly PMNs, decreased glucose	Partially-treated bacterial meningitis Listeria Herpes (HSV-1) encephalitis Tuberculosis (early/beginning therapy) Sarcoidosis	Parameningeal infection Septic emboli 2° to endocarditis Amebic meningoencephalitis Syphilis (early) Posterior-fossa syndrome
Predominantly lymphocytes, normal glucose	Partially-treated bacterial meningitis Sarcoidosis Lyme's disease HIV Leptospirosis Rocky Mountain Spotted Fever	Viral meningitis Viral encephalitis Parameningeal infection TB/fungal meningitis Parasitic meningitis Meningeal carcinomatosis
Predominantly lymphocytes, decreased glucose	Partially-treated bacterial meningitis TB/fungal meningitis Sarcoidosis Lymphocytic choriomeningitis (LCM) Mumps	Enteroviral meningitis Listeria Leptospirosis Syphilis Meningeal carcinomatosis
Red blood cells	Traumatic tap CNS bleed/tumor Listeria Leptospirosis	TB meningitis Amebic meningoencephalitis Herpes (HSV-1) encephalitis Anthrax

Table 7. Clinical Use of the Sputum Gram Stain

Gram Stain	Organism	Comments
Gram-positive diplococci	S. pneumoniae	Coffee bean configuration (lancet-shaped) diplococci (not streptococci)
Gram-positive cocci (grape-like clusters)	S. aureus	Clusters predominant. Short chains or pairs may also be present
Gram-positive cocci (short chains or pairs)	Group A streptococci	Virulence inversely proportional to length of streptococci. Clusters not present
Gram-positive comma-shaped organisms	Nocardia	Sometimes appears like Chinese letters on Gram stain
Gram-negative cocco-bacillary organisms	H. influenzae	Plump and encapsulated (pleomorphic)
Gram-negative bacilli	Klebsiella P. aeruginosa	Plump and encapsulated Thin and often arranged in end-to-end pairs
Gram-negative diplococci	Moraxella (Branhamella) catarrhalis Neisseria meningitidis	Kidney bean-shaped diplococci

Table 8. Clinical Use of the Urine Gram Stain

Gram Stain	Organism	Comments
Gram-positive cocci (clusters)*	S. aureus S. epidermidis S. saprophyticus	Skin flora contaminant Skin flora contaminant Uropathogen

Gram-positive cocci (chains)	Group B streptococci
	Group D streptococci
	    E. faecalis
	    E. faecium
		Uropathogen
		Uropathogen
		May represent colonization or infection
		May represent colonization or infection

Gram-negative bacilli*	Coliform bacilli	Uropathogen; may represent colonization or infection
Gram-negative diplococci*	N. gonorrhoeae N. meningitidis	Gonococcal urethritis Rare cause of urethritis

* Staphylococci (except S. saprophyticus), S. pneumoniae, and B. fragilis are *not* uropathogens

Table 9. Clinical Use of the Fecal Gram Stain

Gram Stain	Possible Organisms	
Fecal leukocytes present	Enteropathogenic E. coli (EPEC) Shigella Yersinia Campylobacter Salmonella Vibrio parahaemolyticus Vibrio vulnificus	Aeromonas hydrophila Chlamydia trachomatis Plesiomonas shigelloides Neisseria gonorrhoeae Herpes simplex virus (HSV-1) *Noninfectious:* Ulcerative colitis
No fecal leukocytes	Enterovirus Rotavirus Coronavirus Enterotoxigenic E. coli (ETEC) S. aureus Clostridium perfringens Adenovirus	Norwalk virus Vibrio cholerae Bacillus cereus Giardia lamblia Isospora belli Cryptosporidia Strongyloides stercoralis
Fecal leukocytes variable	Clostridium difficile Enterohemorrhagic E. coli (EHEC)	Cytomegalovirus (CMV) Herpes simplex virus (HSV-1)
Red blood cells present	Shigella Salmonella Campylobacter EPEC EHEC Enteroinvasive E. coli (EIEC)	Clostridium difficile Cytomegalovirus (CMV) Yersinia Plesiomonas shigelloides *Noninfectious:* Ulcerative colitis

REFERENCES AND SUGGESTED READINGS

Aridan S, Paetznick V, Rex JH. Comparative evaluation of disk diffusion with microdilution assay in susceptibility of caspofungin against Aspergillus and fusarium isolates. Antimicrob Agents Chemother 46:3084-7, 2002.

Bachmann SP, Patterson TF, Lopez-Ribot JL. In vitro activity of caspofungin (MK-0991) against Candida albicans clinical isolates displaying different mechanisms of azole resistance. J Clin Microbiol 46:2228-30, 2002.

Baldis MM, Keidich SD, Mukhejee PK, et al. Mechanisms of fungal resistance: an overview. Drugs 62:1025-40, 2002.

Bartlett JG. Antibiotic-associated diarrhea. N Engl J Med 346:334-9, 2002.

Bingen E, Leclercq R, Fitoussi F, et al. Emergence of group A streptococcus strains with different mechanisms of macrolide resistance. Antimicrob Agents Chemother 46:1199-203, 2002.

Bouza E, Cercenado E. Klebsiella and enterobacter: antibiotic resistance and treatment implications. Semin Respir Infect 17:215-30, 2002.

Brueggemann AB, Coffmen SL, Rhomberg P, et al.

Fluoroquinolone resistance in Streptococcus pneumoniae in United States. Antimicrob Agents Chemother 46:680-8, 2002.

Chryssanthou E, Cuenca-Estrella M. Comparison of the antifungal susceptibility testing subcommittee of the European committee on antibiotic susceptibility testing proposed standard and the E-test with the NCCLS broth microdilution method for voriconazole and caspofungin susceptibility testing of yeast species. J Clin Microbiol 40:3841-4, 2002.

Cunha BA. MRSA & VRE: In vitro susceptibility versus in vivo efficacy. Antibiotics for Clinicians 4:31-32, 2000.

Cunha BA. The significance of antibiotic false sensitivity testing with in vitro testing. J Chemother 9:25-35, 1997.

Cunha BA. Clinical relevance of penicillin-resistant Streptococcus pneumoniae. Semin Respir Infect. 17:204-14, 2002.

Cunha BA. Pseudomonas aeruginosa: resistance and therapy. Semin Respir Infect 17:231-9, 2002.

Espinel-Ingroff A, Chaturvedi V, Fothergill A, et al. Optimal testing conditions for determining MICs and minimum fungicidal concentrations of new and established antifungal agents for uncommon molds: NCCLS collaborative study. J Clin Microbiol 40:3776-81, 2002.

Fuchs PC, Barry AL, Brown SD. Selection of zone size interpretive criterial for disk diffusion susceptibility tests of three antibiotics against Streptococcus pneumoniae, using the new guidelines of the National Committee for Clinical Laboratory Standards. Antimicrob Agents Chemother 46:398-401, 2002.

Fuchs PC, Barry AL, Brown SD. In vitro activity of telithromycin against Streptococcus pneumoniae resistant to other antibiotics, including cefotaxime. J Antimicrob Chemother 49:399-401, 2002.

Ginocchio CC. Role of NCCLS in antimicrobial susceptibility testing and monitoring. Am J Health Syst Pharm 59(Suppl 3):S4-6, 2002.

Hoban DJ, Doern GV, Fluit AC, et al. Worldwide prevalence of antimicrobial resistance in Streptococcus pneumoniae, Haemophilus influenzae, and Moraxella catarrhalis in the SENTRY Antimicrobial Surveillance Program, 1997-1999. Clin Infect Dis 32 (Suppl 2):S81-93, 2001.

Hoban D, Felmingham D. The PROTEKT surveillance study: antimicrobial susceptibility of Haemophilus influenzae and Moraxella catarrhalis from community-acquired respiratory tract infections. J Antimicrob Chemother 50 (Suppl S1):49–59, 2002.

Holleman DB, Kelly LM, Credito K, et al. In vitro antianaerobic activity of ertapenem (MK-0826) compared to seven other compounds. Antimicrob Agents Chemother 46:220-4, 2002.

Jones RN, Kirby JT, Beach ML, et al. Geographic variations in activity of broad-spectrum beta-lactams against Pseudomonas aeruginosa: summary of the worldwide SENTRY antimicrobial surveillance program (1997-2000). Diagn Microbiol Infect Dis 43:239-43, 2002.

Karakoc B, Gerceker AA. In-vitro activities of various antibiotics, alone and in combination with amikacin against Pseudomonas aeruginosa. Int J Antimicrob Agents 18:567-70, 2001.

Kays MB, Wack MF, Smith DW. Azithromycin treatment failure in community-acquired pneumonia caused by a 23S rRNA mutation. Diagn Microbiol Infect Dis 42:163-5, 2002.

King A, Bathgate T, Phillips I. Erythromycin susceptibility of viridans streptococci from the normal throat flora of patients treated with azithromycin or clarithromycin. Clin Microbiol Infect 8:85-92, 2002.

Kingston M, Carlin E. Treatment of sexually transmitted infections with single-dose therapy: a double-edged sword. Drugs 62:871-8, 2002.

Kocazeybek B, Arabaci U, Erenturk S. Investigation of various antibiotic combinations using the E-Test method in multiresistant Pseudomonas aeruginosa strains. Chemotherapy 48:31-5, 2002.

Kontoyiannis DP, Lewis RE. Antifungal drug resistance in pathogenic fungi. Lancet 359:1135-44, 2002.

Kralovic SM, Danko LH, Roselle GA. Laboratory reporting of Staphylococcus aureus with reduced susceptibility to vancomycin in United States Department of Veterans Affairs facilities. Emerg Infect Dis 8:402-7, 2002.

Kremery V, Barnes AJ. Non-albicans Candida spp. causing fungaemia: pathogenicity and antifungal resistance. J Hosp Infect 50:243-60, 2002.

Laverdiere M, Hoban D, Restieri C, et al. In vitro activity of three new triazoles and one echinocandin against Candida bloodstream isolates from cancer patients. J Antimicrob Chemother 50:119-23, 2002.

Linden PK. Treatment options for vancomycin-resistant enterococcal infections. Drugs 62:425-41, 2002.

Linder JA, Stafford RS. Erythromycin-resistant group A streptococci. N Engl J Med 347:614-5, 2002.

Lonks JR, Garau J, Gomez L, et al. Failure of macrolide antibiotic treatment in patients with bacteremia due to erythromycin-resistant Streptococcus pneumoniae. Clin Infect Dis 35:556-64, 2002.

Malbruny B, Nagai K, Coquemont M, et al. Resistance to macrolides in clinical isolates of Streptococcus pyogenes due to ribosomal mutations. J Antimicrob Chemother 49:935-9, 2002.

Midolo PD, Matthews D, Fernandez CD, et al. Detection of extended spectrum beta-lactamases in the routine clinical microbiology laboratory. Pathology 34:362-4, 2002.

Mohammed MJ, Marston CK, Popovic T, et al. Antimicrobial susceptibility testing of Bacillus anthracis: comparison of results obtained by using the National Committee for Clinical Laboratory Standards broth microdilution reference and E-test agar gradient diffusion methods. J Clin Microbiol 40:1902-7, 2002.

Mollering RC Jr. Problems with antimicrobial resistance in gram-positive cocci. Clin Infect Dis 26:1177-8, 1998.

Murray BE. Vancomycin-resistant enterococcal infections. N Engl J Med 342:710-721, 2000.

Nagai K, Appelbaum PC, Davies TA, et al. Susceptibilities to telithromycin and six other agents and prevalence of macrolide resistance due to L4 ribosomal protein mutation among 992 Pneumococci from 10 central and Eastern European countries. Antimicrob Agents Chemother 46:371-7, 2002.

Nagai K, Appelbaum PC, Bavies ATA, et al. Susceptibility to telithromycin in 1,011 Streptococcus pyogenes isolates from 10 central and Eastern European countries. Antimicrob Agents Chemother 46:546-9, 2002.

Nishijima S, Kurokawa I, Nakaya H. Susceptibility change to antibiotics of Staphylococcus aureus strains isolated from skin infections between July 1994 and November 2000. J Infect Chemother 8:187-9, 2002.

Pankuch GA, Davies TA, Jacobs MR, et al. Antipneumococcal activity of ertapenem (MK-0826) compared to those of other agents. Antimicrob Agents Chemother 46:42-6, 2002.

Pelaez T, Alcala L, Alonso R, et al. Reassessment of Clostridium difficile susceptibility to metronidazole and vancomycin. Antimicrob Agents Chemother 46:1647-50,

2002.

Pendland SL, Messick CR, Jung R. In vitro synergy testing of levofloxacin, ofloxacin, and ciprofloxacin in combination with aztreonam, ceftazidime, or piperacillin against Pseudomonas aeruginosa. Diagn Microb Infect Dis 42:75-8, 2002.

Perri MB, Hershberger E, Ionescu M, et al. In vitro susceptibility of vancomycin-resistant enterococci (VRE) to fosfomycin. Diagn Microbiol Infect Dis 42:269-71, 2002.

Pfaller MA, Diekema DJ, Jones RN, et al. Trends in antifungal susceptibility of Candida spp. isolated from pediatric and adult patients with bloodstream infections: SENTRY Antimicrobial Surveillance Program 1997 to 2000. J Clin Microbiol 40:852-6, 2002.

Rex JH, Pfaller MA, Walsh TJ, et al. Antifungal susceptibility testing: practical aspects and current challenges. Clin Microbiol Rev 14:643-658, 2002.

Rex JH, Rinaldi MG, Pfaller MA. Resistance of Candida species to fluconazole. Antimicrob Agents Chemother 39:1-8, 1995.

Safdar A, Chaturvedi V, Koll BS, et al. Prospective, multicenter surveillance study of Candida glabrata: fluconazole and itraconazole susceptibility profiles in bloodstream, invasive, and colonizing strains and differences between isolates from three urban teaching hospitals in New York City (Candida Susceptibility Trends Study, 1998 to 1999). Antimicrob Agents Chemother 46:3268-72, 2002.

Sanglard D, Okks FC. Resistance of Candida species to antifungal agents: molecular mechanisms. Lancet Infect Dis 2:73-85, 2002.

Schaeffer AJ. The expanding role of fluoroquinolones. Am J Med 113 (Suppl 1A):45A-54S, 2002.

Sichito GC, Georgopoulos A, Prieto J. Antibacterial activity of oral antibiotics against community-acquired respiratory pathogens from three European countries. J Antimicrob Chemother 50(TOPIC T 1):7-11, 2002.

Smith CJ. What constitutes an extended-spectrum beta-lactamase? Antimicrob Agents Chemother 46:600-1, 2002.

Syndman DR, Jacobut NV, McDermott LA, et al. National survey on the susceptibility of Bacteroides fragilis: report and analysis of trends for 1997-2000. Clin Infect Dis 35(Suppl 1):S126-34, 2002.

Syndman DR, Jacobus NV, McDermott LA, et al. In vitro activities of newer quinolones against bacteroides group organisms. Antimicrob Agents Chemother 46:3276-9, 2002.

Tallent SM, Bischoff T, Climo M, et al. Vancomycin susceptibility of oxacillin-resistant Staphylococcus aureus isolates causing nosocomial bloodstream infections. J Clin Microbiol 40:2249-50, 2002.

Tomioka H, Sato K, Shimizu T, et al. Anti-Mycobacterium tuberculosis activities of new fluoroquinolones in combination with other antituberculous drugs. J Infect 44:160-5, 2002.

Trunak MR, Bandak SI, Bouchillon SK, et al. Antimicrobial susceptibilities of clinical isolates of Haemophilus influenzae and Moraxella catarrhalis collected during 1999-2000 from 13 countries. Clin Microbiol Infect 7:671-7, 2001.

White RL, Enzweiler KA, Friedrich LV, et al. Comparative activity of gatifloxacin and other antibiotics against 4009 clinical isolates of Streptococcus pneumoniae in the United States during 1999-2000. Diagn Microbiol Infect Dis 43:207-17, 2002.

Yong D, Lee K, Yum JH, et al. Imipenem-EDTA disk method for differentiation of metallo-beta-lactamase-producing clinical isolates of Pseudomonas spp. and Acinetobacter spp. J Clin Microbiol 40:3798-801, 2002.

TEXTBOOKS

Anaissie EJ, McGinnis MR, Pfaller MA (eds). Clinical Mycology. Churchill Livingstone, New York, 2003.

Forbes BA, Sahm DF, Weissfeld AS, et al. (eds). Bailey & Scott's Diagnostic Microbiology. St. Louis, Mosby, 2002.

Koneman EW, Allen SD, Janda WM, et al (eds). Color Atlas and Textbook of Diagnostic Microbiology, 5th Edition. Lippincott-Raven Publishers, Philadelphia, 1997.

Murray PR, Baron EJ, Phaller MA, et al. (eds). Manual of Clinical Microbiology, 8th Edition. Washington, DC, ASM Press, 2003.

Scholar EM Pratt WB (eds). The Antimicrobial Drugs, 2nd Edition, Oxford University Press, New York, 2000.

Chapter 4

Parasites, Fungi, Unusual Organisms

Kenneth F. Wagner, DO
Burke A. Cunha, MD
John H. Rex, MD

Parasites, Fungi, Unusual Organisms in Blood

Microfilaria in Blood

Subset	Pathogen	Preferred Therapy	Alternate Therapy
Filariasis	Brugia malayi	Diethylcarbamazine: day 1: 50 mg (PO) day 2: 50 mg (PO) q8h day 3: 100 mg (PO) q8h days 4-14: 2 mg/kg (PO) q8h	Ivermectin 400 mcg/kg (PO) x 1 dose ± albendazole 400 mg (PO) x 1 dose
	Wuchereria bancrofti	Diethylcarbamazine: day 1: 50 mg (PO) day 2: 50 mg (PO) q8h day 3: 100 mg (PO) q8h days 4-14: 2 mg/kg (PO) q8h	Ivermectin 400 mcg/kg (PO) x 1 dose ± albendazole 400 mg (PO) x 1 dose

Brugia malayi
Clinical Presentation: May present as an obscure febrile illness, chronic lymphedema, lymphangitis, or cutaneous abscess. "Filarial fevers" usually last 1 week and spontaneously remit
Diagnostic Considerations: Diagnosis by demonstrating microfilaria on Giemsa's stained thick blood smear or by using the concentration method; yield is increased by passing blood through a Millipore filter before staining. Several smears should be taken over 24 hours. Common infection in Southeast Asia (primarily China, Korea, India, Indonesia, Malaysia, Philippines, Sri Lanka). Most species have nocturnal periodicity (microfilaria in blood at night). Eosinophilia is most common during periods of acute inflammation
Pitfalls: Genital manifestations—scrotal edema, epididymitis, orchitis, hydrocele—are frequent with W. bancrofti, but rare with B. malayi
Prognosis: Related to state of health and extent of lymphatic obstruction. No satisfactory treatment is available. Single-dose ivermectin is effective treatment for microfilaremia, but does not kill the adult worm (although diethylcarbamazine kills some). If no microfilaria in blood, full-dose diethylcarbamazine (2 mg/kg q8h) can be started on day one. Antihistamines or corticosteroids may decrease allergic reactions from disintegration of microfilaria

Wuchereria bancrofti
Clinical Presentation: May present as an obscure febrile illness, chronic lymphedema, lymphangitis, or cutaneous abscess. Genital (scrotal) lymphatic edema, groin lesions, epididymitis, orchitis, hydroceles are characteristic. Chyluria may occur. "Filarial fevers" usually last 1 week and spontaneously remit
Diagnostic Considerations: Diagnosis by demonstrating microfilaria on Giemsa's stained thick blood smear or by using the concentration method; yield is increased by passing blood through a Millipore filter before staining. Several smears should be taken over 24 hours. W. bancrofti is the most common human filarial infection, particularly in Asia (China, India, Indonesia, Japan, Malaysia, Philippines), Southeast Asia, Sri Lanka, Tropical Africa, Central/South America, and Pacific Islands. Most species have nocturnal periodicity (microfilaria in blood at night). Eosinophilia is common
Pitfalls: Differentiate from "hanging groins" of Loa Loa, which usually do not involve the scrotum
Prognosis: Related to state of health and extent of lymphatic obstruction. No satisfactory treatment is available. Single-dose ivermectin is effective treatment for microfilaremia, but does not kill the adult worm (although diethylcarbamazine kills some). If no microfilaria in blood, full-dose diethylcarbamazine (2 mg/kg q8h) can be started on day one. Antihistamines or corticosteroids decrease allergic reactions from disintegration of microfilaria

Trypanosomes in Blood

Subset	Pathogen	Preferred Therapy	Alternate Therapy
Chagas' disease (American trypanosomiasis)	Trypanosoma cruzi	Nifurtimox 8-10 mg/kg/day (PO) in 3-4 divided doses x 3-4 months	Benznidazole 2.5-3.5 mg/kg (PO) q12h x 2 months
Sleeping sickness *West African trypanosomiasis*	Trypanosoma brucei gambiense	<u>Hemolymphatic stage</u> Pentamidine 4 mg/kg (IM) q24h x 10 days <u>Late disease with CNS involvement</u> Melarsoprol 2.2 mg/kg (IV) q24h x 10 days	<u>Hemolymphatic stage</u> Suramin 200 mg test dose (IV), then 1 gm (IV) on days 1,3,7,14 and 21 **or** Eflornithine 100 mg/kg (IV) q6h x 2 weeks <u>Late disease with CNS involvement</u> None
East African trypanosomiasis	Trypanosoma brucei rhodesiense	<u>Hemolymphatic stage</u> Suramin 200 mg test dose (IV), then 1 gm (IV) on days 1,3,7,14 and 21 <u>Late disease with CNS involvement</u> Melarsoprol 2–3.6 mg/kg (IV) q24h x 3 days. After 1 week, give 3.6 mg/kg (IV) q24h x 3 days; repeat again in 10-21 days	<u>Hemolymphatic stage</u> Eflornithine, pentamidine (see doses above) variably effective <u>Late disease with CNS involvement</u> None

Chagas' Disease (Trypanosoma cruzi) American Trypanosomiasis

Clinical Presentation: Presents acutely after bite of infected reduvid bug with unilateral painless edema of the palpebrae/periocular tissues (Romaña's sign), or as an indurated area of erythema and swelling with local lymph node involvement (chagoma). Fever, malaise, and edema of the face and lower extremities may follow. Generalized lymphadenopathy and mild hepatosplenomegaly sometimes occur. Patients with chronic disease may develop cardiac involvement (cardiomyopathy with arrhythmias, heart block, heart failure, thromboembolism) or GI involvement (megaesophagus/megacolon)

Diagnostic Considerations: Common in Central and South America. Acquired from infected reduvid bug, which infests mud/clay parts of primitive dwellings. Diagnosis in acute disease by detecting parasites in wet prep of anticoagulated blood or buffy coat smear, Giemsa-stained smears, bone marrow or lymph node aspirates, or by xenodiagnosis. rCRP ELISA is the best antigen-based test for Chagas' disease (high sensitivity/specificity)

Pitfalls: Do not overlook the diagnosis in patients from endemic areas with unexplained heart block. Avoid tetracycline and steroids with benznidazole

Prognosis: Related to extent of cardiac/GI involvement

Sleeping Sickness (T. brucei gambiense/rhodesiense) West African/East African Trypanosomiasis

Clinical Presentation: Sleeping sickness from T. brucei gambiense is milder than sleeping sickness from T. brucei rhodesiense, which is usually a fulminant infection. A few days to weeks after bite of tsetse fly, patients progress through several clinical stages:

* *Chancre stage:* Trypanosomal chancre occurs at bite site and lasts several weeks
* *Blood/lymphatic stage:* Blood parasitemia is associated with intermittent high fevers, headaches and insomnia, followed by generalized adenopathy. Posterior cervical lymph node enlargement (Winterbottom's sign) is particularly prominent with T. brucei gambiense. Hepatosplenomegaly and transient edema/pruritus/irregular circinate rash are common. Myocarditis (tachycardia unrelated to fevers) occurs early (before CNS involvement) and is responsible for acute deaths from T. brucei rhodesiense
* *CNS stage:* Occurs after a few months of non-specific symptoms, and is characterized by increasing lethargy, somnolence (sleeping sickness), and many subtle CNS findings. Coma and death ensue without treatment. With melarsoprol, use prednisolone 1 mg/kg (PO) q24h

Diagnostic Considerations: Diagnosis by demonstrating trypanosomes in blood, chancre, or lymph nodes aspirates by Giemsa-stained thin and thick preparations, light microscopy, or buffy coat concentrates with acridine orange

Pitfalls: Do not miss other causes of prominent bilateral posterior cervical lymph node enlargement (e.g., lymphoma, EBV)

Prognosis: Related to extent of cardiac/CNS involvement. Relapse may occur

Spirochetes in Blood

Subset	Pathogen	Preferred Therapy	Alternate Therapy
Relapsing fever *Louse-borne (LBRF)* *Tick-borne (TBRF)*	Borrelia recurrentis. At least 15 Borrelia species (U.S.: B. hermsi; Africa: B. duttonii; Africa/Middle East: B. crocidurae)	<u>LBRF</u> Erythromycin 500 mg (IV or PO) q6h x 7 days <u>TBRF</u> Doxycycline 200 mg (PO) x 3 days, then 100 mg (PO) q12h x 7 days	<u>TBRF with CNS involvement</u> Penicillin G 2 mu (IV) q4h x 2 weeks **or** Ceftriaxone 1 gm (IV) q12h x 2 weeks **or** Cefotaxime 3 gm (IV) q6h x 2 weeks
Rat bite fever	Spirillum minus	Penicillin G 4 mu (IV) q4h. Can switch to amoxicillin 1 gm (PO) q8h for total therapy of 2 weeks **or** Doxycycline 200 mg (IV or PO) q12h x 3 days, then 100 mg (IV or PO) q12h x 11 days	Erythromycin 500 mg (IV or PO) q6h x 2 weeks **or** Chloramphenicol 500 mg (IV) q6h x 2 weeks

Relapsing Fever, Louse-Borne (LBRF) / Tick-Borne (TBRF)

Clinical Presentation: Abrupt onset of "flu-like" illness with high fever, rigors, headache, myalgias, arthralgias, tachycardia, dry cough, abdominal pain after exposure to infected louse or tick. Truncal petechial rash and conjunctival suffusion are common. Hepatosplenomegaly/DIC may occur. Bleeding complications are more common in LBRF. Fevers last ~ 1 week, remit for a week, and usually relapse only once in LBRF, but several times in TBRF. Relapses usually last 2-3 days. Fevers are often higher in TBRF

Diagnostic Considerations: Borreliae are found in > 70% of infected febrile patients when wet blood smears are examined by dark field, Giemsa, or Wright-stained thick and thin peripheral blood smears. LBRF is endemic in South American Andes, Central and East Africa, and is associated with crowded, unhygienic conditions. TBRF is seen throughout the world, and is endemic in Western U.S., British Columbia, Mexico, Central/South America, Mediterranean, Central Asia, and Africa

Pitfalls: Spirochetes are most likely to be seen during febrile periods. Some treatment failures occur in TBRF with single-dose therapy

Prognosis: Good if treated early. Usually no permanent sequelae

Rat Bite Fever (Spirillum minus)

Clinical Presentation: Infection develops 1-4 weeks following bite of wild rat. Healed rat bite becomes red, painful, swollen and ulcerated, with regional lymphangitis/adenopathy. Relapsing fever occurs in 2-4 day fever cycles. Fevers are usually accompanied by chills, headache, photophobia, nausea, vomiting. Rash on palms/soles develops in > 50%. Arthritis, myalgias, and SBE are rare

Diagnostic Considerations: Short thick spirochetes are seen in peripheral blood smears, exudate, or lymph node tissue examined by dark field, Giemsa, or Wright's stain. Mostly seen in Asia. Differential diagnosis includes Borrelia, malaria, and lymphoma. VDRL is positive

Pitfalls: May be confused with syphilis, due to rash on palms/soles and false-positive syphilis serology in 50%. SBE occurs with S. moniliformis, not S. minus (unless there is preexisting valvular disease). Bite wound ulcerates in S. minus, not S. moniliformis

Prognosis: Patients with arthritis have a protracted course

Intracellular Inclusion Bodies in Blood

Subset	Pathogen	Preferred Therapy	Alternate Therapy
Babesiosis	Babesia microti	Azithromycin 1 gm (PO) q24h x 3 days, then 500 mg (PO) q24h x 7 days **plus** Atovaquone (suspension) 750 mg (PO) q12h x 7-10 days	Clindamycin 600 mg (PO) q8h x 7 days **plus** Quinine 650 mg (PO) q8h x 7 days
Ehrlichiosis *Human monocytic (HME)* *Human granulocytic (HGE)*	Ehrlichia chaffeensis Ehrlichia phagocytophilia/ equi	Doxycycline 200 mg (IV or PO) q12h x 3 days, then 100 mg (IV or PO) q12h x 1-2 weeks total	Any once-daily quinolone (IV or PO) x 1-2 weeks **or** Ciprofloxacin 400 mg (IV) q12h or 750 mg (PO) q12h x 1-2 weeks **or** Chloramphenicol 500 mg (IV or PO) q6h x 1-2 weeks

Intracellular Inclusion Bodies in Blood (cont'd)

Subset	Pathogen	Preferred Therapy	Alternate Therapy
Malaria		<u>Chloroquine-sensitive strains</u>	<u>Chloroquine-resistant strains</u>
Benign tertian	Plasmodium ovale Plasmodium vivax	Chloroquine phosphate 1 gm (600 mg base) (PO) x 1 dose, then 500 mg (300 mg base) (PO) at 6, 24, and 48	<u>*Mild/moderately ill*</u> Quinine sulfate 650 mg (500 mg base) (PO) q8h x 7 days
Malignant tertian	Plasmodium falciparum	hours **or**	**plus** Doxycycline 200 mg (PO) q12h x 3 days, then
Quartan	Plasmodium malariae	Quinidine gluconate 10 mg/kg (maximum 600 mg) (IV) over 1-2 hours, followed by continuous IV infusion of 0.02 mg/kg/min until parasitemia < 1% or for 72 hours	100 mg (PO) q12h x 4 days **or monotherapy** **with** Atovaquone/proguanil (250/100 mg tab) 4 tabs as a single dose (PO) q24h x 3 days
		or Chloroquine phosphate 10 mg (base)/kg (IV) over 4 hours, then 5 mg (base)/kg (IV) over 2 hours q12h (total dose not to exceed 25 mg/kg)	<u>*Critically ill*</u> Quinidine gluconate 15 mg/kg (IV) over 1-2 hours, followed by either 7.5 mg/kg (IV) over 1-2 hours q8h or 1-1.5 mg/kg/hr constant (IV) infusion until parasitemia
		or Artemether 3.2 mg/kg (IM) x 1 dose, then 1.6 mg/kg (IM) q24h x 5-7 days	< 1%. Then complete 7 days of total therapy with an oral agent(s), listed above **or**
		<u>For P. vivax or P. ovale, add:</u> Primaquine phosphate 26.3 mg (15 mg base) (PO) q24h x 2 weeks	Quinine dihydrochloride 20 mg (salt)/kg (IV) over 4 hours (in D$_5$W), then 10 mg (salt)/kg (IV) over 2 hours q8h until able to take oral medication. Then use oral agent(s) listed above to complete 7 days total therapy

Babesiosis (Babesia microti)

Clinical Presentation: "Malarial-like illness" with malaise, fever, shaking chills, myalgias, arthralgias, headaches, abdominal pain, relative bradycardia, and splenomegaly. Laboratory abnormalities include anemia, atypical lymphocytes in peripheral smear, lymphopenia, thrombocytopenia, mildly elevated LFTs, ↑ LDH, proteinuria, and hemoglobinuria. Transmitted by infected Ixodes ticks

Diagnostic Considerations: Characteristic "tetrad" when examined by Giemsa or Wright-stained thick and thin peripheral blood smears. IFA serology ≥ 1:256 is diagnostic of acute infection. Hyposplenic patients may have profound hemolytic anemia and life-threatening infection

Pitfalls: Co-infection with Lyme disease may occur. No serological cross-reactivity between Babesia and Borrelia (Lyme disease)

Prognosis: Severe/fatal in patients with decreased or absent splenic function. Exchange transfusions may be life saving

Ehrlichiosis, Human Monocytic (HME) / Human Granulocytic (HGE)

Clinical Presentation: Acute febrile illness with chills, headache, malaise, myalgias, leukopenia, thrombocytopenia, ↑ LFTs. No vasculitis. Resembles Rocky Mountain spotted fever (RMSF), but rash much less frequent

Diagnostic Considerations: Characteristic "morulae" (spherical, basophilic, Mulberry-shaped, cytoplasmic inclusion bodies) seen in peripheral blood neutrophils in HGE. PCR from blood is 86% sensitive and highly specific for early diagnosis. Obtain acute and convalescent IFA serology. Vector is I. scapularis tick. Co-infection with B. burgdorferi (Lyme Disease) is uncommon, but may occur

Pitfalls: Morulae are not seen in HME, so blood smears are unhelpful. Rash occurs in > 90% in Rocky Mountain spotted fever, but is uncommon in HME and rare in HGE

Prognosis: Excellent if treated early

Malaria (Plasmodium ovale/vivax/falciparum/malariae)

Clinical Presentation: Presents acutely with fever/chills, severe headaches, cough, nausea/vomiting, diarrhea, abdominal/back pain. Typical "malarial paroxysm" consists of chills, fever and profuse sweating, followed by extreme prostration. There are a paucity of physical findings, but most have tender hepatomegaly/splenomegaly and relative bradycardia. Anemia, thrombocytopenia, atypical lymphocytes, and ↑ LDH/LFTs are common

Diagnostic Considerations: Diagnosis by demonstrating Plasmodium on thick and thin Giemsa or Wright-stained smears

Pitfalls: Be wary of diagnosing malaria without headache/anemia. Assume all P. falciparum are chloroquine-resistant. Chloroquine-resistant P. vivax are now seen in South America, New Guinea, and Oceania (Indonesia). Chloroquine-sensitive strains are acquired in Central America (north of Panama Canal), Haiti, and parts of the Middle East (although chloroquine-resistant strains have been reported in Yemen, Oman, Saudi Arabia, and Iran). Check for severe G6PD deficiency before starting therapy

Prognosis: Related to species. P. falciparum with high-grade parasitemia is most severe, and may be complicated by coma, hypoglycemia, renal failure, or non-cardiogenic pulmonary edema. If parasitemia exceeds 15%, consider exchange transfusions

Fungi/Mycobacterium in Blood

See histoplasmosis (pp. 251, 258), Mycobacterium tuberculosis (treat as pulmonary TB, pp. 248, 254), Mycobacterium avium-intracellulare (pp. 251, 258)

Parasites, Fungi, Unusual Organisms in CSF/Brain

Cysts/Mass Lesions in CSF/Brain

Subset	Pathogens	Preferred Therapy	PO Therapy
Cerebral nocardiosis	Nocardia sp.	Preferred IV Therapy TMP-SMX (TMP 5 mg/kg, SMX 15 mg/kg) (IV) q6h until clinical improvement followed by (PO) therapy Alternate IV Therapy Minocycline 200 mg (IV) q12h until clinical improvement followed by (PO) therapy	Preferred PO Therapy TMP-SMX 1 DS tablet (PO) q12h x 6 months Alternate PO Therapy Minocycline 200 mg (PO) q12h x 6 months

Cysts/Mass Lesions in CSF/Brain (cont'd)

Subset	Pathogens	Preferred Therapy	Alternate Therapy
Cerebral amebiasis	Entamoeba histolytica	Metronidazole 750 mg (PO) q8h x 10 days **or** Tinidazole 600 mg (PO) q12h x 5 days	
Primary amebic meningo-encephalitis	Naegleria fowleri	See p. 21	
Granulomatous amebic encephalitis	Acanthamoeba	See p. 22	
Cerebral echinococcosis (hydatid cyst disease)	Echinococcus granulosus	Surgical resection plus albendazole 400 mg* (PO) q12h until cured	Surgical resection plus mebendazole 50 mg/kg (PO) q24h until cured
	Echinococcus multilocularis	Surgical resection plus albendazole 400 mg* (PO) q12h until cured	Surgical resection plus mebendazole 50 mg/kg (PO) q24h until cured
Cerebral gnathostomiasis	Gnathostoma spinigerum	Surgical resection	Albendazole 400 mg (PO) q12h x 3 weeks
Cerebral coenurosis	Taenia multiceps	Surgical resection	
Neuro-cysticercosis	Taenia solium	Praziquantel 17 mg/kg (PO) q8h x 4 weeks	Albendazole 400 mg* (PO) q12h x 4 weeks
Cerebral paragonimiasis (lung fluke)	Paragonimus westermani	Praziquantel 25 mg/kg (PO) q8h x 2 days	Bithionol 50 mg/kg (PO) q48h x 10-15 doses
Cerebral toxoplasmosis	Toxoplasmosis gondii	See p. 249	
Cryptococcomas/meningitis	Cryptococcus neoformans	See p. 249	
Chagas' disease (American trypanosomiasis)	Trypanosoma cruzi	Nifurtimox 2 mg/kg (PO) q6h x 4 months	Benznidazole 3.5 mg/kg (PO) q12h x 2 months

* If < 60 kg, give albendazole 7.5 mg/kg

Cerebral Nocardiosis

Clinical Presentation: CNS mass lesion resembling brain tumor/abscess. Symptoms are highly variable, and result from local effects of granulomas/abscesses on CNS. Up to 40% of patients with systemic nocardiosis have associated mass lesions in CNS

Diagnostic Considerations: Diagnosis by demonstrating Nocardia in brain biopsy specimens. Notify laboratory for AFB specimen staining/aerobic cultures if suspect Nocardia. Nocardia are weakly acid-fast and aerobic

Pitfalls: Usually not limited to brain. Look for Nocardia in lungs or liver. Use in-vitro susceptibility data to guide therapy for refractory cases. IV regimens are recommended for critically ill patients. HIV/AIDS patients require life-long suppression with TMP-SMX

Prognosis: Related to health of host, degree of immunosuppression, and extent of lesions

Cerebral Amebiasis (Entamoeba histolytica)

Clinical Presentation: Rare cause of brain abscess. Onset is frequently abrupt with rapid progression. Suspect in patients with a history of amebiasis and altered mental status/focal neurologic signs. If present, meningeal involvement resembles acute bacterial meningitis. CT/MRI shows focal lesions. CSF eosinophilia is not a feature of CNS involvement

Diagnostic Considerations: Diagnosis by demonstrating E. histolytica trophozoites from aspirated brain lesions under CT guidance. Worldwide distribution. Mass lesions may be single or multiple, and more commonly involve the left hemisphere. Most patients have concomitant liver ± lung abscesses

Pitfalls: Trophozoites/eggs in stool are not diagnostic of CNS disease. E. histolytica serology is often positive, but is nonspecific. E. histolytica trophozoites are not present in CSF

Prognosis: Related to size/location of CNS lesions

Primary Amebic Meningoencephalitis (Naegleria fowleri) (see p. 23)

Granulomatous Amebic Encephalitis (Acanthamoeba) (see p. 23)

Cerebral Echinococcosis (Echinococcus granulosus) Hydatid Cyst Disease

Clinical Presentation: Most cysts are asymptomatic. Mass lesions may cause seizures, cranial nerve abnormalities, other focal neurologic symptoms

Diagnostic Considerations: CT/MRI typically shows a single large cyst without edema or enhancement. Multiple cysts are rare. Diagnosis by demonstrating protoscolices in "hydatid sand" in cysts. Usually associated with liver/lung hydatid cysts

Pitfalls: E. granulosus serology lacks specificity

Prognosis: Related to size/location of CNS cysts. Treatment consists of surgical removal of total cyst after instilling cysticidal agent (hypertonic saline, iodophor, ethanol) into cyst plus albendazole

Cerebral Echinococcosis (Echinococcus multilocularis) Hydatid Cyst Disease

Clinical Presentation: Frequently associated with hydatid bone cysts (may cause spinal cord compression), liver/lung cysts. Peripheral eosinophilia occurs in 50%, but eosinophils are not seen in the CSF

Diagnostic Considerations: E. multilocularis ELISA is sensitive and specific

Pitfalls: Praziquantel is ineffective for CNS hydatid cyst disease. Imaging studies suggest carcinoma/sarcoma. Diagnosis is frequently not made until brain biopsy

Prognosis: If treatment is effective, improvement of CNS lesions is evident in 8 weeks (2/3 improve). Brain/bone cysts are difficult to cure

Cerebral Gnathostomiasis (Gnathostoma spinigerum)

Clinical Presentation: Nausea, vomiting, increased salivation, skin flushing, pruritus, urticaria, and upper abdominal pain 1-6 days after exposure. Cerebral form presents as eosinophilic meningitis with radiculomyeloencephalitis, with headache and severe sharp/shooting pains in extremities often followed by paraplegia and coma. Any cranial nerve may be involved. The most characteristic feature is changing/migratory neurological findings. Intense peripheral eosinophilia occurs in 90% of patients. CSF has eosinophilic pleocytosis and may have RBCs

Diagnostic Considerations: In cases with ocular involvement, the worm may be seen in the anterior chamber of eye. Specific Gnathostoma serology of CSF is helpful in establishing the diagnosis. Acquired from infected cat/dog feces. Most cases occur in Southeast Asia. Few other CNS infections have both

RBCs and eosinophils in the CSF
Pitfalls: Do not miss associated eye involvement
Prognosis: Related to invasion of medulla/brainstem

Cerebral Coenurosis (Taenia multiceps)

Clinical Presentation: CNS mass lesion with seizures/cranial nerve abnormalities, often presenting as a posterior-fossa syndrome. Common sites of CNS involvement include paraventricular and basal subarachnoid spaces
Diagnostic Considerations: Diagnosis by demonstrating protoscolices in brain specimens. Worldwide distribution. Transmitted via dog feces
Pitfalls: Do not miss associated ocular lesions, which mimic intraocular neoplasms/granulomas
Prognosis: Related to size/extent of CNS lesions

Neurocysticercosis (Taenia solium)

Clinical Presentation: Chronic meningitis/mass lesions with seizures. Hydrocephalus is common. Spinal involvement may result in paraplegia. Cerebral cysts are usually multiple
Diagnostic Considerations: CT/MRI shows multiple enhancing and non-enhancing unilocular cysts. Diagnosis by specific T. solium serology of serum/CSF. Neurocysticercosis is the most common CNS parasite. Worldwide in distribution, but most common in Eastern Europe, Asia, and Latin America
Pitfalls: Cranial nerve abnormalities are uncommon
Prognosis: Related to extent/location of CNS lesions. Adjunctive therapy includes corticosteroids, anti-epileptics, and shunt for hydrocephalus

Cerebral Paragonimiasis (Paragonimus westermani) Lung Fluke

Clinical Presentation: Can resemble epilepsy, cerebral tumors, or brain embolism. Primary focus of infection is pulmonary, with pleuritic chest pain, cough, and night sweats. CNS findings are a manifestation of extrapulmonary (ectopic) organ involvement
Diagnostic Considerations: Diagnosis by demonstrating operculated eggs in sputum, pleural fluid, or feces. Multiple sputum samples are needed to demonstrate P. westermani eggs. Charcot-Leyden crystals are seen in sputum. Endemic in Far East, India, Africa, and Central/South America
Pitfalls: Extrapulmonary (ectopic) organ involvement (cerebral, subcutaneous, abdominal) is common. Up to 20% of patients have normal chest x-rays
Prognosis: Related to size/location of CNS cysts and extent of lung involvement

Cerebral Toxoplasmosis (T. gondii) (see p. 254)

Cerebral Cryptococcosis (C. neoformans) (see p. 255)

Chagas' Disease (Trypanosoma cruzi) American Trypanosomiasis

Clinical Presentation: Acute unilateral periorbital cellulitis (Romaña's sign) or regional adenopathy and edema of extremity at site of infected reduviid bug (Chagoma). Chronic disease manifests as myocarditis/heart block or megaesophagus/megacolon. Hepatosplenomegaly is common. Overt CNS signs are frequently absent. If meningoencephalitis develops, the prognosis is very poor. In immunosuppressed patients (especially AIDS), recrudescence of disease occurs with development of T. cruzi brain abscesses
Diagnostic Considerations: Diagnosis in acute disease by demonstrating parasite in wet prep of anticoagulated blood/Buffy coat smear, Giemsa-stained smear, bone marrow/lymph node aspirate, or by xenodiagnosis. Serology (mostly used for chronic disease) has limited value in endemic areas due to lack of specificity, but is useful in non-endemic areas. Common in Central/South America. Acquired from infected reduviid bugs, which infest mud/clay/stone parts of primitive dwellings. Infection in humans occurs only in areas containing reduviids that defecate during or immediately after a blood

meal

Pitfalls: Do not overlook diagnosis in persons from endemic areas with unexplained heart block. For children ages 11-16 years, use nifurtimox 3.5 mg/kg (PO) q6h x 3 months. For children < 11 years, use nifurtimox 5 mg/kg (PO) q6h x 3 months

Prognosis: Related to extent of GI/cardiac involvement. The addition of gamma interferon to nifurtimox x 20 days may shorten the acute phase of the disease

Parasites, Fungi, Unusual Organisms in Lungs

Pulmonary Cystic Lesions/Masses

Subset	Pathogens	Preferred Therapy	Alternate Therapy
Alveolar echinococcosis	Echinococcus multilocularis	Operable cases Wide surgical resection plus albendazole 400 mg* (PO) q12h or mebendazole 50 mg/kg (PO) q24h until cured	Inoperable cases Albendazole 400 mg* (PO) q12h x 1 month, then repeat therapy after 2 weeks x 3 cycles (i.e., 4 total months of albendazole)
Pulmonary amebiasis	Entamoeba histolytica	Metronidazole 750 mg (PO) q8h x 10 days	Tinidazole 600 mg (PO) q12h x 5 days
Pulmonary paragonimiasis (lung fluke)	Paragonimus westermani	Praziquantel 25 mg/kg (PO) q8h x 2 days	Bithionol 50 mg/kg (PO) q48h x 4 weeks (14 doses)

* If < 60 kg, give albendazole 7.5 mg/kg

Alveolar Echinococcosis (Echinococcus multilocularis)

Clinical Presentation: Slowly growing cysts remain asymptomatic for 5-20 years, until space-occupying effect elicits symptoms. Rupture or leak into bronchial tree can cause cough, chest pain, and hemoptysis

Diagnostic Considerations: Diagnosis is suggested by typical "Swiss cheese calcification" findings on chest x-ray, and confirmed by specific E. multilocularis serology (which does not cross react with E. granulosus). Most common in Northern forest areas of Europe, Asia, North America, and Arctic. Acquired by ingestion of viable parasite eggs in food. Tapeworm-infected canines/cats or wild rodents are common vectors. Less common than infection with E. granulosus

Pitfalls: Do not confuse central cavitary lesions with squamous cell carcinoma

Prognosis: Related to severity/extent of cysts

Pulmonary Amebiasis (Entamoeba histolytica)

Clinical Presentation: Cough, pelvic pain, fever, and right lung/pleural mass mimicking pneumonia or lung abscess. Bronchopleural fistulas may occur. Sputum has "liver-like" taste if cyst ruptures into bronchus. Bacterial co-infection is rare. Amebic lung lesions are associated with hepatic liver abscesses, and invariably involve the right lobe of lung/diaphragm

Diagnostic Considerations: Diagnosis by aspiration of lungs cysts, which may be massive. Amebic serology is sensitive and specific. Worldwide distribution. Acquired by ingesting amebic cysts. Key to diagnosis is concomitant liver involvement; liver abscess presents years after initial diarrheal episode

Pitfalls: Lung involvement is rarely the sole manifestation of amebic infection, and is usually due to direct extension of amebic liver abscess (10-20% of amebic liver abscesses penetrate through the diaphragm and into the lungs). Follow metronidazole with paromomycin 500 mg (PO) q8h x 7 days to eliminate intestinal focus

Prognosis: Related to severity/extent of cysts

Pulmonary Paragonimiasis (Paragonimus westermani) Lung Fluke

Clinical Presentation: Mild infection; may be asymptomatic. Acute phase of infection is accompanied by abdominal pain, diarrhea and urticaria, followed by pleuritic chest pain. Chronic symptoms occur within 6 months after exposure, with dyspnea/dry cough leading to productive cough ± hemoptysis. Complications include pleural effusion, lung abscess, bronchiectasis, cough, and night sweats. Eosinophilia may be evident acutely

Diagnostic Considerations: Oriental lung fluke acquired by ingestion of freshwater crayfish/crabs. After penetration of the gut/peritoneal cavity, the fluke migrates through the diaphragm/pleural space and invades lung parenchyma. Incubation period is 2-20 days. Diagnosis by demonstrating operculated eggs in sputum, pleural fluid, or feces. Multiple sputum samples are needed to demonstrate P. westermani eggs. Charcot-Leyden crystals are seen in sputum, and characteristic chest x-ray findings of ring-shaped/crescent infiltrates with "thin-walled" cavities are evident in ~ 60%. Endemic in Asia, Africa, and Latin America. Chest x-ray findings take months to resolve

Pitfalls: May have extrapulmonary (ectopic) organ involvement (e.g., cerebral, subcutaneous, abdominal). Up to 20% have normal chest x-rays

Prognosis: Related to degree of lung damage (e.g., bronchiectasis) and extrapulmonary organ involvement, especially CNS

Pulmonary Coin Lesions

Subset	Pathogens	Preferred Therapy	Alternate Therapy
Dog heartworm	Dirofilaria immitis	No therapy necessary	
Aspergilloma	Aspergillus	No therapy if asymptomatic. Surgery for massive hemoptysis	Itraconazole 200 mg (PO) solution q24h x 3-6 months **or** Voriconazole 400 mg (PO) q12h x 1 day, then 200 mg (PO) q12h x 3-6 months

Dog Heartworm (Dirofilaria immitis)

Clinical Presentation: Asymptomatic "coin lesion" after bite of infected mosquito transmits parasite from dogs to humans. Differential diagnosis includes granulomas and malignancy

Diagnostic Considerations: Diagnosis by specific serology or pathological demonstration of organism in granuloma, usually when a coin lesion is biopsied to rule out malignancy. Worldwide distribution. Acquired from pet dogs. Dirofilariasis causes dog heartworm in carrier, but presents as a solitary lung nodule in humans

Pitfalls: Often confused with malignancy

Prognosis: Excellent

Pulmonary Aspergilloma

Clinical Presentation: Coin lesion(s) ± productive cough, hemoptysis, wheezing. May be asymptomatic. Usually occurs in pre-existing cavitary lung lesions, especially TB with cavity > 2 cm

Diagnostic Considerations: Diagnosis by chest x-ray appearance of fungus ball in cavity and Aspergillus precipitins/biopsy. May present with "crescent sign" on chest x-ray (white fungus ball silhouetted against black crescent of the cavity)

Pitfalls: Role of itraconazole or voriconazole as therapy is unclear

Prognosis: Related to degree of hemoptysis

Pulmonary Infiltrates/Mass Lesions

Subset	Pathogens	Preferred Therapy	Alternate Therapy
Pulmonary blastomycosis	Blastomyces dermatitidis	Itraconazole 200 mg (PO)* solution q12h until cured <u>Severely ill</u> Amphotericin B deoxycholate 0.7-1 mg/kg (IV) q24h until 1-2 grams given	Fluconazole 400-800 mg (PO) q24h until cured
Pulmonary histoplasmosis	Histoplasma capsulatum	<u>Immunocompetent</u> Itraconazole 200 mg (PO)* solution q24h until cured <u>Immunocompromised or severely ill</u> Amphotericin B deoxycholate 1 mg/kg (IV) q24h x 7 days† or 0.8 mg/kg q48h until 2-2.5 grams given	<u>Immunocompetent</u> Itraconazole (see below) **or** Fluconazole 1600 mg (PO) x 1 dose, then 800 mg (PO) q24h until cured <u>Immunocompromised or severely ill</u> Itraconazole 200 mg (IV) q12h x 7-14 days, then 200 mg (PO) solution q12h until cured
Pulmonary paracoccidioido-mycosis (South American blastomycosis)	Paracoccidioides brasiliensis	Itraconazole 200 mg (PO) solution q24h x 6 months **or** Ketoconazole 400 mg (PO) q24h x 18 months	Amphotericin B 0.5 mg/kg (IV) q24h until 1.5-2.5 grams given
Pulmonary actinomycosis	Actinomyces israelii	Amoxicillin 1 gm (PO) q8h x 6 months **or** Doxycycline 100 mg (PO) q12h x 6 months	Clindamycin 300 mg (PO) q8h x 6 months **or** Chloramphenicol 500 mg (PO) q6h x 6 months
Pulmonary aspergillosis *BPA*	Aspergillus	Systemic oral steroids	Itraconazole 200 mg (PO) solution q12h x 8 months
Acute invasive pneumonia	Aspergillus	See p. 249	
Chronic pneumonia	Aspergillus	Itraconazole 200 mg (PO)* solution q12h until cured **or** Caspofungin 70 mg (IV) x 1 dose, then 50 mg (IV) q24h until improved†	Amphotericin B 1 mg/kg (IV) q24h x 7 days† or until 2-3 grams given **or** Voriconazole 6 mg/kg (IV) q12h x 1 day, then 4 mg/kg (IV) q12h or 200 mg (PO) q12h until cured. If < 40 kg, use 100 mg instead of 200 mg (PO) maintenance dose

BPA = bronchopulmonary aspergillosis
* Initiate therapy with itraconazole 200 mg (IV) q12h x 7-14 days
† Follow with itraconazole 200 mg (PO) solution q12h until cured

Pulmonary Infiltrates/Mass Lesions (cont'd)

Subset	Pathogens	Preferred Therapy	Alternate Therapy
Pulmonary sporotrichosis	Sporothrix schenckii	Amphotericin B deoxycholate 0.5 mg/kg (IV) q24h until 1-2 grams given **or** Lipid-associated formulation of amphotericin B (p. 297) (IV) q24h x 3 weeks	Itraconazole 200 mg (PO)* solution q12h until cured **or** Fluconazole 800 mg (IV or PO) x 1 dose, then 400 mg (PO) q24h x 6 months, then 200 mg (PO) q12h until cured
Pulmonary coccidioido-mycosis	Coccidioides immitis	Itraconazole 200 mg (PO)* solution q12h until cured **or** Fluconazole 800 mg (IV or PO) x 1 dose, then 400 mg (PO) q24h until cured	Amphotericin B deoxycholate 1 mg/kg (IV) q24h x 7 days†
Pulmonary nocardiosis	Nocardia asteroides	TMP-SMX 1 DS tablet (PO) q12h until cured	Minocycline 100 mg (PO) q12h until cured
Pulmonary cryptococcosis	Cryptococcus neoformans	Fluconazole 800 mg (IV or PO) x 1 dose, then 400 mg (PO) q24h until cured	Amphotericin B deoxycholate 0.5 mg/kg (IV) q24h until 1-2 grams given **or** Lipid-associated formulation of amphotericin B (p. 297) (IV) q24h x 3 weeks
Pulmonary zygomycosis (mucor-mycosis)	Rhizopus/ Mucor/Absidia	Lipid-associated formulation of amphotericin B (p. 297) (IV) q24h x 1-2 weeks† or x 3 wks **or** Amphotericin B deoxycholate 1-1.5 mg/kg (IV) q24h x 1-2 wks† or until 2-3 grams given	Itraconazole 200 mg (PO)* solution q12h until cured
Pulmonary pseudall-escheriasis	Pseudallescheria boydii/ Scedosporium apiospermum	Voriconazole 6 mg/kg (IV) q12h x 1 day, then 4 mg/kg (IV) q12h or 200 mg (PO) q12h until cured. If < 40 kg, use 100 mg instead of 200 mg (PO) maintenance dose	Itraconazole 200 mg (PO)* solution q12h until cured

* Initiate therapy with itraconazole 200 mg (IV) q12h x 7-14 days
† Follow with itraconazole 200 mg (PO) solution q12h until cured

Pulmonary Blastomycosis (Blastomyces dermatitidis)
Clinical Presentation: Highly variable. May present as a chronic/non-resolving pneumonia with fever/cough and characteristic "right-sided perihilar infiltrate" ± small pleural effusion
Diagnostic Considerations: May be recovered from sputum or demonstrated in lung tissue specimens. Usual sites of dissemination include skin, bones and prostate, not CNS or adrenals
Pitfalls: Dissemination to extra-pulmonary sites may occur years after pneumonia

Prognosis: Related to severity/extent of infection. One-third of cases are self-limited and do not require treatment

Pulmonary Histoplasmosis (Histoplasma capsulatum)
Clinical Presentation: Acute primary infection presents as self-limiting flu-like illness with fever, headache, nonproductive cough, chills, and chest pain. Minority of patients become overtly ill with complicated respiratory or progressive pulmonary infection. Can cause arthralgias, E. nodosum, E. multiforme, or pericarditis. May occur in outbreak. Chronic infection presents as chronic pneumonia resembling TB or chronic disseminated infection
Diagnostic Considerations: May be recovered from sputum or demonstrated in lung tissue specimens. Worldwide distribution, but most common in Central/South Central United States. Acute disseminated histoplasmosis suggests HIV/AIDS
Pitfalls: Pleural effusion is uncommon. Do not treat old/inactive/minimal histoplasmosis, histoplasmosis pulmonary calcification, or histoplasmosis fibrosing mediastinitis. Differentiate from TB
Prognosis: Related to severity/extent of infection. No treatment is needed for self-limiting acute histoplasmosis presenting as flu-like illness. HIV/AIDS patients should receive life-long suppressive therapy with itraconazole

Pulmonary Paracoccidioidomycosis (South American Blastomycosis)
Clinical Presentation: Typically presents as a chronic pneumonia syndrome with productive cough, blood-tinged sputum, dyspnea, and chest pain. May also develop fever, malaise, weight loss, mucosal ulcerations in/around mouth and nose, dysphagia, changes in voice, cutaneous lesions on face/limbs, or cervical adenopathy. Can disseminate to prostate, epididymis, kidneys, or adrenals
Diagnostic Considerations: Characteristic "pilot wheel" shaped yeast in sputum. Diagnosis by culture and stain (Gomori) of organism from clinical specimen. Found only in Latin American. One-third of cases have only pulmonary involvement. Skin test is non-specific/non-diagnostic
Pitfalls: No distinguishing radiologic features. No clinical adrenal insufficiency, in contrast to TB or histoplasmosis. Hilar adenopathy/pleural effusions are uncommon
Prognosis: Related to severity/extent of infection. HIV/AIDS require life-long suppression with TMP-SMX 1 DS tablet (PO) q24h or itraconazole 200 mg (PO) solution q24h

Pulmonary Actinomycosis (Actinomyces israelii)
Clinical Presentation: Indolent, slowly progressive infiltrates involving the pulmonary parenchyma ± pleural space. Presents with fever, chest pain, weight loss. Cough/hemoptysis are less common. Chest wall sinuses frequently develop. Chest x-ray shows adjacent dense infiltrate. "Sulfur granules" are common in sinus drainage fluid
Diagnostic Considerations: Diagnosis by stain/culture of drainage from sinuses or lung/bone biopsy specimens. Actinomyces are non-acid fast and anaerobic
Pitfalls: No CNS lesions, but bone erosion is common with chest lesions. Prior antibiotic therapy may interfere with isolation of organism
Prognosis: Excellent when treated until lesions resolve. Use IV regimen in critically ill patients, then switch to oral regimen

Bronchopulmonary Aspergillosis (BPA / ABPA)
Clinical Presentation: Migratory pulmonary infiltrates in chronic asthmatics. Eosinophilia is common, and sputum shows Charcot-Leyden crystals/brown flecks containing Aspergillus
Diagnostic Considerations: Diagnosis by Aspergillus in sputum and high-titers of Aspergillus precipitins in serum. BPA is an allergic reaction in chronic asthmatics, *not* an infectious disease. Pulmonary infiltrates with peripheral eosinophilia in chronic asthmatics suggests the diagnosis
Pitfalls: Correct diagnosis is important since therapy is steroids, not antifungals

Prognosis: Related to severity/duration of asthma and promptness of steroid therapy

Acute Invasive Aspergillus Pneumonia (see p. 254)

Chronic Aspergillus Pneumonia
Clinical Presentation: Occurs in patients with AIDS, chronic granulomatous disease, alcoholism, diabetes, and those receiving steroids for chronic pulmonary disease. Usual features include chronic productive cough ± hemoptysis, low-grade fever, weight loss, and malaise. Chronic Aspergillus pneumonia resembles TB, histoplasmosis, melioidosis
Diagnostic Considerations: Diagnosis by lung biopsy demonstrating septate hyphae invading lung parenchyma. Aspergillus may be in sputum, but is not diagnostic of Aspergillus pneumonia
Pitfalls: May extend into chest wall, vertebral column, or brachial plexus
Prognosis: Related to severity/extent of infection

Pulmonary Sporotrichosis (Sporothrix schenckii)
Clinical Presentation: Occurs in normal hosts, alcoholics, and patients with concomitant medical illness (TB, diabetes, sarcoidosis, steroid use). Usually presents as productive cough, low-grade fever, and weight loss. Chest x-ray shows cavitary thin-walled lesions with associated infiltrate. Hemoptysis is unusual. Differential diagnosis includes other thin-walled cavitary lung lesions (e.g., histoplasmosis, coccidioidomycosis, TB, atypical TB, paragonimiasis)
Diagnostic Considerations: Diagnosis by lung biopsy demonstrating invasive lung disease, not broncho-alveolar lavage. Usually a history of puncture/traumatic wound involving an extremity. May be associated with septic arthritis/osteomyelitis
Pitfalls: Sporotrichosis in lungs implies disseminated disease. May need repeated attempts at culture
Prognosis: Related to extent of infection/degree of immunosuppression

Pulmonary Coccidioidomycosis (Coccidioides immitis)
Clinical Presentation: Usually presents as a solitary, peripheral, thin-walled cavitary lesion in early or later stage of primary infection. May present as a solitary pulmonary nodule. E. nodosum and bilateral hilar adenopathy are common (in contrast to sporotrichosis). Hemoptysis is unusual
Diagnostic Considerations: Diagnosis by biopsy/Coccidioides serology. Increased incidence of dissemination in Filipinos, Blacks, and American Indians. May be associated with chronic meningitis/osteomyelitis
Pitfalls: Dissemination is preceded by ↓ Coccidioides titers/disappearance of E. nodosum
Prognosis: Related to extent of infection/degree of immunosuppression

Pulmonary Nocardiosis (Nocardia asteroides)
Clinical Presentation: Usually presents as a dense lower lobe lung mass without cavitation. May have associated mass lesions in CNS. Chest wall sinuses are more common with Actinomycosis
Diagnostic Considerations: Diagnosis by demonstrating organisms by stain/culture of lung specimens. Nocardia are weakly acid-fast and aerobic
Pitfalls: Use IV regimens in critically ill patients. HIV/AIDS require life-long suppressive therapy with TMP-SMX or minocycline
Prognosis: Related to extent of infection/degree of immunosuppression

Pulmonary Cryptococcosis (Cryptococcus neoformans)
Clinical Presentation: Individual focus of infection is usually inapparent/minimal when patient presents with disseminated cryptococcal infection. Pneumonia is typically a minor part of disseminated disease; CNS manifestations usually predominate (e.g., headache, subtle cognitive changes, occasional meningeal signs, focal neurological deficits)
Diagnostic Considerations: Diagnosis by demonstrating organisms in sputum/lung specimens

Pitfalls: Clinical presentation of isolated cryptococcal pneumonia is rare. HIV/AIDS patients require life-long suppressive therapy with fluconazole
Prognosis: Related to extent of dissemination/degree of immunosuppression

Pulmonary Zygomycosis (Mucormycosis) (Rhizopus/Mucor/Absidia)

Clinical Presentation: Progressive pneumonia with fever, dyspnea, and cough unresponsive to antibiotic therapy. Usually seen only in compromised hosts. Chest x-ray is not characteristic, but shows infiltrate with consolidation in > 50% of patients. Cavitation occurs in 40% as neutropenia resolves
Diagnostic Considerations: Diagnosis by demonstrating organisms in lung biopsy. Pleural effusion is not a feature of pulmonary mucormycosis
Pitfalls: Causes rhinocerebral mucormycosis in diabetics, pneumonia in leukopenic compromised hosts
Prognosis: Related to degree of immunosuppression and underlying disease

Pulmonary Pseudallescheriasis (P. boydii/S. apiospermum)

Clinical Presentation: Progressive pulmonary infiltrates indistinguishable from Aspergillosis or Mucor. Usually seen only in compromised hosts (e.g., prolonged neutropenia, high-dose steroids, bone marrow or solid organ transplants, AIDS). Manifests as cough, fever, pleuritic pain, and often hemoptysis. No characteristic chest x-ray appearance
Diagnostic Considerations: Diagnosis by demonstrating organism in lung biopsy. Hemoptysis is common in patients with cavitary lesions. CNS involvement is rare
Pitfalls: One of few invasive fungi unresponsive to amphotericin B deoxycholate. Cause of sinusitis in diabetics, and pneumonia in leukopenic compromised hosts
Prognosis: Related to severity/extent of infection and degree of immunosuppression. Cavitary lesions causing hemoptysis often require surgical excision. Disseminated infection is often fatal

Parasites, Fungi, Unusual Organisms in Liver

Liver Flukes

Subset	Pathogens	Preferred Therapy	Alternate Therapy
Fascioliasis	Fasciola hepatica Fasciola gigantica	Triclabendazole 10 mg/kg (PO) x 1 dose	Bithionol 30-50 mg/kg (PO) q48h x 10-15 doses
Clonorchiasis/ Opisthorchiasis	Clonorchis sinensis Opisthorchis viverrini	Praziquantel 25 mg/kg (PO) q8h x 3 doses	C. sinensis Albendazole 400 mg (PO) q12h x 7 days O. viverrini None

Hepatic Fascioliasis (F. hepatica/F. gigantica)

Clinical Presentation: Frequently asymptomatic, but may present acutely with fever, right upper quadrant pain, nausea, diarrhea, wheezing, urticaria, hepatomegaly, eosinophilia, anemia. Chronic disease is associated with gallstones, cholecystitis, cholangitis, liver abscess, generalized adenopathy. Subacute nodules, hydrocele, lung/brain abscess can be seen in ectopic forms. "Linear echogenic structures" are evident on liver ultrasound
Diagnostic Consideration: Diagnosis by F. hepatica/F. gigantica eggs in stool. Endemic in sheep-raising areas (sheep liver flukes). Acquired from freshwater plants (watercress). Not associated with cholangiocarcinoma
Pitfalls: May present as Katayama syndrome resembling schistosomiasis, with high fever, eosinophilia,

and hepatosplenomegaly. Unlike other trematodes, praziquantel is ineffective
Prognosis: Related to extent/location of liver damage

Hepatic Clonorchiasis (C. sinensis) / Opisthorchiasis (O. viverrini)

Clinical Presentation: Frequently asymptomatic, but may present 2-4 weeks after ingestion of fluke with fever, tender hepatomegaly, rash, and eosinophilia. Chronically presents as recurrent cholangitis, chronic cholecystitis, or pancreatitis. Associated with cholangiocarcinoma (unlike fascioliasis)
Diagnostic Considerations: Diagnosis by demonstrating C. sinensis/O. viverrini eggs in stool. Clonorchiasis is acquired from ingesting raw/inadequately cooked infected freshwater (Cyprinoid) fish in Southeast Asia. Opisthorchiasis is acquired from ingesting raw/inadequately cooked infected freshwater fish/crayfish from Laos, Cambodia, or Thailand
Pitfalls: Cholecystitis with eosinophilia should suggest clonorchiasis
Prognosis: Related to extent/location of hepatic damage. Associated with cholangiocarcinoma

Cystic Masses in Liver

Subset	Pathogens	Preferred Therapy	Alternate Therapy
Hepatic amebiasis	Entamoeba histolytica	Metronidazole 750 mg (PO) q8h x 7-10 days	Tinidazole 2 gm/day (PO) in 3 divided doses x 3 days
Hepatic echinococcosis (hydatid cyst disease)	Echinococcus granulosus	<u>Operable</u> Surgical resection **plus** Albendazole 400 mg* (PO) q12h x 1-6 months	<u>Inoperable</u> Albendazole 400 mg* (PO) q12h x 1-6 months

* If < 60 kg, give albendazole 7.5 mg/kg

Hepatic Amebiasis (Entamoeba histolytica)

Clinical Presentation: Presents insidiously with weight loss and night sweats, or acutely ill with fever, nausea, vomiting, right upper quadrant pain. Typically, amebic liver abscesses are single, affect the posterior right lobe of liver, and do not show air/fluid levels. (In contrast, bacterial liver abscesses are usually multiple, distributed in all lobes of liver, and often show air/fluid levels.) Amebic liver abscesses do not calcify like hydatid cysts
Diagnostic Considerations: Diagnosis by E. histolytica serology/E. histolytica in cyst walls. Worldwide distribution. Acquired by ingesting amebic cysts. Amebic liver abscess usually presents years after initial mild amebic dysenteric episode
Pitfalls: Amebic abscess fluid ("Anchovy paste") contains no PMNs or amebas; amebas are found only in cyst walls. Eosinophilia is not a feature of amebiasis
Prognosis: Related to health of host/extrapulmonary spread

Hepatic Echinococcosis (Echinococcus granulosus) Hydatid Cyst Disease

Clinical Presentation: Right upper quadrant pain/mass when cysts enlarge enough to cause symptoms. Hepatic cysts are unilocular in 70%, multilocular in 30%
Diagnostic Considerations: Diagnosis by demonstrating E. granulosus in cyst. Serology is unreliable. Worldwide distribution in sheep/cattle raising areas. Acquired by ingestion of eggs from dogs
Pitfalls: Eosinophilia not a feature of hydatid cyst disease. Hydatid cysts are multifaceted, loculated, and calcified
Prognosis: Related to location/extent of extrahepatic cysts. Large cysts are best treated by surgical removal after injection with hypertonic saline, alcohol, or iodophor to kill germinal layer/daughter cysts. Percutaneous drainage under ultrasound guidance plus albendazole may be effective

Hepatomegaly

Subset	Pathogen	Preferred Therapy	Alternate Therapy
Visceral leishmaniasis (Kala-azar)	Leishmania donovani	Antimony stibogluconate or meglumine antimonate 10 mg/kg (IM) q12h x 28 days **or** Miltefosine 50 mg (PO) q12h x 21 days **or** Amphotericin B deoxycholate 0.5-1 mg/kg (IV) q48h up to 8 weeks **or** Lipid-associated formulation of amphotericin B (p. 297) (IV) x 5 days	Pentamidine 4 mg/kg (IM or IV) q48h x 15 doses
Schistosomiasis	Schistosoma mansoni	Praziquantel 20 mg/kg (PO) q12h x 2 doses	Oxamniquine 15 mg/kg (PO) x 1 dose. In Africa, give 20 mg/kg (PO) q24h x 3 days
	Schistosoma japonicum	Praziquantel 20 mg/kg (PO) q8h x 3 doses	None

Visceral Leishmaniasis (Leishmania donovani) Kala-azar
Clinical Presentation: Subacute or chronic systemic cases manifest months to years after initial exposure to Leishmania, most often with fever, weight loss, anemia, hepatosplenomegaly ± generalized adenopathy. Laboratory abnormalities include leukopenia, anemia, and polyclonal gammopathy on SPEP. Incubation period is usually 3-8 months. May have atypical presentation in HIV/AIDS (e.g., no splenomegaly). Acutely can mimic malaria with chills/temperature spikes. Post–Kala-azar dermatitis may resemble leprosy, and is persistent/common on face
Diagnostic Considerations: Double quotidian fever (double daily temperature spike) in persons from endemic areas with hepatosplenomegaly suggests the diagnosis. Diagnosis by liver/bone marrow biopsy demonstrating Leishmania bodies or specific L. donovani serology. Most common in Southern Europe, Middle East, Asia, Africa, and South America. Facial lesion is a clue to the diagnosis
Pitfalls: In acute cases, can mimic malaria with chills and temperature spikes, but no thrombocytopenia or atypical lymphocytes. Antimony resistance is common in India
Prognosis: Related to degree of liver/spleen involvement

Hepatic Schistosomiasis (Schistosoma mansoni/japonicum)
Clinical Presentation: May present acutely with Katayama fever (serum sickness-like illness with wheezing and eosinophilia) 4-8 weeks after exposure. May be accompanied or followed by fever/chills, headache, cough, abdominal pain, diarrhea, generalized lymphadenopathy, or hepatosplenomegaly. Laboratory abnormalities include leukocytosis, eosinophilia, and polyclonal gammopathy on SPEP. Resolves spontaneously after 2-4 weeks. After 10-15 years, may present chronically as hepatosplenic schistosomiasis, with pre-sinusoidal portal hypertension, hepatomegaly (L > R lobe enlargement), no jaundice, and intact liver function
Diagnostic Considerations: Diagnosis by S. mansoni/S. japonicum eggs in stool/liver biopsy. Serology is good for acute (not chronic) schistosomiasis. CT/MRI of liver shows "turtle back" septal calcifications. Rare complications include cor pulmonale and protein-losing enteropathy. Increased incidence of hepatitis B/C and chronic Salmonella infections. Renal complications include glomerulonephritis and nephrotic syndrome

Pitfalls: Chronic schistosomiasis is not associated with eosinophilia. S. hematobium does not infect the liver/spleen. Oxamniquine is contraindicated in pregnancy
Prognosis: Related to egg burden

Parasites, Fungi, Unusual Organisms in Stool/Intestines

Intestinal Protozoa

Subset	Pathogens	Preferred Therapy	Alternate Therapy
Amebiasis	E. histolytica	See p. 67	
Giardiasis	Giardia lamblia	See p. 67	
Isosporiasis	Isospora belli	TMP-SMX 1 DS tablet (PO) q12h x 10 days. If immunocompromised, give TMP-SMX 1 DS tablet (PO) q6h x 3 weeks	Ciprofloxacin 500 mg (PO) q12h x 7 days **or** Pyrimethamine 75 mg (PO) q24h + folinic acid 10 mg (PO) q24h x 2 weeks
Dientamoebiasis	Dientamoeba fragilis	Doxycycline 100 mg (PO) q12h x 10 days	Iodoquinol 650 mg (PO) q8h x 20 days **or** Paromomycin 8-12 mg/kg (PO) q8h x 7 days **or** Metronidazole 500-750 mg (PO) q8h x 10 days
Blastocystis	Blastocystis hominis	Metronidazole 750 mg (PO) q8h x 10 days	Iodoquinol 650 mg (PO) q8h x 20 days
Cyclospora	Cyclospora	See p. 67	
Cryptosporidiosis	Cryptosporidia	See p. 67 (for HIV/AIDS, see p. 250)	
Balantidiasis	Balantidium coli	Doxycycline 100 (PO) q12h x 10 days	Iodoquinol 650 mg (PO) q8h x 20 days **or** Metronidazole 750 mg (PO) q8h x 5 days

Amebiasis (Entamoeba histolytica) (see p. 69)

Giardiasis (Giardia lamblia) (see p. 69)

Isosporiasis (Isospora belli)
Clinical Presentation: Acute/subacute onset of diarrhea. Isospora belli is the only protozoa to cause diarrhea with eosinophils in stool

Diagnostic Considerations: Diagnosis by demonstrating organism in stool/intestinal biopsy specimen. Associated with HIV, immigration from Latin America, daycare centers, and mental institutions. If stool exam is negative, "string test"/duodenal aspirate and biopsy may be helpful
Pitfalls: Difficult to eradicate; may last months. Multiple stool samples may be needed for diagnosis. Add folinic acid 10 mg (PO) q24 if pyrimethamine is used. In HIV/AIDS, may need life-long suppressive therapy with TMP-SMX 1-2 DS tablet (PO) q24h (pp. 251, 257)
Prognosis: Related to adequacy of treatment/degree of immunosuppression

Dientamoebiasis (Dientamoeba fragilis)
Clinical Presentation: Acute/subacute onset of diarrhea. No cyst stage. Lives only as trophozoite
Diagnostic Considerations: Diagnosis by demonstrating organism in stool/intestinal biopsy specimen. Mucus in diarrheal stools, not blood. May have abdominal pain. Diarrhea may last for months/years
Pitfalls: Frequently associated with pinworm (Enterobius vermicularis) infection
Prognosis: Related to adequacy of fluid replacement/underlying health of host

Blastocystis (Blastocystis hominis)
Clinical Presentation: Acute/subacute onset of diarrhea
Diagnostic Considerations: Diagnosis by demonstrating organism in stool/intestinal biopsy specimen. Trichrome stain reveals characteristic "halo" (slime capsule) in stool specimens
Pitfalls: Uncommon GI pathogen. Consider as cause of diarrhea only after other pathogens excluded
Prognosis: Related to adequacy of fluid replacement/underlying health of host

Cyclospora (see p. 69)

Cryptosporidiosis (see p. 69; for HIV/AIDS, see p. 257)

Balantidiasis (Balantidium coli)
Clinical Presentation: Acute/subacute onset of diarrhea. Fecal WBCs only with mucosal invasion. Largest intestinal protozoa and only ciliated protozoa to infect humans
Diagnostic Considerations: Diagnosis by demonstrating organism in stool/intestinal biopsy specimen. Identifying features include darkly staining "kidney shaped" nucleus and large size. Fulminant dysentery seen only in debilitated/compromised hosts
Pitfalls: Stools not bloody. Diarrhea may be intermittent
Prognosis: Related to adequacy of fluid replacement/underlying health of host

Intestinal Nematodes (Roundworms)

Subset	Pathogens	Preferred Therapy	Alternate Therapy
Capillariasis	Capillaria philippinensis	Mebendazole 200 mg (PO) q12h x 20 days	Albendazole 400 mg (PO) q24h x 10 days
Angiostrongyliasis (rodent lung/ intestinal worm)	Angiostrongylus costaricensis	Mebendazole 200-400 mg (PO) q8h x 10 days	Thiabendazole 25 mg/kg (PO) x q8h x 3 days (max. 3 gm/day)
Hookworm	Necator americanus/ Ancylostoma duodenale	Albendazole 400 mg (PO) x 1 dose **or** Mebendazole 100 mg (PO) q12h x 3 days or 500 mg (PO) x 1 dose	Pyrantel pamoate 11 mg/kg (PO) q24h x 3 days (max. 1 gm/day)

Intestinal Nematodes (Roundworms) (cont'd)

Subset	Pathogens	Preferred Therapy	Alternate Therapy
Strongyloidiasis	Strongyloides stercoralis	Ivermectin 200 mcg/kg (PO) q24h x 2 days **or** Thiabendazole 25 mg/kg (PO) q12h x 2 days (max. 3 gm/day)	Albendazole 400 mg (PO) q24h x 3 days
Ascariasis	Ascaris lumbricoides	Albendazole 400 mg (PO) x 1 dose **or** Mebendazole 100 mg (PO) q12h x 3 days or 500 mg (PO) x 1 dose	Pyrantel pamoate 11 mg/kg (PO) x 1 dose (max. 1 gm)
Trichostrongyliasis	Trichostrongylus orientalis	Pyrantel pamoate 11 mg/kg (PO) x 1 dose (max. 1 gm)	Albendazole 400 mg (PO) x 1 dose **or** Mebendazole 100 mg (PO) q12h x 3 days
Pinworm	Enterobius vermicularis	Pyrantel pamoate 11 mg/kg (PO) x 1 dose (max. 1 gm); repeat in 2 weeks **or** Albendazole 400 mg (PO) x 1 dose; repeat in 2 weeks	Mebendazole 100 mg (PO) x 1 dose; repeat in 2 weeks
Whipworm	Trichuris trichiura	Mebendazole 100 mg (PO) q12h x 3 days, or 500 mg (PO) x 1 dose	Albendazole 400 mg (PO) x 1 dose

Capillariasis (Capillaria philippinensis)

Clinical Presentation: Intermittent voluminous watery diarrhea ± malabsorption. Fever is uncommon
Diagnostic Considerations: Diagnosis by demonstrating ova or parasite in stools. Resembles Trichuris, but C. philippinensis ova are larger and have a "pitted shell" with prominent polar plugs. Peripheral eosinophilia is uncommon until after therapy
Pitfalls: Serology is positive in 85%, but cross-reacts with other parasites
Prognosis: Related to severity of malabsorption/extra-intestinal disease

Angiostrongyliasis (A. costaricensis) Rodent Lung/Intestinal Worm

Clinical Presentation: Presents as appendicitis (worm resides and deposits eggs in arteries/arterioles around ileocecum/appendix)
Diagnostic Considerations: Diagnosis by demonstrating organism in biopsied/excised tissue. May involve proximal small bowel, liver, CNS
Pitfalls: Can present as RLQ mass/fever resembling regional enteritis (Crohn's disease), but with eosinophilia and leukocytosis
Prognosis: Related to severity of malabsorption and extra-intestinal disease

Hookworm (Necator americanus/Ancylostoma duodenale)

Clinical Presentation: Pruritic, vesicular eruptions at site of filariform larval entry ("ground itch"). Pulmonary symptoms and transient eosinophilia may occur during migratory phase to intestines. Later, abdominal pain, diarrhea, weight loss, hypoalbuminemia, and anemia develop

Diagnostic Considerations: Diagnosis by demonstrating eggs/larvae in stool specimens. N. americanus can ingest 0.3 ml of blood/worm/day, much greater than A. duodenale. Anemia may be severe with heavy infestation (up to 100 mL/day)

Pitfalls: Eggs in fresh stool, not rhabditiform larvae

Prognosis: Related to severity of anemia/malabsorption

Strongyloidiasis (Strongyloides stercoralis)

Clinical Presentation: Pruritic, papular, erythematous rash. Pulmonary symptoms (cough, asthma) may occur during lung migration phase. May develop Loeffler's syndrome (pulmonary infiltrates with eosinophilia) or ARDS in heavy infections. Intestinal phase associated with colicky abdominal pain, diarrhea, and malabsorption

Diagnostic Considerations: Diagnosis by demonstrating larvae in stool specimens/duodenal fluid. Usually asymptomatic in normal hosts, but causes "hyperinfection syndrome" in compromised hosts. CNS strongyloides (part of hyperinfection syndrome) should suggest diagnosis of HIV in non-immunosuppressed patients. Diarrhea/abdominal pain mimics regional enteritis (Crohn's disease) or ulcerative colitis. Malabsorption is common and mimics tropical sprue. Anemia is usually mild

Pitfalls: Usually rhabditiform larvae (not eggs) in stools

Prognosis: Related to severity of malabsorption

Ascariasis (Ascaris lumbricoides)

Clinical Presentation: Pulmonary symptoms (cough, asthma) may occur during lung migration phase. May develop Loeffler's syndrome (pulmonary infiltrates with eosinophilia), as with hookworm/Strongyloides. Intestinal symptoms develop late. Usually asymptomatic until intestinal/biliary obstruction occurs. Can obstruct the appendix/pancreatic duct

Diagnostic Considerations: Diagnosis by demonstrating eggs in stool specimens. Abdominal ultrasound can detect obstruction from adult worms. Most infections are asymptomatic; symptoms are related to "worm burden"/ectopic migration. Each female worm may produce up to 250,000 eggs/day

Pitfalls: Lung involvement (bronchospasm, bronchopneumonia, lung abscess) is prominent in HIV/AIDS

Prognosis: Related to worm burden/extra-intestinal organ invasion

Trichostrongyliasis (Trichostrongylus orientalis)

Clinical Presentation: Mild intestinal symptoms with persistent eosinophilia

Diagnostic Considerations: Diagnosis by demonstrating eggs in stool specimens. Most prevalent in the Middle East and Asia. Mild anemia. Eosinophilia is usually > 10%

Pitfalls: Must differentiate eggs from hookworm, and rhabditiform larvae from Strongyloides. T. orientalis eggs have "pointed ends"

Prognosis: Related to extent of disease/underlying health of host

Pinworm (Enterobius vermicularis)

Clinical Presentation: Primarily affects children. Perianal pruritus is the main symptom. Worm lives in the cecum, but patients do not have intestinal symptoms

Diagnostic Considerations: Scotch tape of anus at night can be used to detect eggs left by migrating female worms (Scotch tape test). Number of E. vermicularis in stool is low

Pitfalls: Abdominal pain and diarrhea should prompt search for Dientamoeba fragilis, since co-infection is common

Prognosis: Excellent

Whipworm (Trichuris trichiura)

Clinical Presentation: May present as "chronic appendicitis." Severe infestation may cause bloody diarrhea/abdominal pain ("Trichuris dysentery syndrome"), rectal prolapse

Diagnostic Considerations: Diagnosis by demonstrating large eggs with bile-stained, triple-layered eggshell walls and doubly operculated transparent plugs. Most patients are asymptomatic or mildly anemic

Pitfalls: Commonly co-exists with Ascaris, hookworm, or E. histolytica

Prognosis: Related to severity/extent of dysentery. May need retreatment if heavy infection

Intestinal Cestodes (Tapeworms)

Subset	Pathogens	Preferred Therapy	Alternate Therapy
Beef tapeworm	Taenia saginata	Praziquantel 5-10 mg/kg (PO) x 1 dose	Niclosamide 2 gm (PO) x 1 dose
Pork tapeworm	Taenia solium	Praziquantel 5-10 mg/kg (PO) x 1 dose	Niclosamide 2 gm (PO) x 1 dose
Dwarf tapeworm	Hymenolepis nana	Praziquantel 25 mg/kg (PO) x 1 dose	None
Fish tapeworm	Diphyllobothrium latum	Praziquantel 10 mg/kg (PO) x 1 dose	Niclosamide 2 gm (PO) x 1 dose

Beef Tapeworm (Taenia saginata) / Pork Tapeworm (Taenia solium)

Clinical Presentation: Usually mild symptoms (weight loss, anemia), since most infections are caused by a single tapeworm

Diagnostic Considerations: Diagnosis by demonstrating tapeworm in stool. Taenia eggs in stool cannot be speciated; all are brown and spherical with a radially-striated inner shell. T. saginata may survive for 10 years, T. solium for 25 years

Pitfalls: Severe cases may cause appendicitis, intestinal obstruction/perforation

Prognosis: Related to severity of malabsorption/intestinal obstruction

Dwarf Tapeworm (Hymenolepis nana)

Clinical Presentation: Usually asymptomatic

Diagnostic Considerations: Diagnosis by demonstrating typical eggs in stool, with two shells enclosing inner oncosphere with hooklets. ELISA is positive in 85%, but cross-reacts with Taenia/Cysticercosis. GI symptoms develop with stool egg counts > 15,000/gm

Pitfalls: Abdominal pain and diarrhea in heavy infestations

Prognosis: Related to severity of malabsorption/underlying health of host

Fish Tapeworm (Diphyllobothrium latum)

Clinical Presentation: Symptoms secondary to macrocytic anemia from vitamin B_{12} deficiency. Most infestations are asymptomatic

Diagnostic Considerations: Diagnosis by demonstrating eggs/proglottides in stool

Pitfalls: Vitamin B_{12} deficiency anemia requires prolonged infection (> 3 years)

Prognosis: Related to severity of B_{12} deficiency anemia/underlying health of host

Intestinal Trematodes (Flukes/Flatworms)

Subset	Pathogens	Preferred Therapy
Fasciolopsiasis	Fasciolopsis buski	Praziquantel 25 mg/kg (PO) q8h x 3 doses
Heterophyiasis	Heterophyes heterophyes Metagonimus yokogawai	Praziquantel 25 mg/kg (PO) q8h x 3 doses

Fasciolopsiasis (Fasciolopsis buski)
Clinical Presentation: Diarrhea with copious mucus in stool. Most cases are asymptomatic
Diagnostic Considerations: Diagnosis by demonstrating eggs in stool. May have eosinophilia, low-grade fever ± malabsorption. Intestinal obstruction is the most serious complication
Pitfalls: Mimics peptic ulcer disease with upper abdominal pain relieved by food
Prognosis: Related to severity/extent of malabsorption/intestinal obstruction

Heterophyiasis (Heterophyes heterophyes / Metagonimus yokogawai)
Clinical Presentation: Usually asymptomatic or mild intestinal symptoms. Embolization of eggs may result in myocarditis, myocardial fibrosis, or cerebral hemorrhage. Eosinophilia may be present
Diagnostic Considerations: Diagnosis by demonstrating eggs in stool. Small intestinal fluke
Pitfalls: Difficult to differentiate from Clonorchis sinensis
Prognosis: Related to extent/severity of extra-intestinal dissemination to heart, lungs, CNS

Other Intestinal Infections

Subset	Pathogen	Preferred Therapy
Whipple's disease	Tropheryma whippelii	Ceftriaxone 1-2 gm (IV) q24h x 2 weeks plus streptomycin 1 gm (IM) q24h x 2 weeks. Follow with TMP-SMX 1 DS tablet (PO) q12h x 1 year

Whipple's Disease (Tropheryma whippelii)
Clinical Presentation: Diarrhea, fever, encephalopathy/dementia, weight loss, polyarthritis, myocarditis, pericarditis, general lymphadenopathy ± malabsorption
Diagnostic Considerations: Diagnosis by demonstrating organism by stain/culture from macrophages in small bowel biopsy specimens
Pitfalls: May present with dementia mimicking Alzheimer's disease, or FUO mimicking celiac disease or lymphoma. Optimum length of treatment is unknown. Relapses occur
Prognosis: Related to severity/extent of extra-intestinal disease

Parasites, Fungi, Unusual Organisms in Skin/Muscle

Infiltrative Skin/Subcutaneous Lesions

Subset	Pathogens	Preferred Therapy
Cutaneous leishmaniasis Old World	Leishmania major Leishmania tropica	Sodium stibogluconate 20 mg/kg (IV or IM) q24h x 20-28 days **or** Pentamidine 4 mg/kg (IV) q48h x 4 doses **or** Fluconazole 200 mg (PO) q24h x 6 weeks (L. major)
New World	Leishmania mexicana Leishmania braziliense	Sodium stibogluconate 20 mg/kg (IV or IM) q24h x 20-28 days **or** Pentamidine 4 mg/kg (IV) q48h x 4 doses **or** Miltefosine 2.25 mg/kg (PO) q24h x 3-4 weeks
Leprosy Lepromatous	Mycobacterium leprae	Dapsone 100 mg (PO) q24h x 1-2 years + clofazimine 50 mg (PO) q24h x 1-2 years + rifampin 600 mg (PO) monthly x 1-2 years
Non-lepromatous	Mycobacterium leprae	Dapsone 100 mg (PO) q24h x 6 months + rifampin 600 mg (PO) monthly x 6 months
Erythrasma	Corynebacterium minutissimum	Erythromycin 250 mg (PO) q6h x 2 weeks

Cutaneous Leishmaniasis (Old World/New World)

Clinical Presentation: Variable presentation. Typically, a nodule develops then ulcerates, with a raised/erythematous outer border and a central area of granulation tissue. May be single or multiple. Usually non-pruritic/non-painful. Occurs weeks after travel to endemic areas (New World leishmaniasis: Latin America; Old World leishmaniasis: Central Asia)

Diagnostic Considerations: Diagnosis by demonstrating Leishmania amastigotes or promastigotes in biopsy specimen

Pitfalls: Most skin lesions undergo spontaneous resolution. However, treatment is advisable for lesions caused by L. braziliensis or related species causing mucosal leishmaniasis

Prognosis: Excellent

Lepromatous Leprosy (Mycobacterium leprae)

Clinical Presentation: Diffuse, symmetrical, red or brown skin lesions presenting as macules, papules, plaques, or nodules. May also present as diffuse thickening of skin, especially involving ear lobes, face, and extremities. Loss of eyebrows/body hair may occur

Diagnostic Considerations: Diagnosis by demonstrating organism in tissue specimens. Afebrile bacteremia is frequent, with blood culture buffy coat smears positive for M. leprae. E. nodosum and polyclonal gammopathy on SPEP are common, and lepromin skin test/PPD are negative (anergic). When present, peripheral neuropathy is often symmetrical and acral in distribution

Pitfalls: Differential diagnosis is large. Consider leprosy in patients with unexplained skin diseases
Prognosis: Good if treated early

Non-Lepromatous Leprosy (Mycobacterium leprae)

Clinical Presentation: Small number of asymmetrical, hypopigmented skin lesions, which are often scaly with sharp borders and associated anesthesia. Asymmetric peripheral nerve trunk involvement is common
Diagnostic Considerations: Diagnosis by demonstrating granulomas with few acid-fast bacilli. Differentiate from cutaneous leishmaniasis by skin biopsy. Lepromin skin test/PPD are positive and SPEP is normal (in contrast to lepromatous leprosy)
Pitfalls: Wide spectrum of presentations depending on immune status and duration of disease. Differential diagnosis is large. Consider leprosy in patients with unexplained skin diseases
Prognosis: Good if treated early

Erythrasma (Corynebacterium minutissimum)

Clinical Presentation: Reddened/raised skin lesions on face/trunk. Not hot or pruritic
Diagnostic Considerations: Differentiated from Tinea versicolor by culture. C. minutissimum skin lesions fluoresce red under UV light
Pitfalls: Resembles Tinea versicolor, but lesions primarily involve the face, not trunk
Prognosis: Excellent

Infiltrative Skin Lesions ± Ulcers/Sinus Tracts/Abscesses

Subset	Pathogens	Preferred Therapy
Cutaneous histoplasmosis	Histoplasma capsulatum	Amphotericin B deoxycholate 0.5-1 mg/kg (IV) q24h x 7 days, then 0.8 mg/kg (IV) q48h or 3x/week until total of 10-15 mg/kg. Follow with suppressive therapy with itraconazole 200 mg (PO) solution q24h x 6-24 months (or indefinitely if HIV/AIDS) _Mild or moderate symptoms, no need for hospitalization_ Itraconazole 200 mg (PO) solution q12h x 2 days, then 200 mg (PO) solution q24h x 9 months
Cutaneous blastomycosis	Blastomyces dermatitidis	Treat the same as pulmonary infection (p. 198)
Cutaneous coccidioidomycosis	Coccidioides immitis	Treat the same as pulmonary infection (p. 199)
Cutaneous actinomycosis	Actinomyces israelii	Treat the same as pulmonary infection (p. 198)
Cutaneous nocardiosis	Nocardia sp.	Treat the same as pulmonary infection (p. 199)
Cutaneous amebiasis	Entamoeba histolytica	Treat the same as pulmonary infection (p. 196)

Infiltrative Skin Lesions ± Ulcers/Sinus Tracts/Abscesses (cont'd)

Subset	Pathogens	Preferred Therapy
Cutaneous mycobacteria *Scrofula*	Mycobacterium tuberculosis	INH 300 mg (PO) q24h + rifampin 600 mg (PO) q24h x 6 months
	Mycobacterium scrofulaceum	Surgical excision is curative
M. fortuitum-chelonae	Mycobacterium fortuitum-chelonae	Surgical excision + clarithromycin 500 mg (PO) q12h x 6 months
Swimming pool granuloma	Mycobacterium marinum	TMP-SMX 1 DS tablet (PO) q12h + ethambutol 15 mg/kg (PO) q24h x 6-12 weeks **or** Minocycline or doxycycline 100 mg (PO) q12h x 6-12 weeks
Buruli ulcer	Mycobacterium ulcerans	TMP-SMX 1 DS tablet (PO) q12h + ethambutol 15 mg/kg (PO) q24h x 6 weeks
Cutaneous MAI	Mycobacterium avium-intracellulare	Ethambutol 15 mg/kg (PO) q24h + azithromycin 1200 mg (PO) weekly x 6 months

Cutaneous Histoplasmosis (Histoplasma capsulatum)
Clinical Presentation: Chronic, raised, verrucous lesions
Diagnostic Considerations: Diagnosis by demonstrating organism by culture/tissue staining
Pitfalls: Skin nodules represent disseminated histoplasmosis, not isolated skin infection. Look for histoplasmosis elsewhere (e.g., lung, liver, bone marrow)
Prognosis: Related to extent of infection/degree of immunosuppression

Cutaneous Blastomyces (Blastomyces dermatitidis)
Clinical Presentation: Painless, erythematous, well-circumscribed, hyperkeratotic, crusted nodules or plaques that enlarge over time. Some may ulcerate and leave an undermined edge
Diagnostic Considerations: Diagnosis by demonstrating organism by culture/tissue staining. Blastomyces dermatitidis affects many organs
Pitfalls: When found in skin, look for Blastomyces elsewhere (e.g., lungs, prostate)
Prognosis: Related to extent of infection/degree of immunosuppression

Cutaneous Coccidioidomycosis (Coccidioides immitis)
Clinical Presentation: Skin lesions take many forms, including raised verrucous lesions, cold subcutaneous abscesses, indolent ulcers, or small papules
Diagnostic Considerations: Diagnosis by demonstrating organism by culture/tissue staining
Pitfalls: Skin nodules represent disseminated coccidioidomycosis, not isolated skin infection. Look for Coccidioides elsewhere (e.g., CNS, bone, lungs)
Prognosis: Related to extent of infection/degree of immunosuppression

Cutaneous Actinomycosis (Actinomyces israelii)
Clinical Presentation: Erythematous, uneven, indurated, woody, hard, cervicofacial tumor. Localized single/multiple sinus tracts in chest wall, abdominal wall, or inguinal/pelvic area may be present
Diagnostic Considerations: Diagnosis by demonstrating organism by culture/tissue staining

Pitfalls: Look for underlying bone involvement
Prognosis: Good with early/prolonged treatment

Cutaneous Nocardia (Nocardia brasiliensis)
Clinical Presentation: Subcutaneous abscesses may rupture to form chronically draining fistulas
Diagnostic Considerations: Diagnosis by demonstrating organism by culture/tissue staining. May present as "Madura foot"
Pitfalls: Look for underlying immunosuppressive disorder
Prognosis: Related to extent of infection/degree of immunosuppression

Cutaneous Amebiasis (Entamoeba histolytica)
Clinical Presentation: Ulcers with ragged edges, sinus tracts, amebomas, and strictures may develop around the anus/rectum or abdominal wall
Diagnostic Considerations: Diagnosis by demonstrating organism by culture/tissue staining
Pitfalls: If abdominal sinus tract is present, look for underlying ameboma and evidence of infection in other organs (e.g., CNS, lung, liver)
Prognosis: Related to extent of infection/degree of organ damage

Scrofula (Mycobacterium tuberculosis)
Clinical Presentation: Cold, chronic, anterior cervical adenopathy ± sinus tracts. Usually in children
Diagnostic Considerations: Diagnosis by culture of node/drainage for speciation
Pitfalls: Cured by antibiotic therapy alone. No need for surgical excision
Prognosis: Excellent with treatment

Scrofula (Mycobacterium scrofulaceum)
Clinical Presentation: Cold, chronic, anterior cervical adenopathy ± sinus tracts. Usually in adults
Diagnostic Considerations: Diagnosis by culture of node/drainage for speciation
Pitfalls: Highly resistant to anti-TB therapy
Prognosis: Excellent with surgical excision

Cutaneous Mycobacterium fortuitum-chelonae
Clinical Presentation: Usually associated with chronic foreign body infection, especially infected breast implants. May present as cold abscess
Diagnostic Considerations: Diagnosis by demonstrating organism by acid fast smear or culture of drainage/infected prosthetic material
Pitfalls: Highly resistant to anti-TB therapy, but sensitive to clarithromycin and azithromycin
Prognosis: Good with surgical excision/treatment with clarithromycin or azithromycin

Swimming Pool Granuloma (Mycobacterium marinum)
Clinical Presentation: Begins as erythema with tenderness at inoculation site, followed by a papule or violaceous nodule that ulcerates and drains pus. May have sporotrichoid spread. Presents as a skin lesion unresponsive to antibiotics after abrasive water exposure (e.g., cutting finger or scraping knee in swimming pool/lake)
Diagnostic Considerations: Diagnosis by demonstrating organism by acid-fast smear/culture
Pitfalls: Resistant to INH/pyrazinamide. Surgical excision is an option
Prognosis: Good with prolonged therapy

Buruli Ulcer (Mycobacterium ulcerans)
Clinical Presentation: Begin as a firm, painless, movable, subcutaneous nodule. In 1-2 months, nodule becomes fluctuant, ulcerates, and develops an undermined edge. May have edema around lesion and in extremity (if involved)

Diagnostic Considerations: Diagnosis by acid-fast culture of punch biopsy of ulcer rim. Patient is usually from Africa, but M. ulcerans also exists in Asia, Australia, and Central/South America
Pitfalls: Steroids/skin grafting sometimes needed
Prognosis: Good with surgical excision

Cutaneous MAI (Mycobacterium avium-intracellulare)
Clinical Presentation: Nodules, abscesses, ulcers, plaques, ecthyma and draining sinuses can occur, but are uncommon in normal hosts and usually only seen in immunosuppressed patients
Diagnostic Considerations: Diagnosis by demonstrating organism by acid-fast staining of tissue biopsy specimens
Pitfalls: Usually represents disseminated infection. Look for non-cutaneous evidence of infection (e.g., lungs, bone marrow, liver/spleen)
Prognosis: Related to extent of organ damage/degree of immunosuppression

Skin Vesicles/Bullae

Subset	Pathogens	Preferred Therapy
Herpes simplex	Herpes simplex virus (HSV)	See p. 102 (for HIV/AIDS, see pp. 252, 258)
Herpes zoster	Varicella zoster virus (VZV)	See pp. 102-103 (for HIV/AIDS, see pp. 252, 259)

Subcutaneous Serpiginous Lesions

Subset	Pathogens	Preferred Therapy
Cutaneous larva migrans (creeping eruption)	Ancylostoma braziliense	Ivermectin 150 mcg/kg (PO) q24h x 2 days **or** Albendazole 200 mg (PO) q12h x 3 days
Guinea worm	Dracunculus medinensis	Surgical removal of worm near skin surface. Metronidazole 250 mg (PO) q8h x 10 days facilitates worm removal
Cutaneous gnathostomiasis	Gnathostoma spinigerum	Surgical removal **or** Albendazole 400 mg (PO) q12-24h x 3 weeks **or** Ivermectin 200 mcg/kg (PO) q24h x 2 days

Cutaneous Larva Migrans (Ancylostoma braziliense) Creeping Eruption
Clinical Presentation: Intensely pruritic, migratory, subcutaneous, raised serpiginous lesions
Diagnostic Considerations: Diagnosis by clinical appearance
Pitfalls: Must be differentiated from "swimmer's itch" caused by schistosomal cercariae
Prognosis: Excellent with treatment

Guinea Worm (Dracunculus medinensis)
Clinical Presentation: Serpiginous, raised, subcutaneous tract overlying worm
Diagnostic Considerations: Diagnosis by demonstrating Dracunculus worm when surgically removed
Pitfalls: Resembles cutaneous larva migrans, but worm is visible below the skin and lesions are serpiginous with Dracunculus
Prognosis: Excellent with treatment. Soaking extremity in warm water promotes emergence/removal of worm. Metronidazole can also be used to decrease inflammation and facilitate worm removal. Mebendazole 200-400 mg (PO) q12h x 6 days may kill worms directly

Cutaneous Gnathostomiasis (Gnathostoma spinigerum)

Clinical Presentation: Painful, intermittent, subcutaneous swelling with local edema, intense pruritus, and leukocytosis with eosinophilia. Acquired by eating undercooked fish, frogs, and other intermediate larvae-containing hosts

Diagnostic Considerations: Diagnosis by demonstrating Gnathostoma in tissue specimens. Relatively common infection in Thailand and parts of Japan, South America, and Southeast Asia

Prognosis: Good if limited to the skin and surgically removed. Poor with CNS involvement

Skin Papules/Nodules/Abscesses

Subset	Pathogens	Preferred Therapy
Bacillary angiomatosis, peliosis hepatis	Bartonella henselae Bartonella quintana	Treat until cured with either doxycycline 100 mg (PO) q12h or azithromycin 250 mg (PO) q24h or any quinolone (PO)
Cutaneous Alternaria	Alternaria alternata	Amphotericin B* 1.5 mg/kg (IV) q24h x 2-3 grams
Entomophthoro-mycosis	E. basidiobolus E. conidiobolus	Amphotericin B* 1.5 mg/kg (IV) q24h x 1-2 grams **or** TMP-SMX 1 DS tablet (PO) q24h until cured
Chromomycosis	Fonsecaea pedrosoi, compactum Phialophora verrucosa, others	Few small lesions: Wide/deep surgical excision or cryosurgery with liquid nitrogen Larger lesions: Itraconazole 200 mg (PO) solution q24h until lesions regress ± cryosurgery
Cutaneous Fusarium	Fusarium solani	Amphotericin B* 1.5 mg/kg (IV) q24h x 2-3 grams **or** Voriconazole 6 mg/kg (IV) q12h x 1 day, then 4 mg/kg (IV) q12h or 200 mg (PO) q12h until cured. If < 40 kg, use 100 mg instead of 200 mg (PO) maintenance dose
Cutaneous Penicillium	Penicillium marneffei	Amphotericin B* 0.6 mg/kg (IV) q24h x 14 days, then itraconazole 200 mg (IV) q12 x 2 days followed by 200 mg (PO) q12h x 10 weeks. For HIV/AIDS, continue with itraconazole 200 mg (PO) solution q24h indefinitely
Cutaneous Prototheca	Prototheca wickerhamii	Surgical excision. If excision is incomplete, add either amphotericin B* 1.5 mg/kg (IV) q24h x 2-3 grams or itraconazole 200 mg (PO)† solution q12h until cured
Trichosporon	Trichosporon beigelii	Amphotericin B* 1.5 mg/kg (IV) q24h x 2-3 grams
Cutaneous aspergillosis	Aspergillus sp.	Voriconazole 6 mg/kg (IV) q12h x 1 day, then 4 mg/kg (IV) q12h or 200 mg (PO) q12h until cured. If < 40 kg, use 100 mg instead of 200 mg (PO) maintenance dose **or** Itraconazole 200 mg (IV) q12h x 7-14 days, then 200 mg (PO) solution q12h until cured **or** Caspofungin 70 mg (IV) x 1 dose, then 50 mg (IV) q24h until improved, then give itraconazole 200 mg (PO) solution q12h until cured

* *Amphotericin B deoxycholate*
† *Initiate therapy with itraconazole 200 mg (IV) q12h x 7-14 days*

Skin Papules/Nodules/Abscesses (cont'd)

Subset	Pathogens	Preferred Therapy
Cutaneous mucormycosis	Mucor/Rhizopus/Absidia	Amphotericin B* 1-1.5 mg/kg (IV) q24h x 2-3 grams Alternate therapy Lipid-associated formulation of amphotericin B (p. 297) (IV) q24h x 3-4 weeks
Cutaneous coccidioido-mycosis	Coccidioides immitis	Fluconazole 800 mg (PO) x 1 dose, then 400 mg (PO) q24h until cured **or** Itraconazole 200 mg (PO)† solution q12h until cured Alternate therapy Amphotericin B* 1 mg/kg (IV) q24h x 7 days, then 0.8 mg/kg (IV) q48h x 2-3 grams total dose
Cutaneous histoplasmosis	Histoplasmosis capsulatum	See p. 212
Cutaneous cryptococcosis	Cryptococcus neoformans	Amphotericin B* 0.5 mg/kg (IV) q24h x 1-2 grams **or** Lipid-associated formulation of amphotericin B (p. 297) (IV) q24h x 3 weeks, **then follow with** Fluconazole 800 mg (PO) x 1 dose, then 400 mg (PO) q24h x 8-10 weeks
Cutaneous sporotrichosis	Sporothrix schenckii	Itraconazole 200 mg (PO) solution q24h x 6 months. If HIV/AIDS, continue therapy until cured
Nodular/pustular candidiasis	Candida sp.	Treat as disseminated infection (see Candida sepsis, p. 120)
Cutaneous onchocerciasis	Onchocerca volvulus	Ivermectin 150 mcg/kg (PO) x 1 dose, repeated q6-12 months until asymptomatic **plus** doxycycline 100 mg (PO) q12h x 6 weeks

* Amphotericin B deoxycholate
† Initiate therapy with itraconazole 200 mg (IV) q12h x 7-14 days

Bacillary Angiomatosis (Bartonella henselae/quintana) Peliosis Hepatis
Clinical Presentation: Skin lesions resemble Kaposi's sarcoma. Liver lesions resemble CMV hepatitis in HIV/AIDS patients
Diagnostic Considerations: Diagnosis by demonstrating organism by stain/culture of skin lesions or by blood culture after lysis-centrifugation
Pitfalls: Requires life-long suppressive therapy
Prognosis: Related to extent of infection/degree of immunosuppression

Cutaneous Alternaria (Alternaria alternata)
Clinical Presentation: Bluish/purple papules that are often painful and non-pruritic. Usually seen only in leukopenic compromised hosts
Diagnostic Considerations: Diagnosis by demonstrating organism by stain/culture in tissue specimen
Pitfalls: Skin lesions usually represent disseminated disease in compromised hosts, not local infection
Prognosis: Poor/fair. Related to degree of immunosuppression

Cutaneous Entomophthoromycosis (E. basidiobolus / E. conidiobolus)

Clinical Presentation: E. conidiobolus infection presents as swelling of nose, paranasal tissues and mouth, accompanied by nasal stuffiness, drainage, and sinus pain. Begins as swelling of inferior nasal turbinates and extends until generalized facial swelling occurs. Subcutaneous nodules can be palpated in tissue. E. basidiobolus infection presents as a non-painful, firm, slowly progressive, subcutaneous nodule of the trunk, arms, legs, or buttocks

Diagnostic Considerations: Diagnosis by demonstrating organism by stain/culture in tissue specimen. Skin lesions usually represent disseminated disease in compromised hosts, not localized infection

Pitfalls: Unlike Mucor, E. basidiobolus does not usually invade blood vessels, although tissue infarction/necrosis is occasionally seen in diabetics and immunocompromised patients

Prognosis: May spontaneously resolve. Surgical removal of accessible nodules and reconstructive surgery may be helpful for disfigurement

Cutaneous Chromomycosis (F. pedrosoi/compactum, P. verrucosa, others)

Clinical Presentation: Warty papule/nodule that enlarges slowly to form a scarred, verrucous plaque. May also begin as a pustule, plaque, or ulcer. Over time, typical papule/nodule ulcerates, and the center becomes dry/crusted with raised margins. Lesions can be pedunculated/cauliflower-like

Diagnostic Considerations: Diagnosis by demonstrating organism by stain/culture in tissue specimen. Chromomycosis remains localized within cutaneous/subcutaneous tissues

Pitfalls: May resemble other fungal diseases. Sclerotic bodies in tissue and exudate distinguish chromomycosis from other related fugal diseases

Prognosis: Related to degree of organ damage

Cutaneous Fusarium (Fusarium solani)

Clinical Presentation: Presents in compromised hosts as multiple papules or painful nodules, initially macular with central pallor, which then become raised, erythematous, and necrotic. Seen mostly in leukopenic compromised hosts (especially acute leukemia and bone marrow transplants). Also a cause of mycetoma/onychomycosis

Diagnostic Considerations: Diagnosis by demonstrating organism by stain/culture from blood/tissue

Pitfalls: Skin lesions usually represent disseminated disease, not localized infection

Prognosis: Poor/fair. Related to degree of immunosuppression. Amphotericin B lipid formulation (p. 297), colony-stimulating granulocyte factor, and granulocyte transfusions may be useful

Cutaneous Penicillium (Penicillium marneffei)

Clinical Presentation: Papules, pustules, nodules, ulcers, or abscesses. Mostly seen in HIV/AIDS (requires life-long suppressive therapy with itraconazole)

Diagnostic Considerations: Diagnosis by demonstrating organism by stain/culture in tissue specimen. Affects residents/visitors of Southeast Asia/Southern China

Pitfalls: Lesions commonly become umbilicated and resemble molluscum contagiosum

Prognosis: Poor/fair. Related to degree of immunosuppression

Cutaneous Prototheca (Prototheca wikermanii)

Clinical Presentation: Most common presentation is a single plaque or papulonodular lesion of the skin or subcutaneous tissue. Lesions are usually painless, slowly progressive (enlarge over weeks to months without healing), well-circumscribed, and may become eczematoid/ulcerated

Diagnostic Considerations: Diagnosis by demonstrating organism by stain/culture in tissue specimen. Skin lesions in HIV/AIDS are not different from normal hosts

Pitfalls: Lesions are usually painless and may resemble eczema

Prognosis: Poor/fair. Related to degree of immunosuppression. Surgical excision has been successful

Cutaneous Trichosporon (Trichosporon beigelii)

Clinical Presentation: Seen mostly in leukopenic compromised hosts (especially in acute leukemia, but also in HIV/AIDS, burn wounds, and organ transplants). Usually presents as multiple red-bluish/purple papules, which are often painful and non-pruritic

Diagnostic Considerations: Diagnosis by demonstrating organism by stain/culture in tissue specimen

Pitfalls: Skin lesions usually represent disseminated disease, not localized infection

Prognosis: Related to extent of infection/degree of immunosuppression

Cutaneous Aspergillosis (Aspergillus fumigatus)

Clinical Presentation: Seen at site of IV catheter insertion or adhesive dressing applied to skin in leukopenic, compromised hosts. Lesion is similar to pyoderma gangrenosum. May also invade burn wounds and cause rapidly progressive necrotic lesions

Diagnostic Considerations: Diagnosis by demonstrating organism by stain/culture in tissue specimen

Pitfalls: Infiltrative/ulcerative skin lesions usually represent disseminated disease in compromised hosts, not localized infection. May cause invasive dermatitis/skin lesions in HIV/AIDS

Prognosis: Related to extent of infection/degree of immunosuppression

Cutaneous Mucormycosis/Rhizopus/Absidia

Clinical Presentation: Necrotic skin lesion secondary to vascular invasion. Involves epidermis and dermis. Black eschars are evident

Diagnostic Considerations: Diagnosis by demonstrating broad, non-septate hyphae with branches at right angles by stain/culture in tissue specimen

Pitfalls: Skin lesions usually represent disseminated disease in compromised hosts, not localized infection. Contaminated elastic bandages have been associated with cutaneous Mucor

Prognosis: Related to extent of infection/degree of immunosuppression

Cutaneous Coccidioidomycosis (Coccidioides immitis)

Clinical Presentation: Skin lesions may take many forms, including verrucous granulomas, cold subcutaneous abscesses, indolent ulcers, or small papules

Diagnostic Considerations: Diagnosis by demonstrating organism by stain/culture in tissue specimen

Pitfalls: Skin lesions usually represent disseminated disease in compromised hosts, not local infection

Prognosis: Related to extent of infection/degree of immunosuppression

Cutaneous Histoplasmosis (Histoplasma capsulatum)

Clinical Presentation: Common cutaneous findings include maculopapular eruption, petechiae, and ecchymosis. Histopathology reveals necrosis around superficial dermal vessels

Diagnostic Considerations: Diagnosis by demonstrating organism by stain/culture in tissue specimen

Pitfalls: Skin lesions usually represent disseminated disease in compromised hosts, not local infection

Prognosis: Related to extent of infection/degree of immunosuppression

Cutaneous Cryptococcosis (Cryptococcus neoformans)

Clinical Presentation: May present as single or multiple papules, pustules, erythematous indurated plaques, soft subcutaneous masses, draining sinus tracts, or ulcers with undermined edges

Diagnostic Considerations: Diagnosis by demonstrating organism by stain/culture in tissue specimen

Pitfalls: Skin lesions usually represent disseminated disease in compromised hosts, not localized infection. In AIDS patients, umbilicated papules resemble molluscum contagiosum. In organ transplants, cellulitis with necrotizing vasculitis may occur

Prognosis: Related to extent of infection/degree of immunosuppression

Cutaneous Sporotrichosis (Sporothrix schenckii)

Clinical Presentation: Primary cutaneous lymphatic sporotrichosis starts as a small, firm, movable, subcutaneous nodule, which then becomes soft and breaks down to form a persistent, friable ulcer. Secondary lesions usually develop proximally along lymphatic channels, but do not involve lymph nodes. Plaque form does not spread locally

Diagnostic Considerations: Diagnosis by demonstrating organism by stain/culture in tissue specimen. Cutaneous disease arises at sites of minor trauma with inoculation of fungus into skin. Skin lesions usually represent disseminated disease in compromised hosts, not localized infection

Pitfalls: HIV/AIDS patients with CD_4 < 200 may have widespread lymphocutaneous disease that ulcerates and is associated with arthritis. Unusual in axilla due to increased temperature

Prognosis: Related to extent of infection/degree of immunosuppression

Nodular/Pustular Candidiasis (see sepsis in chronic steroids, p. 122)

Cutaneous Onchocerciasis (Onchocerca volvulus)

Clinical Presentation: Early manifestation is pruritic, papular rash with altered pigmentation. Later, papules, scaling, edema, and depigmentation may develop. Nodules develop in deep dermis/ subcutaneous tissue (especially over bony prominences) or in deeper sites near joints, muscles, bones

Diagnostic Considerations: Diagnosis by serology/demonstration of microfilaria in tissue specimens. Intradermal edema produces "peau d'orange" effect with pitting around hair follicles/sebaceous glands

Pitfalls: Ivermectin is effective against microfilaria, not adult worms

Prognosis: Related to location/extent of organ damage

Rickettsias (Fever/Petechial Skin Rash)

Subset	Pathogens	Preferred Therapy	Alternate Therapy
Rocky Mountain spotted fever (RMSF)	Rickettsia rickettsii	Doxycycline 200 mg (IV or PO) q12h x 3 days, then 100 mg (IV or PO) x 4 days	Any quinolone (IV or PO) x 7 days **or** Chloramphenicol 500 mg (IV or PO) q6h x 7 days
Epidemic (louse-borne) typhus, flying squirrel typhus	Rickettsia prowazekii	Same as RMSF	Same as RMSF
Murine (flea-borne) typhus	Rickettsia typhi	Same as RMSF	Same as RMSF
Scrub (chigger mite-borne) typhus (Tsutsugamushi fever)	Rickettsia tsutsugamushi	Same as RMSF	Rifampin 600-900 mg (PO) q24h x 7 days
Rickettsialpox	Rickettsia akari	Same as RMSF	Same as RMSF
Tick typhus fevers (Mediterranean spotted fever, Boutonneuse fever, Israeli spotted fever)	Rickettsia conorii	Same as RMSF	Same as RMSF
African tick bite fever	Rickettsia africae	Same as RMSF	Same as RMSF

Rocky Mountain Spotted Fever (Rickettsia rickettsia) RMSF

Clinical Presentation: Fever with relative bradycardia, severe frontal headache, severe myalgias of abdomen/back/legs 3-12 days after tick bite. Rash begins as erythematous macules on wrists and ankles 3-5 days after tick bite, and progresses to petechiae/palpable purpura with confluent areas of ecchymosis. Periorbital edema, conjunctival suffusion, acute deafness, and edema of the dorsum of the hands/feet are important early signs. Abdominal pain can mimic acute abdomen, and meningismus and headache can mimic meningitis. Hepatosplenomegaly, cough, and coma may develop late. Laboratory findings include normal leukocyte count, thrombocytopenia, ↑ LFTs, and pre-renal azotemia. Hypotension/shock may occur secondary to myocarditis, which is the most common causes of death. Primary vector in United States is the Dermacentor tick; primary animal reservoir is small wild animals

Diagnosis: Primarily a clinical diagnosis requiring a high index of suspicion and early empiric therapy. Early/rapid diagnosis can be made by DFA of biopsy specimen of rash. Specific R. rickettsii IFA, complement fixation, ELISA antibody titers are confirmatory. Include RMSF in differential diagnosis of any patient with fever and potential tick exposure, especially during the summer months

Pitfalls: Most cases occur in eastern and southeastern United States, not Rocky Mountain area. Many cases go unrecognized due to nonspecific early findings. Early antibiotic therapy may blunt/eliminate serologic response. Patients with signs/symptoms of RMSF but without a rash should be considered as having ehrlichiosis ("spotless RMSF") until proven otherwise. Early therapy is essential; begin empiric therapy as soon as RMSF is suspected. Other adjunctive measures may be required

Prognosis: Late (after day 5) initiation of treatment increases the risk of death by 5-fold. Adverse prognostic factors include myocarditis and severe encephalitis

Epidemic (Louse-Borne) Typhus (Rickettsia prowazekii)

Clinical Presentation: High fever with relative bradycardia, chills, headache, conjunctival suffusion, and myalgias. A macular, rubella-like, truncal rash develops in most on the fifth febrile day, which may become petechial and involve the extremities, but spares the palms/soles. Facial swelling/flushing occurs at end of first week, along with CNS symptoms (e.g., tinnitus, vertigo, delirium) and GI complaints (diarrhea, constipation, nausea, vomiting, abdominal pain). Hypotension, pneumonia, renal failure, gangrene, cerebral infarction may develop late. Laboratory findings include normal leukocyte count, thrombocytopenia, and ↑ serum creatinine/LFTs. Primary vector is the human body louse; primary reservoir is humans

Diagnosis: Primarily a clinical diagnosis requiring a high index of suspicion and early empiric therapy. Specific R. prowazekii antibody titers are confirmatory. Consider epidemic (louse-borne) typhus in febrile impoverished persons infested with lice, especially in Africa and parts of Latin America. Rarely seen in the United States. Milder recrudescent form (Brill-Zinsser disease) is also rare

Pitfalls: Many cases go unrecognized due to nonspecific early findings. Early therapy is essential

Prognosis: Gangrene of nose, ear lobes, genitalia, toes, and fingers may develop in severe cases. Death occurs in 10-50% of untreated patients

Murine (Flea-Borne) Typhus (Rickettsia typhi)

Clinical Presentation: Similar to epidemic typhus but less severe, with fever in most, and headache, myalgias, and a macular rash in half. Laboratory findings include a normal leukocyte count, mild thrombocytopenia, and mildly ↑ LFTs. Primary vector is the Asian rat flea (Xenopsylla cheopis); primary reservoir is the commensal rat (Rattus genus). Uncommon in United States; most cases from Texas, California, Florida, Hawaii

Diagnosis: Primarily a clinical diagnosis requiring a high index of suspicion. More common during summer and fall. Specific R. typhi antibody titers are confirmatory

Pitfalls: Many cases go unrecognized due to nonspecific findings. Rash becomes maculopapular, compared to epidemic typhus, which remains macular

Prognosis: Good if treated early. Death occurs in < 1%

Scrub Typhus (Rickettsia tsutsugamushi) Tsutsugamushi Fever

Clinical Presentation: Fever, chills, headache, myalgias, arthralgias, GI symptoms, other nonspecific complaints. Eschar at mite bite site (tache noire) ± regional adenopathy. A macular, truncal rash develops in most, usually in the first week, and may progress to involve the extremities and face, but spares the palms/soles. Vasculitis may lead to cardiopulmonary, CNS, hematologic abnormalities during the second week. Hepatosplenomegaly is common. Primary vector/reservoir is the larval (chigger) trombiculid mite. Endemic areas include northern Australia, southeastern Asia, Indian subcontinent
Diagnosis: Presumptive diagnosis is clinical. Specific R. tsutsugamushi serology is confirmatory
Pitfalls: Incomplete therapy frequently results in relapse
Prognosis: Excellent if treated early

Rickettsialpox (Rickettsia akari)

Clinical Presentation: Milder illness than other rickettsioses, with initial eschar at bite site, high fever, and generalized rash (usually erythematous papules which become vesicular and spares the palms/soles). Fever peak is usually < 104°F, occurs 1-3 weeks after mite bite, and lasts ~ 1 week without therapy. Headache, photophobia, marked diaphoresis, sore throat, GI complaints (nausea/vomiting following initial headache) may occur. Most labs are normal, although leukopenia may be present. Primary vector is the mouse mite; primary animal reservoir is the house mouse. Rare in the United States
Diagnosis: Presumptive diagnosis by clinical presentation. Specific R. akari serology is confirmatory
Pitfalls: Do not confuse with African tick-bite fever, which may also have a vesicular rash
Prognosis: Excellent even without therapy

Tick Typhus Fevers (Rickettsia conorii) Mediterranean Spotted Fever, Boutonneuse Fever, Israeli Fever

Clinical Presentation: Similar to RMSF with fever, chills, myalgias, but less severe. Unlike RMSF, an eschar is usually present at the site of the tick bite ± regional adenopathy. Leukocyte count is normal and thrombocytopenia is common. Transmitted by the brown dog tick, Rhipicephalus sanguineus
Diagnosis: Presumptive diagnosis by clinical presentation. Specific R. conorii serology is confirmatory
Pitfalls: Suspect in travelers from endemic areas with a RMSF-like illness. Consider different diagnosis in absence of an eschar
Prognosis: Good with early treatment. Prostration may be prolonged even with proper therapy

African Tick Bite Fever (Rickettsia africae)

Clinical Presentation: Similar to murine typhus with fever, chills, myalgias, but regional adenopathy and multiple eschars are common. Incubation period ~ 6 days. Amblyomma hebreum/variegatum tick vectors frequently bite humans multiple times
Diagnosis: Presumptive diagnosis by clinical presentation. Specific R. africae serology is confirmatory
Pitfalls: Rash is transient, and may be vesicular or absent
Prognosis: Good even without therapy; excellent with therapy

Other Skin Lesions

Subset	Pathogens	Topical Therapy	PO Therapy
Tinea versicolor (pityriasis)	Malassezia furfur (Pityrosporum orbiculare)	Clotrimazole cream (1%) *or* miconazole cream (2%) *or* ketoconazole cream (2%) daily x 7 days	Ketoconazole 200 mg (PO) q24h x 7 days **or** Itraconazole 200 mg (PO) solution q24h x 7 days **or** Fluconazole 400 mg (PO) x 1 dose

Other Skin Lesions (cont'd)

Subset	Pathogens	Preferred Therapy
Eosinophilic folliculitis	Malassezia furfur (Pityrosporum orbiculare)	Ketoconazole cream (2%) topically x 2-3 weeks ± ketoconazole 200 mg (PO) q24h x 2-3 weeks

Tinea Versicolor/Pityriasis (Malassezia furfur)
Clinical Presentation: Hyper– or hypopigmented scaling papules (0.5-1 cm), which may coalesce into larger plaques. Most commonly affects the upper trunk and arms. May be asymptomatic or pruritic
Diagnostic Considerations: M. furfur also causes eosinophilic folliculitis in HIV/AIDS, and catheter-acquired sepsis mostly in neonates or immunosuppressed patients. Diagnosis is clinical
Pitfalls: Skin pigmentation may take months to return to normal after adequate therapy
Prognosis: Excellent

Eosinophilic Folliculitis (Malassezia furfur)
Clinical Presentation: Intensely pruritic folliculitis, usually on lower extremities
Diagnostic Considerations: Tissue biopsy shows eosinophilic folliculitis. Diagnosis by demonstrating organism by culture on Sabouraud's agar overlaid with olive oil
Pitfalls: Resembles folliculitis, but lesions are concentrated on lower extremities (not on trunk as with cutaneous candidiasis)
Prognosis: Related to degree of immunosuppression. Use oral therapy if topical therapy fails

Myositis

Subset	Pathogens	Preferred Therapy
Chromomycosis	Cladosporium/Fonsecaea	Itraconazole 200 mg (PO) solution q24h until cured **or** Terbinafine 250 mg (PO) q24h until cured
Trichinosis	Trichinella spiralis	Albendazole 400 mg (PO) q12h x 8-14 days **or** Mebendazole 5 mg/kg (PO) q12h x 2 weeks

Chromomycosis (Cladosporium/Fonsecaea)
Clinical Presentation: Subcutaneous/soft tissue nodules or verrucous lesions
Diagnostic Considerations: Diagnosis by demonstrating organism by culture/tissue biopsy specimen
Pitfalls: May resemble Madura foot or cause ulcerative lesions in muscle
Prognosis: Related to degree of immunosuppression

Trichinosis (Trichinella spiralis)
Clinical Presentation: Muscle tenderness, low-grade fevers, peripheral eosinophilia, conjunctival suffusion
Diagnostic Considerations: Diagnosis by Trichinella serology or by demonstrating larvae in muscle biopsy
Pitfalls: ESR is very low (near zero), unlike other causes of myositis, which have elevated ESRs
Prognosis: Excellent with early treatment. Short-term steroids may be useful during acute phase. Therapy is ineffective against calcified larvae in muscle

REFERENCES AND SUGGESTED READINGS

Arathoon EG, Gotuzzo E, Noriega LM, et al. Randomized, double-blind, multicenter study of caspofungin versus amphotericin B for treatment of oropharyngeal and esophageal candidiasis. Antimicrob Agents Chemother 46:451-7, 2002.

Arikan S, Lozano-Chiu M, Paetznick V, et al. In vitro synergy of caspofungin and amphotericin B against Aspergillus and Fusarium spp. Antimicrob Agents Chemother 46:245-7, 2002.

Asciogul S, Rex JH, DePauw B, et al. Defining opportunistic invasive fungal infections in immunocompromised patients with cancer: An international consensus. Clin Infect Dis 34:7-14, 2002.

Aubry A, Chosidow O, Caumes E, et al. Sixty-three cases of Mycobacterium marinum infection: clinical features, treatment, and antibiotic susceptibility of causative isolates. Arch Intern Med 162:1746-52, 2002.

Avulunov A, Klaus S, Vardy D. Fluconazole for the treatment of cutaneous leishmaniasis. N Engl J Med 347:370-1, 2002.

Castiglioni B, Sutton DA, Rinaldi MG, et al. Pseudallescheria boydii (Anamorph Scedosporium apiospermum). Infection in solid organ transplant recipients in a tertiary medical center and review of the literature. Medicine (Baltimore) 81:333-48, 2002.

Chen XM, Keithly JS, Paya CV, et al. Cryptosporidiosis. N Engl J Med 346:1723-1731, 2002.

Croft SL, Yardley V. Chemotherapy of leishmaniasis. Curr Pharm Des. 8:319-42, 2002.

Gardon J, Boussinesq J, Kamgno J, et al. Effects of standard and high doses of ivermectin on adult worms of Onchocerca volvulus: a randomised controlled trial. Lancet 360:203-10, 2002.

Haque R, Huston CD, Hughes M et al. Amebiasis. N Engl J Med 348:1565-73, 2003.

Kauffman MA. Endemic mycoses in patients with hematologic malignancies. Semin Respir Infect 17:106-12, 2002.

Kremery V, Barnes AJ. Non-albicans Candida spp. causing fungaemia: pathogenicity and antifungal resistance. J Hosp Infect 50:243-60, 2002.

Lionakis MS, Kontoyiannis DP. Glucocorticoids and invasive fungal infections. Lancet 362:1828-38, 2003.

Lok AS. Chronic hepatitis B. N Engl J Med 346:1682-3, 2002

Perea S, Patterson TF. Invasive Aspergillus infections in hematologic malignancy patients. Semin Respir Infect 17:99-105, 2002.

Rao R, Well GJ. In vitro effects of antibiotics on Brugia malayi worm survival and reproduction. J Parasitol 88:199, 2002.

Ross AGP, Bartley PB, Sleigh AC, et al. Schistosomiasis. N Engl J Med 346:1212-1220, 2002.

Rubin MA, Carroll KC, Cahill BC. Caspofungin in combination with itraconazole for the treatment of invasive aspergillosis in humans. Clin Infect Dis 34:1160-1, 2002.

Ryan ET, Wilson ME, Kain KC. Illness after international travel. N Engl J Med 347:505-516, 2002.

Sharkey PK, Kauffman CA, Graybill JR, et al. Itraconazole treatment of sporotrichosis. Am J Med 95:279-285, 1993.

Sundar S, Jha TK, Thakur CP, et al. Oral miltefosine for Indian visceral leishmaniasis. N Engl J Med 347:1739-45, 2002.

Tomioka H, Sato K, Shimizu T, et al. Anti-Mycobacterium tuberculosis activities of new fluoroquinolones in combination with other antituberculous drugs. J Infect 44:160-5, 2002.

Zerouali K, Elmdaghri N, Boudouma, et al. Serogroups, serotypes, serosubtypes and antimicrobial susceptibility of Neisseria meningitidis isolates in Casablanca, Morocco. Eur J Clin Microbiol Infect Dis 21:483-5, 2002.

GUIDELINES

Chapman SW, Bradsher RW Jr, Campbell GD Jr, et al. Practice guidelines for the management of patients with blastomycosis. Infectious Diseases Society of America. Clin Infect Dis. 30:679-83, 2000.

Galgiani JN, Ampel NM, Catanzaro A. et al. Practice guidelines for the treatment of coccidiomycosis. Infectious Diseases Society of America. Clin Infect Dis 30:658-61, 2000.

Kauffman CA, Hajjeh R, Chapman SW. Practice guidelines for the management of patients with sporotrichosis. For the Mycoses Study Group. Infectious Diseases Society of America. Clin Infect Dis 30:684-7, 2000.

Rex JH, Walsh TJ, Sobel JD, et al. Practice guidelines for the treatment of candidiasis. Infectious Diseases Society of America. 30:662-78, 2000.

Saag MS, Graybill RJ, Larsen RA, Pappas PG, et al. Practice guidelines for the management of cryptococcal disease. Infectious Diseases Society of America. Clin Infect Dis 30:710-8, 2000.

Sobel JD. Practice guidelines for the treatment of fungal infections. For the Mycoses Study Group. Infectious Diseases Society of America. Clin Infect Dis. 30:652, 2000.

Stevens DA, Kan VL, Judson MA, et al. Practice guidelines for diseases caused by Aspergillus. Infectious Diseases Society of America. Clin Infect Dis 30:696-709, 2000.

Wheat J, Sarosi G, McKinsey D, Hamill R, et al. Practice guidelines for the management of patients with histoplasmosis. Infectious Diseases Society of America. Clin Infect Dis. 30:688-95, 2000.

TEXTBOOKS

Anaissie EJ, McGinnis MR, Pfaller MA (eds). Clinical Mycology. Churchill Livingstone, New York, 2003.

Andriole VT, Bodey GP (eds). Systemic Antifungal Therapy. Scientific Therapeutic Information, Springfield, NJ 1994

Arikan S and Rex JH. Antifungal Drugs. In: Manual of Clinical Microbiology, 8th Edition, 2003.

Beran GW (ed). Handbook of Zoonoses, 2nd Edition. Section B: Viral. CRC Press, Boca Raton, 1994.

Beran GW (ed). Handbook of Zoonoses, 2nd Edition. Section A: Bacterial, Rickettsial, Chlamydial, and Mycotic. CRC Press, Boca Raton, 1994.

Bodey GP, Fainstein V (eds). Candidiasis. New York, Raven Press, 1985.

Calderone RA (ed). Candida and Candidiasis. Washington DC, ASM Press, 2002.

Cohen DM, Rex JH. Antifungal Therapy. In: Scholssberg DM (ed). Current Therapy of Infectious Diseases, 1996.

Cook GC (ed). Manson's Tropical Diseases, 20th Edition. WB Saunders Company, Ltd., London, 1996.

Cunha BA (ed). Tick-Borne Infectious Diseases. Marcel Dekker, New York, 2000.

Despommier DD, Gwadz RW, Hotez PJ, Knirsch CA (eds). Parasitic Diseases, 4th Edition. Apple Trees Productions, LLC, New York, 2000.

Drugs for Parasitic Infections, Med Letter, March, 2000

Emmons CW, Binford CH, Utz JP, Kwon-Chung KJ (eds). Medical Mycology, 3rd Edition. Lea & Febiger, Philadelphia, 1977.

Frey D, Oldfield RJ, Bridger RC (eds). Color Atlas of Pathogenic Fungi. Year Book Medical Publishers, Chicago, 1979.

Garcia LS (ed). Diagnostic Medical Parasitology, 4th Edition. ASM Press, Washington, DC, 2001.

Gilles HM (ed). Protozoal Diseases. Arnold Publishers, London, 1999.

Goldsmith R, Heyneman (eds). Tropical Medicine and Parasitology. Appleton & Lange, Norwalk, 1989.

Guerrant RL, Walker DH, Weller PF (eds). Tropical Infectious Disease: Principles, Pathogens & Practice. Churchill Livingstone, Philadelphia, 1999.

Gutierrez Y (ed). Diagnostic Pathology of Parasitic Infections with Clinical Correlations, 2nd Edition. Oxford University Press, New York, 2000.

Howard DH (ed). Pathogenic Fungi in Humans and Animals. 2nd Edition. New York, Marcel Dekker, 2003.

Knipe DM, Howley PM (eds). Fields Virology, 4th Edition. Lippincott Williams & Wilkins, Philadelphia, 2001.

Martins MD, Rex JH. Antifungal Therapy. In: Parillo JE (ed). Current Therapy in Critical Care Medicine, 3rd Edition. 1997.

Merck & Co. Introduction to Medical Mycology. North Whales Press, North Whales, PA, 2001.

Pappas PG, Rex JH. Therapeutic Approaches to Candida Sepsis. In: Mandell GL and Tunkel A (eds), Current Infectious Diseases Reports, 1:245-252, 2000.

Porterfield JS (ed). Exotic Viral Infections. Chapman & Hall Medical, London, 1995.

Rex JH, Pappas PG. Hematogenously Disseminated Fungal Infections. In: Anaissie EJ, Pfaller MA, McGinnis M (eds). Clinical Mycology, Churchill-Livingstone, Edinburgh, 2003.

Rex JH. Approach to the Treatment of Systemic Fungal Infections. In: Kelley WN (ed). Kelley's Textbook of Internal Medicine, 4th Edition, 2000.

Rex JH, Sobel JD, Powderly WB. Candida Infections. In: Yu VL, Jr., Merigan TC, Jr., and Barriere SL (eds.). Antimicrobial Therapy & Vaccines. Williams & Wilkins, Baltimore, MD. 1998.

Richman DD, Whitley RJ, Hayden FG (eds). Clinical Virology, 2nd Edition. ASM Press, Washington, DC, 2002.

Rippon JW (ed). Medical Mycology, 3rd Edition. W. B. Saunders, Philadelphia, 1988.

Sarosi GA, Davies SF (eds). Fungal Diseases of the Lung. Grune & Stratton, New York, 1986.

Strickland GT (ed). Hunter's Tropical Medicine and Emerging Infectious Diseases, 8th Edition. W.B. Saunders Company, Philadelphia, 2000.

Sun T (ed). Parasitic Disorders: Pathology, Diagnosis, and Management, 2nd Edition. Williams & Wilkens, Baltimore, 1999.

Walker DH (ed). Biology of Rickettsial Diseases I. CRC Press, Boca Raton, 2000.

Walker DH (ed). Biology of Rickettsial Diseases II. CRC Press, Boca Raton, 2000.

Warren KS, Mahmoud AAF (eds). Tropical and Geographical Medicine, 2nd Edition. McGraw-Hill Information Services Co., New York, 1990.

Chapter 5

HIV Infection

Paul E. Sax, MD

HIV Infection

Paul E. Sax, M.D.

Infection with Human Immunodeficiency Virus (HIV-1) leads to a chronic and usually fatal infection characterized by progressive immunodeficiency, a long clinical latency period, and opportunistic infections. The hallmark of HIV disease is infection and viral replication within T-lymphocytes expressing the CD_4 antigen (helper-inducer lymphocytes), a critical component of normal cell-mediated immunity. Qualitative defects in CD_4 responsiveness and progressive depletion in CD_4 cell counts increase the risk for opportunistic infections such as Pneumocystis carinii pneumonia, and neoplasms such as lymphoma and Kaposi's sarcoma. HIV infection can also disrupt blood monocyte, tissue macrophage, and B-lymphocyte (humoral immunity) function, predisposing to infection with encapsulated bacteria. Direct attack of CD_4-positive cells in the central and peripheral nervous system can cause HIV meningitis, peripheral neuropathy, and dementia. Nearly 1 million people in the United States and 40 million people worldwide are infected with HIV. Without treatment, the average time from acquisition of HIV to an AIDS-defining opportunistic infection is about 10 years; survival then averages 1-2 years. There is tremendous individual variability in these time intervals, with some patients progressing from acute HIV infection to death within 1-2 years, and others not manifesting HIV-related immunosuppression for > 20 years after HIV acquisition. Antiretroviral therapy and prophylaxis against opportunistic infections have markedly improved the overall prognosis of HIV disease. The approach to HIV infection is shown in Figure 1.

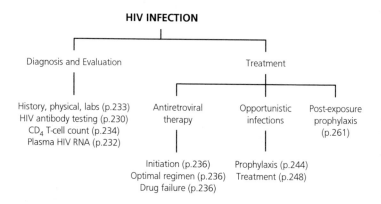

Figure 1. Diagnosis, Evaluation, and Treatment of HIV Infection

STAGES OF HIV INFECTION

A. Viral Transmission. HIV infection is acquired primarily by sexual intercourse (anal, vaginal, infrequently oral), exposure to contaminated blood (primarily needle transmission), or maternal-fetus (perinatal) transmission. Sexual practices with the highest risk of transmission include unprotected receptive anal intercourse (especially with mucosal tearing), unprotected receptive vaginal intercourse (especially during menses), and unprotected rectal/vaginal intercourse in the presence of genital ulcers (e.g., primary syphilis, genital herpes, chancroid). Lower risk sexual practices include insertive anal/vaginal intercourse and oral-genital contact. The risk of transmission after a single encounter with an HIV source has been estimated to be 1 in 150 with needle sharing, 1 in 300 with occupational percutaneous exposure, 1 in 300-1000 with receptive anal intercourse, 1 in 500-1250 with receptive vaginal intercourse, 1 in 1000-3000 with insertive vaginal intercourse, and 1 in 3000 with insertive anal intercourse. Transmission risk increases with the number of encounters and with higher HIV RNA plasma levels. The mode of transmission does not affect the natural history of HIV disease.

B. Acute (Primary) HIV Infection (p. 229). Acute HIV occurs 1-4 weeks after transmission, and is accompanied by a burst of viral replication with a decline in CD_4 cell count. Most patients manifest a symptomatic flu-like syndrome, which is often overlooked. Acute HIV infection is confirmed by demonstrating a high HIV RNA in the absence of HIV antibody. Some experts believe that antiretroviral therapy is indicated, although the optimal duration of therapy and role of intermittent treatment await definition.

C. Seroconversion. Development of a positive HIV antibody test usually occurs within 4 weeks of acute infection, and invariably (with few exceptions) by 6 months.

D. Asymptomatic HIV Infection lasts a variable amount of time (average 8-10 years), and is accompanied by a gradual decline in CD_4 cell counts and a relatively stable HIV RNA level (sometimes referred to as the viral "set point").

E. Symptomatic HIV Infection. Previously referred to as "AIDS Related Complex (ARC)," findings include thrush or vaginal candidiasis (persistent, frequent, or poorly responsive to treatment), cervical dysplasia/carcinoma in-situ, herpes zoster (recurrent episodes or involving multiple dermatomes), oral hairy leukoplakia, peripheral neuropathy, diarrhea, or constitutional symptoms (e.g., low-grade fevers, weight loss).

F. AIDS is defined by a CD_4 cell count < 200/mm^3, a CD_4 cell percentage of total lymphocytes <14%, or one of several AIDS-related opportunistic infections. Common opportunistic infections include Pneumocystis carinii pneumonia, cryptococcal meningitis, recurrent bacterial pneumonia, Candida esophagitis, CNS toxoplasmosis, tuberculosis, and non-Hodgkin's lymphoma. Other AIDS indicators in HIV-infected patients include candidiasis of the bronchi, trachea, or lungs; disseminated/extrapulmonary coccidiomycosis, cryptococcosis, or histoplasmosis; chronic (>1 month) intestinal cryptosporidiosis or isosporiasis; Kaposi's sarcoma; lymphoid interstitial pneumonia/pulmonary lymphoid hyperplasia; disseminated/extrapulmonary Mycobacterium (avium-intracellular, kansasii, other species) infection; progressive multifocal leukoencephalopathy (PML); recurrent Salmonella septicemia; or HIV wasting syndrome.

G. **Advanced HIV Disease** is diagnosed when the CD_4 cell count is < 50/mm^3. Most AIDS-related deaths occur at this point. Common late stage opportunistic infections are caused by CMV disease (retinitis, colitis) or disseminated Mycobacterium avium complex (MAC).

ACUTE (PRIMARY) HIV INFECTION

A. **Description.** Acute clinical illness associated with primary acquisition of HIV, occurring 1-4 weeks after viral transmission (range: 6 days to 6 weeks). Symptoms develop in 50-90%, but are often mistaken for the flu, mononucleosis, or other nonspecific viral syndrome. More severe symptoms may correlate with more rapid HIV disease progression. Even without therapy, most patients recover, reflecting development of a partially effective immune response and depletion of susceptible CD_4 cells.

B. **Differential Diagnosis** includes **EBV, CMV**, viral hepatitis, enteroviral infection, 2° syphilis, toxoplasmosis, HSV with erythema multiforme, drug reaction, Behcet's disease, acute lupus.

C. **Signs and Symptoms** usually reflect hematogenous dissemination of virus to lymphoreticular and neurologic sites:
   - Fever (97%)
   - Pharyngitis (73%). Typically non-exudative (unlike EBV, which is usually exudative)
   - Rash (77%). Maculopapular viral exanthem of the face and trunk is most common, but can involve the extremities, palms and soles
   - Arthralgia/myalgia (58%)
   - Neurologic symptoms (12%). Headache is most common. Neuropathy, Bell's palsy, and meningoencephalitis are rare, but may predict worse outcome
   - Oral/genital ulcerations, thrush, nausea, vomiting, diarrhea, weight loss

D. **Laboratory Findings**
   1. **CBC.** Lymphopenia followed by lymphocytosis (common). Atypical lymphocytosis is absent/mild (unlike EBV, where atypical lymphocytosis may be 20-30% or higher). Thrombocytopenia occurs in some
   2. **Elevated transaminases** in some but not all patients
   3. **Depressed CD_4 cell count.** Can rarely be low enough to induce opportunistic infections
   4. **HIV antibody.** Usually negative, although persons with prolonged symptoms of acute HIV may have positive antibody tests if diagnosed late during the course of illness

E. **Confirming the Diagnosis of Acute HIV Infection**
   1. **Obtain HIV antibody** after informed consent to exclude prior disease
   2. **Order viral load test (HIV RNA PCR),** preferably RT-PCR (lower limit 400 copies/mL).

HIV RNA confirms acute HIV infection prior to seroconversion. Most individuals will have very high HIV RNA (>100,000 copies/mL). Be suspicious of a false-positive test if the HIV RNA is low (< 20,000 copies/mL). For any positive test, follow-up antibody testing at 1, 3, and 6 months is mandatory to confirm HIV infection. p24 antigen can also be used to establish the diagnosis, but is less sensitive than HIV RNA PCR

3. **Order other tests/serologies if HIV RNA test is negative.** Order throat cultures for bacterial/viral respiratory pathogens, EBV VCA IgM/IgG, CMV IgM/IgG, HHV-6 IgM/IgG, and hepatitis serologies as appropriate to establish a diagnosis for patient's symptoms

4. **Repeat HIV serology** is recommended at 1, 3, and 6 months to document seroconversion in patients who are HIV RNA positive but HIV antibody negative

F. Management of Acute HIV Infection

1. **Initiate antiretroviral therapy.** Patients with acute HIV infection should be referred to an HIV specialist, who ideally will enroll the patient into a clinical study. Most experts recommend antiretroviral therapy, although no long-term clinical studies comparing treatment vs. observation have been conducted. The optimal duration of therapy and role of intermittent treatment are under investigation

2. **Obtain HIV resistance genotype (p. 239)** because of a rising background prevalence of transmission of antiretroviral therapy-resistant virus. A genotype resistance test is preferred; therapy can be started pending results of the test

3. **Rationale for treatment of acute HIV infection.** Hastens resolution of symptoms (possibly); reduces dissemination of virus to other organs (unlikely); reduces viral transmission (sometimes); lowers virologic "set point" (possibly); preserves virus-specific CD_4 response to slow disease progression (likely); eradicates HIV (extremely unlikely)

APPROACH TO HIV TESTING (Figure 2)

A. HIV Antibody Tests. Most patients produce antibody to HIV within 6-8 weeks of exposure; half will have a positive antibody test in 3-4 weeks, and nearly 100% will have detectable antibody by 6 months

1. **ELISA.** Usual screening test. All positives must be confirmed with Western blot or other more specific tests

2. **Western blot.** CDC criteria for interpretation:
   a. **Positive:** At least two of the following bands: p24, gp41, gp160/120
   b. **Negative:** No bands
   c. **Indeterminate:** Any HIV band, but does not meet criteria for positivity

3. **Test performance.** Standard method is ELISA screen with Western blot confirmation
   a. **ELISA negative:** Western blot is not required (ELISA sensitivity 99.7%, specificity 98.5%). Obtain HIV RNA if acute HIV infection is suspected
   b. **ELISA positive:** Confirm with Western blot. Probability that ELISA and Western blot are both false-positives is extremely low (< 1 per 140,000). Absence of p31 band could be a clue to a false positive Western blot
   c. **Unexpected ELISA/Western blot:** Repeat test to exclude clerical/computer error

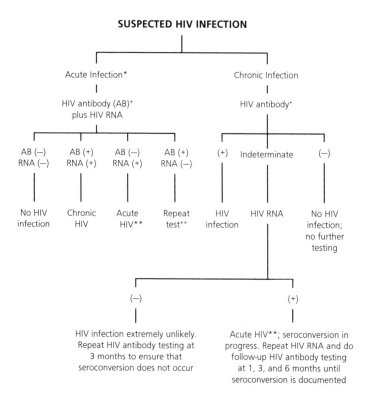

SUSPECTED HIV INFECTION

Figure 2. Approach to HIV Testing

(−) = negative test; (+) = positive test

* Occurs 1-4 weeks after viral transmission. Most patients manifest a viral syndrome (fever, pharyngitis ± rash/arthralgias), which is often mistaken for the flu and therefore overlooked

** HIV RNA in acute HIV infection should be very high (usually > 100,000 copies/mL)

+ All positive ELISA tests must be confirmed by Western Blot; usually this is done automatically in clinical laboratories

++ May be long-term non-progressor or laboratory error

4. **Indeterminate Western Blot.** Common clinical problem, affecting 4-20% of reactive ELISAs. Usually due to a single p24 band or weak other bands. Causes include seroconversion in progress, advanced HIV disease with loss of antibody response, cross-reacting antibody from pregnancy, blood transfusions, organ transplantation, autoantibodies from collagen vascular disease, infection with HIV-2, influenza vaccination, or recipient of HIV vaccine. In low-risk patients, an indeterminate result almost never represents true HIV infection; options include repeating the test in 2-3 and 6 months (if still indeterminate, reassure) or ordering a HIV RNA test (if negative, reassure; if HIV RNA is high, seroconversion is in progress).

B. Quantitative Plasma HIV RNA (HIV Viral Load Assays)

1. **Description.** Measures amount of HIV RNA in plasma. High sensitivity of assays allows detection of virus in most patients not on antiviral therapy. Used to diagnose acute HIV infection and more commonly to monitor the response to antiretroviral therapy.

2. **Uses of HIV RNA Assay**

   a. **Confirms diagnosis of acute HIV infection.** A high HIV RNA with a negative HIV antibody test confirms acute HIV infection prior to seroconversion.

   b. **Helpful in initial evaluation of HIV infection.** Establishes baseline HIV RNA and helps (along with CD_4 cell count) determine whether to initiate or defer therapy.

   c. **Identifies potential "long-term non-progressors"** (no universally accepted definition; one sometimes used is 10 or more years of HIV infection without immunologic decline even without antiretroviral therapy). Such patients almost invariably have HIV RNA assays consistently < 5000 (usually < 1000).

   d. **Monitors response to antiviral therapy.** HIV RNA changes rapidly decline 2-4 weeks after starting or changing effective antiretroviral therapy, with slower decline thereafter. Patients with the greatest HIV RNA response have the best clinical outcome. No change in HIV RNA suggests therapy will be ineffective.

   e. **Estimates risk for opportunistic infection.** For patients with similar CD_4 cell counts, the risk of opportunistic infections is higher with higher HIV RNAs.

3. **Assays and Interpretation**

   a. **Tests, sensitivities, and dynamic range**. Three main assays, each with advantages and disadvantages, are widely used. Any assay can be used to diagnose acute HIV infection and guide/monitor therapy, but the same test should be used to follow patients longitudinally.

      1. **RT-PCR Amplicor** (Roche): Sensitivity = 400 copies/mL; dynamic range = 400-750,000 copies/mL

      2. **RT-PCR Ultrasensitive 1.5** (Roche): Sensitivity = 50 copies/mL; dynamic range = 50-75,000 copies/mL

      3. **bDNA Versant 3.0** (Bayer): Sensitivity = 75 copies/mL; dynamic range = 50-500,000 copies/mL

   b. **Correlation between HIV RNA and CD_4.** HIV RNA assays correlate inversely with CD_4 cell counts, but do so imperfectly (e.g., some patients with high CD_4 counts have relatively high HIV RNA levels, and vice versa.) For any given CD_4, higher HIV RNA levels correlate with more rapid disease progression. In response to antiretroviral therapy, changes in HIV RNA generally precede changes in CD_4 cell count.

c. **Significant change in HIV RNA assay** is defined by at least a 2-fold (0.3 log) change in viral RNA (accounts for normal variation in clinically stable patients), or a 3-fold (0.5 log) change in response to new antiretroviral therapy (accounts for intra-laboratory and patient variability). For example, if a HIV RNA result = 50,000 copies/mL, then the range of possible actual values = 25,000-100,000 copies/mL, and the value needed to demonstrate antiretroviral activity is $\leq$ 17,000 copies/mL.

4. **Indications for HIV RNA Testing.** Usually performed in conjunction with CD_4 cell counts. Indicated for the diagnosis of acute HIV infection, and for initial evaluation of newly diagnosed HIV. Also recommended 2-8 weeks after initiation of antiretroviral therapy and every 3-4 months in all HIV patients.

5. **When to Avoid HIV RNA Testing**
   a. **During acute illnesses and immunizations.** Patients with acute opportunistic infections may experience significant (> 5-fold) rises in HIV RNA, which return to baseline 1-2 months after recovery; similar patterns have been reported for bacterial pneumonia and HSV recurrences. Although data are conflicting, many studies show at least a transient increase in HIV RNA levels following influenza and other immunizations, which return to baseline after 2 months
   b. **When results of test would not influence therapy.** Frequent scenario in patients with advanced disease who have no antiretroviral options or cannot tolerate therapy
   c. **To diagnose HIV infection**, except if acute (primary) HIV disease is suspected during the HIV antibody window (i.e., first 3-6 weeks after viral transmission)

INITIAL ASSESSMENT OF HIV-INFECTED PATIENTS

A. **Clinical Evaluation.** History and physical exam should focus on diagnoses associated with HIV infection. Compared to patients without HIV, the severity, frequency, and duration of these conditions are usually increased in HIV disease.

1. **Dermatologic:** Severe herpes simplex (oral/anogenital); herpes zoster (especially recurrent, cranial nerve, or disseminated); molluscum contagiosum; staphylococcal abscesses; tinea nail infections; Kaposi's sarcoma (from HHV-8 infection); petechiae (from ITP); seborrheic dermatitis; new or worsening psoriasis; eosinophilic pustular folliculitis; severe cutaneous drug eruptions (especially sulfonamides)
2. **Oropharyngeal:** Oral candidiasis; oral hairy leukoplakia (from EBV); Kaposi's sarcoma (frequently on palate/gums); gingivitis/periodontitis; warts; aphthous ulcers (especially esophageal/perianal)
3. **Constitutional symptoms:** Fatigue, fevers, chronic diarrhea, weight loss
4. **Lymphatic:** Persistent, generalized lymphadenopathy
5. **Others:** Active TB (especially extrapulmonary); non-Hodgkin's lymphoma (especially CNS); unexplained leukopenia, anemia, thrombocytopenia (especially ITP); myopathy; miscellaneous neurologic conditions (cranial/peripheral neuropathies, Guillain-Barre syndrome, mononeuritis multiplex, aseptic meningitis, cognitive impairment)

B. **Baseline Laboratory Testing (Table 1)**

C. CD$_4$ Cell Count (lymphocyte subset analysis)
   1. **Overview.** Acute HIV infection is characterized by a decline in CD$_4$ cell count, followed by a gradual rise associated with clinical recovery. Chronic HIV infection shows progressive declines (~ 50-80 cells/year) in CD$_4$ cell count without treatment, followed by more rapid decline 1-2 years prior to opportunistic infection (AIDS-defining diagnosis). Cell counts remain stable over 5-10 years in 5% of patients, while others may show rapid declines (> 300 cells/year). Since variability exists within individual patients and between laboratories, it is useful to *repeat any value before making management decisions.*
   2. **Uses of CD$_4$ Cell Count**
      a. **Gives context of degree of immunosuppression** for interpretation of symptoms/signs (Table 2)
      b. **Used to guide therapy.** Most guidelines support CD$_4$ < 200/mm^3 as a threshold for initiating treatment, regardless of HIV RNA or symptoms; treatment should be considered for CD$_4$ < 350/mm^3. For prophylaxis against PCP, toxoplasmosis, and MAC/CMV infection, CD$_4$ cell counts of 200/mm^3, < 100/mm^3, and < 50/mm^3 are used as threshold levels, respectively
      c. **Provides estimate of risk of death.** CD$_4$ cell counts < 50/mm^3 are associated with a markedly increased risk of death (median survival 1 year), although some patients with low counts survive > 3 years even without antiretroviral therapy. Prognosis is heavily influenced by HIV RNA, presence/history of opportunistic infections or neoplasms, performance status, and the immune reconstitution response to antiretroviral therapy

D. HIV RNA Assay (HIV RNA PCR) (p. 232)

Table 1. Baseline Laboratory Testing for HIV-Infected Patients

Test	Rationale
Repeat HIV serology (ELISA/confirmatory Western blot)	Indicated for patients unable to document a prior positive test, and for "low risk" individuals with a positive test (to detect computer/clerical error). Repeat serology is now less important since HIV RNA testing provides an additional means of confirming HIV infection
CBC with differential, platelets	Detects cytopenias (e.g., ITP) seen in HIV. Needed to calculate CD$_4$ cell count
Chemistry panel ("SMA 20")	Detects renal dysfunction and electrolyte/LFT abnormalities, which may accompany HIV and associated infections (e.g., HIV nephropathy, HCV)
CD$_4$ cell count	Determines the need for antiretroviral therapy and opportunistic infection (OI) prophylaxis. Best test for defining risk of OIs and prognosis
"HIV RNA" assay (plasma HIV RNA)	Provides a marker for the pace of HIV disease progression. Determines indication for and response to antiretroviral therapy
Tuberculin skin test (standard 5 TU of PPD)	Detects latent TB infection and targets patients for preventive therapy. Anergy skin tests are no longer indicated due to poor predictive value. HIV is the most powerful co-factor for the development of active TB
PAP smear	Risk of cervical cancer is nearly twice as high in HIV-positive women compared to uninfected controls

Table 1. Baseline Laboratory Testing for HIV-Infected Patients (cont'd)

Test	Rationale
Toxoplasmosis serology (IgG)	Identifies patients at risk for subsequent cerebral/systemic toxoplasmosis and the need for prophylaxis. Those with negative tests should be counseled on how to avoid infection
Syphilis serology (VDRL or RPR)	Identifies co-infection with syphilis, which is epidemiologically-linked to HIV. Disease may have accelerated course in HIV patients
Hepatitis C serology (anti-HCV)	Identifies HCV infection and usually chronic carriage. If positive, follow with HCV genotype and HCV viral load assay. If the patient is antibody-negative and at high-risk for hepatitis, order HCV RNA to exclude a false-negative result
Hepatitis B serologies (HBsAb, HBcAb, HBsAg)	Identifies patients who are immune to hepatitis B (HBsAb) or chronic carriers (HBsAg). If all three are negative, hepatitis B vaccine is indicated
G6PD screen	Identifies patients at risk for dapsone or primaquine-associated hemolysis
CMV serology (IgG)	Identifies patients who should receive CMV-negative or leukocyte-depleted blood if transfused
VZV serology (IgG)	Identifies patients at risk for varicella (chickenpox), and those who should avoid contact with active varicella or herpes zoster patients. Serology-negative patients exposed to chickenpox should receive varicella-zoster immune globulin (VZIG)
Chest x-ray	Sometimes ordered as a baseline test for future comparisons. May detect healed granulomatous diseases/other processes. Indicated in all tuberculin skin test positive patients

Table 2. Use of CD$_4$ Cell Count for Interpretation of Patient Signs/Symptoms

CD$_4$ Cell Count (cells/mm^3)	Associated Conditions
> 500	Most illnesses are similar to those in HIV-negative patients. Some increased risk of bacterial infections (pneumococcal pneumonia, sinusitis), herpes zoster, tuberculosis, skin conditions
200-500*	Bacterial infections (especially pneumococcal pneumonia, sinusitis), cutaneous Kaposi's sarcoma, vaginal candidiasis, ITP
50-200*	Thrush, oral hairy leukoplakia, classic HIV-associated opportunistic infections (e.g., P. carinii pneumonia, cryptococcal meningitis, toxoplasmosis). For patients receiving prophylaxis, most opportunistic infection do not occur until CD$_4$ cell counts fall significantly below 100/mm^3
< 50*	"Final common pathway" opportunistic infections (disseminated M. avium-intracellulare, CMV retinitis), HIV-associated wasting, neurologic disease (neuropathy, encephalopathy)

* Patients remain at risk for all processes noted in earlier stages

ANTIRETROVIRAL THERAPY

A. **Initiation of Antiretroviral Therapy (Figure 3).** Advances in antiretroviral therapy have led to dramatic reductions in HIV-related morbidity and mortality for patients with severe immunosuppression ($CD_4 < 200$) or a prior AIDS-defining illness. Treatment of asymptomatic patients is far more controversial, many of whom live years before developing any HIV-related symptom. Potential benefits of starting antiretroviral therapy with relatively high CD_4 cell counts include control of viral replication, reduction in HIV RNA, prevention of immunodeficiency, delayed time to onset of AIDS, decreased risk of drug toxicity, viral transmission, and selecting resistant virus. Potential risks of early antiretroviral therapy include reduced quality of life (from side effects/inconvenience), earlier development of drug resistance (with consequent transmission of resistant virus and limitation in future antiretroviral choices), unknown long-term toxicity of antiretroviral drugs, and unknown duration of effectiveness. The primary goals of therapy are prolonged suppression of viral replication to undetectable levels (HIV RNA < 50-75 copies/mL), restoration/preservation of immune function, and improved clinical outcome. Once initiated, antiretroviral therapy is usually continued indefinitely.

B. **Choice of Initial Antiretroviral Therapy (Tables 3-5, Figure 4).** Specific regimens are chosen to improve the length and quality of life by reducing the HIV RNA to undetectable levels. These include NNRTI-based regimens, PI-based regimens, and triple NRTI regimens (Table 4). No single regimen is ideal for all patients. At least 3 active agents are required.

C. **Antiretroviral Treatment Failure (Figure 4).** There are several overlapping definitions of drug failure, including virologic failure, immunologic failure, and clinical failure (pp. 238-239). Virologic failure generally precedes immunologic failure, and immunologic failure generally precedes clinical failure. Before changing therapy, it is important to distinguish drug toxicity from drug failure. For drug toxicity, single drug substitutions from the same drug class may be appropriate. For drug failure, most cases require ≥ 2 new drugs or a new drug regimen. It is also important to determine the cause of drug failure (e.g, viral resistance, drug interactions, malabsorption, poor patient compliance). Treatment of mental health disorders and other measures to improve compliance may obviate the need to change therapy.

HIV-INFECTED PATIENT

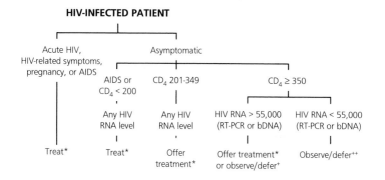

Figure 3. Indications for Initiating Antiretroviral Therapy

*   See Table 4 (p. 241), Figure 4 (below)

+   Some experts would initiate therapy, given the high (>30%) 3-year risk of AIDS in untreated patients. Without very high plasma HIV RNA, some would defer therapy and monitor CD_4 and HIV RNA frequently

++ Many experts would defer therapy and observe, given the relatively lower (<15%) 3-year risk of AIDS

Adapted from: Guidelines for the Use of Antiretroviral Agents for HIV-1-infected Adults and Adolescents: recommendations of the Panel on Clinical Practices for Treatment of HIV Infection;: www.aidsinfo.gov/guidelines/, November 10, 2003

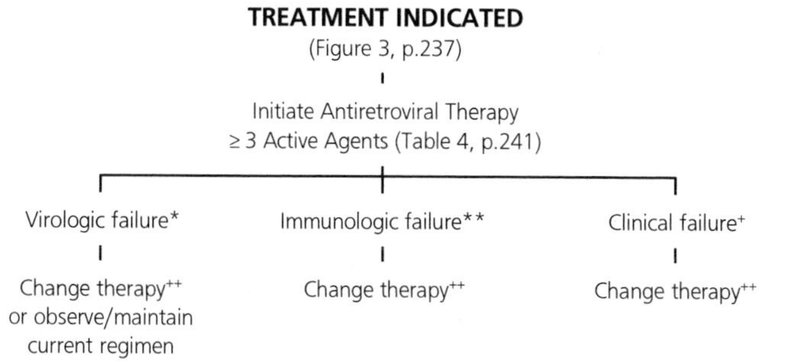

TREATMENT INDICATED
(Figure 3, p.237)

Initiate Antiretroviral Therapy
≥ 3 Active Agents (Table 4, p.241)

Virologic failure*	Immunologic failure**	Clinical failure+
Change therapy++ or observe/maintain current regimen	Change therapy++	Change therapy++

Figure 4. Approach to Antiretroviral Therapy

*   See next page for criteria

** 30% decline in CD_4 cell count or 3% decline in CD_4% from baseline, confirmed on repeat testing

+   Disease progression (constitutional symptoms, opportunistic infection, recurrent bacterial pneumonia)

++ Based on resistance testing and previous antiretroviral regimen

1. **Virologic failure.** HIV RNA fails to reach undetectable levels or rebounds. Drug failure is confirmed by significant increases in viremia on repeat testing not caused by a transient stimulus (e.g., acute illness, immunization), regardless of CD$_4$ cell counts.

   a. **Criteria for virologic failure** are based on demonstrating either a suboptimal reduction in viremia after starting therapy, re-emergence of viremia after suppression to undetectable levels, or a significant increase in viremia from the nadir of suppression.

      1. **Less than a 0.5-0.75 log reduction in plasma HIV RNA by 4 weeks** after starting therapy, or < 1 log reduction by 8 weeks

      2. **Failure to suppress plasma HIV RNA to undetectable levels within 4-6 months of starting therapy.** The degree of initial decrease in plasma HIV RNA and overall trend in decreasing viremia should be considered before changing therapy. For example, a patient with a HIV RNA >750,000 copies/mL before therapy who stabilizes after 6 months of therapy at a level that is detectable but <10,000 copies/mL may not warrant an immediate change in therapy, so long as the trend is still downward

      3. **Repeated detection of virus in plasma after initial suppression to undetectable levels**, suggesting the development of resistance. The degree of plasma HIV RNA increase should be considered. For example, it may be reasonable to consider close, short-term observation in a patient whose plasma HIV RNA increases from undetectable to low-level detectability (50-5000 copies/mL)

      4. **Any reproducible significant (≥ 3-fold) increase from the nadir of plasma HIV RNA** not caused by intercurrent infection, vaccination, or test methodology

   b. **Risk factors for virologic failure** include low drug levels (due to poor adherence, enhanced metabolism, or diminished absorption), high baseline HIV RNA or low baseline CD$_4$ cell counts (patients with advanced disease are at greater risk of failing therapy), slow HIV RNA response, genetic factors (heterozygotes for mutant CCR5 may be more likely to respond), baseline viral resistance (due to prior antiretroviral therapy or primary acquisition of a highly drug-resistant strain), and double nucleoside therapy or other non-preferred therapy.

   c. **Management of virologic failure in patients who are otherwise doing well** is not well established. One approach is to change therapy as soon as virologic failure is evident, since continued treatment with "non-suppressive" regimens selects for additional resistance mutations. Another approach is to change therapy only for immunologic or clinical failure, given the discordance between virologic failure and clinical failure ("CD$_4$/HIV RNA disconnect"), increased pill burden/side effects associated with subsequent regimens, the perception that changing treatment too soon may exhaust future options, and lack of guarantee that changing regimens improves prognosis. We recommend early regimen changes for virologic failure when there are still viable treatment options. This should be guided by resistance testing. For patients with no alternative treatment options, continued monitoring on the virologically failing regimen is usually warranted.

2. **Immunologic Failure.** Progressive decline in CD$_4$ cell count. Change in therapy is recommended based on results of resistance testing and previous antiretroviral regimen.

3. **Clinical Failure.** HIV disease progression (e.g., constitutional symptoms, opportunistic infections, recurrent bacterial pneumonia) or death. Change in therapy is recommended based on results of resistance testing and previous antiretroviral regimen.

4. **Resistance Testing and Selection of New Antiretroviral Therapy.** Genotypic assays characterize nucleotide sequences of the reverse transcriptase/protease portions of the virus, and identify resistance mutations associated with various drugs. Phenotypic assays attempt to grow the virus in the presence of drugs, providing a more intuitively applicable measurement of resistance (similar to that done with bacteria). Compared to phenotypic assays, genotypic assays are faster (1-2 weeks vs. 2-4 weeks for results), less expensive ($400 vs. $1000), and have less inter-laboratory variability; however, mutations do not always correlate with resistance and results are difficult to interpret.

5. **Use of Enfuvirtide for Treatment Failure.** Enfuvirtide is the only fusion inhibitor to be approved by the FDA. This agent interferes with entry of HIV-1 into cells by blocking fusion of HIV-1 and CD_4 cellular membranes. Enfurvitide is effective in heavily antiretroviral-experienced patients experiencing treatment failure, further increasing CD_4 cell counts and decreasing HIV-1 RNA levels when given with an optimized background regimen. It does not have any cross-resistance with any other antiretroviral agents. Enfuvirtide is useful for selected patients with treatment failure; ideal candidates are patients with extensive antiretroviral experience, documented resistance on genotype or phenotype testing, but with 1 or more active drugs available to use in the optimized background regimen (N Engl J Med 2003;348:2175-85). Enfuvirtide requires twice daily subcutaneous injection, needs extensive pre-treatment education, and is expensive. Optimal use in patients with higher CD4 cell counts and less immediate risk of HIV disease progression awaits definition.

D. **Body Shape Changes and Metabolic Abnormalities Associated with HIV Therapy**

1. **Lipodystrophy Syndrome.** Prevalence varies widely (5%-75%), depending on the definition used. Features are similar to Syndrome X, with truncal obesity, insulin resistance, and hyperlipidemia (especially in patients on protease inhibitors). Other features include peripheral fat wasting from the face and limbs, breast enlargement in women (sometimes gynecomastia in men), and dorsocervical fat pad. Frank diabetes mellitus and diabetic ketoacidosis have been reported; close monitoring of patients with pre-existing diabetes is recommended, especially if protease inhibitors are used. Risk factors include advanced HIV disease, older age, total duration of antiretroviral therapy and treatment with protease inhibitors or certain nucleoside reverse transcriptase inhibitors (NRTIs), especially D4T. Optimal treatment awaits definition. Experimental options include liposuction, polylactate injections for fat atrophy, anabolic steroids, growth hormone, metformin, or aggressive treatment of hyperlipidemia. Since hypertriglyceridemia is often marked, initial use of a fibrate (gemfibrozil 600 mg q12h or fenofibrate 67 mg q24h) is recommended, followed if necessary by a statin. Pravastatin starting at 20 mg daily is the preferred statin for patients on protease inhibitors. If pravastatin is ineffective, administer atorvastatin starting at 10 mg daily. Atazanavir, the only once-daily protease inhibitor, is unique among protease inhibitors in its neutral effect on plasma lipids. This has been shown both in prospective studies comparing it with other protease inhibitors, as well as in a "switch" study where patients

receiving nelfinavir were switched to atazanavir and had a subsequent reduction in plasma lipids. Even when given as a boosted protease inhibitor with 100 mg daily of ritonavir, lipid elevations appear to be lower than with other boosted-protease inhibitor regimens.

2. **Lactic Acidosis/Hepatomegaly with Hepatic Steatosis** is a rare but potentially fatal complication, most often associated with prolonged use of NRTIs. Clinical presentation includes nonspecific GI complaints (abdominal distension/pain, nausea, vomiting), weakness, weight loss, and sometimes dyspnea. In addition to elevated serum lactate levels, patients may have an anion gap metabolic acidosis, and elevated liver transaminases, CPK, LDH, lipase, and amylase. For symptomatic lactic acidosis, immediate cessation of antiretroviral therapy is indicated, along with supportive care (bicarbonate, hemodialysis, intubation) as needed.

3. **Bone Disorders.** Two syndromes have been described: 1) osteopenia/osteoporosis; 2) avascular necrosis (most commonly of the hip). Relationship to antiretroviral therapy is not clear.

4. **Increased Bleeding in Hemophilia.** Spontaneous bleeding is increased in hemophilia patients on protease inhibitors. Joint/soft tissue bleeding is most common, but intracranial and GI bleeding have occurred.

5. **Rash.** Mild rashes are relatively common with NNRTIs. Severe rashes (including Stevens-Johnson syndrome) may rarely develop in a small percentage of patients.

Table 3. Antiretroviral Agents for HIV Infection

Drug Class	Drugs	
Nucleoside analogue reverse transcriptase inhibitors (NRTIs)	Abacavir (Ziagen) Didanosine (ddI, Videx) Emtricitabine (Emtriva) Lamivudine (3TC, Epivir) Stavudine (d4T, Zerit) Zalcitabine (ddC, Hivid)	Zidovudine (AZT, ZDV, Retrovir) Zidovudine + lamivudine (Combivir) Zidovudine + lamivudine + abacavir (Trizivir)
Non-nucleoside reverse transcriptase inhibitors (NNRTIs)	Delavirdine (Rescriptor) Efavirenz (Sustiva)	Nevirapine (Viramune)
Protease inhibitors (PIs)	Amprenavir (Agenerase) Atazanavir (Reyataz) Fosamprenavir (Lexiva) Indinavir (Crixivan) Lopinavir + ritonavir (Kaletra)	Nelfinavir (Viracept) Ritonavir (Norvir) Saquinavir (hard-gel [Invirase]; soft-gel [Fortovase])
Nucleotide analogue	Tenofovir (Viread)	
Fusion inhibitor	Enfurvirtide (Fuzeon)	

Table 4. Antiretroviral Regimens Recommended for Treatment of HIV-1 Infection in Antiretroviral Naive Patients[†]

	NNRTI–Based Regimens
Preferred	• Efavirenz + lamivudine + (zidovudine or tenofovir DF or stavudine*)[‡]
Alternative	• Efavirenz + emtricitabine + (zidovudine or tenofovir DF or stavudine*)[‡] • Efavirenz + (lamivudine or emtricitabine) + didanosine[‡] • Nevirapine + (lamivudine or emtricitabine) + (zidovudine or stavudine* or didanosine)
	PI–Based Regimens
Preferred	• Kaletra (lopinavir/ritonavir) + lamivudine + (zidovudine or stavudine)
Alternative	• Amprenavir/ritonavir[††] + (lamivudine or emtricitabine) + (zidovudine or stavudine) • Atazanavir + (lamivudine or emtricitabine) + (zidovudine or stavudine*) • Indinavir + (lamivudine or emtricitabine) + (zidovudine or stavudine*) • Indinavir/ritonavir[††] + (lamivudine or emtricitabine) + (zidovudine or stavudine*) • Kaletra (lopinavir/ritonavir) + emtricitabine + (zidovudine or stavudine*) • Nelfinavir[§] + (lamivudine or emtricitabine) + (zidovudine or stavudine*) • Saquinavir (SGC or HGC)/ritonavir[††] + (lamivudine or emtricitabine) + (zidovudine or stavudine)
	Triple NRTI Regimen (only when NNRTI- or PI- based regimen cannot or should not be used as first-line therapy)
Alternative[¥]	• Abacavir + lamivudine + zidovudine (or stavudine*)

HGC = saquinavir hard-gel capsule (Invirase), NNRTI = non-nucleoside reverse transcriptase inhibitor, NRTI = nucleoside reverse transcriptase inhibitor, PI = protease inhibitor, SGC = saquinavir soft-gel capsule (Fortovase). See Chapter 7 for individual drug summaries

†   Guidelines for HIV-infected patients with no prior experience with HIV therapy, based on the totality of virologic, immunologic, and toxicity data. Regimens should be individualized based on variables such as pill burden, dosing frequency, toxicities, drug-drug interactions, pregnancy status, co-morbid conditions, and plasma HIV RNA level. In some cases, based on individual patient characteristics, an "alternative" regimen may actually be the preferred regimen for a selected patient. Guidelines for initiation of antiretroviral therapy in HIV-1 infected pregnant patients can be found at www.aidsinfo.nih.gov/guidelines/. From: Guidelines for the Use of Antiretroviral Agents for HIV-1-infected Adults and Adolescents: recommendations of the Panel on Clinical Practices for Treatment of HIV Infection; www.aidsinfo.gov/guidelines/, November 10, 2003

*   Higher incidence of lipoatrophy, hyperlipidemia, and mitochondrial toxicities reported with stavudine than with other NRTIs

‡   Regimen not recommended for pregnant women or women with pregnancy potential (i.e., women who want to conceive or those who are not using effective contraception)

†† Low-dose (100-400 mg) ritonavir

§   Nelfinavir available in 250 mg or 625 mg tablet

¥   Only as alternative to NNRTI- or PI-based regimen

Table 5. Advantages and Disadvantages of Common Antiretroviral Agents/Combinations

Agent/Combination	Advantages	Disadvantages
NRTI COMBINATIONS		
Zidovudine 300 mg (PO) q12h + lamivudine150 mg (PO) q12h	Fixed-dose combination tablet (Combivir) reduces pill burden. AZT especially effective in treating ITP and has relatively good CNS penetration	AZT has highest rate of subjective side effects (nausea, GI disturbance, headache) in NRTI class and is the most marrow suppressive
Stavudine 40 mg (PO) q12h + lamivudine 150 mg (PO) q12h or emtricitabine 200 mg (PO) q24h	Excellent initial tolerability	d4T-based regimes associated in some studies with higher rates of hyperlipidemia, neuropathy, lipodystrophy
Zidovudine 300 mg (PO) q12h + lamivudine 150 mg (PO) q12h + abacavir 300 mg (PO) q12h	Defers protease inhibitor and NNRTI regimens. Fixed-dose combination tablet (Trizivir) has lowest pill burden (1 pill q12h) for a complete triple-drug regimen	Abacavir hypersensitivity in 3-8%. As triple therapy, may have lower efficacy in patients with baseline HIV RNA > 100,000 copies/mL and compared with efavirenz-based regimens
Lamivudine 300 mg (PO) q24h (or emtricitabine 200 mg [PO] q24h) + didanosine 400 mg (PO) q24h	Once-daily dosing, low pill burden (2 per day)	Limited long-term data. ddI must be taken on an empty stomach
Lamivudine 300 mg (PO) q24h (or emtricitabine 200 mg [PO] q24h) + tenofovir 300 mg (PO) q24h	Advantages: As effective as d4T/3TC when used as part of triple therapy and causes less hyperlipidemia. Once-daily dosing, low pill burden (2 per day); tenofovir/emtricitabine likely available as co-formulated tablet soon Disadvantages: Lowers atazanavir levels	
Lamivudine 300 mg (PO) q24h + abacavir 300 mg (PO) q12h (or 600 mg [PO] q24)	Low pill burden; likely approved for combination tablet soon (1 pill/day)	Abacavir hypersensitivity; limited long-term data
PROTEASE INHIBITORS		
Lopinavir + ritonavir (Kaletra) 3 caps (400 mg/100 mg) (PO) q12h	More effective than nelfinavir when combined with d4T and 3TC in randomized, double-blind trial (Walmsley, N Engl J Med;346:2039, 2002). Generally well tolerated	Associated with hyperlipidemia (especially hypertriglyceridemia). Diarrhea and nausea are the most common adverse effects
Indinavir 800 mg (PO) q8h	Longest follow-up data showing viral suppression (MK-035 study)	Q8h dosing on empty stomach is required. Nephrolithiasis, paronychia, dry skin are unique side effects to this agent. Can be given with low-dose ritonavir for twice-daily dosing (indinavir 800 mg plus ritonavir 100 mg q12h), but optimal dose is not clear and adverse effects are often increased

Table 5. Advantages and Disadvantages of Common Antiretroviral Agents/Combinations

Agent/Combination	Advantages	Disadvantages
PROTEASE INHIBITORS (cont.)		
Nelfinavir 1250 mg (PO) q12h	Early virologic failure often associated with unique D30N mutation, allowing "salvage" with other protease inhibitors	Diarrhea may be incapacitating for some patients
Ritonavir 400 mg (PO) q12h + saquinavir 400 mg (PO) q12h	Some studies show this combination to be more effective than single protease inhibitors	High pill burden (6 large caps q12h). Ritonavir is associated with relatively high rates of GI toxicity. Most likely to produce elevations in triglycerides and cholesterol. Alternative dose (ritonavir 100 mg q12 + saquinavir 1000 q12h) better tolerated
Atazanavir 400 mg (PO) q24h (or 300 mg q24h + ritonavir 100 mg q24h with efavirenz or tenofovir, or in PI-experienced patients)	Only once daily protease inhibitor, low pill burden; neutral or minimal effect on plasma lipids (even when given with 100 mg daily of ritonavir)	Mild indirect hyperbilirubinemia frequent; when given unboosted (without ritonavir), may be less active than lopinavir/ritonavir in protease-inhibitor experienced patients; first-degree AV block may occur (not advanced heart block)
Fosamprenavir: *PI naive*: 1400 mg q12h (or 1400 mg q24h with ritonavir 200 mg q24h). *PI experienced*: 700 mg q12h with ritonavir 100 mg q12h	More active than nelfinavir in head-to head study; relatively low rates of GI side effects	Rash may occur somewhat more commonly than with other PIs; should not be used with Kaletra due to bidirectional drug interaction
NNRTIs		
Efavirenz 600 mg (PO) q24h	Long half-life (60 hours) allows once-daily dosing. Superior to indinavir in open label head-to-head trial (NEJM 1999;341: 1865). Proven efficacy in patients with high HIV RNA and advanced disease	Near-universal CNS disturbances (vivid dreams, daytime somnolence, dizziness) at outset of therapy (usually abates with time). Rash in ~ 20% (can generally can treat through). Not to be used in pregnancy (teratogenic in monkeys). Single mutation leads to high-level resistance
Nevirapine 200 mg (PO) q24h x 14 days, then 200 mg (PO) q12h	Low pill-burden. Can be taken with or without food	Relatively high rate of hepatotoxicity and severe dermatologic/ systemic reactions, more commonly in women (use with caution in pregnancy). Rate of Stevens-Johnson syndrome ~ 1%). Single mutation leads to high-level resistance
Delavirdine 400 mg (PO) q8h	Can be taken with or without food. Inhibits p450 enzymes and can act as a pharmaco-kinetic booster for some protease inhibitors, most notably indinavir	Highest pill burden and most frequent dosing in drug class. Rash in 18%, though usually mild. Single mutation leads to high-level resistance

Table 5. Advantages and Disadvantages of Common Antiretroviral Agents/Combinations

Agent/Combination	Advantages	Disadvantages
FUSION INHIBITOR		
Enfuvirtide 90 mg (SQ) q12h	Useful for treatment failures (drug resistance to NRTIs, NNRTIs, PIs). Produces further ↑ in CD₄ and ↓ in HIV-1 RNA in multiple-treatment experienced patients when given with an optimized background regimen. No cross resistance with other antiretrovirals.	Requires twice-daily subcutaneous injection; induces injection site reactions of varying severity; associated in clinical trials with increased risk of pneumonia (cause unclear); expensive
NUCLEOTIDE ANALOGUE		
Tenofovir 300 mg (PO) q24h with food	Low pill burden, well-tolerated, once-daily therapy. As effective as d4T in naive patients in combination with 3TC and efavirenz, with less effect on lipids. Few drug interactions	Shares cross-resistance pattern with NRTIs (certain NRTI mutations do not respond as well). Increases ddI levels by 30%; monitor for ddI toxicity (neuropathy, pancreatitis) and consider a lower dose of ddI (from 400 mg to 250 mg daily)

OPPORTUNISTIC INFECTIONS IN HIV DISEASE

Patients with HIV disease are at risk for infectious complications not otherwise seen in immunocompetent patients. Such opportunistic infections occur in proportion to the severity of immune system dysfunction (reflected by CD₄ cell count depletion). While community acquired infections (e.g., pneumococcal pneumonia) can occur at any CD₄ cell count, "classic" HIV-related opportunistic infections (PCP, toxoplasmosis, cryptococcus, disseminated M. avium- intracellulare, CMV) do not occur until CD₄ cell counts are dramatically reduced. Specifically, it is rare to encounter PCP in HIV patients with CD₄ > 200/mm³, and CMV and disseminated MAC occur at median CD₄ cell counts < 50/mm³. The U.S. Public Health Service/Infectious Diseases Society of America 2001 guidelines for the prevention of opportunistic infections in persons infected with HIV can be found at www.hivatis.org/trtgdlns.html#Opportunistic

Table 6. Overview of Prophylaxis (See Table 7 [pp. 245-247] for details)

Infection	Indication	Intervention	Infection	Indication	Intervention
PCP	CD₄ < 200/mm³	TMP-SMX	Hepatitis B	Susceptible patients	Hepatitis B vaccine
TB (M. tuberculosis)	PPD > 5 mm (current or past) or contact with active case	INH	Hepatitis A	HCV (+) and HA Ab (–); HCV (–) and HA Ab (–) gay men and travelers to endemic areas, chronic liver disease	Hepatitis A vaccine
Toxoplasma	IgG Ab (+) and CD₄ < 100/mm³	TMP-SMX	Influenza	All patients	Annual flu vaccine
MAC	CD₄ < 50/mm³	Azithromycin or clarithromycin	VZV	Exposure to chickenpox or shingles; no prior history	VZIG
S. pneumoniae	CD₄ > 200/mm³	Pneumococcal vaccine	*Abbreviations: Ab = antibody; HA = Hepatitis A; HCV = Hepatitis C virus; VZIG = varicela-zoster immune globulin; VZV = varicela- zoster virus; other abbreviations (p. 1)*		

Table 7. Prophylaxis of Opportunistic Infections in HIV

Infection	Indications and Prophylaxis	Comments
P. jiroveci (formerly carinii) pneumonia (PCP)	Indications: $CD_4 < 200/mm^3$, oral thrush, constitutional symptoms, or previous history of PCP Preferred prophylaxis: TMP-SMX 1 DS tablet (PO) q24h or 1 SS tablet (PO) q24h. 1 DS tablet (PO) 3x/week is also effective, but daily dosing may be slightly more effective based on 1 comparative study Alternate prophylaxis: Dapsone 100 mg (PO) q24h (preferred as second-line by most; more effective than aerosolized pentamidine when CD_4 cell count < 100 **or** Atovaquone 1500 mg (PO) q24h (comparably effective to dapsone and aerosolized pentamidine; more GI toxicity vs. dapsone, but less rash) **or** Aerosolized pentamidine 300 mg via Respirgard II nebulizer once monthly (exclude active pulmonary TB first to avoid nosocomial transmission)	Without prophylaxis, 80% of AIDS patients develop PCP, and 60-70% relapse within one year after the first episode. Prophylaxis with TMP-SMX also reduces the risk for toxoplasmosis and possibly bacterial infections. Among patients with prior non-life-threatening reactions to TMP-SMX, 55% can be successfully rechallenged with 1 SS tablet daily, and 80% can be rechallenged with gradual dose escalation using TMP-SMX elixir (8 mg TMP + 40 mg SMX/mL) given as 1 mL x 3 days, then 2 mL x 3 days, then 5 mL x 3 days, then 1 SS tablet (PO) q24h. Macrolide-regimens for MAC (azithromycin, clarithromycin) add to efficacy of PCP prophylaxis. Primary and secondary prophylaxis may be discontinued if CD_4 cell counts increase to > 200 cells/mm^3 for 3 months or longer in response to antiretroviral therapy (i.e., immune reconstitution). Prophylaxis should be resumed if the CD_4 cell count decreases to < 200/mm^3
Toxoplasmosis	Indications: $CD_4 < 100/mm^3$ with positive toxoplasmosis serology (IgG) Preferred prophylaxis: TMP-SMX 1 DS tablet (PO) q24h Alternate prophylaxis: Dapsone 50 mg (PO) q24h + pyrimethamine 50 mg weekly + folinic acid 25 mg (PO) weekly **or** Dapsone 100 mg/pyrimethamine 50 mg twice weekly (no folinic acid) **or** Atovaquone 1500 mg (PO) q24h	Incidence of toxoplasmosis in seronegative patients is too low to warrant chemoprophylaxis. Primary prophylaxis can be discontinued if CD_4 cell counts increase to > 200/mm^3 for at least 3 months in response to antiretroviral therapy. Secondary prophylaxis (chronic maintenance therapy) may be discontinued in patients who responded to initial therapy, remain asymptomatic, and whose CD_4 counts increase to > 200/mm^3 for 6 months or longer in response to antiretroviral therapy. Prophylaxis should be restarted if the CD_4 count decreases to < 200/mm^3. Some experts would obtain an MRI of the brain as part of the evaluation prior to stopping secondary prophylaxis

Table 7. Prophylaxis of Opportunistic Infections in HIV (cont'd)

Infection	Indications and Prophylaxis	Comments
Tuberculosis (M. tuberculosis)	<u>Indications:</u> Any CD_4 cell count with PPD induration ≥ 5 mm or history of positive PPD without prior treatment, or close contact with active case of TB. Must exclude active disease (chest x-ray mandatory) <u>Preferred prophylaxis:</u> INH 300 mg (PO) q24h x 9 months + pyridoxine 50 mg (PO) q24h x 9 months <u>Alternate prophylaxis:</u> Rifampin 600 mg (PO) q24h x 2 months + pyrazinamide 20 mg/kg (PO) q24h x 2 months. Rifampin should not be given to patients receiving amprenavir, indinavir, lopinavir + ritonavir, nelfinavir, saquinavir, or delavirdine	Consider prophylaxis for skin test negative patients when the probability of prior TB exposure is > 10% (e.g., patients from developing countries, IV drug abusers in some cities, prisoners). However, a trial testing this strategy in the U.S. did not find a benefit for empiric prophylaxis. INH prophylaxis delayed progression to AIDS and prolonged life in Haitian cohort with positive PPD treated x 6 months. Rifampin plus pyrazinamide x 2 months was effective in a multinational clinical trial (but the combination may ↑ hepatotoxicity). Rifabutin may be substituted for rifampin in rifampin-containing regimens (see p. 248 for dosing)
M. avium intracellulare complex (MAC)	<u>Indications:</u> $CD_4 < 50/mm^3$ <u>Preferred prophylaxis:</u> Azithromycin 1200 mg (PO) once a week (fewest number of pills; fewest drug interactions; may add to efficacy of PCP prophylaxis) **or** Clarithromycin 500 mg (PO) q12h (more effective than rifabutin; associated with survival advantage; resistance detected in some breakthrough cases) <u>Alternate prophylaxis:</u> Rifabutin (less effective). See TB (p. 248) for dosing	Macrolide options (azithromycin, clarithromycin) preferable to rifabutin. Azithromycin is preferred for patients on protease inhibitors (fewer drug interactions). Primary prophylaxis may be discontinued if CD_4 cell counts increase to > 100/mm³ and HIV RNA suppresses for 3-6 months or longer in response to antiretroviral therapy. Secondary prophylaxis may be discontinued for CD_4 cell counts that increase to > 100/mm³ x 6 months or longer in response to antiretroviral therapy if patients have completed 12 months of MAC therapy and have no evidence of disease. Resume MAC prophylaxis for $CD_4 < 100/mm^3$
Pneumococcus (S. pneumoniae)	<u>Indications:</u> $CD_4 > 200/mm^3$ <u>Preferred prophylaxis:</u> Pneumococcal polysaccharide (23 valent) vaccine.* Re-vaccinate x 1 at 5 years	Incidence of invasive pneumococcal disease is > 100-fold higher in HIV patients. Re-immunize if initial vaccine is given when $CD_4 < 200/mm^3$, but is now > 200/mm³ due to antiretroviral therapy
Influenza	<u>Indications:</u> Generally recommended for all patients <u>Preferred prophylaxis:</u> Influenza vaccine (inactivated whole virus and split virus vaccine)*	Give annually (optimally October–January). Some experts do not give vaccine if CD_4 is < 100/mm³ (antibody response is poor). New intranasal live virus vaccine is contraindicated in immunosuppressed patients

Table 7. Prophylaxis of Opportunistic Infections in HIV (cont'd)

Infection	Indications and Prophylaxis	Comments
Hepatitis B	<u>Indications:</u> All susceptible (anti-HBcAb negative and anti-HBsAg negative) patients <u>Preferred prophylaxis:</u> Hepatitis B recombinant DNA vaccine*	Response rate is lower than in HIV-negative controls. Repeat series if no response, especially if CD_4 was low during initial series and is now increased
Hepatitis A	<u>Indications:</u> All susceptible patients who are also infected with hepatitis C; HAV-susceptible seronegative gay men or travelers to endemic areas; any chronic liver disease <u>Preferred prophylaxis:</u> Hepatitis A vaccine*	Response rate is lower than in HIV-negative controls
Measles, mumps, rubella	<u>Indications:</u> Patients born after 1957 and never vaccinated; patients vaccinated between 1963-1967 <u>Preferred prophylaxis:</u> MMR (measles, mumps, rubella) vaccine*	Single case of vaccine-strain measles pneumonia in severely immuno-compromised adult who received MMR; vaccine is therefore contraindicated in patients with severe immunodeficiency ($CD_4 < 200$)
H. influenzae	<u>Indications:</u> Not generally recommended for adults <u>Preferred prophylaxis:</u> H. influenzae type B polysaccharide vaccine*	Incidence of H. influenzae disease is increased in HIV patients, but 65% are caused by non-type B strains. Unclear whether vaccine offers protection
Travel vaccines*	<u>Indications:</u> Travel to endemic areas	All considered safe except oral polio, yellow fever, and live oral typhoid–each a live virus vaccine

* Same dose as for normal hosts (see pp. 283-284). If possible, give vaccines early in course of HIV infection, while immune system may still respond. Alternatively, to increase the likelihood of response in patients with advanced HIV disease, vaccines may be administered after 6-12 months of effective antiretroviral therapy. Vaccines should be given when patients are clinically stable, not acutely ill (e.g., give during a routine office visit, rather than during hospitalization for an opportunistic infection). Live vaccines (e.g., oral polio, oral typhoid, Yellow fever) are generally contraindicated, but measles vaccine is well-tolerated in children, and MMR vaccine is recommended for adults as described above

TREATMENT OF OPPORTUNISTIC INFECTIONS (Table 8)

Antiretroviral therapy (ART) and specific antimicrobial prophylaxis regimens have led to a dramatic decline in HIV-related opportunistic infections. Today, opportunistic infections occur predominantly in patients not receiving ART (due to undiagnosed HIV infection or nonacceptance of therapy), or in the period after starting ART (due to lack of immune reconstitution or from eliciting a previously absent inflammatory host response). Despite high rates of virologic failure, the rate of opportunistic infections in patients compliant with ART remains low, presumably due to continued immunologic response despite virologic failure, a phenomenon that may be linked to impaired "fitness" (virulence) of resistant HIV strains. For patients on or off ART, the absolute CD_4 cell count provides the best marker of risk for opportunistic infections.

Table 8. Treatment of Opportunistic Infections in HIV (see comments, pp. 253-259)

RESPIRATORY TRACT OPPORTUNISTIC INFECTIONS IN HIV		
Infection	**Preferred Therapy**	**Alternate Therapy**
Pneumocystis jiroveci (formerly carinii) pneumonia (PCP) *Mild disease (p0$_2$ > 70 mmHg, A-a gradient < 35)*	TMP-SMX 2 DS tablets (PO) q6-8h x 3 weeks	TMP 300 mg (PO) q8h + dapsone 100 mg (PO) q24h x 3 weeks (less leukopenia/hepatitis vs. TMP-SMX) **or** Clindamycin 450 mg (PO) q6h (or 600 mg q8h) + primaquine 30 mg (PO) q24h x 3 weeks **or** Atovaquone suspension 750 mg (PO) q12h with food x 3 weeks **or** Aerosolized pentamidine 600 mg q24h x 3 weeks (least effective)
Moderate/severe disease (p0$_2$ < 70 mmHg, A-a gradient > 35)	TMP-SMX (5 mg/kg TMP) (IV) q6h x 3 weeks **plus** Prednisone 40 mg (PO) q12h x 5 days, then 40 mg (PO) q24h x 5 days, then 20 mg (PO) q24h until end of therapy	Pentamidine 4 mg/kg (IV) q24h x 3 weeks + prednisone (see preferred therapy) **or** Trimetrexate 45 mg/m^2 (IV) q24h + folinic acid 20 mg/m^2 (PO or IV) q6h x 3 weeks, plus prednisone
Bacterial pneumonia	<u>Inpatient:</u> Azithromycin 500 mg (IV or PO) q24h *plus either* ceftriaxone 2 gm (IV) q24h *or* cefotaxime 1 gm (IV) q8h x 7-14 days. Alternative: IV or PO quinolone x 7-14 days	<u>Outpatient:</u> Gatifloxacin 400 mg (PO) q24h *or* levofloxacin 500 mg (PO) q24h *or* moxifloxacin 400 mg (PO) q24h x 7-14 days
Tuberculosis (M. tuberculosis) (For isolates found to be susceptible to INH and rifampin)	<u>Patients **NOT** on protease inhibitors (PIs) or NNRTIs</u> INH 300 mg (PO) q24h + rifampin 600 mg (PO) q24h + pyrazinamide 25 mg/kg (PO) q24h + ethambutol 15-20 mg/kg (PO) q24h x 8 weeks. Then continue INH + rifampin at same daily doses x 18 weeks. May substitute streptomycin 15 mg/kg (IM) q24h for ethambutol during 8-week induction	<u>Patients **ON** PIs or NNRTIs</u> INH 300 mg (PO) q24h + rifabutin*[†] + pyrazinamide 25 mg/kg (PO) q24h + ethambutol 15-20 mg/kg (PO) q24h x 8 weeks. Then continue INH + rifabutin at same daily doses x 18 weeks <u>Intolerant to rifabutin[†]</u> INH 300 mg (PO) q24h + streptomycin 15 mg/kg (IM) q24h + ethambutol 15-20 mg/kg (PO) q24h + pyrazinamide 25 mg/kg (PO) q24h x 8 weeks. Then continue INH + SM + PZA at same doses 2-3x/week x 30 weeks

* *Rifabutin is contraindicated in patients receiving delavirdine or hard-gel saquinavir. For concurrent use with nelfinavir, indinavir, or amprenavir, decrease rifabutin to 150 mg (PO) q24h. For concurrent use with ritonavir, decrease rifabutin to 150 mg (PO) q48h or 3x/week. For concurrent use with efavirenz, increase rifabutin to 450-600 mg (PO) q24h. (The dose of PIs or NNRTIs may need to be increased by 20-25%.) Monitor carefully for rifabutin drug toxicity (arthralgia, uveitis, leukopenia)*

† *Rifampin can be used with ritonavir, ritonavir + saquinavir, efavirenz, and possibly nevirapine*

Table 8. Treatment of Opportunistic Infections (cont'd) (see comments, pp. 253-259)

RESPIRATORY TRACT OPPORTUNISTIC INFECTIONS IN HIV

Infection	Preferred Therapy	Alternate Therapy
Invasive pulmonary aspergillosis	Voriconazole: loading dose of 6 mg/kg (IV) q12h x 2 doses, then either 4 mg/kg (IV) q12h or 200 mg (PO) q12h x 6-18 months **or** Amphotericin B deoxycholate 1-1.5 mg/kg (IV) q24h until 2-3 gm total dose given (duration of therapy poorly defined)	Itraconazole 200 mg (IV) q12h x 2 days, then itraconazole 200 mg (PO) solution q12h x 6-18 months **or** Caspofungin 70 mg (IV) x 1 dose, then 50 mg (IV) q24h x 6-18 months **or** Amphotericin B lipid formulation (p. 297) (IV) q24h x 6-18 months

CNS OPPORTUNISTIC INFECTIONS IN HIV

Infection	Preferred Therapy	Alternate Therapy
Toxoplasma encephalitis (T. gondii)	Sulfadiazine 1.5-2 gm (PO) q6h + pyrimethamine 200 mg (PO) x 1 dose then 50 mg (PO) q24h + folinic acid 10 mg (PO) q24h x 6-8 weeks until good clinical response. Follow with life-long suppressive therapy* with sulfadiazine 0.5-1 gm (PO) q12h + pyrimethamine 50 mg (PO) q24h + folinic acid 10 mg (PO) q24h	Clindamycin 600 mg (IV or PO) q6h + pyrimethamine 200 mg (PO) x 1 dose then 50 mg (PO) q6h + folinic acid 10 mg (PO) q24h x 6-8 weeks until good clinical response. Follow with life-long suppressive therapy* *with either* clindamycin 300 mg (PO) q6h + pyrimethamine 50 mg (PO) q24h + folinic acid 10 mg (PO) q24h *or* TMP-SMX 5 mg/kg (PO or IV) q12h
Cryptococcal meningitis (C. neoformans)	Amphotericin B deoxycholate 0.7-1 mg/kg (IV) q24h x 2-3 weeks + 5-FC (optional) 25 mg/kg (PO) q6h x 2-3 weeks. Follow with fluconazole 800 mg (IV or PO) x 1 dose followed by 400 mg (PO) q24h indefinitely* (if stable after 10 weeks of 400 mg q24h, can reduce maintenance dose to 200 mg q24h)	Fluconazole 800 mg (IV or PO) q24h x 6-8 weeks, then 400 mg (PO) q24h indefinitely* **or** Amphotericin B lipid formulation (p. 297) (IV) q24h x 2-3 weeks, then fluconazole 800 mg (IV or PO) x 1 dose followed by 400 mg (PO) q24h indefinitely*
CMV encephalitis or polyradiculitis	Ganciclovir 5 mg/kg (IV) q12h ≥ 3 weeks followed by valganciclovir 900 mg (PO) q24h indefinitely†. For severe cases, consider ganciclovir + foscarnet	Foscarnet 60 mg/kg (IV) q8h or 90 mg/kg (IV) q12h x 3 weeks ± ganciclovir 5 mg/kg (IV) q12h x 3 weeks. Follow with valganciclovir 900 mg (PO) q24h indefinitely†
Progressive multifocal leukoencephalopathy (PML)	Antiretroviral therapy with immune reconstitution	May attempt treatment with cidofovir 5 mg/kg (IV) once weekly x 2, then every 2 weeks for total of 24 weeks. Give probenecid 2 gm (PO) 3 hours before and 1 gm (PO) 2 and 8 hours after cidofovir

* *Consider discontinuation of therapy if CD_4 > 200 for ≥ 6 months in response to antiretroviral therapy*
† *Consider discontinuation of therapy if CD_4 > 100-150 for ≥ 6 months in response to antiretroviral therapy*

Table 8. Treatment of Opportunistic Infections (cont'd) (see comments, pp. 253-259)

GI TRACT OPPORTUNISTIC INFECTIONS IN HIV		
Infection	**Preferred Therapy**	**Alternate Therapy**
Oral thrush (Candida) *Acute infection*	Fluconazole 200 mg (PO) x 1 dose, then 100 mg (PO) q24h until symptoms resolve (usually 5-10 days). Patients with multiple prior courses may require a higher dose	Clotrimazole oral troches 10 mg 5x/day until symptoms resolve **or** Itraconazole (PO) solution 100 mg q12h or 200 mg q24h until symptoms resolve <u>Refractory to oral therapy</u> Caspofungin 70 mg (IV) x 1, then 50 mg (IV) q24h until symptoms resolve (↓ dose to 35 mg q24h with moderate hepatic insufficiency) **or** Amphotericin B‡ 0.3-0.5 mg/kg (IV) q24h until symptoms resolve
Maintenance therapy to prevent frequent relapses	Fluconazole 100 mg (PO) q24h to once weekly indefinitely*, depending on need	Amphotericin B‡ 1 mg/kg (IV) once weekly indefinitely*
Candida esophagitis *Initial infection*	Fluconazole 200-400 mg (PO) x 1 dose, then 200 mg (PO) x 1-3 weeks	Same as for oral thrush (except for clotrimazole oral troches) x 1-3 weeks
Maintenance therapy to prevent frequent relapses	Fluconazole 100 mg (PO) q24h to once weekly indefinitely*, depending on need	Amphotericin B‡ 1 mg/kg (IV) once weekly indefinitely*
CMV esophagitis/ colitis	Valganciclovir 900 mg (PO) q12h x 3-6 weeks **or** Ganciclovir 5 mg/kg (IV) q12h x 3-6 weeks	<u>Ganciclovir failure</u> Foscarnet 60 mg/kg (IV) q8h or 90 mg/kg (IV) q12h x 3-6 weeks <u>Foscarnet failure</u> Ganciclovir + foscarnet x 3-6 weeks <u>Relapsing disease</u> Valganciclovir 900 mg (PO) q24h indefinitely*
Salmonella enteritis with bacteremia†	Ciprofloxacin 750 mg (PO) q12h x 2 weeks. If relapse upon discontinuation, give ciprofloxacin 500 mg (PO) q12h indefinitely	Azithromycin 1 gm (PO) x 1, then 500 mg (PO) q24h x 6 days. If relapse, continue azithromycin 250 mg (PO) q24h indefinitely
Cryptosporidia enteritis	Nitazoxamide 500 mg (PO) q6h x 4-6 weeks then q12h indefinitely **or** Paromomycin 1 gm (PO) q12h x 2-4 weeks, then 500 mg (PO) q12h indefinitely*. Most important treatment is antiretroviral therapy with immune reconstitution	Paromomycin 1 gm (PO) q12h + azithromycin 600 mg (PO) q24h x 4 weeks, then paromomycin 500 mg (PO) q12h indefinitely*

* *Consider discontinuation of therapy if CD_4 > 200 for ≥6 months in response to antiretroviral therapy*
† *Consider using AZT as part of antiretroviral regimen (activity against Salmonella)*
‡ *Amphotericin B deoxycholate*

Table 8. Treatment of Opportunistic Infections (cont'd) (see comments, pp. 253-259)

GI TRACT OPPORTUNISTIC INFECTIONS IN HIV

Infection	Preferred Therapy	Alternate Therapy
Microsporidia enteritis	Albendazole 400-800 mg (PO) q12h x 2-4 weeks. Patients with low CD_4 cell counts prone to relapsing disease may require treatment indefinitely*. Most important treatment is antiretroviral therapy with immune reconstitution	Metronidazole 500 mg (PO) q8h x 2-4 weeks; some may require treatment indefinitely* **or** Atovaquone 750 mg (PO) q8h x 2-4 weeks; some may require treatment indefinitely*
Isospora enteritis	TMP-SMX 2 DS tablets (PO) q12h or 1 DS tablet (PO) q8h x 2-4 weeks. Follow with TMP-SMX 1-2 DS tablet(s) (PO) q24h indefinitely*	Ciprofloxacin 500 mg (PO) q12h x 2-4 weeks, or combination therapy with pyrimethamine 50-75 mg (PO) q24h + folinic acid 5-10 mg (PO) q24h x 2-4 weeks. Follow with pyrimethamine 25 mg (PO) q24h + folinic acid 5 mg (PO) q24h indefinitely*
Antibiotic-associated diarrhea/colitis (C. difficile)	Metronidazole 500 mg (PO) q8h x 10-14 days. Avoid use of other antibacterials if possible	Vancomycin 125 mg (PO) q6h x 10-14 days

OTHER OPPORTUNISTIC INFECTIONS IN HIV

Infection	Preferred Therapy	Alternate Therapy
Disseminated M. avium complex (MAC)	Life-long therapy† with: Clarithromycin 500 mg (PO) q12h + ethambutol 15-25 mg/kg (PO) q24h (usually 800 or 1200 mg daily) + rifabutin 300 mg (PO) q24h. (See pulmonary TB [p. 248] for rifabutin dosing with antiretroviral therapy)	Preferred therapy **plus either** Amikacin 15 mg/kg (IV) q24h x 1-2 months **or** Levofloxacin 500 mg (PO) q24h indefinitely
Extrapulmonary TB (M. tuberculosis)	Treat the same as pulmonary TB (p. 248). May require longer duration of therapy based on clinical response	
Histoplasmosis, disseminated *Initial therapy*	Severe disease Amphotericin B deoxycholate 0.5-1 mg/kg (IV) x 7-14 days until able to take PO meds, then itraconazole 200 mg (PO) solution q12h x 12 weeks Mild disease Itraconazole 300 mg (PO) solution q12h x 3 days, then 200 mg (PO) solution q12h x 12 weeks	Fluconazole 800 mg (PO) q24h x 12 weeks

* Consider discontinuation of therapy if $CD_4 > 200$ for ≥ 6 months in response to antiretroviral therapy
† May discontinue if good response to ≥ 1 year of therapy plus $CD_4 > 100$ for ≥ 6 months

Table 8. Treatment of Opportunistic Infections (cont'd) (see comments, pp. 253-259)

OTHER OPPORTUNISTIC INFECTIONS IN HIV		
Infection	**Preferred Therapy**	**Alternate Therapy**
Histoplasmosis, disseminated *Maintenance therapy (all patients)*	Itraconazole 100 mg (PO) solution q12h indefinitely.** Give loading dose of 200 mg (IV) q12h x 2 days if treated initially with amphotericin B deoxycholate	Amphotericin B deoxycholate 1 mg/kg (IV) once a week indefinitely** **or** Fluconazole 800 mg (IV or PO) x 1 dose, then 400 mg (PO) q24h indefinitely**
Herpes simplex (genital/oral) *Mild infection*	Acyclovir 400 mg (PO) q8h x 7-10 days **or** Famciclovir 250 mg (PO) q8h x 7-10 days **or** Valacyclovir 1 gm (PO) q12h x 7-10 days	<u>Failure to respond</u> Famciclovir 500 mg (PO) q8h x 7 days **or** Valacyclovir 1 gm (PO) q8h x 7 days
Severe or refractory infection	Acyclovir 5 mg/kg (IV) q8h x 2-7 days. If improvement, switch to acyclovir 400 mg (PO) q8h to complete 7-10 days	<u>Acyclovir-resistant strain</u> Foscarnet 60 mg/kg (IV) q12h x 3 weeks
Frequent recurrences (≥ 6/year)	Acyclovir 400 mg (PO) q12h indefinitely*	Famciclovir 125-250 mg (PO) q12h indefinitely* **or** Valacyclovir 500 mg (PO) q12h or 1 gm (PO) q24h indefinitely*
Herpes zoster (VZV) *Localized*	Famciclovir 500 mg (PO) q8h x 7 days or until lesions crust **or** Valacyclovir 1 gm (PO) q8h x 7 days or until lesions crust **or** Acyclovir 800 mg (PO) 5x/day x 7 days or until lesions crust	Acyclovir 10 mg/kg (IV) q8h, with transition to oral therapy when clinical improvement is evident **or** Foscarnet 60 mg/kg (IV) q12, with transition to oral therapy when clinical improvement is evident
Disseminated, ophthalmic nerve or visceral involvement	Acyclovir 10-12 mg/kg (IV) q8h x 7 days or longer	Foscarnet 60 mg/kg (IV) q12h x 7 days or longer
Acyclovir-resistant strains	Foscarnet 60 mg/kg (IV) q12h x 7 days or longer	Not applicable

*   *Consider discontinuation of therapy if CD₄ > 200 for ≥6 months in response to antiretroviral therapy*
** *Consider discontinuation of therapy if CD₄ > 100 for ≥6 months in response to antiretroviral therapy*

Table 8. Treatment of Opportunistic Infections (cont'd) (see comments, pp. 253-259)

OTHER OPPORTUNISTIC INFECTIONS IN HIV		
Infection	Preferred Therapy	Alternate Therapy
CMV retinitis *Initial therapy*	<u>Initiate systemic CMV therapy pending ophthalmology consult</u> Valganciclovir 900 mg (PO) q12h x 3 weeks **or** Ganciclovir 5 mg/kg (IV) q12h x 3 weeks	<u>Initiate systemic CMV therapy pending ophthalmology consult</u> Foscarnet 60 mg/kg (IV) q8h or 90 mg/kg (IV) q12h x 3 weeks **or** Cidofovir 5 mg/kg (IV) once weekly x 2, then every 2 weeks. Give probenecid 2 gm (PO) 3 hours before and 1 gm (PO) 2 and 8 hours after cidofovir to preserve renal function
Maintenance therapy	Valganciclovir 900 mg (PO) q24h indefinitely[†] **plus** Intraocular ganciclovir release device (Vitrasert), if needed[‡]	<u>Vitrasert failure</u> Foscarnet 90 mg/kg (IV) q24h indefinitely[†]
Candida vaginitis *Initial infection*	Intravaginal miconazole suppository 200 mg q24h x 3 days or miconazole cream (2%) x 7 days **or** Fluconazole 150 mg (PO) x 1 dose (higher dose/longer course sometimes required)	Clotrimazole cream (1%) x 7 days or clotrimazole tablets 100 mg (PO) q24h x 7 days (or 100 mg q12h x 3 days, or 500 mg x 1 dose)
Frequent relapses	Fluconazole 100 mg (PO) q24h or 200 mg (PO) once weekly indefinitely.* Higher dose sometimes required	Not applicable

*   Consider discontinuation of therapy if $CD_4 > 200$ for ≥6 months in response to antiretroviral therapy
†   Consider discontinuation of therapy if $CD_4 > 100$-150 for ≥6 months in response to antiretroviral therapy, in consultation with ophthalmologist
‡   Intraocular ganciclovir insert is rarely needed if $CD_4 > 100$ in response to antiretroviral therapy

Pneumocystis carinii Pneumonia (PCP)

Clinical Presentation: Fever, cough, dyspnea; often indolent presentation. Physical exam is usually normal. Chest x-ray is variable, but commonly shows a diffuse interstitial pattern. Elevated LDH and exercise desaturation are highly suggestive of PCP

Diagnostic Considerations: Diagnosis by immunofluorescent stain of induced sputum or bronchoscopy specimen. Check ABG if O_2 saturation is abnormal or respiratory rate is increased

Pitfalls: Slight worsening of symptoms is common after starting therapy, especially if not treated with steroids. Do not overlook superimposed bacterial pneumonia or other secondary infections while on pentamidine. Patients receiving second-line agents for PCP prophylaxis—in particular aerosolized pentamidine—may present with atypical radiographic findings, including apical infiltrates, multiple small-walled cysts, pleural effusions, pneumothorax, or single/multiple nodules

Therapeutic Considerations: Outpatient therapy is possible for mild disease, but only when close follow-up is assured. Adverse reactions to TMP-SMX (rash, fever, GI symptoms, hepatitis, hyperkalemia, leukopenia, hemolytic anemia) occur in 25-50% of patients, many of whom will need a second-line regimen to complete therapy (e.g., trimethoprim-dapsone or atovaquone). Unless an adverse reaction to TMP-SMX is particularly severe (e.g., Stevens-Johnson syndrome or other life-threatening problem), TMP-SMX may be considered for PCP prophylaxis, since prophylaxis requires a much lower dose (only 10-15% of treatment dose). Patients being treated for severe PCP who do not improve after one week may be switched to pentamidine, although there are no prospective data to confirm this approach. In general, patients receiving antiretroviral therapy when PCP develops should have their treatment continued, since intermittent antiretroviral therapy can lead to drug resistance. For newly-diagnosed or antiretroviral-naive HIV patients, treatment of PCP may be completed before starting antiretroviral therapy. Steroids should be tapered (p. 248), not discontinued abruptly. Adjunctive steroids increase the risk of thrush/herpes simplex infection, but probably not CMV, TB, or disseminated fungal infection
Prognosis: Usually responds to treatment. Adverse prognostic factors include ↑ A-a gradient, hypoxemia, ↑ LDH

Bacterial Pneumonia (see p. 49)

Pulmonary Tuberculosis (TB) (Mycobacterium tuberculosis)
Clinical Presentation: May present atypically. HIV patients with high (> 500) CD_4 cell counts are more likely to have a typical pulmonary presentation, but patients with advanced HIV disease may have a diffuse interstitial pattern, hilar adenopathy, or a normal chest x-ray. Tuberculin skin testing (TST) is reliable if positive, but unreliable if negative
Diagnostic Considerations: In many urban areas, TB is one of the most common HIV-related respiratory illnesses. In other areas, HIV-related TB occurs infrequently except in immigrants or patients arriving from highly TB endemic areas. Maintain a high Index of suspicion for TB in HIV patients with unexplained fevers/pulmonary infiltrates
Pitfalls: Extrapulmonary and pulmonary TB often coexist, especially in advanced HIV disease
Therapeutic Considerations: Duration of therapy should be extended if response at end of 8-week induction is delayed (failure of sputum culture to convert to negative, lack of clinical response)
Prognosis: Usually responds to treatment. Relapse rates are related to the degree of immunosuppression and local risk of re-exposure to TB

Invasive Pulmonary Aspergillosis
Clinical Presentation: Pleuritic chest pain, hemoptysis, cough in a patient with advanced HIV disease
Diagnostic Considerations: Diagnosis by bronchoscopy with biopsy/culture. Open lung biopsy (usually video-assisted thorascopic surgery) is sometimes required. Radiographic appearance includes cavitation, nodules, sometimes focal consolidation. Dissemination to CNS may occur, and manifests as focal neurological deficits
Pitfalls: Positive sputum culture for Aspergillus in advanced HIV disease should heighten awareness of possible infection
Therapeutic Considerations: Decrease/discontinue corticosteroids, if possible. Consider granulocyte-colony stimulating factor (G-CSF) if neutropenic
Prognosis: Poor unless immune deficits can be corrected

Toxoplasma Encephalitis (Toxoplasma gondii)
Clinical Presentation: Wide spectrum of neurologic symptoms, including sensorimotor deficits, seizures, confusion, ataxia. Fever/headache are common
Diagnostic Considerations: Diagnosis by characteristic radiographic appearance and response to empiric therapy in a Toxoplasma seropositive patient
Pitfalls: Use folinic acid 10 mg (PO) daily with pyrimethamine-containing regimens, not folate. Radiographic improvement may lag behind clinical response

Therapeutic Considerations: Alternate agents include atovaquone, azithromycin, clarithromycin, minocycline (all with pyrimethamine if possible). Decadron 4 mg (PO or IV) q6h is useful for edema/mass effect

Prognosis: Usually responds to treatment if able to tolerate drugs. Clinical response is evident by 1 week in 70%, by 2 weeks in 90%. Radiographic improvement is usually apparent by 2 weeks. Neurologic recovery is variable

Cryptococcal Meningitis (Cryptococcus neoformans)

Clinical Presentation: Often indolent onset of fever, headache, subtle cognitive deficits. Occasional meningeal signs and focal neurologic findings, though non-specific presentation is most common

Diagnostic Considerations: Diagnosis by CSF cryptococcal antigen; India ink stain is less sensitive. Diagnosis is essentially excluded with a negative serum cryptococcal antigen (sensitivity of test in AIDS patients approaches 100%). If serum cryptococcal antigen is positive, CSF antigen may be negative in disseminated disease without spread to CNS/meninges. Brain imaging is often normal, but CSF analysis is usually abnormal with a markedly elevated opening pressure

Pitfalls: Be sure to obtain a CSF opening pressure, since reduction of increased intracranial pressure is mandatory for successful treatment. Remove sufficient CSF during the initial lumbar puncture (LP) to reduce closing pressure to < 200 mm H_2O or 50% of opening pressure. Increased intracranial pressure requires repeat daily LPs (until CSF pressure stabilizes), placement of a lumbar drain, or ventriculo-peritoneal shunting. Adjunctive corticosteroids are not recommended

Therapeutic Considerations: Optimal total dose/duration of amphotericin B deoxycholate prior to fluconazole switch is unknown (2-3 weeks is reasonable if patient is doing well). Treatment with 5-FC is optional; however, since 5-FC is associated with more rapid sterilization of CSF, it is reasonable to start 5-FC and then discontinue it for toxicity (neutropenia, nausea). Fluconazole is preferred over itraconazole for life-long maintenance therapy

Prognosis: Variable. Mortality up to 40%. Adverse prognostic factors include increased intracranial pressure, abnormal mental status

CMV Encephalitis/Polyradiculitis

Clinical Presentation: Encephalitis presents as fever, mental status changes, and headache evolving over 1-2 weeks. True meningismus is rare. CMV encephalitis occurs in advanced HIV disease (CD_4 < 50/mm³), often in patients with prior CMV retinitis. Polyradiculitis presents as rapidly evolving weakness/sensory disturbances in the lower extremities, often with bladder/bowel incontinence. Anesthesia in "saddle distribution" with reduced sphincter tone may be present

Diagnostic Considerations: CSF may show lymphocytic or neutrophilic pleocytosis; glucose is often decreased. For CMV encephalitis, characteristic findings on brain MRI include confluent periventricular abnormalities with variable degrees of enhancement. Diagnosis is confirmed by CSF CMV PCR (preferred), CMV culture, or brain biopsy

Pitfalls: For CMV encephalitis, a wide spectrum of radiographic findings are possible, including mass lesions (rare). Obtain ophthalmologic evaluation to exclude active retinitis. For polyradiculitis, obtain sagittal MRI of the spinal cord to exclude mass lesions, and CSF cytology to exclude lymphomatous involvement (can cause similar symptoms)

Therapeutic Considerations: Ganciclovir plus foscarnet may be beneficial as initial therapy for severe cases. Consider discontinuation of valganciclovir maintenance therapy if CD_4 increases to > 100-150/mm³ x 6 months or longer in response to antiretroviral therapy

Prognosis: Unless immune reconstitution occurs, response to therapy is usually transient, followed by progression of symptoms

Progressive Multifocal Leukoencephalopathy (PML)

Clinical Presentation: Hemiparesis, ataxia, aphasia, other focal neurologic defects, which may progress over weeks to months. Usually alert without headache or seizures on presentation

Diagnostic Considerations: Demyelinating disease caused by reactivation of latent papovavirus (JC strain most common). Diagnosis by clinical presentation and MRI showing patchy demyelination of white matter ± cerebellum/brainstem. JC virus PCR of CSF is useful for non-invasive diagnosis. Biopsy may be needed to distinguish PML from other opportunistic infections or CNS lymphoma. Affects ~ 1-3% of AIDS patients

Pitfalls: Primary HIV-related encephalopathy has a similar appearance on MRI

Therapeutic Considerations: Most effective therapy is antiretroviral therapy with immune reconstitution. May attempt cidofovir (placebo-controlled trial showed no benefit)

Prognosis: Rapid progression to death over weeks to months is common. Best chance for survival is immune reconstitution in response to antiretroviral therapy

Oral Thrush (Candida)

Clinical Presentation: Dysphagia/odynophagia. More common/severe in advanced HIV disease

Diagnostic Considerations: Pseudomembranous (most common), erythematous, and hyperplastic (leukoplakia) forms. Pseudomembranes (white plaques on inflamed base) on buccal muscosa/tongue/gingiva/palate scrape off easily, hyperplastic lesions do not. Diagnosis by clinical appearance ± KOH/gram stain of scraping showing yeast/pseudomycelia. Other oral lesions in AIDS patients include herpes simplex, aphthous ulcers, Kaposi's sarcoma, oral hairy leukoplakia

Pitfalls: Patients may be asymptomatic

Therapeutic Considerations: Fluconazole is superior to topical therapy in preventing relapses of thrush and treating Candida esophagitis. Continuous treatment with fluconazole may lead to fluconazole-resistance, which is best treated initially with itraconazole suspension and, if no response, with IV caspofungin or amphotericin. Chronic suppressive therapy is usually only considered for severely immunosuppressed patients

Prognosis: Improvement in symptoms are often seen within 24-48 hours

Candida Esophagitis

Clinical Presentation: Dysphagia/odynophagia, almost always in the setting of oropharyngeal thrush. Fever is uncommon

Diagnostic Considerations: Most common cause of esophagitis in HIV disease. For persistent symptoms despite therapy, endoscopy with biopsy/culture is recommended to confirm diagnosis and assess azole-resistance. Other causes of esophagitis include CMV, herpes simplex, aphthous ulcers

Pitfalls: May extend into stomach. Kaposi's sarcoma, non-Hodgkin's lymphoma, zidovudine, dideoxycytidine, and other infections may cause esophageal symptoms

Therapeutic Considerations: Systemic therapy is preferred over topical therapy. Failure to improve on empiric therapy mandates endoscopy to look for other causes, especially herpes viruses/aphthous ulcers. Consider maintenance therapy with fluconazole for frequent relapses, although the risk of fluconazole resistance is increased. Continuous treatment with fluconazole may lead to fluconazole-resistance, which is best treated initially with itraconazole suspension and, if no response, with IV caspofungin or amphotericin

Prognosis: Relapse rate related to degree of immunosuppression

CMV Esophagitis/Colitis

Clinical Presentation: Localizing symptoms, including odynophagia, abdominal pain, diarrhea, sometimes bloody stools

Diagnostic Considerations: Diagnosis by finding CMV inclusions on biopsy. CMV can affect the entire GI tract, resulting in oral/esophageal ulcers, gastritis, and colitis (most common). CMV colitis varies greatly in severity, but typically causes fever, abdominal cramping, and sometimes bloody stools

Pitfalls: CMV colitis may cause colonic perforation and should be considered in any AIDS patient presenting with an acute abdomen, especially if radiography demonstrates free intraperitoneal air

Therapeutic Considerations: Consider chronic suppressive therapy for recurrent disease. Screen for CMV retinitis

Prognosis: Relapse rate is greatly reduced with immune reconstitution due to antiretroviral therapy

Salmonella Enteritis
Clinical Presentation: Patients with HIV are at markedly increased risk of developing salmonellosis. Three different presentations may be seen: (1) self-limited gastroenteritis, as typically seen in immunocompetent hosts; (2) a more severe and prolonged diarrheal disease, associated with fever, bloody diarrhea, and weight loss; or (3) Salmonella septicemia, which may present with or without gastrointestinal symptoms
Diagnostic Considerations: The diagnosis is established through cultures of stool and blood. Given the high rate of bacteremia associated with Salmonella gastroenteritis–especially in advanced HIV disease–blood cultures should be obtained in any HIV patient presenting with diarrhea and fever
Pitfalls: A distinctive feature of salmonella bacteremia in patients with AIDS is its propensity for relapse (rate > 20%)
Therapeutic Considerations: The mainstay of treatment is a fluoroquinolone (greatest experience with ciprofloxacin). For uncomplicated salmonellosis in an HIV patient with CD_4 cell counts > 200, 1-2 weeks of treatment is reasonable to reduce extraintestinal spread. For patients with advanced HIV disease (CD_4 < 200) or who have salmonella bacteremia, at least 4-6 weeks of treatment is required. Chronic suppressive therapy, given for several months or until antiretroviral therapy-induced immune reconstitution ensues, is indicated for patients who relapse after cessation of therapy
Prognosis: Usually responds well to treatment

Cryptosporidia Enteritis
Clinical Presentation: High-volume watery diarrhea with weight loss and electrolyte disturbances, especially in advanced HIV disease
Diagnostic Considerations: Spore-forming protozoa. Diagnosis by AFB smear of stool demonstrating characteristic oocyte. Malabsorption may occur
Pitfalls: No fecal leukocytes
Therapeutic Considerations: Anecdotal reports of antimicrobial success. Newest agent nitazoximide may be effective in some settings. Immune reconstitution in response to antiretroviral therapy is the most effective therapy, and may induce prolonged remissions. Anti-diarrheal agents (Lomotil, Pepto-Bismol) are useful to control symptoms. Hyperalimentation may be required for severe cases
Prognosis: Related to degree of immunosuppression/response to antiretroviral therapy

Microsporidia Enteritis
Clinical Presentation: Intermittent chronic diarrhea without fever/fecal leukocytes
Diagnostic Considerations: Spore-forming protozoa (S. intestinalis, E. bieneusi). Diagnosis by modified trichrome or fluorescent antibody stain of stool. Microsporidia can rarely disseminate to sinuses/cornea. Severe malabsorption may occur
Pitfalls: Cannot be detected by routine microscopic examination of stool due to small size
Therapeutic Considerations: Albendazole is less effective for E. bieneusi than S. intestinalis, but speciation is usually not possible
Prognosis: Related to degree of immunosuppression/response to antiretroviral therapy

Isospora Enteritis
Clinical Presentation: Severe chronic diarrhea without fever/fecal leukocytes
Diagnostic Considerations: Spore-forming protozoa (Isospora belli). Oocyst on AFB smear of stool larger that Cryptosporidium (20-30 microns vs. 4-6 microns). More common in HIV patients from the Tropics (e.g., Haiti). Less common than Cryptosporidium or Microsporidia. Malabsorption may occur
Pitfalls: Multiple relapses are possible
Therapeutic Considerations: Chronic suppressive therapy may be required
Prognosis: Related to degree of immunosuppression/response to antiretroviral therapy

Antibiotic-Associated Diarrhea/Colitis (Clostridium difficile) (see p. 68)

Disseminated Mycobacterium avium-complex (MAC)

Clinical Presentation: Typically presents as a febrile wasting illness in advanced HIV disease ($CD_4 < 50/mm^3$). Focal invasive disease is possible, especially in patients with advanced immunosuppression after starting antiretroviral therapy. Focal disease likely reflects restoration of pathogen-specific immune response to subclinical infection ("immune reconstitution" syndrome), and typically manifests as lymphadenitis (mesenteric, cervical, thoracic) or rarely disease in the spine mimicking Pott's disease. Immune reconstitution syndrome usually occurs within weeks to months after starting antiretroviral therapy for the first time, but may occur a year or more later

Diagnostic Considerations: Diagnosis by isolation of organism from a normally sterile body site (blood, lymph node, bone marrow, liver biopsy). Lysis centrifugation (DuPont isolators) is the preferred blood culture method. Anemia/↑ alkaline phosphatase are occasionally seen

Pitfalls: Isolator blood cultures may be negative, especially in immune reconstitution syndrome

Therapeutic Considerations: Some studies suggest benefit for addition of rifabutin 300 mg (PO) q24h, others do not. Rifabutin is contraindicated in patients receiving delavirdine or hard-gel saquinavir. For concurrent use with nelfinavir, indinavir, or amprenavir, decrease rifabutin to 150 mg (PO) q24h. For concurrent use with ritonavir, decrease rifabutin to 150 mg (PO) 2-3x/week. For concurrent use with efavirenz, increase rifabutin to 450-600 mg (PO) q24h. The dose of PIs or NNRTIs may need to be increased by 20-25%. Monitor carefully for rifabutin drug toxicity (arthralgias, uveitis, leukopenia). Treat immune reconstitution syndrome the same as for disseminated MAC; corticosteroids may be necessary to control fevers. Optimal long-term management is unknown

Prognosis: Depends on immune reconstitution in response to antiretroviral therapy. Adverse prognostic factors include high-grade bacteremia or severe wasting

Extrapulmonary Tuberculosis

Clinical Presentation: Multiple presentations possible (e.g., lymphadenitis, osteomyelitis, meningitis, hepatitis). Dissemination is more common in patients with low CD_4 counts ($< 100/mm^3$)

Diagnostic Considerations: Diagnosis by isolator blood cultures or tissue biopsy

Pitfalls: Patients with disseminated disease frequently have pulmonary disease, which has implications for infection control

Therapeutic Considerations: Response to therapy may be slower than in normal hosts

Prognosis: Usually responsive to therapy

Non-meningeal Cryptococcus (see index for site-specific disease)

Disseminated Histoplasmosis

Clinical Presentation: Two general forms: Mild disease with fever/lymph node enlargement (e.g., cervical adenitis), or severe disease with fever, wasting ± diarrhea/meningitis/GI ulcerations

Diagnostic Considerations: Diagnosis by urine/serum histoplasmosis antigen, sometimes by culture of bone marrow/liver or isolator blood cultures. May occur in patients months to years after having lived/moved from an endemic area

Pitfalls: Relapse is common after discontinuation of therapy; cultures may take 7-21 days to turn (+)

Therapeutic Considerations: Initial therapy depends on severity of illness on presentation. Extremely sick patients should be started on amphotericin B deoxycholate. Mildly ill patients can be started on itraconazole. All patients require chronic suppressive therapy, with possible discontinuation for immune reconstitution with CD_4 counts $> 100/mm^3$ for at least 6 months

Prognosis: Usually responds to treatment, except in fulminant cases

Herpes Simplex (genital/oral)

Clinical Presentation: Painful, grouped vesicles on an erythematous base that rupture, crust, and heal within 2 weeks. Lesions may be chronic, severe, ulcerative with advanced immunosuppression

Diagnostic Considerations: Diagnosis by Herpes culture of swab from lesion base/roof of blister

Pitfalls: Acyclovir prophylaxis is not required in patients receiving ganciclovir or foscarnet

Therapeutic Considerations: In refractory cases, consider acyclovir resistance and treat with foscarnet. Topical trifluridine ophthalmic solution (Viroptic 1%) may be considered for direct application to small, localized areas of refractory disease; clean with hydrogen peroxide, then debride lightly with gauze, apply trifluridine, and cover with bacitracin/polymyxin ointment and nonadsorbent gauze; topical cidofovir (requires compounding) also may be tried

Prognosis: Responds well to treatment except in severely immunocompromised patients, in whom acyclovir resistance may develop

Herpes Zoster (Varicella-Zoster Virus, VZV)

Clinical Presentation: Primary varicella (chickenpox) presents as clear vesicles on an erythematous base that heal with crusting and sometimes scarring. Zoster usually presents as painful tense vesicles on an erythematous base in a dermatomal distribution. In AIDS, primary varicella is more severe/prolonged, and zoster is more likely to involve multiple dermatomes/disseminate

Diagnostic Considerations: Diagnosis is clinical. Immunofluorescence can be used to distinguish herpes zoster from herpes simplex

Pitfalls: Extend duration of therapy for slowly responsive lesions

Therapeutic Considerations: IV therapy is generally indicated for severe disease/cranial nerve zoster

Prognosis: Usually responds slowly to treatment

CMV Retinitis

Clinical Presentation: Blurred vision, scotomata, field cuts common. Often bilateral, even when initial symptoms are unilateral

Diagnostic Considerations: Diagnosis by characteristic hemorrhagic ("tomato soup and milk") retinitis on funduscopic exam. Consult ophthalmology in suspected cases

Pitfalls: May develop immune reconstitution vitreitis after starting antiretroviral therapy

Therapeutic Considerations: Oral valganciclovir is now an option for initial therapy and maintenance. Life-long maintenance therapy for CMV retinitis is required for CD_4 counts < 100, but may be discontinued if CD_4 counts increase to > 100-150 for 6 or more months in response to antiretroviral therapy (in consultation with ophthalmologist)

Prognosis: Good initial response to therapy. High relapse rate

Candida Vaginitis

Clinical Presentation: White, cheesy, vaginal discharge or vulvar rash ± itching/pain

Diagnostic Considerations: Local infection. Not a manifestation of disseminated disease

Pitfalls: Women with advanced AIDS receiving fluconazole may develop fluconazole-resistant Candida

Therapeutic Considerations: For recurrence, consider maintenance with daily or weekly fluconazole

Prognosis: Good response to therapy. Relapses common

FEVER OF UNKNOWN ORIGIN (FUO)

A. **Differential Diagnosis.** Fever without localizing symptoms or signs is common in HIV disease. Infectious causes of fever in patients with CD_4 cell counts > 500/mm^3 are similar to immunocompetent hosts. With CD_4 cell counts of 200-500/mm^3, the most common causes of fever include respiratory bacterial infections (especially S pneumoniae, H. influenzae), TB, and complications of IV drug use. Patients with advanced HIV disease can have any cause of fever listed in Table 9, including typical opportunistic infections and non-infectious causes, such as neoplasm (especially non-Hodgkin's lymphoma) or drug fever. Common causes of drug fever include sulfonamides, dapsone, beta-lactams, phenytoin, carbamazepine, thalidomide, and pentamidine. NNRTIs such as nevirapine, delavirdine, and efavirenz can also cause fevers ± rash. Abacavir hypersensitivity reactions occur in ~ 3%, and are usually associated with fever and multisystem complaints (GI disturbances, rash, respiratory symptoms); rechallenge is contraindicated (can be fatal).

B. Key Historical Features. Level of immunosuppression; travel/residence history; medication history (new agents, prophylaxis); need for central venous access; intravenous drug use; prior opportunistic infections.

C. Diagnostic Approach. Begin with non-invasive tests and become more invasive if fevers persist, weight loss is evident, or the illness appears to be progressing. Physical examination/labs should focus on possible clues suggesting a diagnosis, including skin rashes (disseminated fungal infections; Cryptococcus may cause a molluscum-like rash), oral ulcerations (histoplasmosis, CMV), new or regional lymphadenopathy (lymphoma, immune reconstitution MAC), retinal lesions (CMV), hepatosplenomegaly (histoplasmosis, MAC, disseminated Pneumocystis carinii), new cytopenias (bone marrow infiltrative process), ↑ LDH (lymphoma, Pneumocystis carinii), ↑ alkaline phosphatase (liver infiltrative process), hilar adenopathy on chest x-ray (histoplasmosis, TB, lymphoma). Abdominal CT scan often shows mesenteric adenopathy in MAC disease, and chest CT may show faint infiltrates of early PCP not evident on plain films. Routine blood cultures are useful for detecting endocarditis, Salmonella bacteremia, or line infections, and isolator blood cultures are useful for detecting disseminated MAC, other mycobacterium, or histoplasmosis. Serum cryptococcal antigen, urine histoplasmosis antigen, and CMV antigenemia studies may be appropriate. Yields from liver/bone marrow biopsy range from 20-80%. In general, ↑ alkaline phosphatase increases the likelihood of a diagnostic liver biopsy.

Table 9. Causes of Pulmonary, CNS, Diarrheal Disease and FUO in HIV Disease

	Very Common	Somewhat Common	Rare
Respiratory disease	PCP, S. pneumoniae, H. influenzae, M. tuberculosis[†]	Enteric gram (−) rods, H. capsulatum, C. neoformans, CMV, Aspergillus, pulmonary lymphoma, heart failure, Kaposi's sarcoma	N. asteroides, Legionella spp., MAC, T. gondii, Cryptosporidia, R. equii, primary pulmonary hypertension
CNS disease	C. neoformans, T. gondii*, drug reactions, psychiatric illness, HIV, PML*, CNS lymphoma*	M. tuberculosis[†], CMV, bacterial brain abscess*	N. asteroides*, H. capsulatum, C. immitis, Aspergillus sp.*, L. monocytogenes, VZV, HSV* , T. pallidum, Acanthamoeba*, T. cruzi
Diarrheal disease	CMV, C. difficile, Salmonella, MAC, Giardia, protease inhibitors	Shigella, Campylobacter, Microsporidia, Cryptosporidia, Isospora, Cyclospora	Amebiasis, S. stercoralis GI lymphoma, Kaposi's sarcoma, entero-aggregative E. coli
Fever of unknown origin (FUO)	MAC, M. tuberculosis[†], CMV, drug fever, sinusitis, central line infection, early PCP, HIV	C. neoformans, H. capsulatum, endocarditis, lymphoma	Extrapulmonary PCP, B. henselae, C. immitis, M. kansasii, P. marneffei, Leishmania sp., T. gondii

† Incidence dependent on local rates of TB;   * Generally characterized by focal lesions on MRI/CT

POST-EXPOSURE PROPHYLAXIS (PEP)

The CDC estimates > 600,000 significant exposures to blood-borne pathogens occur yearly. Of 56 confirmed cases of HIV acquisition in healthcare workers, more than 90% involved percutaneous exposure, with the remaining cases due to mucous membrane/skin exposure. Estimates of HIV seroconversion rates after percutaneous and mucous membrane exposure to HIV-infected blood are 0.3% and 0.09%, respectively; lower rates of transmission occur after nonintact skin exposure. (By comparison, the risks of seroconversion after percutaneous exposure to Hepatitis B and Hepatitis C viruses are 30% and 3%, respectively.) Risk factors for increased risk of HIV transmission after percutaneous exposure include deep injury (odds ratio 16.1), visible blood on device (odds ratio 5.2), source patient is terminally ill (odds ratio 6.4), or needle was in source patient's artery/vein (odds ratio 5.1); AZT prophylaxis reduces the risk of transmission (OR 0.2). All guidelines suggest PEP should be administered as soon as possible after exposure, but there is no absolute window (e.g., within 1-2 weeks) after which PEP should be withheld following serious exposure. Because clear-cut efficacy data for patient selection and PEP regimens are lacking, most experts rely on CDC guidelines, which emphasize the type of exposure and potential infectivity of the source patient (Tables 10, 11). There are no formal guidelines for non-occupational PEP, but it is reasonable to consider PEP for serious exposures (e.g., rape victims, shared needle use, HIV-infected partner and broken condom). The latest U.S. Public Health Service (USPHS) guidelines for the management of occupational exposure to HIV and postexposure prophylaxis are summarized below and are detailed in Morbidity Mortality Weekly Review 50(RR11):1-52, June 29, 2001, or at www.cdc.gov/mmwr/preview/mmwrhtml/rr5011a1.htm. Other occupational exposure resources include the National Clinicians' Postexposure Prophylaxis Hotline (www.ucsf.edu/hivcntr), Needlestick! (www.needlestick.mednet.ucla,edu), and HIV Antiretroviral Pregnancy Registry (www.glaxowellcome.com/preg[underscore]reg/antiretroviral). Occupationally acquired HIV infections and PEP failures can be reported to the CDC at (800) 893-0485.

Recommendations from the updated 2001 USPHS guidelines include:
*   Initiate PEP as soon as possible after exposure (preferably within hours), and continue PEP for 4 weeks if tolerated (Tables 10, 11)
*   Seek expert consultation if viral resistance is suspected
*   Offer pregnancy testing to all women of childbearing age not known to be pregnant
*   Advise exposed persons to seek medical evaluation for any acute illness during follow-up
*   Perform HIV-antibody testing and HIV RNA testing for any illness compatible with an acute retroviral syndrome (e.g., pharyngitis, fever, rash, myalgia, fatigue, malaise, lymphadenopathy)
*   Perform HIV-antibody testing for at least 6 months postexposure (at baseline, 6 weeks, 3 months, and 6 months)
*   Advise exposed persons to use precautions to prevent secondary transmission during follow-up, especially during the first 6-12 weeks, when most HIV-infected patients will seroconvert. Precautions include sexual abstinence or use of condoms, refrain from

donating blood, plasma, organs, tissue or semen, and discontinuation of breast-feeding after high-risk exposures
• Evaluate exposed persons taking PEP within 72 hours after exposure, and monitor for drug toxicity for at least 2 weeks. Approximately 50% will experience nausea, malaise, headache, or anorexia, and about one-third will discontinue PEP due to drug toxicity. Lab monitoring should include (at a minimum) a CBC, serum creatinine, liver function tests, serum glucose (if receiving a protease inhibitor to detect hyperglycemia), and monitoring for crystalluria, hematuria, hemolytic anemia, and hepatitis (if indinavir is prescribed). Serious adverse events should be reported to the FDA's MedWatch Program

Table 10. Recommendations for HIV Postexposure Prophylaxis
(see Table 11 for basic and expanded PEP regimens)

Exposure Type	Infection Status of Source Patient				
	HIV (+) Class 1*	HIV (+) Class 2*	HIV status unknown[†]	Unknown source[††]	HIV (−)
Percutaneous injuries *Less severe*[+]	Recommend basic 2-drug PEP	Recommend expanded 3-drug PEP	Generally no PEP warranted; consider basic 2-drug PEP[†††] for source with HIV risk factors**	Generally no PEP warranted; consider basic 2-drug PEP[†††] if exposure to HIV-infected persons is likely	No PEP warranted
More severe[+]	Recommend expanded 3-drug PEP	Recommend expanded 3-drug PEP			
Mucous membrane/ nonintact skin exposure *Small volume*[++]	Consider basic 2-drug PEP	Recommend basic 2-drug PEP			
Large volume[++]	Recommend expanded 3-drug PEP	Recommend expanded 3-drug PEP			

HIV (+) = HIV-positive, HIV (−) = HIV-negative, PEP = postexposure prophylaxis
*   Class 1: Asymptomatic HIV infection or known low HIV RNA (e.g., < 1500 RNA copies/mL)
     Class 2: Symptomatic HIV infection, AIDS, acute seroconversion, or known high HIV RNA. If drug resistance is a concern, obtain expert consultation; do not delay PEP pending consultation
**   Source with HIV risk factors: If PEP is administered and the source patient is later determined to be HIV-negative, PEP should be discontinued
†   HIV status unknown: for example, source patient is deceased with no samples available for HIV testing
††   Unknown source: for example, a needle from a sharps disposal container (percutaneous injury), or a splash from inappropriately disposed blood (mucous membrane/nonintact skin exposure)
††† PEP is optional; discuss with patient and individualize decision
+   Less severe: for example, a solid needle and superficial injury. More severe: for example, a large-bore hollow needle, deep puncture, visible blood on device, or needle used in patient's artery/vein
++   Small volume: a few drops. Large volume: major blood splash
From: Updated U.S. Public Health Service Guidelines for the Management of Occupational Exposures to HBV, HCV, and HIV and Recommendations for Postexposure Prophylaxis, MMWR, 50 (RR11) June 29, 2001 (www.cdc.gov/mmwr/preview/mmwrhtml/rr5011a1.htm)

**Table 11. Basic and Expanded HIV Postexposure Prophylaxis Regimens
(see Table 10 for patient selection guidelines)**

Regimen	Dosage	Comments
Basic regimen *Preferred*	Combivir (zidovudine 300 mg + lamivudine 150 mg) 1 tablet (PO) q12h x 4 weeks	Most experience; serious toxicity rare; side effects common but usually manageable with antimotility/antiemetic agents; probably safe during pregnancy; source patient virus may be resistant
Alternate	Lamivudine 150 mg (PO) q12h + stavudine 40 mg (PO) q12h* x 4 weeks	Well-tolerated; good adherence; serious toxicity rare; source patient virus may be resistant
	Didanosine 400 mg (PO) q24h** on empty stomach + stavudine 40 mg (PO) q12h* x 4 weeks	Likely to be effective against HIV strains from source patients taking zidovudine and lamivudine; serious toxicity may occur (e.g., neuropathy, pancreatitis, hepatitis); careful monitoring required; side effects common (anticipate diarrhea and low adherence)
Expanded regimen *(basic regimen plus one of the following drugs)*	Indinavir 800 mg (PO) q8h on empty stomach x 4 weeks	Potent HIV inhibitor; serious toxicity may occur (e.g., nephrolithiasis); 8 glasses of fluid required per day; hyperbilirubinemia is common; avoid during late pregnancy; cannot be co-administered with didanosine in chewable/dispersible buffered tablet formulation (doses must be separated by at least 1 hour); many drug interactions possible
	Nelfinavir 750 mg (PO) q8h or 1250 mg (PO) q12h with food x 4 weeks	Potent HIV inhibitor; may accelerate clearance of certain drugs, including oral contraceptives; many drug interactions possible
	Efavirenz 600 mg (PO) q24h at bedtime x 4 weeks	Once daily dosing may improve adherence; may cause severe rash with rare progression to Stevens-Johnson syndrome; CNS side effects common (e.g., dizziness, somnolence, insomnia, abnormal dreaming); severe psychiatric symptoms possible; avoid during pregnancy; many drug interactions possible
	Abacavir 300 mg (PO) q12h x 4 weeks	Potent HIV inhibitor; well-tolerated; severe hypersensitivity reactions may occur; available as combination tablet (Trizivir = abacavir 300 mg + lamivudine 150 mg + zidovudine 300 mg)
For PEP only with expert consultation	Ritonavir, saquinavir, amprenavir, delavirdine, lopinavir + ritonavir, atazanavir, fosamprenavir	Many drug interactions

*   If < 60 kg, give 30 mg (PO) q12h
** If < 60 kg, give 125 mg (PO) q12h
Adapted from: U.S. Public Health Service Guidelines. MMWR 50(RR11):47-52, June 29, 2001,
www.cdc..gov/mmwr/preview/mmwrhtml/rr5011a4.htm

REFERENCES AND SUGGESTED READINGS

Albrecht MA, Bosch RJ, Hammer SM, et al. Nelfinavir, efavirenz, or both after the failure of nucleoside treatment of HIV infection. N Engl J Med 345:398-407, 2001.

Ammassari A, Scoppettuolo G, Murri R, et al. Changing disease patterns in focal brain lesion-causing disorders in AIDS. J Acquir Immune Defic Syndr Hum Retroviral 18:365, 1998.

Antinori A, Giancola MI, Griserri S, et al. Factors influencing virological response to antiretroviral drugs in cerebrospinal fluid of advanced HIV-1-infected patients. AIDS 16:1867-76, 2002.

Armstrong WS, Katz JT, Kazanjian PH. Human immunodeficiency virus-associated fever of unknown origin: a study of 70 patients in the United States and review. Clin Infect Dis 28:341, 1999.

Barbut F, Meynard JL, Guiguet M, et al. Clostridium difficile-associated diarrhea in HIV-infected patients: epidemiology and risk factors. J Acquir Immune Defic Syndr Hum Retroviral 16:176, 1997.

Barreiro P, Soriano V, Blanco F, et al. Risks and benefits of replacing protease inhibitors by nevirapine in HIV-infected subjects under long-term successful triple combination therapy. AIDS 14:807-812, 2000.

Bartlett JG. Pneumonia in the patient with HIV infection. Infect Dis Clin North Am 12:807, 1998.

Bayard PJ, Berger TG, Jacobson MA. Drug hypersensitivity reactions and human immunodeficiency virus disease. J Acquir Immune Defic Syndr 5:1237, 1992.

Benson CA, Deeks SG, Brun SC, et al. Safety and antiviral activity at 48 weeks of lopinavir/ritonavir plus nevirapine and 2 nucleoside reverse-transcriptase inhibitors in human immunodeficiency virus type 1-infected protease inhibitor-experienced patients. J Infect Dis 185:599-607, 2002.

Berasconi E, Boubaker K, Junghans C, et al. Abnormalities of body fat distribution in HIV-infected persons treated with antiretroviral drugs: The Swiss HIV Cohort Study. J Acquir Immune Defic Syndr 31:50-5, 2002.

Borck C. Garlic supplements and saquinavir. Clin Infect Dis 35:343, 2002.

Bozzette SA, Sattler FR, Chiu J, et al. A controlled trial of early adjunctive treatment with corticosteroids for Pneumocystis carinii pneumonia in the acquired immunodeficiency syndrome. California Collaborative Treatment Group. N Engl J Med 323:1451, 1990.

Bozzette SA, Finkelstein DM, Spector SA, et al. A randomized trial of three antipneumocystis agents in patients with advanced human immunodeficiency virus infection. NIAID AIDS Clinical Trials Group. N Engl J Med 332:693, 1995.

Brosgart CL, Louis TA, Hillman DW, et al. A randomized, placebo-controlled trial of the safety and efficacy of oral ganciclovir for prophylaxis of cytomegalovirus disease in HIV-infected individuals. AIDS 12:269-77, 1998.

Cardiello PF, van Heeswijk RP, Hassink EA, et al. Simplifying protease inhibitor therapy with once-daily dosing of saquinavir soft-gelatin capsules/ritonavir (1600/100 mg): HIVNAT 001.3 study. J Acquir Immune Defic Syndr 29:464-70, 2002.

Carr A, Workman C, Smith DE, et al. Abacavir substitution for nucleoside analogs in patients with HIV lipotropin. A randomized trial. JAMA 288:207-15, 2002.

Carr A, Marriott D, Field A, et al. Treatment of HIV-1-associated microsporidiosis and cryptosporidiosis with combination antiretroviral therapy. Lancet 351:256, 1998.

Carr A, Samara K, Thorisdottir A, et al. Diagnosis, prediction, and natural course of HIV-1 protease-inhibitor associated lipodystrophy, hyperlipidaemia, and diabetes mellitus: a cohort study. Lancet 353:2093-2099, 1999.

Cascade Collaboration. Determinants of survival following HIV-1 seroconversion after the introduction of HAART. Lancet 362:1267-74, 2003.

Centers for Disease Control and Prevention. Notice to Readers: Updated guidelines for the use of rifabutin or rifampin for the treatment and prevention of tuberculosis among HIV-infected patients taking protease inhibitors or nonnucleoside reverse transcriptase inhibitors. MMWR 49:183-9, 2000.

Centers for Disease Control and Prevention. 1993 revised classification system for HIV infection and expanded surveillance case definition for AIDS among adolescents and adults. MMWR 41:1-19, 1992.

Chaisson RE, Keruly JC, Moore RD. Association of initial CD4 cell count and viral load with response to highly active antiretroviral therapy. J Am Med Assoc 284:3128-3129, 2000.

Cinque P, Scarpellini P, Vago L, et al. Diagnosis of central nervous system complications in HIV-infected patients: cerebrospinal fluid analysis by the polymerase chain reaction [editorial]. Aids 11:1, 1997.

Clotet B, Ruiz L, Martinez-Picado J, et al. Prevalence of HIV protease mutations on failure of nelfinavir-containing HAART: a retrospective analysis of four clinical studies and two observational cohorts. HIV Clin Trials 3:316-23, 2002.

Cohen C, Hunt S, Sension M, et al. Phenotypic resistance testing significantly improves response to therapy: A randomized trial (VIRA3001). In: 7th Conference on Retrovirus and Opportunistic Infections. San Francisco: Abstract 237, 2000.

Cohn JA, McMeeking A, Cohen W, et al. Evaluation of the policy of empiric treatment of suspected Toxoplasma encephalitis in patients with the acquired immunodeficiency syndrome. Am J Med 86:521, 1989.

Colson AE and Sax PE. Primary HIV-1 infection. In: UpToDate in Medicine (a CD-ROM textbook) 1998. Revised October, 1999.

Cunha BA. Community-acquired pneumonia in HIV patients. Clinical Infectious Diseases 28:410, 1999.

Cunha BA. Fever of unknown origin in HIV/AIDS patients. Drugs for Today 35:429, 1999.

Cunha BA. Community-acquired pneumonia in patients with HIV. Drugs for Today 31:739, 1998.

Currier JS, Williams PL, Koletar SL, et al. Discontinuation of Mycobacterium avium complex prophylaxis in patients with antiretroviral therapy-induced increases in CD4+ cell count. A randomized, double-blind, placebo-controlled trial. AIDS Clinical Trials Group 362 Study Team. Ann Intern Med 133:493, 2000.

Deeks SG, Barbour JD, Martin JN, et al. Sustained CD4+ T cell response after virologic failure of protease inhibitor-based regimens in patients with human immunodeficiency virus infection. J Infect Dis 181:946, 2000.

Deeks SG. Treatment of antiretroviral-drug-resistant HIV-1 infection. Lancet 362:2002-11, 2003.

DeSimone JA, Pomerantz RJ, Babinchak TJ. Inflammatory reactions in HIV-1-infected persons after initiation of highly active antiretroviral therapy. Ann Intern Med 133:447, 2000.

Detels R, Munoz A, McFarlane G, et al. Effectiveness of potent antiretroviral therapy on time to AIDS and death in men with known HIV infection duration. Multicenter AIDS Cohort Study Investigators. JAMA 280:1497, 1998.

Dietrich CG, Geier A, Matern S, Gartung C. Multidrug resistance and response to antiretroviral treatment. Lancet 359:2114, 2002.

Dube MP, Stein JH, Aberg JA. Guidelines for the evaluation and management of dyslipidemia in human immunodeficiency virus (HIV)-infected adults receiving antiretroviral therapy: recommendations of the HIV Medical Association of the Infectious Disease Society of America and the Adult AIDS Clinical Trials Group. Clin Infect Dis 37:613-27, 2003.

Durat J, Clevenbergh P, Halfon P, et al. Drug-resistance genotyping in HIV-1 therapy: the VIRADAPT randomized controlled trial. Lancet 353:2195-2199, 1999.

Egger M, May M, Chene G, et al. Prognosis of HIV-1-infected patients starting highly active antiretroviral therapy: a collaborative analysis of prospective studies. Lancet 360:119-29, 2002.

El-Sadr WM, Burman WJ, Grant LB, et al. Discontinuation of prophylaxis for mycobacterium avium complex disease in HIV-infected patients who have a response to antiretroviral therapy. N Engl J Med 342:1085-95, 2000.

Ensing G. Cardiac complications with vertically transmitted HIV infection. Lancet 360:350-1, 2002.

Epstein BJ, Little SJ, Richman DD. Drug resistance among patients recently infected with HIV. N Engl J Med 347:1889-90, 2002.

FDA notifications. FDA changes information for stavudine label. Aids Alert 17:67, 2002.

Fellay J, Marzolini C, Meaden ER, et al. Response to antiretroviral treatment in HIV-infected individuals with allele variants of the multidrug resistance transporter 1: a pharmacogenetics study. Lancet 359:30-6, 2002

Furrer H, Oparavil M, Bernasconi E, et al. Stopping primary prophylaxis in HIV-1 infected patients at high risk of toxoplasma encephalitis. Lancet 355:2217-8, 2000.

Gallant JE, Chaisson RE, Moore RD. The effect of adjunctive corticosteroids for the treatment of Pneumocystis carinii pneumonia on mortality and subsequent complications. Chest 114:1258, 1998.

Garcia-Benayas T, Blanco F, Soriano V. Weight loss in HIV-infected patients. N Engl J Med 347:1287-8, 2002.

Garcia-Ordonez MA, Colmenero JD, Jimenez-Onate F, et al. Diagnostic usefulness of percutaneous liver biopsy in HIV-infected patients with fever of unknown origin. J Infect 38:94, 1999.

Gildenberg PL, Gathe JC, Jr., Kim JH. Stereotactic biopsy of cerebral lesions in AIDS. Clin Infect Dis 30:491, 2000.

Graybill JR, Sobel J, Saag M, et al. Diagnosis and management of increased intracranial pressure in patients with AIDS and cryptococcal meningitis. The NIAID Mycoses Study Group and AIDS Cooperative Treatment Groups. Clin Infect Dis 30:47, 2000.

Hammer SM, Vaida F, Bennett KK, et al. Dual vs single protease inhibitor therapy following antiretroviral treatment failure: a randomized trial. JAMA 288:169-80, 2002.

Hammer SM. Increasing choices for HIV therapy. N Engl J Med 346:2002-3, 2002.

Hardy WD, Feinberg J, Finkelstein DM, et al., for the AIDS Clinical Trials Group. A controlled trial of trimethoprim-sulfamethoxazole or aerosolized pentamidine for secondary prophylaxis of Pneumocystis carinii pneumonia in patients with the acquired immunodeficiency syndrome: AIDS Clinical Trials Group protocol 021. N Engl J Med 327:1842-8, 1992.

Haubrich RH, Kemper CA, Hellmann NS, et al. The clinical relevance of non-nucleoside reverse transcriptase inhibitor hypersusceptibility: a prospective cohort analysis. AIDS 16:F33-F40, 2002.

Havlir DV, Dube MP, Sattler FR, et al. Prophylaxis against disseminated Mycobacterium avium complex with weekly azithromycin, daily rifabutin, or both. N Engl J Med 335:392-8, 1996.

HIV Trialists' Collaborative Group. Zidovudine, didanosine, and zalcitabine in the treatment of HIV infection: meta-analyses of the randomised evidence. Lancet 353:2014-2025, 1999.

Jackson JB, Musoke P, Fleming T et al. Intrapartum and neonatal single-dose nevirapine compared with zidovudine for prevention of mother-to-child transmission of HIV-1 in Kampala, Uganda: 18 month follow-up of the HIVNET 012 randomized trial. Lancet 362:859-68, 2003.

Jacobson MA, Hahn SM, Gerberding JL, et al. Ciprofloxacin for Salmonella bacteremia in the acquired immunodeficiency syndrome (AIDS). Ann Intern Med 110:1027, 1989.

Johnson S, Chan J, Bennett CL. Hepatotoxicity after prophylaxis with a nevirapine-containing antiretroviral regimen. Ann Intern Med 137:146-7, 2002.

Joly V, Flandre P, Meiffredy V, et al. Efficacy of zidovudine compared to stavudine, both in combination with lamivudine and indinavir, in human immunodeficiency virus-infected nucleoside-experienced patients with no prior exposure to lamivudine, stavudine, or protease inhibitors (Novavir trial). Antimicrob Agents Chemother 46:1906-13, 2002.

Kaiser L, Wat C, Mills T et al. Impact of oseltamivir treatment of influenza-related lower respiratory tract complications and hospitalizations. Arch Intern Med 163:1667-1672, 2003.

Kartalija M, Sande MA. Diarrhea and AIDS in the era of highly active antiretroviral therapy. Clin Infect Dis 28:701-5, 1999.

Kitabwalla M, Ruprecht RM. RNA interference–a new weapon against HIV and beyond. N Engl J Med 24;347,2002.

Kopp JB, Falloon J, Filie A, et al. Indinavir-associated intestinal nephritis and urothelial inflammation: clinical and cytologic findings. Clin Infect Dis 34:1122-8, 2002

Kourtis AP, Bulterys M, Nesheim SR, et al., Understanding the timing of HIV transmission from mother to infant. JAMA 285:709-712, 2001.

Ledergerber B, Egger M, Opravil M, et al. Clinical progression and virological failure on highly active antiretroviral therapy in HIV-1 patients: A prospective cohort study. Swiss HIV Cohort Study. Lancet 353:863, 1999.

Leenders AC, Reiss P, Portegies P, et al. Liposomal amphotericin B (AmBisome) compared with amphotericin B both followed by oral fluconazole in the treatment of AIDS-associated cryptococcal meningitis. AIDS 11:1463, 1997.

Little SJ, Holte S, Routy JP, et al. Antiretroviral-drug resistance among patients recently infected with HIV. N Engl J Med 347:385-94, 2002.

Lonergan JT, Behling C, Pfander H, et al. Hyperlactatemia and hepatic abnormalities in 10 human immunodeficiency virus-infected patients receiving nucleoside analogue combination regimens. Clin Infect Dis 31:162-166, 2000.

Lopez JC, Miro JM, Pena JM, Podzamczer D, and the GESIDA 04-98 Study Group. A randomized trial of the discontinuation of primary and secondary prophylaxis against Pneumocystis carinii pneumonia after HAART in patients with HIV infection. N Engl J Med 344:159-167, 2001.

Maggi P, Larocca AM, Quarto M, et al. Effect of antiretroviral therapy on cryptosporidiosis and microsporidiosis in patients infected with human immunodeficiency virus type 1. Eur J Clin Microbiol Infect Dis 19:213, 2000.

Manabe YC, Clark DP, Moore RD, et al. Cryptosporidiosis in patients with AIDS: correlates of disease and survival. Clin Infect Dis 27:536, 1998.

Martin DF, Kupperman BD, Wolitz RA, et al. Oral ganciclovir for patients with cytomegalovirus retinitis treated with a ganciclovir implant. N Engl J Med 340:1063-70, 1999.

Martinez E, Arnaiz JA, Podzamczer D, et al. Substitution of nevirapine, efavirenz, of abacavir for protease inhibitions in patients with human immunodeficiency virus infection. N Engl J Med 349:1036-46, 2003.

Max B, Sherer R. Management of the adverse effects of antiretroviral therapy and medication adherence. Clin Infect Dis 30 Suppl 2:S96-S116, 2000.

Mendelson MH, Gurtman A, Szabo S, et al. Pseudomonas aeruginosa bacteremia in patients with AIDS. Clin Infect Dis 18:886, 1994.

Meraviglia P, Angeli E, Del Sorbo F, et al. Risk factors for indinavir-related renal colic in HIV patients: predicative value of indinavir dose-body mass index. AIDS 16:2089-2093, 2002.

Mikhail N. Insulin resistance and HIV-related lipoatrophy. JAMA 288:1716, 2002.

Montaner JS, Reiss P, Cooper D, et al. A randomized, double-blind trial comparing combinations of nevirapine, didanosine, and zidovudine for HIV-infected patients: the INCAS trial (Italy, The Netherlands, Canada and Australia Study). JAMA 279:930-937, 1998.

Murphy RL, Brun S, Hicks C, et al. ABT-378/ritonavir plus stavudine and lamivudine for the treatment of antiretroviral-naive adults with HIV-1 infection: 48-week results. AIDS 15:F1-9, 2001.

Mwinga A, Nunn A, Ngwira B, et al. Mycobacterium vaccine (SRL 172) immunotherapy as an adjunct to standard antituberculosis treatment in HIV-infected adults with pulmonary tuberculosis randomised placebo-controlled trial. Lancet 360:1050-5, 2002.

Negredo E, Cruz L, Paredes R, et al. Virological, immunological, and clinical impact of switching from protease inhibitors to nevirapine or to efavirenz in patients with human immunodeficiency virus infection and long-lasting viral suppression. Clin Infect Dis 34:504-510, 2002.

Negredo E, Ribalta J, Paredes R, et al. Reversal of atherogenic lipoprotein profile in HIV-1 infected patients with lipodystrophy after replacing protease inhibitors by nevirapine. AIDS 16:1383-9, 2002.

Nicholson KG, Wood JM, Zambon M. Influenza. Lancet 362:1733-45, 2003.

Osmond DH, Buchbinder S, Cheng A. Prevalence of Kaposi sarcoma-associated herpesvirus infection in homosexuals beginning of and during the HIV epidemic. JAMA 287:221-5, 2002.

Palella FJ, Jr., Delaney KM, Moorman AC, et al. Declining morbidity and mortality among patients with advanced human immunodeficiency virus infection. HIV Outpatient Study Investigators. N Engl J Med 338:853-860, 1998.

Pierce M, Crampton S, Henry D, et al. A randomized. trial of clarithromycin as prophylaxis against disseminated Mycobacterium avium complex infection in patients with advanced acquired immunodeficiency syndrome. N Engl J Med 335:384, 1996.

Piliero PJ. Interaction between ritonavir and statins. Am J Med 112:510-1, 2002.

Powderly WG, Mayer KH. Centers for Disease Control and Prevention revised guidelines for human immunodeficiency virus (HIV) counseling, testing, and referral: targeting HIV specialists. Clin Infect Dis 37:813-9, 2003.

Racoosin JA, Kessler CM. Bleeding episodes in HIV-positive patients taking HIV protease inhibitors: a case series. Haemophilia 5:266-269, 1999.

Rathbun RC, Rossi DR. Low-dose ritonavir for protease inhibitor pharmacokinetic enhancement. Ann Pharmacother 36:702-6, 2002.

Robbins GK, De Gruttola V, Shafer RW et al. Comparison of Sequential three-drug regimens as initial therapy for HIV-1 infection. N Engl J Med 349:2293-303, 2003.

Robbins KG, De Gruttola V, Snyder SW. Comparison of Four-drug regimens and pairs of sequential three-drug regimens as initial therapy for HIV-1 infection. N Engl J Med 349:2293-303, 2003.

Sax PE. Opportunistic infections in HIV disease: down but not out. Infectious Disease Clinics of North America 15:433-455, 2001.

Sax PE. Managing long-term complications of HIV care. Infectious Disease Special Edition 3:115-118, 2000.

Schacker T, Zeh J, Hu HL, et al. Frequency of symptomatic and asymptomatic herpes simplex virus type 2 reactivations among human immunodeficiency virus-infected men. J Infect Dis 178:1616-22, 1998.

Schacker T, Collier AC, Hughes J, et al. Clinical and epidemiologic features of primary HIV infection. Ann Intern Med 125:257-264, 1996.

Schneider MME, Hoepelman AIM, Schattenkerk JKME, et al., and the Dutch AIDS Treatment Group. A controlled trial of aerosolized pentamidine or trimethoprim-sulfamethoxazole as primary prophylaxis against Pneumocystis carinii pneumonia in patients with human immunodeficiency virus infection. N Engl J Med 327:1836-41, 1992.

Shafer RW, Smeaton LM, Robbins GK, et. al. Comparison of four-drug regimens and pairs of sequential three-drug regimens as initial therapy for HIV-1 infection. N Engl J Med 349:2304-15, 2003.

Sherman DS, Fish DN. Management of protease inhibitor-associated diarrhea. Clin Infect Dis 30:908, 2000.

Smith NH, Cron S, Valdez LM, et al. Combination drug therapy for cryptosporidiosis in AIDS. J Infect Dis 178:900, 1998.

Staszewski S, Morales-Ramirez J, Tashima KT, et al. Efavirenz plus zidovudine and lamivudine, efavirenz plus indinavir, and indinavir plus zidovudine and lamivudine in the treatment of HIV-1 Infection in adults. N Engl J Med 341:1865-1873, 1999.

Staszewski S, Keiser P, Mantaner J, et al. Abacavir-lamivudine-zidovudine vs. indinavir-lamivudine-zidovudine in antiretroviral-naive HIV-infected adults: a randomized equivalence trial. JAMA 285:1155-63, 2001.

Sterling TR, Vlahov D, Astemborski J, et al. Initial HIV-1 RNA level and progression to AIDS in women and men. N Engl J Med 344:720-725, 2001.

Tassie JM, Gasnault J, Bentata M, et al. Survival improvement of AIDS-related progressive multifocal leukoencephalopathy in the era of protease inhibitors. Clinical Epidemiology Group. French Hospital Database on HIV. AIDS 13:1881, 1999.

The Antiretroviral Therapy (ART) Cohort Collection. Prognostic importance of initial response in HIV-1 infected patients starting potent antiretroviral therapy: analysis of prospective studies. Lancet 362:679-86, 2003.

The Data Collection of Adverse Events of Anti-HIV Drugs (DAD) Study Group. Combination antiretroviral therapy and the risk of myocardial infarction. N Engl J Med 349:1993-2003, 2003.

Van Damme L, Ramjee G, Alary M, et al. Effectiveness of COL-1492, a nonoxynol-9 vaginal gel, on HIV-1 transmission female sex workers: a randomised controlled trial. Lancet 360:917-7, 2002.

Watts DH. Management of human immunodeficiency virus infections in pregnancy. N Engl J Med 346:1879, 2002.

Weber T. Cerebrospinal fluid analysis for the diagnosis of human immunodeficiency virus-related neurologic diseases. Semin Neurol 19:223, 1999.

Weverling GJ, Mocroft A, Ledergerber B, et al. Discontinuation of Pneumocystis carinii pneumonia prophylaxis after start of highly active antiretroviral therapy in HIV-1 infection. EuroSIDA Study Group. Lancet 353:1293-1298, 1999.

Yeni PG, Hammer SM, Carpenter CC, et al. Antiretroviral treatment for adult HIV infection in 2002; updated recommendations of the International AIDS Society-USA Panel. JAMA 288:222-35, 2002.

GUIDELINES

Guidelines for the Use of Antiretroviral Agents in HIV-Infected Adults and Adolescents - November 10, 2003. www.aidsinfo.nih.gov/guidelines/default_db2.asp?id=50.

Guidelines for the Use of Antiretroviral Agents in Pediatric HIV Infection Nov 26, 2003. www.aidsinfo.nih.gov/guidelines/default_db2.asp?id=51.

Guidelines for using antiretroviral agents among HIV-infected adults and adolescents: recommendations of the Panel on Clinical Practices for Treatment of HIV. MMWR 51 (RR-7), May 17, 2002.

Public Health Service Task Force Recommendations for Use of Antiretroviral Drugs in Pregnant HIV-1-Infected Women for Maternal Health and Interventions to Reduce Perinatal HIV-1 Transmission in the United States Nov 26, 2003. www.aidsinfo.nih.gov/guidelines/.

Treatment of Tuberculosis - June 20, 2003. www.aidsinfo.nih.gov/guidelines/.

Guidelines for preventing opportunistic infections among HIV-infected persons - 2002: recommendations of the U.S. Public Health Service and the Infectious Diseases Society of America. MMWR 51 (RR-8), June 14, 2002.

Saag MS, Graybill RJ, Larsen RA, et al. Practice guidelines for the management of cryptococcal disease. Infectious Diseases Society of America. Clin Infect Dis 30:710, 2000.

Updated U.S. Public Health Service Guidelines for the management of occupational exposures to HBV, HCV, and HIV and recommendations for postexposure prophylaxis. MMWR 50(RR-11); 1-42, June 29, 2001.

USPHS Task Force Recommendations for use of antiretroviral drugs in pregnant HIV-1-infected women for maternal health and interventions to reduce perinatal HIV-1 transmission in the United States. MMWR 51(RR18):1-38, November 22, 2002. http://hivatis.org/trtgdlns.html.

TEXTBOOKS

Bartlett JG (ed). The Johns Hopkins Hospital Guide to Medical Care of Patients with HIV Infection, 10th edition, Lippincott Williams & Wilkins, Philadelphia, 2002.

Dolin R, Masur H, Saag MS (eds). AIDS Therapy, 2nd edition. Churchill Livingstone, New York, 2003.

Chapter 6

Antibiotic Prophylaxis and Immunizations*

Pierce Gardner, MD
Burke A. Cunha, MD

* For prophylaxis of opportunistic infections in HIV/AIDS, see Chapter 5, pp. 244-247

ANTIBIOTIC PROPHYLAXIS

Antibiotic prophylaxis is designed to prevent infection for a defined period of time. Prophylaxis is most likely to be effective when given for a short duration against a single pathogen with a known sensitivity pattern, and least likely to be effective when given for a long duration against multiple organisms with varying/unpredictable sensitivity patterns (Table 1). It is a common misconception that antibiotics used for prophylaxis should not be used for therapy and vice versa. The only difference between prophylaxis and therapy is the inoculum size and the duration of antibiotic administration: In prophylaxis, there is no infection, so the inoculum is minimal/none and antibiotics are administered only for the duration of exposure/surgical procedure. With therapy, the inoculum is large (infection already exists), and antibiotics are continued until the infection is eradicated.

Table 1. Factors Affecting the Efficacy of Surgical Antibiotic Prophylaxis

Number of Organisms	Susceptibility Pattern	Duration of Protection	Efficacy of Prophylaxis
Single organism	Predictable	Short	Excellent
Multiple organisms	Predictable	Short	Excellent
Single organism	Unpredictable	Short	Good
Single organism	Predictable	Long	Good
Multiple organisms	Unpredictable	Long	Poor/none

SURGICAL PROPHYLAXIS

Antibiotic prophylaxis is designed to achieve maximum antibiotic serum/tissue concentrations at the time of initial surgical incision, and is maintained throughout the "vulnerable period" of the procedure (i.e., time between skin incision and skin closure) to protect against transient bacteremias (Table 2). If prophylaxis is given too early, antibiotic levels will be suboptimal/nonexistent when protection is needed. Appropriate pre-operative prophylaxis is mandatory, since antibiotics given after skin closure are unlikely to be effective. When no infection exists prior to surgery (clean/clean contaminated surgery), single-dose prophylaxis is preferred. When infection is present/likely prior to surgery ("dirty" surgery, e.g., perforated colon, TURP in the presence of positive urine cultures, repair of open fracture), antibiotics are given for > 1 day and represent early therapy, not true prophylaxis. Parenteral cephalosporins are commonly used for surgical prophylaxis, and ordinarily given as a bolus injection/rapid IV infusion 15-30 minutes prior to the procedure. Prophylaxis with vancomycin or gentamicin is given by slow IV infusion over 1 hour, starting ~ 1 hour prior to the procedure.

Table 2. Surgical Prophylaxis

Procedure	Usual Organisms	Preferred Prophylaxis	Alternate Prophylaxis	Comments
CNS shunt (VP/VA) placement, craniotomy, open CNS trauma	S. epidermidis S. aureus	<u>MRSA/MRSE unlikely</u> Ceftriaxone 1 gm (IV) x 1 dose <u>MRSA/MRSE likely</u> Linezolid 600 mg (IV) x 1 dose	<u>MRSA/MRSE unlikely</u> Cefotaxime 2 gm (IV) x 1 dose **or** Ceftizoxime 2 gm (IV) x 1 dose <u>MRSA/MRSE likely</u> Linezolid 600 mg (PO) x 1 dose **or** Vancomycin 1 gm (IV) x 1 dose **or** Minocycline 200 mg (IV) x 1 dose	Administer immediately prior to procedure. Vancomycin protects against wound infections, but may not prevent CNS infections. Give vancomycin slowly IV over 1 hour prior to procedure
Thoracic (non-cardiac) surgery	S. aureus (MSSA)	Ceftriaxone 1 gm (IV) x 1 dose **or** Cefazolin 1 gm (IV) x 1 dose	Cefotaxime 2 gm (IV) x 1 dose **or** Ceftizoxime 2 gm (IV) x 1 dose	Administer immediately prior to procedure
Cardiac valve replacement surgery	S. epidermidis (MSSE/MRSE) S. aureus (MSSA/MRSA) Enterobacter	Vancomycin 1 gm (IV) x 1 dose **plus** Gentamicin 240 mg (IV) x 1 dose	Linezolid 600 mg (IV) x 1 dose **plus** Gentamicin 240 mg (IV) x 1 dose	Administer vancomycin and gentamicin slowly IV over 1 hour prior to procedure
Coronary artery bypass graft (CABG) surgery	S. aureus (MSSA)	Ceftriaxone 1 gm (IV) x 1 dose **or** Cefazolin 2 gm (IV) x 1 dose	Cefotaxime 2 gm (IV) x 1 dose **or** Ceftizoxime 2 gm (IV) x 1 dose	Administer immediately prior to procedure. Repeat dose intraoperatively for procedures lasting > 3 hours
Biliary tract surgery	E. coli Klebsiella Enterococci	Ampicillin 1 gm (IV) x 1 dose **plus either** Ceftriaxone 1 gm (IV) x 1 dose **or** Cefazolin 1 gm (IV) x 1 dose	Meropenem 1 gm (IV) x 1 dose **or** Ampicillin/sulbactam 3 gm (IV) x 1 dose **or** Any quinolone (IV) x 1 dose	Administer immediately prior to procedure (anaerobic coverage unnecessary)

Table 2. Surgical Prophylaxis (cont'd)

Procedure	Usual Organisms	Preferred Prophylaxis	Alternate Prophylaxis	Comments
Hepatic surgery	E. coli Klebsiella Enterococci B. fragilis	Ampicillin/ sulbactam 3 gm (IV) x 1 dose **or** Piperacillin/ tazobactam 4.5 gm (IV) x 1 dose	Meropenem 1 gm (IV) x 1 dose **or** Moxifloxacin 400 mg (IV) x 1 dose	Administer immediately prior to procedure
Stomach, upper small bowel surgery	S. aureus Group A streptococci	Ceftriaxone 1 gm (IV) x 1 dose **or** Cefazolin 1 gm (IV) x 1 dose	Cefotaxime 2 gm (IV) x 1 dose **or** Ceftizoxime 2 gm (IV) x 1 dose	Administer immediately prior to procedure (anaerobic coverage unnecessary)
Distal small bowel, colon surgery	E. coli Klebsiella B. fragilis Enterococci	Ceftriaxone 1 gm (IV) x 1 dose **plus** Metronidazole 1 gm (IV) x 1 dose	Metronidazole 1 gm (IV) x 1 dose **plus either** Gatifloxacin 400 mg (IV) x 1 dose **or** Levofloxacin 500 mg (IV) x 1 dose **or** Gentamicin 240 mg (IV) x 1 dose	Administer immediately prior to procedure. Give gentamicin slowly IV over 1 hour
Pelvic (OB/GYN) surgery	Aerobic gram-negative bacilli Anaerobic streptococci B. fragilis	Ceftriaxone 1 gm (IV) x 1 dose **plus** Metronidazole 1 gm (IV) x 1 dose	Cefotetan 2 gm (IV) x 1 dose **or** Cefoxitin 2 gm (IV) x 1 dose **or** Ceftizoxime 2 gm (IV) x 1 dose	Administer immediately prior to procedure
Orthopedic prosthetic implant surgery (total hip/knee replacement)	S. epidermidis S. aureus	<u>MRSA/MRSE unlikely</u> Cefazolin 2 gm (IV) x 1 dose <u>MRSA/MRSE likely</u> Vancomycin 1 gm (IV) x 1 dose	<u>MRSA/MRSE unlikely</u> Ceftriaxone 1 gm (IV) x 1 dose <u>MRSA/MRSE likely</u> Linezolid 600 mg (IV) x 1 dose	Administer immediately prior to procedure. Post-operative doses are ineffective and unnecessary
Arthroscopy	S. aureus Enteric gram-negative bacilli	Ceftriaxone 1 gm (IV) x 1 dose **or** Cefazolin 1 gm (IV) x 1 dose	Cefotaxime 2 gm (IV) x 1 dose **or** Ceftizoxime 2 gm (IV) x 1 dose	Pre-procedure prophylaxis is usually unnecessary in clean surgical procedures

Table 2. Surgical Prophylaxis (cont'd)

Procedure	Usual Organisms	Preferred Prophylaxis	Alternate Prophylaxis	Comments
Orthopedic surgery (open fracture)	S. aureus Aerobic gram negative bacilli	Ceftriaxone 1 gm (IV) x 3-7 days	Clindamycin 600 mg (IV) q8h x 3-7 days **plus** Gentamicin 240 mg (IV) q24h x 3-7 days	Represents early therapy, not true prophylaxis. Duration of post-op antibiotics depends on severity of infection
Urological implant surgery	S. aureus Enteric gram negative bacilli	Ceftriaxone 1 gm (IV) x 1 dose	Cefotaxime 2 gm (IV) x 1 dose **or** Ceftizoxime 2 gm (IV) x 1 dose	Administer immediately prior to procedure
TURP, cystoscopy	P. aeruginosa P. cepacia P. maltophilia E. faecalis Enteric gram negative bacilli	Piperacillin/ tazobactam 4.5 gm (IV) x 1 dose **or** Ciprofloxacin 400 mg (IV) x 1 dose	Gatifloxacin 400 mg (IV) x 1 dose **or** Levofloxacin 500 mg (IV) x 1 dose	Prophylaxis given to TURP patients with positive pre-op urine cultures. Represents early therapy, not true prophylaxis. No prophylaxis required for TURP if pre-op urine culture is negative
	E. faecium (VRE)	Linezolid 600 mg (IV) x 1 dose	Quinupristin/ dalfopristin 7.5 mg/kg (IV) x 1 dose	

MSSA/MRSA = methicillin-sensitive/resistant S. aureus; MSSE/MRSE = methicillin-sensitive/resistant S. epidermidis.

POST-EXPOSURE MEDICAL PROPHYLAXIS (Table 3)

Some infectious diseases can be prevented by post-exposure prophylaxis (PEP). To be maximally effective, PEP should be administered within 24 hours of the exposure, since the effectiveness of prophylaxis > 24 hours after exposure decreases rapidly in most cases. PEP is usually reserved for persons with close face-to-face/intimate contact with an infected individual. Casual contact usually does not warrant PEP.

Table 3. Post-Exposure Medical Prophylaxis

Exposure	Usual Organisms	Preferred Prophylaxis	Alternate Prophylaxis	Comments
Meningitis	N. meningitidis	Any quinolone (PO) x 1 dose	Minocycline 100 mg (PO) q12h x 2 days **or** Rifampin 600 mg (PO) q12h x 2 days	Must be administered within 24 hours of close face-to-face exposure to be effective. Otherwise, observe and treat if infection develops. Avoid tetracyclines in children ≤ 8 years
	H. influenzae	Rifampin 600 mg (PO) q24h x 3 days	Any quinolone (PO) x 3 days	Must be administered within 24 hours of close face-to-face exposure to be effective. H. influenzae requires 3 days of prophylaxis
Viral influenza	Influenza virus, type A or B	Oseltamivir (Tamiflu) 75 mg (PO) for duration of outbreak (or at least 7 days after close contact to an infected person). For CrCl 10-30 cc/min, give 75 mg (PO) q48h	Rimantadine 100 mg (PO) q12h* for duration of outbreak (or at least 7-10 days after close contact to infected person) **or** Amantidine 200 mg (PO) q24h† for duration of outbreak (or at least 7-10 days after close contact to infected person)	Give to non-immunized contacts and high-risk contacts even if immunized. Begin at onset of outbreak or within 2 days of close contact to an infected person. Oseltamivir is active against both influenza A and B; rimantadine and amantadine are only active against influenza A
Pertussis	B. pertussis	Erythromycin 500 mg (PO) q6h x 2 weeks	TMP-SMX 1 SS tablet (PO) q12h x 2 weeks **or** Levofloxacin 500 mg (PO) q24h x 2 weeks	Administer as soon as possible after exposure. Effectiveness is greatly reduced after 24 hours

*   For elderly, severe liver dysfunction, or CrCl < 10 cc/min, give 100 mg (PO) q24h

†   For age ≥ 65 years, give 100 mg (PO) q24h. For renal dysfunction, give 200 mg (PO) load followed by 100 mg q24h (CrCl 30-50 cc/min), 100 mg q48h (CrCl 15-29 cc/min), or 200 mg weekly (CrCl < 15 cc/min)

Table 3. Post-Exposure Medical Prophylaxis (cont'd)

Exposure	Usual Organisms	Preferred Prophylaxis	Alternate Prophylaxis	Comments
Diphtheria	C. diphtheriae	Erythromycin 500 mg (PO) q6h x 1 week **or** Benzathine penicillin 1.2 mu (IM) x 1 dose	Azithromycin 500 mg (PO) q24h x 3 days	Administer as soon as possible after exposure. Effectiveness is greatly reduced after 24 hours
TB	M. tuberculosis	INH 300 mg (PO) q24h x 9 months	Rifampin 600 mg (PO) q24h x 4 months	For INH, monitor SGOT/SGPT weekly x 4, then monthly x 3. Mild elevations are common and resolve spontaneously. INH should be stopped for SGOT/SGPT levels ≥ 5 x normal
Gonorrhea	N. gonorrhoeae	Ceftriaxone 125 mg (IM) x 1 dose	Spectinomycin 2 gm (IM) x 1 dose **or** Any oral quinolone x 1 dose	Administer as soon as possible after sexual exposure ($\leq$ 72 hours). Ceftriaxone also treats incubating syphilis
Syphilis	T. pallidum	Benzathine penicillin 2.4 mu (IM) x 1 dose	Doxycycline 100 mg (PO) q12h x 1 week	Administer as soon as possible after sexual exposure. Obtain HIV serology
Chancroid	H. ducreyi	Ceftriaxone 250 mg (IM) x 1 dose	Azithromycin 1 gm (PO) x 1 dose **or** Any oral quinolone x 3 days	Administer as soon as possible after sexual exposure. Obtain HIV and syphilis serologies
Non-gonococcal urethritis (NGU)	C. trachomatis U. urealyticum M. genitalium	Azithromycin 1 gm (PO) x 1 dose **or** Doxycycline 100 mg (PO) q12h x 1 week	Any oral quinolone x 1 week	Administer as soon as possible after sexual exposure. Also test for gonorrhea/Ureaplasma

Table 3. Post-Exposure Medical Prophylaxis (cont'd)

Exposure	Usual Organisms	Preferred Prophylaxis	Alternate Prophylaxis	Comments
Varicella (chicken-pox)	VZV	Varicella-zoster immune globulin (VZIG) 625 mcg (IM) x 1 dose. For exposure > 72 hours in pregnancy with respiratory symptoms (esp. smokers), consider acyclovir 800 mg (PO) 5x/day x 5-10 days	Varicella vaccine 0.5 mL (SC) x 1 dose. Repeat in 4 weeks	Administer as soon as possible after exposure (< 72 hours). Varicella vaccine is a live attenuated vaccine and should not be given to immunocompromised or pregnant patients. If varicella develops, start acyclovir treatment immediately
Hepatitis B (HBV)	Hepatitis B virus	<u>Unvaccinated</u> Hepatitis B immune globulin (HBIG) 0.06 mL/kg (IM) x 1 dose **plus** HBV vaccine (40 mcg HBsAg/mL) deep deltoid (IM) at 0, 1, 6 months (can use 10-mcg dose in healthy adults < 40 years)	<u>Previously vaccinated</u> *Known responder* (anti-HBsAg antibody levels ≥ 10 IU/mL): No treatment *Known non-responder* (anti-HBsAg antibody levels < 10 IU/mL): Treat as if unvaccinated *Antibody status unknown*: Obtain HBsAg antibody levels to determine immunity status. If testing is not possible or results are not available within 24 hours of exposure, give HBIG plus 1 dose of HBV vaccine (booster)	
Hepatitis A (HAV)	Hepatitis A virus	HAV vaccine 1 mL (IM) x 1 dose	Immune serum globulin (IG) 0.02 mL/kg (IM) x 1 dose	Give HAV vaccine plus IG if > 72 hours after exposure
Rocky Mountain spotted fever	R. rickettsia	Doxycycline 100 mg (PO) q12h x 1 week	Any oral quinolone x 1 week	Administer prophylaxis after removal of Dermacentor tick
Lyme disease	B. burgdorferi	Doxycycline 200 mg (PO) x 1 dose **or** Amoxicillin* 1 gm (PO) q8h x 3 days	Any oral 1st gen. cephalosporin* x 3 days **or** Azithromycin* 500 mg (PO) q24h x 3 days	If tick is in place ≥ 72 hours or is grossly engorged, prophylaxis may be given after tick is removed. Otherwise, prophylaxis is usually not recommended
		* Although experience is limited, single-dose prophylaxis with these agents is probably also effective		

Table 3. Post-Exposure Medical Prophylaxis (cont'd)

Exposure	Usual Organisms	Preferred Prophylaxis	Alternate Prophylaxis	Comments
Zoonotic diseases (plague, anthrax)	B. anthracis Y. pestis	Doxycycline 100 mg (PO) q12h for duration of exposure	Any oral quinolone for duration of exposure	Continued for the duration of a naturally-acquired exposure/outbreak. See p. 277 for bioterrorist plague/anthrax recommendations
Rabies	Rabies virus	<u>No Previous Immunization</u> HRIG 20 IU/kg* **plus either** PCEC 1 mL (IM) in deltoid **or** RVA 1 mL (IM) in deltoid **or** HDCV 1 mL (IM) in deltoid PCEC, RVA, HDCV given on days 0, 3, 7, 14, and 28 post-exposure	<u>Previous Immunization</u> PCEC 1 mL (IM) in deltoid on days 0 and 3 **or** RVA 1 mL (IM) in deltoid on days 0 and 3 **or** HDCV 1 mL (IM) in deltoid on days 0 and 3	Following unprovoked or suspicious dog or cat bite, immediately begin prophylaxis if animal develops rabies during a 10-day observation period. If dog or cat is suspected of being rabid, begin vaccination sequence immediately. Raccoon, skunk, bat, fox and most wild carnivore bites should be regarded as rabid, and bite victims should be vaccinated against rabies immediately (contact local health department regarding rabies potential of animals in your area). All potential rabies wounds should immediately be thoroughly cleaned with soap and water. Do not inject rabies vaccine IV (may cause hypotension/shock). Serum sickness may occur with HDCV

HDCV = human diploid cell vaccine, HRIG = human rabies immune globulin, PCEC = purified chick embryo cells, RVA = rabies vaccine absorbed

*   All or as much of the full dose of HRIG should be injected into the wound, and the remaining vaccine should be injected IM into the deltoid. Do not give HRIG at the same site or through the same syringe with PCEC, RVA, or HDCV

Table 3. Post-Exposure Medical Prophylaxis (cont'd)

Exposure	Usual Organisms	Preferred Prophylaxis	Alternate Prophylaxis	Comments
BIOTERRORIST AGENTS				
Anthrax *Inhalation/ cutaneous*	B. anthracis	Doxycycline 100 mg (PO) q12h x 60 days **or** Ciprofloxacin 500 mg (PO) q12h x 60 days **or** Gatifloxacin 400 mg (PO) q24h x 60 days **or** Levofloxacin 500 mg (PO) q24h x 60 days	Amoxicillin 1 gm (PO) q8h x 60 days	Duration of anthrax PEP based on longest incubation period of inhaled spores in nares
Tularemia pneumonia	F. tularensis	Doxycycline 100 mg (PO) q12h x 2 weeks	Ciprofloxacin 500 mg (PO) q12h x 2 weeks **or** Gatifloxacin 400 mg (PO) q24h x 2 weeks **or** Levofloxacin 500 mg (PO) q24h x 2 weeks	Duration of PEP for tularemia is 2 weeks, not 1 week as for plague
Pneumonic plague	Y. pestis	Doxycycline 100 mg (PO) q12h x 7 days **or** Ciprofloxacin 500 mg (PO) q12h x 7 days **or** Gatifloxacin 400 mg (PO) q24h x 7 days **or** Levofloxacin 500 mg (PO) q24h x 7 days	Chloramphenicol 500 mg (PO) q6h x 7 days	Pneumonic plague should be considered bioterrorism since most natural cases of plague are bubonic plague
Smallpox	Variola virus	Smallpox vaccine ≤ 4 days after exposure	None	Smallpox vaccine is protective when diluted 1:5

CHRONIC MEDICAL PROPHYLAXIS/SUPPRESSION (Table 4)

Some infectious diseases are prone to recurrence/relapse and may benefit from intermittent or chronic suppressive therapy. The goal of suppressive therapy is to minimize the frequency/severity of recurrent infectious episodes.

Table 4. Chronic Medical Prophylaxis/Suppression

Disorder	Usual Organisms	Preferred Prophylaxis	Alternate Prophylaxis	Comments
Asplenia	S. pneumoniae H. influenzae N. meningitidis	Amoxicillin 1 gm (PO) q24h indefinitely	Levofloxacin 500 mg (PO) q24h indefinitely **or** Gatifloxacin 400 mg (PO) q24h indefinitely **or** Moxifloxacin 400 mg (PO) q24h indefinitely	Chemoprophylaxis is uniformly effective, but needs to be given long-term. Pneumococcal, H. influenzae, and meningococcal vaccines should be given if possible, but are not always protective. Use amoxicillin in children, if possible
UTIs (recurrent)	Gram-negative bacilli Enterococci	Nitrofurantoin 100 mg (PO) q24h x 6 months	Amoxicillin 500 mg (PO) q24h x 6 months **or** TMP-SMX 1 SS tablet (PO) q24h x 6 months	Prophylaxis is indicated for frequent (≥ 3 per year) UTIs caused by reinfection; usually taken at bedtime. Recurrent UTIs of the "relapse" variety (same organism/serotype for each UTI) should be investigated for stones, abscesses, or structural abnormalities
Asymptomatic bacteriuria in pregnancy	Gram-negative bacilli	Nitrofurantoin 100 mg (PO) q24h x 1 week	Amoxicillin 1 gm (PO) q24h x 1 week	Prophylaxis prevents symptomatic infections
Prevention of CMV in organ transplants	CMV	Valganciclovir 900 mg (PO) q24h until CMV antigen levels ↓ to pre-flare levels		Begin pre-emptive therapy when semi-quantitative CMV antigen levels ↑. Pre-emptive therapy prevents CMV flare
Recurrent genital herpes (treatment of episodic recurrences)	H. simplex (HSV-2)	Acyclovir 400 mg (PO) q8h x 5 days **or** Famciclovir 125 mg (PO) q12h x 5 days	Valacyclovir 500 mg (PO) q12h x 3 days	Begin therapy as soon as lesions appear

Table 4. Chronic Medical Prophylaxis/Suppression (cont'd)

Disorder	Usual Organisms	Preferred Prophylaxis	Alternate Prophylaxis	Comments
Recurrent genital herpes *(chronic suppressive therapy)*	H. simplex (HSV-2)	Famciclovir 250 mg (PO) q12h x 1 year **or** Acyclovir 400 mg (PO) q12h x 1 year	Valacyclovir 500 mg (PO) q24h x 1 year; for > 9 episodes/year, use 1 gm (PO) q24h x 1 year	Suppressive therapy is indicated for frequent recurrences (≥ 3/year)
Acute exacerbation of chronic bronchitis (AECB)	S. pneumoniae H. influenzae M. catarrhalis	Moxifloxacin 400 mg or levofloxacin 500 mg or gatifloxacin 400 mg or gemifloxacin 320 mg (PO) q24h x 5 days **or** Amoxicillin/clavulanic acid XR 2 tablets (PO) q12h x 5 days **or** Telithromycin 800 mg (PO) q24h x 5 days **or** Clarithromycin XL 1 gm (PO) q24h x 5 days **or** Doxycycline 100 mg (PO) q12h x 5 days **or** Azithromycin 500 mg (PO) x 3 days		Treat each episode individually
Acute rheumatic fever (ARF)	Group A streptococci	Benzathine penicillin 1.2 mu (IM) monthly until age 30	Amoxicillin 500 mg (PO) q24h until age 30 **or** Azithromycin 500 mg (PO) q72h until age 30	Group A streptococcal pharyngitis and acute rheumatic fever are uncommon after age 30
Neonatal Group B streptococcal (GBS) infection (primary prevention)	Group B streptococci	Ampicillin 2 gm (IV) q4h at onset of labor until delivery	Clindamycin 600 mg (IV) q8h at onset of labor until delivery **or** Vancomycin 1 gm (IV) q12h at onset of labor until delivery	Indicated for previous infant with GBS infection, maternal GBS colonization/infection during pregnancy, or vaginal/rectal culture of GBS after week 35 of gestation. Also indicated for delivery ≤ week 37 of gestation without labor/ruptured membranes, for ruptured membranes ≥ 12 hours, or for intra-partum temp ≥ 100.4°F
Febrile neutropenia	Treat until neutropenia resolves (see p. 123)			

ENDOCARDITIS PROPHYLAXIS (Tables 5-7)

Endocarditis prophylaxis is designed to prevent native/prosthetic cardiac valve infections by preventing procedure-related bacteremias due to cardiac pathogens. For procedures above-the-waist, usual pathogens are viridans streptococci from the mouth. For procedures below-the-waist, usual pathogens are enterococci. Since procedure-related bacteremias are usually asymptomatic and last less than 15 minutes, single-dose oral regimens prior to the procedure provide effective prophylaxis. Parenteral SBE prophylaxis is preferred for patients with previous endocarditis, shunts, or prosthetic heart valves. Regimens vary among the experts, and no regimen is fully protective. Since erythromycin-based regimens have had the highest failure rate in the past, macrolides have not been included in the recommendations.

Table 5. Indications for Infective Endocarditis (IE) Prophylaxis*

Subset	Prophylaxis Recommended (Column A)	Prophylaxis Not Recommended (Column B)
Cardiac conditions	• Ostium primum ASD • Prosthetic heart valves, including bioprosthetic and homograft valves • Previous infective endocarditis • Most congenital cardiac malformations • Rheumatic valve disease • Hypertrophic cardiomyopathy • MVP with valvular regurgitation	• Isolated ostium secundum ASD • Surgical repair without residue beyond 6 months of ostium secundum ASD or PDA • Previous coronary artery bypass surgery • MVP without valvular regurgitation • Physiologic, functional, or innocent murmurs • Previous Kawasaki's cardiac disease or rheumatic fever without valve disease
Procedures	• Dental procedures known to induce gingival/mucosal bleeding, including dental cleaning • Tonsillectomy or adenoidectomy • Surgical operations involving intestinal or respiratory mucosa • Rigid bronchoscopy • Sclerotherapy for esophageal varices • Esophageal dilation • Gallbladder surgery • Cystoscopy or urethral dilation • Urethral catheterization or urinary tract surgery if UTI is present • Prostate surgery • I & D of infected tissue • Vaginal hysterectomy • Vaginal delivery, D & C, IUD insertion/removal, or therapeutic abortion in the presence of infection	• Dental procedures not likely to induce gingival bleeding • Tympanostomy tube insertion • Flexible bronchoscopy ± biopsy • Endotracheal intubation • Endoscopy ± gastrointestinal biopsy • Cesarean section • D & C, IUD insertion/removal, or therapeutic abortion in the absence of infection • Cardiac pacemaker/defibrillator insertion • Coronary stent implantation • Percutaneous transluminal coronary angioplasty (PTCA) • Cardiac catheterization

ASD = atrial septal defect, D & C = dilatation and curettage, I & D = incision and drain, IUD = intrauterine device, MVP = mitral valve prolapse, PDA = patent ductus arteriosus, UTI = urinary tract infection

* Prophylaxis is indicated for patients with cardiac conditions in Column A undergoing procedures in Column A. Prophylaxis is not recommended for patients or procedures in Column B. See Tables 6 and 7 for prophylaxis regimens for above-the-waist and below-the-waist procedures, respectively

Table 6. **Endocarditis Prophylaxis for Above-the-Waist (Dental, Oral, Esophageal, Respiratory Tract) Procedures***

Prophylaxis**	Reaction to Penicillin	Antibiotic Regimen
Oral prophylaxis	None	Amoxicillin 2 gm (PO) 1 hour pre-procedure[†]
	Non-anaphylactoid	Cephalexin 1 gm (PO) 1 hour pre-procedure
	Anaphylactoid	Clindamycin 300 mg (PO) 1 hour pre-procedure[††]
IV prophylaxis	None	Ampicillin 2 gm (IV) 30 minutes pre-procedure
	Non-anaphylactoid	Cefazolin 1 gm (IV) 15 minutes pre-procedure
	Anaphylactoid	Clindamycin 600 mg (IV) 30 minutes pre-procedure

* Endocarditis prophylaxis is directed against Streptococcus viridans, the usual SBE pathogen above the waist. Macrolide regimens are less effective than other regimens; clarithromycin/azithromycin regimens (500 mg PO 1 hour pre-procedure) are of unproven efficacy

** Oral prophylaxis is preferred to IV prophylaxis, except in patients with previous endocarditis, shunts, or prosthetic heart valves

† Some recommend a 3 gm dose of amoxicillin, which is excessive given the sensitivity of viridans streptococci to amoxicillin

†† Some recommend a 600 mg dose of clindamycin, but a 300 mg dose gives adequate blood levels and is better tolerated (less diarrhea)

Table 7. **Endocarditis Prophylaxis for Below-the-Waist (Genitourinary, Gastrointestinal) Procedures***

Prophylaxis**	Reaction to Penicillin	Antibiotic Regimen
Oral prophylaxis	None	Amoxicillin 2 gm (PO) 1 hour pre-procedure
	Non-anaphylactoid, anaphylactoid	Linezolid 600 mg (PO) 1 hour pre-procedure
IV prophylaxis	None	Ampicillin 2 gm (IV) 30 minutes pre-procedure **plus** Gentamicin 80 mg (IM) or (IV) over 1 hour 60 minutes pre-procedure
	Non-anaphylactoid, anaphylactoid	Vancomycin 1 gm (IV) over 1 hour 60 minutes pre-procedure **plus** Gentamicin 80 mg (IM) or (IV) over 1 hour 60 minutes pre-procedure

* Endocarditis prophylaxis is directed against Enterococcus faecalis, the usual SBE pathogen below the waist

** Oral prophylaxis is preferred to IV prophylaxis, except in patients with previous endocarditis, shunts, or prosthetic heart valves

TRAVEL PROPHYLAXIS (Tables 8, 9)

Travelers may acquire infectious diseases from ingestion of fecally-contaminated water/food, exchange of infected body secretions, inhalation of aerosolized droplets, direct inoculation via insect bites, or from close contact with infected birds/animals. Recommendations to prevent infection in travelers consist of general travel precautions (Table 8), and specific travel prophylaxis regimens (Table 9).

Table 8. General Infectious Disease Travel Precautions

Exposure	Risk	Precautions
Unsafe water (fecally-contaminated)	Diarrhea/dysentery, viral hepatitis (HAV)	• Avoid ingestion of unbottled/unpotable water. Be sure bottled water has an unbroken seal and has not been opened/refilled with tap water • Avoid ice cubes made from water of uncertain of origin/handling, and drinking from unclean glasses • Drink only pasteurized bottled drinks. Be sure bottles/cans are opened by you or in your presence • Avoid drinking unpasteurized/warm milk; beer, wine, and pure alcoholic beverages are safe • Eat only canned fruit or fresh fruit peeled by you or in your presence with clean utensils • Avoid eating soft cheeses • Avoid eating raw tomatoes/uncooked vegetables that may have been exposed to contaminated water • Avoid using hotel water for tooth brushing/rinsing unless certain of purity. Many hotels use common lines for bath/sink water that is suitable for drinking • Avoid wading/swimming/bathing in lakes or rivers
Food-borne (fecally-contaminated)	Diarrhea/dysentery	• Eat only seafood/poultry/meats that are freshly cooked and served hot. Avoid eating at roadside stands or small local restaurants with questionable sanitary practices • "Boil it, peel it, or forget it"
Body fluid secretions	Viral hepatitis (HBV, HCV, etc.), STDs, HIV/other retroviruses	• Do not share utensils/glasses/straws or engage in "risky behaviors" involving body secretion exchange • Avoid blood transfusion (use blood expanders instead) • Treat dental problems before travel
Animal bite	Animal bite-associated infections	• Do not pet/play with stray dogs/cats. Rabies and other infections are common in wild (and some urban) animals
Flying insects	Malaria, arthropod-borne infections	• Avoid flying/biting insects by wearing dark protective clothing (long sleeves/pants) and using insect repellent on clothes/exposed skin, especially during evening hours • Minimize dawn-to-dusk outdoor exposure • Use screens/mosquito nets when possible • Do not use perfume, after shave, or scented deodorants/toiletries that will attract flying insects

Table 9. Travel Prophylaxis Regimens

Exposure	Usual Pathogens	Prophylaxis Regimens	Comments
Traveler's diarrhea	E. coli Salmonella Shigella Non-cholera vibrios V. cholerae Aeromonas Plesiomonas Rotavirus Norwalk virus Giardia lamblia Campylobacter Yersinia Cryptosporidium Cyclospora Enteroviruses Amebiasis	Doxycycline 100 mg (PO) q24h for duration of exposure **or** Any quinolone (PO) for duration of exposure **or** TMP-SMX 1 SS tablet (PO) q24h for duration of exposure	Observe without prophylaxis and treat mild diarrhea symptomatically with loperamide (2 mg). Persons with medical conditions adversely affected by dehydration caused by diarrhea may begin prophylaxis after arrival in country and continue for 1 day after returning home. Should severe diarrhea/dysentery occur, continue/switch to a quinolone, maximize oral hydration, and see a physician if possible. Anti-spasmodics may be used for symptomatic relief of mild, watery diarrhea. Bismuth subsalicylate is less effective than antibiotic prophylaxis. Traveler's diarrhea usually presents as acute watery diarrhea with low-grade fever after ingestion of fecally-contaminated water. Most cases are due to enterotoxigenic E. coli. TMP-SMX is active against some bacterial pathogens and Cyclospora, but not against E. histolytica or enteroviral pathogens (e.g., Rotavirus, Norwalk agent). Doxycycline is active against most bacterial pathogens and E. histolytica, but misses Campylobacter, Cryptosporidium, Cyclospora, Giardia, and enteroviral pathogens. Although emerging resistance is a problem, ciprofloxacin is active against most pathogens except Giardia, Cryptosporidium, Cyclospora, E. histolytica, and enteroviral pathogens. All antibiotics are inactive against viral/parasitic pathogens causing diarrhea
Meningococcal meningitis	N. meningitidis	<u>Pre-travel prophylaxis</u> Meningococcal vaccine 0.5 mL (SC) ≥ 1 month prior to travel to outbreak area <u>Post-exposure prophylaxis</u> See p. 273	Acquired via close face-to-face contact (airborne aerosol/droplet exposure). Vaccine is highly protective against N. meningitidis serotypes A, C, Y, and W-135, but misses B serotype

Table 9. Travel Prophylaxis Regimens (cont'd)

Exposure	Usual Pathogens	Prophylaxis Regimens	Comments
Hepatitis A (HAV)	Hepatitis A virus	HAV vaccine 1 mL (IM) prior to travel, then follow with a one-time booster ≥ 6 months later	HAV vaccine is better than immune globulin for prophylaxis. Take care to avoid direct/indirect ingestion of fecally-contaminated water. HAV vaccine is recommended for travel to all developing countries. Protective antibody titers develop after 2 weeks
Typhoid fever	S. typhi	ViCPS vaccine 0.5 mL (IM). Booster every 2 yrs for repeat travelers **or** Oral Ty21a vaccine 1 capsule (PO) q48h x 4 doses. Booster every 5 years for repeat travelers	For the oral vaccine, do not co-administer with antibiotics. Contraindicated in compromised hosts and children ≤ 6 years old. Take oral capsules with cold water. Degree of protective immunity is limited with vaccine. Some prefer chemoprophylaxis the same as for Traveler's diarrhea (p. 283)
Yellow fever	Yellow fever virus	Yellow fever vaccine 0.5 mL (SC). Booster every 10 years for repeat travelers	Vaccine is often required for travel to or from Tropical South America or Tropical Central Africa. Administer 1 month apart from other live vaccines. Contraindicated in children < 4 months old; caution in children ≤ 1 year old. Reactions may occur in persons with egg allergies. Immunity is probably life long, but a booster every 10 years is needed for vaccination certification by some countries
Japanese encephalitis (JE)	Japanese encephalitis virus	JE vaccine 1 mL (SC) on days 0, 7, and 14 or 30. Booster schedule not established	Recommended for travelers planning prolonged (> 3 week) visits during the rainy season to rural, endemic areas of Asia (e.g., Eastern Russia, Indian subcontinent, China, Southeast Asia, Thailand, Korea, Laos, Cambodia, Vietnam, Malaysia, Philippines). Administer ≥ 2 weeks before exposure. Children < 3 years may be given 0.5 mL (SC) on same schedule as adults
Rabies	Rabies virus	HDCV, PCEC, or RVA 1 mL (IM) on days 0, 7, and 21 or 28 prior to travel **or** HDCV 0.1 mL (ID) on days 0, 7, and 21 or 28 prior to travel	Avoid contact with wild dogs/animals during travel. Dose of rabies vaccine for adults and children are the same. A booster dose prior to travel is recommended if antibody levels are measured and are low

Table 9. Travel Prophylaxis Regimens (cont'd)

Exposure	Usual Pathogens	Prophylaxis Regimens	Comments
Malaria	P. vivax P. ovale P. malariae P. falciparum (chloroquine sensitive)	Chloroquine phosphate 500 mg (300 mg base) (PO) weekly **or** Malarone (atovaquone 250 mg + proguanil 100 mg) 1 tablet (PO) q24h **or** Mefloquine 250 mg (228 mg base) (PO) weekly	Acquired from female Anopheles mosquito bites. Avoid mosquito exposure using long-sleeved shirts/long pants at dawn/dusk when mosquitoes feed. Screens/mosquito nets are the best natural protection. DEET/pyrethrin sprays on clothing is helpful. Begin anti-malarial prophylaxis 1 week before travel to malarious areas (most of Africa, Latin America, Indian subcontinent, Southeast Asia), and continue for 4 weeks after returning home. Chemoprophylaxis reduces but does not eliminate the risk of malaria. Malarone prophylaxis may be given 1 day before travel, daily during malaria exposure, and for 1 week after returning home. Malarone is effective against sensitive/resistant P. falciparum strains, but not hepatic stages of P. vivax/P. ovale. Chloroquine-resistant P. falciparum is seen in sub-Saharan Africa, South America (except Chile, Argentina), Indian subcontinent, and Southern Asia (Burma, Thailand, Cambodia). Only areas without chloroquine-resistant P. falciparum are Middle East (except Saudi Arabia), Central America (west of Panama Canal), Haiti, and Dominican Republic. Fansidar resistance is common in chloroquine-resistant areas of Asia, Latin American, Africa. Mefloquine (but not doxycycline) resistance is seen in Thailand. Doxycycline is contraindicated in pregnancy, but chloroquine and proguanil are safe, and mefloquine is probably safe late in pregnancy. If pregnant, try to delay travel to malarial areas until after delivery
	P. falciparum (chloroquine resistant)	Doxycycline 100 mg (PO) q24h **or** Malarone (atovaquone 250 mg + proguanil 100 mg) 1 tablet (PO) q24h **or** Mefloquine 250 mg (228 mg base) (PO) weekly	

HDCV = human diploid cell vaccine, PCEC = purified chick embryo cell vaccine, RVA = rabies vaccine absorbed, RIG = rabies immune globulin

TETANUS PROPHYLAXIS (Table 10)

Current information suggests that immunity lasts for decades/life-time after tetanus immunization. A tetanus booster should not be routinely given for minor wounds, but is recommended for wounds with high tetanus potential (e.g., massive crush wounds, soil-contaminated wounds, or deep puncture wounds).

Table 10. Tetanus Prophylaxis in Routine Wound Management

History of Adsorbed Tetanus Toxoid	Wound Type	Recommendations
Unknown or < 3 doses	Clean, minor wounds	Td‡
	Tetanus-prone wounds†	Td‡ plus TIG
≥ 3 doses	Clean, minor wounds	No prophylaxis needed
	Tetanus-prone wounds†	Td‡ if > 10 years since last dose*

DT = diphtheria and tetanus toxoids adsorbed (pediatrics), DTP = diphtheria and tetanus and pertussis vaccine adsorbed, Td = tetanus and diphtheria toxoids adsorbed (adult), TIG = tetanus immune globulin

† For example, massive crush wounds; wounds contaminated with dirt, soil, feces, or saliva; deep puncture wounds; or significant burn wounds or frostbite
‡ For children < 7 years, DTP (DT if pertussis is contraindicated) is preferred to tetanus toxoid alone. For children ≥ 7 years old and adults, Td is preferred to tetanus toxoid alone
* More frequent booster doses are unnecessary and can increase side effects. Protection lasts > 20 yrs
Adapted from: Centers for Disease Control and Prevention. MMWR Rep 40 (RR-10):1-28, 1991

IMMUNIZATIONS (Tables 11-13)

Immunizations are designed to reduce infections in large populations, and may prevent/decrease the severity of infection in non-immunized individuals. Compromised hosts with altered immune systems may not develop protective antibody titers to antigenic components of various vaccines. Immunizations are not fully protective, but are recommended (depending on the vaccine) for most normal hosts, since some protection is better than none. Post-exposure prophylaxis and travel prophylaxis are described on pp. 272-277 and 282-285.

Table 11. Adult Immunizations

Vaccine	Indications	Dosage	Comments
Bacille Calmette Guérin (BCG)	Possibly beneficial for adults at high-risk of multiple-drug resistant tuberculosis	Primary: 1 dose (intradermal). Booster not recommended	Live attenuated vaccine. PPD remains positive for years/life. Contraindicated in immuno-compromised hosts. Side effects include injection site infection or disseminated infection (rare)

Table 11. Adult Immunizations (cont'd)

Vaccine	Indications	Dosage	Comments
Hemophilus influenzae (type B)	Patients with splenic dysfunction	Primary: 0.5 mL dose (IM). Booster not recommended	Capsular polysaccharide conjugated to diphtheria toxoid. Safety in pregnancy unknown. Mild local reaction in 10%
Hepatitis A (HAV)	Adults at increased risk for HAV	Primary: 1 mL dose (IM). One-time booster ≥ 6 months later	Inactivated whole virus. Pregnancy risk not fully evaluated. Mild soreness at injection site. Occasional headache/malaise
Hepatitis B (HBV)	Household/sexual contact with carrier, IV drug use, multiple sex partners (heterosexual), homosexual male activity, blood product recipients, hemodialysis, occupational exposure to blood, residents/staff of institutions for developmentally disabled, prison inmates, residence ≥ 6 months in areas of high endemicity, others at high risk	Primary (3 dose series): Recombivax 10 mcg (1 mL) or Engerix-B 20 mcg (1 mL) IM in deltoid at 0, 1, and 6 months. Alternate schedule for Engerix-B: 4 dose series at 0, 1, 2, and 12 months. Booster not routinely recommended	Recombinant vaccine comprised of hepatitis B surface antigen. For compromised hosts (including dialysis patients), use specially packaged Recombivax 40-mcg doses (1 mL vial containing 40 mcg/mL). HBsAb titers should be obtained 6 months after 3-dose primary series. Those with non-protective titers (≤ 10 mIU/mL) should receive 1 dose monthly (with subsequent HbsAb testing) up to a maximum of 3 doses. Safety to fetus unknown; pregnancy not a contraindication in high-risk females. Mild local reaction in 10-20%. Occasional fever, headache, fatigue, nausea. Twinrix 1 mL (IM) (combination of Hepatitis A inactivated vaccine and Hepatitis B recombinant vaccine) is available for adults on a 0-, 1-, and 6-month schedule
Influenza	Healthy persons ≥ 50 years, healthcare personnel, adults with high-risk conditions (e.g., heart disease, lung disease, diabetes, renal dysfunction, hemoglobinopathies, immunosuppression)	Annual vaccine. Single 0.5 mL dose (IM) between October and November (before flu season) is optimal, but can be given anytime during flu season	Trivalent inactivated whole and split virus. Contraindications include anaphylaxis to eggs or sensitivity to thimerosal. Mild local reaction in up to 30%. Occasional malaise/myalgia beginning 6-12 hours after vaccination. Neurologic and allergic reactions are rare. For pregnancy, administer in 2nd or 3rd trimester during flu season. A nasally-administered live attenuated influenza vaccine has been approved for healthy individuals aged 5-49 years

Table 11. Adult Immunizations (cont'd)

Vaccine	Indications	Dosage	Comments
Measles	Adults born after 1956 without live-virus immunization or measles diagnosed by a physician or immunologic test. Also indicated for revaccination of persons given killed measles vaccine between 1963-67	Primary: 0.5 mL dose (SC). A second dose (≥ 1 month later) is recommended for certain adults at increased risk of exposure (e.g., healthcare workers, travelers to developing countries)	Live virus vaccine (usually given in MMR). Contraindicated in compromised hosts, pregnancy, history of anaphylaxis to eggs or neomycin. Ineffective if given 3-11 months after blood products. Side effects include low-grade fever 5-21 days after vaccination (5-15%), transient rash (5%), and local reaction in 4-55% of persons previously immunized with killed vaccine (1963-67)
Mumps	Non-immune adults	Primary: 0.5 mL dose (SC)	Live attenuated vaccine (usually given in MMR). Contraindicated in immunocompromised hosts, pregnancy, history of anaphylaxis to eggs or neomycin. Side effects include mild allergic reactions (uncommon), parotitis (rare)
Pneumococcus (S. pneumoniae)	Immunocompetent hosts ≥ 65 years old, or > 2 years old with diabetes, CSF leaks, or chronic cardiac, pulmonary or liver disease. Also for immunocompromised hosts > 2 years old with functional/anatomic asplenia, leukemia, lymphoma, multiple myeloma, widespread malignancy, chronic renal failure, bone marrow/organ transplant, or on immunosuppressive/steroid therapy	Primary: 0.5 mL dose (SC or IM). A one-time booster at 5 years is recommended for immunocompromised hosts > 2 years old and for those who received the vaccine before age 65 for high-risk conditions	Polyvalent vaccine against 23 strains. Revaccination is not recommended for normal hosts previously vaccinated with 23-valent vaccine

Table 11. Adult Immunizations (cont'd)

Vaccine	Indications	Dosage	Comments
Rubella	Non-immune adults, particularly women of childbearing age	Primary: 0.5 mL dose (SC)	Live virus (RA 27/3 strain) vaccine (usually given in MMR). Contraindicated in immuno-compromised hosts, pregnancy, history of anaphylactic reaction to neomycin. Joint pains and transient arthralgias in up to 40%, beginning 3-25 days after vaccination and lasting 1-11 days; frank arthritis in < 2%
Tetanus-diphtheria	Adults	Primary: Two 0.5 mL doses (IM), 1-2 months apart; third dose 6-12 months after second dose. No booster (unless develop a tetanus-prone wound, p. 286)	Adsorbed toxoid vaccine. Contraindicated if hypersensitivity/neurological reaction or severe local reaction to previous doses. Side effects include local reactions, occasional fever, systemic symptoms, Arthus-like reaction in persons with multiple previous boosters, and systemic allergy (rare)
Varicella (VZV) chickenpox	Non-immune adolescents and adults, especially healthcare workers and others likely to be exposed	Primary: Two 0.5 mL doses (SC), 4-8 weeks apart. Vaccine must be stored frozen and used within 30 minutes after thawing and reconstitution. No booster	Live attenuated vaccine. Contraindications include pregnancy, active untreated TB, immunocompromised host, malignancy of bone marrow or lymphatic system, anaphylactic reaction to gelatin/neomycin, or blood product recipient within previous 6 months (may prevent development of protective antibody). Mild febrile illness in 10%. Injection site symptoms in 25-30% (local rash in 3%). Mild diffuse rash in 5%

Recommended Adult Immunization Schedule United States, 2002-2003. MMWR 51(40):904-908, Oct. 11, 2002 (www.cdc.gov/mmwr/PDF/wk/mm5140.pdf) Avery RK. Immunizations in Adult Immunocompromised Patients: Which to Use and Which to Avoid. Cleve Clin J Med 68:337-348,2001. Reid KC, Grizzard TA, Poland GA. Adult Immunizations: Recommendations for Practice. Mayo Clin Proc 74:377-384,1999.

Table 12. Immunizations Before Organ Transplantation

Vaccine	Recommendation
Measles-mumps-rubella (MMR), polio, diphtheria-tetanus-pertussis (DPT), H. influenza (type b)	Complete series
Hepatitis A	Vaccinate, especially pre-liver transplant
Hepatitis B	Vaccinate; give 3rd dose ≥ 2 months after 2nd dose
Influenza	Vaccinate annually
Varicella	Vaccinate seronegative patients
Pneumococcal	Vaccinate high-risk patients with cardiac/pulmonary disease
Meningococcal	Vaccinate young adults

Table 13. Immunizations in Pregnancy

Vaccine	Recommendation
Hepatitis A, Hepatitis B, influenza, tetanus/diphtheria, meningococcal, rabies, typhoid feve (ViCPS), polio (IPV), yellow fever*	Should be considered if otherwise indicated
Measles*, mumps*, rubella*, varicella*, BCG*, vaccinia*, typhoid (oral Ty21a*)	Contraindicated in pregnancy
Pneumococcal, cholera, Japanese encephalitis, plague	Inadequate information for recommendation

* Live attenuated vaccine

REFERENCES AND SUGGESTED READINGS

Adverse events associated with 17D-derived Yellow Fever vaccination-United states, 2001-2002. MMWR.51:989-993, 2002.

Antrum RM, Solomkin JS. A review of antibiotic prophylaxis for open fractures. Orthop Rev 16:246-54, 1987.

Batiuk TD, Bodziak KA, Goldman M. Infectious disease prophylaxis in renal transplant patients: a survey of US transplant centers. Clin Transplant 16:1-8, 2002.

Burroughs, MH. Immunization in transplant patients. Pediatr Infect Dis J 21:158-60, 2002.

Carratala J. Role of antibiotic prophylaxis for the prevention of intravascular catheter-related infection. Clin Microbiol Infect 7 (Suppl 4):83-90, 2001.

Chattopadhyay B. Splenectomy pneumococcal vaccination and antibiotic prophylaxis. Br J Hosp Med 41:172-4, 1989.

Colizza S, Rossi S. Antibiotic prophylaxis and treatment of surgical abdominal sepsis. J Chemother 13 (Spec No 1):193-201, 2001.

Conte JE Jr. Antibiotic prophylaxis: non-abdominal surgery. Curr Clin Top Infect Dis 10:254-305, 1989.

Court-Brown CM. Antibiotic prophylaxis in orthopaedic surgery. Scand J Infect Dis Suppl 70:74-9, 1990.

Cunha BA, Gossling HR, Nightingale C, et al. Penetration characteristics of cefazolin, cephalothin, and cephradine into bone in patients undergoing total hip replacement. Journal of Bone and Surgery 59:856-859, 1977.

Cunha BA, Pyrtek LJ, Quintiliani R. Prophylactic antibiotics in cholecystectomy. Lancet 1:207-8, 1979.

Cunha BA, Ristuccia A, Jonas M, et al. Penetration of ceftizoxime and cefazolin into bile and gallbladder wall. Journal of Antimicrobial Chemotherapy 10:117-120, 1982.

Cunha BA. Antibiotic tissue penetration. Bulletin of the New York Academy of Medicine 59:443-449, 1983.

Cunha BA, Gossling HR, Nightingale CH, et al. Penetration of cefazolin and cefradine into bone in patients undergoing total knee arthroplasty. Infection 2:80-84, 1984

De Lalla F. Surgical prophylaxis in practice. J Hosp Infect 50 (Suppl A):S9-12, 2002.

De Lalla F. Antibiotic prophylaxis in orthopedic prosthetic surgery. J Chemother. 13 Spec No 1:48-53, 2001.

Dellinger EP. Antibiotic prophylaxis in trauma: penetrating abdominal injuries and open fractures. Rev Infect Dis 13 (Suppl 10):S847-57, 1991.

Dennehy PH. Active immunization in the United States: developments over the past decade. Clin Microbiol Rev 14:872-908, 2001.

Dietrich ES, Bieser U, Frank U, et al. Ceftriaxone versus other cephalosporins for perioperative antibiotic prophylaxis: a meta analysis of 43 randomized controlled trials. Chemotherapy 48:49-56, 2002.

Duff P, Park RC. Antibiotic prophylaxis in vaginal hysterectomy: a review. Obstet Gynecol 55(Suppl 5): 193S-202S, 1980.

Esposito S. Is single-dose antibiotic prophylaxis sufficient for any surgical procedure? J Chemother 11:556, 2000.

Faix, RG. Immunization during pregnancy. Clin Obstet Gynecol 45:42-58, 2002.

Faro S. Antibiotic prophylaxis. Obstet Gynecol Clin North Am 16:279-89, 1989.

Galask RP. Changing concepts in obstetric antibiotic prophylaxis. Am J Obstet Gynecol 157:491-7, 1987.

Gall SA. Immunology update: hepatitis B virus immunization today. Infect Dis Obstet Gynecol 9:63-4, 2001.

Gardner P, Eickhoff T. Immunization in adults in the 1990s. Curr Clin To Infect Dis 15:271-300, 1995.

Gardner P, Peter G. Recommended schedules for routine immunization of children and adults. Infect Dis Clin North Am 15:1-8, 2001.

Gardner P, Schaffner W. Immunization of adults. N Engl J Med 328:1252-8, 1993.

Gellin BG, Curlin GT, Rabinovich NR, et al. Adult immunization: principles and practice. Adv Intern Med 44:327-52, 1999.

Grabe M. Perioperative antibiotic prophylaxis in urology. Curr Opin Urol 11:81-5, 2001.

Guaschino S, De Santo D, De Seta F. New perspectives in antibiotic prophylaxis for obstetric and gynecological surgery. J Hosp Infect 50 (Suppl A):SS13-6, 2002.

Guglielmo BJ, Hohn DC, Koo PJ, et al. Antibiotic prophylaxis in surgical procedures. Arch Surg 118:943-55, 1983.

Haines SJ. Antibiotic prophylaxis in neurosurgery. The controlled trials. Neurosurg Clin N Am 3:355-8, 1992.

Hartman BJ. Selective aspects of infective endocarditis: considerations on diagnosis, risk factors, treatment and prophylaxis. Adv Cardiol 39:195-202, 2002.

Hopkins CC. Antibiotic prophylaxis in clean surgery: peripheral vascular surgery, noncardiovascular thoracic surgery, herniorrhaphy, and mastectomy. Rev Infect Dis 13 (Suppl 10):S869-73, 1991.

Jackson LA, Neuzil KM, Yu O et al. Effectiveness of pneumococcal polysaccharide vaccine in older adults. N Engl J Med 348:1747-55, 2003.

Jong EC, Nothdurft HD. Current drugs for antimalarial chemoprophylaxis: a review of efficacy and safety. J Travel Med 8(Supp. 3):S48-56, 2001.

Kain KC, Shanks GD, Keystone JS. Malaria chemoprophylaxis in the age of drug resistance. I. Currently recommended drug regimens. Clin Infect Dis 33:226-34, 2001.

Leaper DJ, Melling AG. Antibiotic prophylaxis in clean surgery: clean non-implant wounds. J Chemother. 13 (Spec No 1):96-101, 2001.

Lewis RT. Oral versus systemic antibiotic prophylaxis in elective colon surgery: a randomized study and meta-analysis send a message from the 1990s. Can J Surg 45:173-80, 2002.

Ling J, Baird JK, Fryauff DJ, et al. Randomized, placebo-controlled trial of atovaquone-proguanil for the prevention of plasmodium falciparum or plasmodium vivax malaria among migrants to Paupa, Indonesia. Clin Infect Dis 35:825-33, 2002.

Love TA. Antibiotic prophylaxis and urologic surgery. Urology 26 (Suppl 5):2-5, 1985.

Malangoni MA, Jacobs DG. Antibiotic prophylaxis for injured patients. Infec Dis Clin North Am 6:627-42, 1992.

McDonnell WM, Askari FK. Immunization. JAMA 278:2000-7, 1997.

Nichols RL. Surgical antibiotic prophylaxis. Med Clin North Am 79:509-22, 1995.

Norden CW. Antibiotic prophylaxis in orthopedic surgery. Rev Infect Dis 13 (Suppl 10):S842-6, 1991.

Overbosch D, Schilthuis H, Bienzle U, et al. Atovaquone-proguanil versus mefloquine for malaria prophylaxis in nonimmune travelers: results from a randomized, double-blind study. Clin Infect Dis 33:1015-21, 2001.

Peter G, Gardner P. Standards for immunization practice for vaccines in children and adults. Infect Dis Clin North Am 15:9-19, 2001.

Phillips P, Chan K, Hogg R, et al. Azithromycin prophylaxis for Mycobacterium avium complex during the era of highly active antiretroviral therapy: evaluation of a provincial program. Clin Infect Dis 34:371-8, 2002.

Pratesi C, Russo D, Dorigo W, et al. Antibiotic prophylaxis in clean surgery: vascular surgery. J Chemother 13 (Spec 1):123-8, 2001.

Randomised trial of efficacy and safety of inhaled zanamivir in treatment of influenza A and B virus infections. The MIST (Management of Influenza in the Southern Hemisphere Trialists) Study Group. Lancet 352:1877-81, 1998.

Rex JH, Sobel JD. Prophylactic antifungal therapy in the intensive care unit. Clin Infect Dis 32:1191-200, 2001.

Ryan Et, Wilson ME, Kain KC. Illness after international travel. N Engl J Med 347:505-516, 2002.

Segreti J. Is antibiotic prophylaxis necessary for preventing prosthetic device infection. Infect Dis Clin North Am 13:871-7, 1999.

Seymour RA, Whitworth JM. Antibiotic prophylaxis for endocarditis, prosthetic joints, and surgery. Dent Clin North Am 46:635-51, 2002.

Sganga G. New perspectives in antibiotic prophylaxis for intra-abdominal surgery. J Hosp Infect 50 (Suppl A):S17-21, 2002.

Sobel JD, Rex JH. Invasive candidiasis: Turning risk into a practical prevention policy? Clin Infect Dis 33:187-190, 2001.

Steinman RM, Dhodapkar M. Active immunization against cancer with dendritic cells: the near future. Int J Cancer 94:459-73, 2001.

Vazquez M, LaRussa PS, Gershon AA, et al. The effectiveness of the varicella vaccine in clinical practice. N Engl J Med 344:955-60, 2001.

Waddell TK, Rotstein OD. Antimicrobial prophylaxis in surgery. Committee on Antimicrobial Agents, Canadian Infectious Disease Society. CMAJ 151:925-31, 1994.

Wendel Jr GD, Sheffield JS, Hollier LM, et al. Treatment of syphilis in pregnancy and prevention of congenital syphilis. Clin Infect Dis 15;35 (Suppl 2):S200-9, 2002.

Wertzel H, Swoboda L, Joos-Wurtemberger A, et al. Perioperative antibiotic prophylaxis in general thoracic surgery. Thorac Cardiovasc Surg 40:326-9, 1992.

Whitney CG, Farley MM, Hadler J et al. Decline in Invasive pneumococcal disease after the introduction of protein-polysaccharide conjugate vaccine. N Engl J Med 348:1737-46, 2003.

Wingard JR. Antifungal chemoprophylaxis after blood and marrow transplantation. Clin Infect Dis 34:1386-90, 2002.

Winstanley PA, Ward SA, Snow RW. Clinical status and implications of antimalarial drug resistance. Microbes Infect 4:157-64, 2002.

Winston DJ, Busuttil RW. Randomized controlled trial of oral itraconazole solution versus intravenous/oral fluconazole for prevention of fungal infections in liver transplant recipients. Transplantation 74:688-95, 2002.

Wistrom J, Norrby R. Antibiotic prophylaxis of travellers' diarrhoea. Scand J Infect Dis Suppl 70:111-29, 1990.

Wittmann DH, Schein M. Let us shorten antibiotic prophylaxis and therapy in surgery. Am J Surg 172:26S-23S, 1996.

Zelenitsky SA, Ariano RE, Harding GK, et al. Antibiotic pharmacodynamics in surgical prophylaxis: an association between intraoperative antibiotic concentrations and efficacy. Antimicrob Agents Chemother 46:3026-30, 2002.

Zimmerman RK, Burns IT. Childhood immunization guidelines: current and future. Prim Care 21:693-715, 1994.

GUIDELINES

Dykewicz CA. Summary of the guidelines for preventing opportunistic infections among hematopoietic stem cell transplant recipients. Clin Infect Dis. 33:139-44, 2001.

Prevention and control of influenza. Recommendations of the Advisory Committee on Immunization Practices (ACIP). MMWR 51(3), April 12, 2002.

Prevention of Perinatal Group B Streptococcal Disease. Revised CDC guidelines. MMWR 51(11), August 12, 2002.

Recommended adult immunization schedule–United States, 2002-2003. MMWR 51(40):904-8, 2002.

Recommended childhood immunization schedule - United States. MMWR 51(02);31, January 1, 2002.

Use of anthrax vaccine in response to terrorism: supplemental recommendations of the Advisory Committee on Immunization Practices. MMWR 51(No. 45);1024, November 15, 2002.

Yellow fever vaccine. Recommendations of the Advisory Committee on Immunization Practices (ACIP). MMWR 51(17), November 8, 2002.

TEXTBOOKS

Conte Jr JE, Jacob LS, Polk Jr JC (eds). Antibiotic Prophylaxis in Surgery. J.B. Lippincott Company, Philadelphia, 1984.

Keystone JS, Kozarski PE, Freedman DO, et al (eds). Travel Medicine. Mosby, Edinburgh, 2004.

Plotkin SA, Orenstein WA (eds). Vaccines 3rd Edition. W.B. Saunders, Philadelphia, 1999.

Yu VL, Merigan Jr, TC, Barriere SL (eds). Antimicrobial Therapy and Vaccines. Williams & Wilkins, Baltimore, 1999.

Chapter 7
Antimicrobial Drug Summaries

Burke A. Cunha, MD
Demary Castanheira, PharmD
Christy Owens, PharmD
Robert C. Owens, Jr., PharmD
John H. Rex, MD
Mark H. Kaplan, MD

This section contains prescribing information pertinent to the clinical use of 130 antimicrobial agents, as compiled from a variety of sources (p. 404). The information provided is not exhaustive, and the reader is referred to other drug information references and the manufacturer's product literature for further information. Clinical use of the information provided and any consequences that may arise from its use are the responsibilities of the prescribing physician. The authors, editors, and publisher do not warrant or guarantee the information contained in this section, and do not assume and expressly disclaim any liability for errors or omissions or any consequences that may occur from such. The use of any drug should be preceded by careful review of the package insert, which provides indications and dosing approved by the U.S. Food and Drug Administration.

Drugs are listed alphabetically by generic name; trade names follow in parentheses. To search by trade name, consult the index. Each drug summary contains the following information:

Usual dose. Represents the usual dose to treat most susceptible infections in adult patients with normal hepatic and renal function. Dosing for special situations is listed under the comments section; additional information can be found in Chapters 2, 4, 5 and the manufacturer's product literature. Loading doses for doxycycline, fluconazole, itraconazole, voriconazole, caspofungin, ganciclovir, and valganciclovir are described in either the usual dose or comments section. Meningeal doses of antimicrobials used for CNS infection are described at the end of the comments section.

Peak serum level. Refers to the peak serum concentration (mcg/ml) after the usual dose is administered. Peak serum level is useful in calculating the "kill ratios," the ratio of peak serum level to minimum inhibitory concentration (MIC) of the organism. The higher the "kill ratio," the more effective the antimicrobial is likely to be against a particular organism.

Bioavailability. Refers to the percentage of the dose reaching the systemic circulation from the site of administration (PO or IM). For PO antibiotics, bioavailability refers to the percentage of dose adsorbed from the GI tract. For IV antibiotics, "not applicable" appears next to bioavailability, since the entire dose reaches the systemic circulation. Antibiotics with high bioavailability (> 90%) are ideal for IV to PO switch therapy. Antibiotics with low bioavailability are effective if their "kill ratios" are favorable.

Excreted unchanged. Refers to the percentage of drug excreted unchanged, and provides an indirect measure of drug concentration in the urine/feces. Antibiotics excreted unchanged in the urine in low percentage are unlikely to be useful for urinary tract infections.

Serum half-life (normal/ESRD). The serum half-life ($T_{1/2}$) is the time (in hours) in which serum concentration falls by 50%. Serum half-life is useful in determining dosing interval. If the half-life of drugs eliminated by the kidneys is prolonged in end-stage renal disease (ESRD), then the total daily dose is reduced in proportion to the degree of renal dysfunction. If the half-life in ESRD is similar to the normal half-life, then the total daily dose does not change.

Plasma protein binding. Expressed as the percentage of drug reversibly bound to serum albumin. It is the unbound (free) portion of a drug that equilibrates with tissues and imparts antimicrobial activity. Plasma protein binding is not typically a factor in antimicrobial effectiveness unless binding exceeds 95%, and then only if the "kill ratio" is relatively low. Decreases in serum albumin (nephrotic syndrome, liver disease) or competition for protein binding from other drugs or endogenously produced substances (uremia, hyperbilirubinemia) will increase the percentage of free drug available for antimicrobial activity, and may require a decrease in dosage. Increases in serum binding proteins (trauma, surgery, critical illness) will decrease the percentage of free drug available for antimicrobial activity, and may require an increase in dosage.

Volume of distribution (V_d). Represents the apparent volume into which the drug is distributed, and is calculated as the amount of drug in the body divided by the serum concentration (in liters/kilogram). V_d is related to total body water distribution (V_d H_2O = 0.7 L/kg). Hydrophilic (water soluble) drugs are restricted to extracellular fluid and have a $V_d \leq 0.7$ L/kg. In contrast, hydrophobic (highly lipid soluble) drugs penetrate most fluids/tissues of the body and have a large V_d. Drugs that are concentrated in certain tissues (e.g., liver) can have a V_d greatly exceeding total body water. V_d is affected by organ profusion, membrane diffusion/permeability, lipid solubility, protein binding, and state of equilibrium between body compartments. For hydrophilic drugs, increases in V_d may occur with burns, heart failure, dialysis, sepsis, cirrhosis, or mechanical ventilation; decreases in V_d may occur with trauma, hemorrhage, pancreatitis (early), or GI fluid losses. Increases in V_d may require an increase in total daily drug dose for antimicrobial effectiveness; decreases in V_d may require a decrease in drug dose. In addition to drug distribution, V_d reflects binding avidity to cholesterol membranes and concentration within organ tissues (e.g., liver).

Mode of elimination. Refers to the primary route of inactivation/excretion of the antibiotic, which impacts dosing adjustments in renal/hepatic failure.

Dosage adjustments. Each grid provides dosing adjustments based on renal and hepatic function. Antimicrobial dosing for hemodialysis (HD)/peritoneal dialysis (PD) patients is the same as indicated for patients with a CrCl < 10 mL/min. Some antimicrobial agents require a supplemental dose immediately after hemodialysis (post–HD)/peritoneal dialysis (post–PD); following the supplemental dose, antimicrobial dosing should once again resume as indicated for a CrCl < 10 mL/min. "No change" indicates no change from the usual dose. "Avoid" indicates the drug should be avoided in the setting described. "None" indicates no supplemental dose is required. "No information" indicates there are insufficient data from which to make a dosing recommendation. Dosing recommendations are based on data, experience, or pharmacokinetic parameters. CVVH dosing recommendations represent general guidelines, since antibiotic removal is dependent on area/type of filter, ultrafiltration rates, and sieving coefficients; replacement dosing should be individualized and guided by serum levels, if possible. Creatinine clearance (CrCl) is used to gauge the degree of renal insufficiency, and can be estimated by the following calculation: CrCl (mL/min) = [(140 – age) x weight (kg)] / [72 x serum creatinine (mg/dL)]. The calculated value is multiplied by 0.85 for females. It is important to recognize that due to age-dependent decline in renal function, elderly patients with "normal" serum creatinines may have low CrCls requiring dosage adjustments. (For example, a 70-year-old, 50-kg female with a serum creatinine of 1.2 mg/dL has an estimated CrCl of 34 mL/min.) "Antiretroviral Dosage Adjustment" grids indicate recommended dosage adjustments when protease inhibitors (PIs) and non-nucleoside reverse transcriptase inhibitor (NNRTIs) are combined or used in conjunction with rifampin or rifabutin. These grids were compiled, in part, from "Guidelines for the Use of Antiretroviral Agents in HIV-Infected Adults and Adolescents," Panel on Clinical Practices for Treatment of HIV Infection, Department of Health and Human Services, MMWR 51(RR-7), May 17, 2002.

Drug interactions. Refers to common/important drug interactions, as compiled from various sources. If a specific drug interaction is well-documented (e.g, antibiotic X with lovastatin), than other drugs from the same drug class (e.g., atorvastatin) may also be listed, based on theoretical considerations. Drug interactions may occur as a consequence of altered absorption (e.g., metal ion chelation of tetracycline), altered distribution (e.g., sulfonamide displacement of barbiturates from serum albumin), altered metabolism (e.g., rifampin–induced hepatic P-450 metabolism of theophylline/warfarin; chloramphenicol inhibition of phenytoin metabolism), or altered excretion (e.g., probenecid competition with penicillin for active transport in the kidney).

Adverse side effects. Common/important side effects are indicated.

Allergic potential. Described as low or high. Refers to the likelihood of a hypersensitivity reaction to a particular antimicrobial.

Safety in pregnancy. Designated by the U.S. Food and Drug Administration's (USFDA) use-in-pregnancy letter code (Table 1).

Table 1. USFDA Use-in-Pregnancy Letter Code

Category	Interpretation
A	**Controlled studies show no risk.** Adequate, well-controlled studies in pregnant women have not shown a risk to the fetus in any trimester of pregnancy
B	**No evidence of risk in humans.** Adequate, well-controlled studies in pregnant women have not shown increased risk of fetal abnormalities despite adverse findings in animals, or, in the absence of adequate human studies, animal studies show no fetal risk. The chance of fetal harm is remote, but remains a possibility
C	**Risk cannot be ruled out.** Adequate, well-controlled human studies are lacking, and animal studies have shown a risk to the fetus or are lacking. There is a chance of fetal harm if the drug is administered during pregnancy, but potential benefit from use of the drug may outweigh potential risk
D	**Positive evidence of risk.** Studies in humans or investigational or post-marketing data have demonstrated fetal risk. Nevertheless, potential benefit from use of the drug may outweigh potential risk. For example, the drug may be acceptable if needed in a life-threatening situation or serious disease for which safer drugs cannot be used or are ineffective
X	**Contraindicated in pregnancy.** Studies in animals or humans or investigational or post-marketing reports have demonstrated positive evidence of fetal abnormalities or risk which clearly outweigh any possible benefit to the patient

Comments. Includes various useful information for each antimicrobial agent.

Cerebrospinal fluid penetration. Indicated as a percentage relative to peak serum concentration. If an antimicrobial is used for CNS infections, then its meningeal dose is indicated directly above CSF penetration. No meningeal dose is given if CSF penetration is inadequate for treatment of meningitis due to susceptible organisms.

Biliary tract penetration. Indicated as a percentage relative to peak serum concentrations. Percentages > 100% reflect concentration within the biliary system. This information is useful for the treatment of biliary tract infections.

Selected references. These references are classic, important, or recent. When available, the website containing the manufacturer's prescribing information/package insert is provided. (The use of any drug should be preceded by careful review of the package insert, which provides indications and dosing approved by the U.S. Food and Drug Administration.) Additional references, guidelines, and textbooks relating to antimicrobial therapy are listed at the back of each chapter.

Lipid-Associated Formulations of Amphotericin B. There are 3 licensed lipid-associated formulations of amphotericin B (LFAB) (Table 2). Although closely related in some ways, these formulations have distinct properties and must be understood separately. The principal advantage of the LFAB over amphotericin B deoxycholate (AMBD) is greater safety. In general, the rates of both acute infection-related toxicities (fever, chills, etc.) and chronic therapy-associated toxicities (principally nephrotoxicity) are reduced with LFAB. However, the LFAB can produce all of the toxicities of AMBD (and in selected patients, LFAB have been more toxic than AMBD). Overall, LAMB (AmBisome) and ABLC (Abelcet) appear to be safer than ABCD (Amphotec, Amphocil). Whichever formulation is selected for therapy, it is important to specify its name carefully when prescribing. The phrase "lipid amphotericin B" should be avoided due to its imprecision. Patients who are tolerating one formulation may develop all the standard infusion-related toxicities if switched inadvertently to a new formulation. In general (and in contrast to the usual preference for generic names), use of trade names is the clearest way to specify the choice of drug in this category. In this handbook, the phrase "lipid-associated formulation of amphotericin B" suggests use of any of the 3 formulations. The issues surrounding the selection of an LFAB for an individual patient are summarized in Table 2 (see comments).

Table 2. Lipid-Associated Formulations of Amphotericin B

Generic name (abbreviation)	Trade names	Licensed (IV) dosages in the United States	Comments
Amphotericin B lipid complex (ABLC)	Abelcet	5 mg/kg/d	Reliable choice; long history of use
Liposomal amphotericin B (LAMB)	AmBisome	3 mg/kg/d (empiric therapy) 3-5 mg/kg/d (systemic fungal infections) 6 mg/kg/d (cryptococcal meningitis in HIV patients)	Reliable choice; best studied LFAB; well-supported dosing recommendations by indication; probably the least nephrotoxic; good data to support increasing the dose safely
Amphotericin B colloidal dispersion, amphotericin B cholesteryl sulfate complex (ABCD)	Amphotec, Amphocil	3-4 mg/kg/d	Infusion-related toxicities have limited its use

References:
Arikan S, Rex JH. Lipid-based antifungal agents: Current status. Curr Pharm Design 7:393-415, 2001.
Groll AH, Walsh TJ. Antifungal drugs. Side Effects of Drugs Annual 26:302-314, 2003.
Ostrosky-Zeichner L, Marr KA, Rex JH, Cohen SH. Amphotericin B: Time for a new "gold standard." Clin Infect Dis 37:415-425, 2003.

Abacavir (Ziagen)

Drug Class: Antiretroviral NRTI (nucleoside reverse transcriptase inhibitor)
Usual Dose: 300 mg (PO) q12h
Pharmacokinetic Parameters:
Peak serum level: 3 mcg/mL
Bioavailability: 83%
Excreted unchanged (urine): 1.2%
Serum half-life (normal/ESRD): 1.5 /8 hrs
Plasma protein binding: 50%
Volume of distribution (V_d): 0.86 L/kg
Primary Mode of Elimination: Hepatic
Dosage Adjustments*

CrCl ~ 40–60 mL/min	No change
CrCl ~ 10–40 mL/min	No change
CrCl < 10 mL/min	No change
Post–HD dose	None
Post–PD dose	None
CVVH dose	No change
Mild hepatic insufficiency	200 mg (PO) q24h
Moderate or severe hepatic insufficiency	Avoid

Drug Interactions: Methadoner (↑ methadone clearance with abacavir 600 mg bid); ethanol (↑ abacavir serum levels/half-life and may ↑ toxicity)
Adverse Effects: *Abacavir may cause severe hypersensitivity reactions (see comments), usually during the first 4-6 weeks of therapy, which may be fatal;* report cases of hypersensitivity syndrome to Abacavir Hypersensitivity Registry at 1-800-270-0425. Drug fever/rash, abdominal pain/diarrhea, nausea, vomiting, anorexia, insomnia, weakness, headache, ↑ SGOT/SGPT, hyperglycemia, hypertriglyceridemia, lactic acidosis with hepatic steatosis (rare, but potentially life-threatening toxicity with use of NRTIs)
Allergic Potential: High (~ 5%)
Safety in Pregnancy: C

Comments: May be taken with or without foods. Discontinue abacavir and **do not restart in patients with signs/symptoms of hypersensitiviy reaction**, which may include fever, rash, fatigue, nausea, vomiting, diarrhea, abdominal pain, anorexia, respiratory symptoms. Effective antiretroviral therapy consists of at least 3 antiretrovirals (same/different classes)
Cerebrospinal Fluid Penetration: 27-33%

REFERENCES:
Carr A, Workman C, Smith DE, et al. Abacavir substitution for nucleoside analogs in patients with HIV lipotropin. A randomized trial. JAMA 288:207-15, 2002.
Katalama C, Clotet B, Plettenberg A, et al. The role of abacavir (AVC, 1592) in antiretroviral therapy-experiences patients: results from randomized, double-blind, trial. CNA3002 European Study Team. AIDS 14:781-9, 2000.
Keating MR. Antiviral agents. Mayo Clin Proc 67:160-78, 1992.
McDowell JA, Lou Y, Symonds WS, et al. Multiple-dose pharmacokinetics and pharmacodynamics of abacavir alone and in combination with zidovudine in human immunodeficiency virus-infected adults. Antimicrob Agents Chemother 44:2061-7, 2000.
Panel on Clinical Practices for Treatment of HIV Infection. Guidelines for the Use of Antiretroviral Agents in HIV-Infected Adults and Adolescents. Department of Health and Human Services. www.aidsinfo.nih.gov/guidelines/. November 10, 2003.
Staszewski S, Keiser P, Mantaner J, et al. Abacavir-lamivudine-zidovudine vs. indinavir-lamivudine-zidovudine in antiretroviral-naive HIV-infected adults: a randomized equivalence trial. JAMA 285:1155-63, 2001.
Website: www.TreatHIV.com

Abacavir + lamivudine + zidovudine (Trizivir)

Drug Class: Antiretroviral NRTI combination
Usual Dose: Trizivir tablet = abacavir 300 mg + lamivudine 150 mg + zidovudine 300 mg. Usual dose = 1 tablet (PO) q12h
Pharmacokinetic Parameters:
Peak serum level: 3/1.5/1.2 mcg/mL
Bioavailability: 86/86/64%
Excreted unchanged (urine): 1.2/90/16%

"Usual dose" assumes normal renal/hepatic function. * For renal insufficiency, give usual dose x 1 followed by maintenance dose per CrCl. For dialysis patients, dose the same as for CrCl < 10 mL/min and give supplemental (post-HD/PD dose) immediately after dialysis. CrCl = creatinine clearance; CVVH = continuous veno-venous hemo-filtration; HD/PD = hemodialysis/peritoneal dialysis. See pp. 293-297 for explanations, p. 1 for abbreviations

Serum half-life (normal/ESRD): [1.5/6/1.1] / 8/20/2.2] hrs
Plasma protein binding: 30/36/20%
Volume of distribution (V_d): 0.86/1.3/1.6 L/kg
Primary Mode of Elimination: Hepatic/renal
Dosage Adjustments*

CrCl < 50 mL/min	Avoid
Post–HD or post-PD	Avoid
CVVH dose	Avoid
Moderate or severe hepatic insufficiency	Not recommended

Drug Interactions: Amprenavir, atovaquone (↑ zidovudine levels); clarithromycin (↓ zidovudine levels); cidofovir (↑ zidovudine levels, flu-like symptoms); doxorubicin (neutropenia); stavudine (antagonistic to zidovudine; avoid combination); TMP-SMX (↑ lamivudine and zidovudine levels); zalcitabine (↓ lamivudine levels)
Adverse Effects: *Abacavir may cause severe/fatal rash/hypersensitivity reaction;* do not restart after reaction. Must not be used in patients with prior abacavir reactions. Most common (>5%): nausea, vomiting, diarrhea, anorexia, insomnia, fever/chills, headache, malaise/fatigue. Others (less common): peripheral neuropathy, myopathy, steatosis, pancreatitis. Lab abnormalities: mild hyperglycemia, anemia, LFT elevations, hypertriglyceridemia, leukopenia
Allergic Potential: High (~5%)
Safety in Pregnancy: C
Comments: Avoid in patients with CrCl < 50 mL/min. May be taken with or without food. HBV hepatitis may relapse if lamivudine is discontinued

REFERENCES:
Havlir DV, Lange JM. New antiretrovirals and new combinations. AIDS 12(Suppl A):S165-74, 1998.
McDowell JA, Lou Y, Symonds WS, et al. Multiple-dose pharmacokinetics and pharmacodynamics of abacavir alone and in combination with zidovudine in human immunodeficiency virus-infected adults. Antimicrob Agents Chemother 44:2061-7, 2000.
Three new drugs for HIV infection. Med Lett Drugs Ther 40:114-6, 1998.

Weverling GJ, Lange JM, Jurriaans S, et al. Alternative multidrug regimen provides improved suppression of HIV-1 replication over triple therapy. AIDS 12:117-22, 1998.
Website: www.TreatHIV.com

Acyclovir (Zovirax)

Drug Class: Antiviral
Usual Dose: <u>HSV</u>: 5 mg/kg (IV) q8h until able to take PO, then 400 mg (PO) 5x/day for 10-day total course. <u>VZV</u>: 10 mg/kg (IV) q8h until able to take PO, then 800 mg (PO) 5x/day for 10-day total course
Pharmacokinetic Parameters:
Peak serum level: 7.7 mcg/mL
Bioavailability: 30%
Excreted unchanged: 70%
Serum half-life (normal/ESRD): 3/5 hrs
Plasma protein binding: 30%
Volume of distribution (V_d): 0.7 L/kg
Primary Mode of Elimination: Renal
Dosage Adjustments* for HSV/VZV

CrCl ~ 10-25 mL/min	No change; 800 mg (PO) q8h
CrCl < 10 mL/min	200 mg (PO) q12h; 800 mg (PO) q12h
Post–HD dose	200 mg (IV/PO); 800 mg (IV/PO)
Post–PD dose	None
CVVH dose	See CrCl 10-25 mL/min
Moderate or severe hepatic insufficiency	No change

Drug Interactions: Cimetidine, probenecid (↑ acyclovir levels); nephrotoxic drugs (↑ nephrotoxicity); zidovudine (lethargy)
Adverse Effects: Seizures/tremors (dose related), crystalluria. Base dose on ideal body weight in the elderly to minimize adverse effects
Allergic Potential: Low
Safety in Pregnancy: C
Comments: Na+ content = 4 mEq/g. CSF levels may be increased with probenecid.

"Usual dose" assumes normal renal/hepatic function. * For renal insufficiency, give usual dose x 1 followed by maintenance dose per CrCl. For dialysis patients, dose the same as for CrCl < 10 mL/min and give supplemental (post-HD/PD dose) immediately after dialysis. CrCl = creatinine clearance; CVVH = continuous veno-venous hemofiltration; HD/PD = hemodialysis/peritoneal dialysis. See pp. 293-297 for explanations, p. 1 for abbreviations

Meningeal dose = VZV/HSV encephalitis dose
Cerebrospinal Fluid Penetration: 50%

REFERENCES:
Keating MR. Antiviral Agents. Mayo Clin Proc 67:160-78, 1992.
Geers TA, Isada CM. Update on antiviral therapy for genital herpes infection. Cleve Clinic J Med 67:567-73, 2000.
Owens RC, Ambrose PG. Acyclovir. Antibiotics for Clinicians 1:85-93, 1997.
Whitley RJ, Gnann JW Jr. Acyclovir: a decade later. N Engl J Med 327:782-3, 1992
Website: www.pdr.net.

Adefovir dipivoxil (Hepsera)

Drug Class: Antiretroviral NRTI (nucleotide reverse transcriptase inhibitor)
Usual Dose: 10 mg (PO) q24h
Pharmacokinetic Parameters:
Peak serum level: 18 ng/mL
Bioavailability: 59%
Excreted unchanged: 45%
Serum half-life (normal/ESRD): 7.5/9 hrs
Plasma protein binding: 4%
Volume of distribution (V_d): 0.4 L/kg
Primary Mode of Elimination: Renal
Dosage Adjustments*

CrCl ≥ 50 mL/min	10 mg (PO) q24h
CrCl ~ 20-49 mL/min	10 mg (PO) q48h
CrCl ~ 10–19 mL/min	10 mg (PO) q72h
Hemodialysis	10 mg (PO) q7d
Post–HD or PD dose	No information
CVVH dose	No information
Moderate or severe hepatic insufficiency	No change

Drug Interactions: No significant interaction with lamivudine, TMP-SMX, acetaminophen, ibuprofen
Adverse Effects: Asthenia, headache, abdominal pain, nausea, flatulence, diarrhea, dyspepsia
Allergic Potential: Low

Safety in Pregnancy: C
Comments: May be taken with or without food. Does not inhibit CP450 isoenzymes. Do not discontinue abruptly to avoid exacerbation of HBV hepatitis
Cerebrospinal Fluid Penetration: No data

REFERENCES:
Cundy KC, Burditch-Crovo P, Walker RE, et al. Clinical pharmacokinetics of adefovir in human HIV-1 infected patients. Antimicrob Agents Chemother 35:2401-2405, 1995.
Davis GL. Update on the management of chronic hepatitis B. Rev Gastroenterol Disord 2:106-15, 2002.
Hadziyannis SJ, Tassopoulos NC, Heathcote E, et al. Adefovir dipivoxil for the treatment of hepatitis B e antigien-negative chonic hepatitis B. N Engl J Med 348:800-7, 2003.
Perillo R, Schiff E, Yoshida E, et al. Adefovir for the treatment of lamivudine-resistant hepatitis B mutants. Hepatology 32:129-34, 2000.
Website: www.hepsera.com

Amantadine (Symmetrel)

Drug Class: Antiviral
Usual Dose: 200 mg (PO) q24h
Pharmacokinetic Parameters:
Peak serum level: 0.5 mcg/mL
Bioavailability: 90%
Excreted unchanged: 90%
Serum half-life (normal/ESRD): 16/192 hrs
Plasma protein binding: 67%
Volume of distribution (V_d): 6.6 L/kg
Primary Mode of Elimination: Renal
Dosage Adjustments*

CrCl ~ 30–50 mL/min	100 mg (PO) q24h
CrCl ~ 15–29 mL/min	100 mg (PO) q48h
CrCl < 15 mL/min	200 mg (PO) qweek
Post–HD	200 mg (PO) qweek
Post–PD	None
CVVH dose	100 mg (PO) q48h
Moderate or severe hepatic insufficiency	No change

Drug Interactions: Alcohol (↑ CNS effects);

benztropine, trihexyphenidyl (↑ interacting drug effect: dry mouth, ataxia); CNS stimulants (additive stimulation); digoxin (↑ digoxin levels); trimethoprim (↑ amantadine and trimethoprim levels); scopolamine (↑ scopolamine effect: blurred vision, slurred speech, toxic psychosis)

Adverse Effects: Confusion/delusions, dysarthria, ataxia, anticholinergic effects (blurry vision, dry mouth, orthostatic hypotension, urinary retention, constipation), livedo reticularis, may ↑ QT_c interval

Allergic Potential: Low

Safety in Pregnancy: C

Comments: May precipitate heart failure. Avoid co-administration with anticholinergics, MAO inhibitors, or antihistamines

Cerebrospinal Fluid Penetration:
Non-inflamed meninges = 15%
Inflamed meninges = 20%

REFERENCES:
Douglas RG, Jr. Prophylaxis and treatment of influenza. N Engl J Med 322:443-50, 1990.
Gubareva LV, Kaiser L, Hayden FG. Influenza virus neuraminidase inhibitors. Lancet 355:827-5, 2000.
Keyers LA, Karl M, Nafziger AN, et al. Comparison of central nervous system adverse effects of amantadine and rimantadine used as sequential prophylaxis of influenza A in elderly nursing home patients. Arch Intern Med 160:1485-8, 2000.
Website: www.pdr.net

Amikacin (Amikin)

Drug Class: Aminoglycoside
Usual Dose: 15 mg/kg or 1 gm (IV) q24h (preferred to q12h dosing)
Pharmacokinetic Parameters:
Peak serum level: 20-30 mcg/mL (q12h dosing); 65-75 mcg/mL (q24h dosing)
Bioavailability: Not applicable
Excreted unchanged: 95%
Serum half-life (normal/ESRD): 2/50 hrs
Plasma protein binding: < 5%
Volume of distribution (V_d): 0.25 L/kg
Primary Mode of Elimination: Renal
Dosage Adjustments*

CrCl ~ 40–60 mL/min	7.5 mg/kg (IV) q24h or 500 mg (IV) q24h
CrCl ~ 10–40 mL/min	7.5 mg/kg (IV) q48h or 500 mg (IV) q48h
CrCl < 10 mL/min	3.75 mg/kg (IV) q48h or 250 mg (IV) q48h
Post–HD dose	7.5 mg/kg (IV) or 500 mg (IV)
Post–PD dose	3.75 mg/kg (IV) or 250 mg (IV)
CVVH dose	7.5 mg/kg (IV) or 500 mg (IV) q12h
Moderate or severe hepatic insufficiency	No change

Drug Interactions: Amphotericin B, cephalothin, cyclosporine, enflurane, methoxyflurane, NSAIDs, polymyxin B, radiographic contrast, vancomycin (↑ nephrotoxicity); cis-platinum (↑ nephrotoxicity, ↑ ototoxicity); loop diuretics (↑ ototoxicity); neuromuscular blocking agents (↑ apnea, prolonged paralysis); non-polarizing muscle relaxants (↑ apnea)

Adverse Effects: Neuromuscular blockade with rapid infusion/absorption. Nephrotoxicity only with prolonged/extremely high serum trough levels; may cause reversible non–oliguric renal failure (ATN). Ototoxicity associated with prolonged/extremely high peak serum levels (usually irreversible): Cochlear toxicity (1/3 of ototoxicity) manifests as decreased high frequency hearing, but deafness is unusual. Vestibular toxicity (2/3 of ototoxicity) develops before ototoxicity (typically manifests as tinnitus)

Allergic Potential: Low

Safety in Pregnancy: D

Comments: Dose for synergy = 7.5 mg/kg (IV) q24h or 500 mg (IV) q24h. Single daily dosing greatly reduces nephrotoxic/ototoxic potential. Incompatible with solutions containing β–lactams, erythromycin, chloramphenicol, furosemide, sodium bicarbonate. IV infusion should be given slowly over 30 minutes. May be given IM. Avoid intraperitoneal infusion due to risk of neuromuscular blockade. Avoid intratracheal/aerosolized intrapulmonary

---

"Usual dose" assumes normal renal/hepatic function. * For renal insufficiency, give usual dose x 1 followed by maintenance dose per CrCl. For dialysis patients, dose the same as for CrCl < 10 mL/min and give supplemental (post-HD/PD dose) immediately after dialysis. CrCl = creatinine clearance; CVVH = continuous veno-venous hemo-filtration; HD/PD = hemodialysis/peritoneal dialysis. See pp. 293-297 for explanations, p. 1 for abbreviations

instillation, which may predispose to antibiotic resistance. V_d increases with edema/ascites, trauma, burns, cystic fibrosis; may require ↑ dose. V_d decreases with dehydration, obesity; may require ↓ dose. Renal cast counts are the best indicator of aminoglycoside nephrotoxicity, not serum creatinine. Dialysis removes ~ 50% of amikacin from serum. Na⁺ content = 1.3 mEq/g

Therapeutic Serum Concentrations:
Peak (q24h/q12h dosing): 65-75/20-30 mcg/mL
Trough (q24h/q12h dosing): 0/4-8 mcg/mL
Intrathecal (IT) dose = 10–20 mg (IT) q24h

Cerebrospinal Fluid Penetration:
Non-inflamed meninges = 15%
Inflamed meninges = 20%

Bile Penetration: 30%

REFERENCES:
Bacopoulou F, Markantonis SL, Pavlou E, et al. A study of once-daily amikacin with low peak target concentrations in intensive care unit patients: pharmacokinetics and associated outcomes. J Crit Care. 18:107-13, 2003.

Cunha BA. Aminoglycosides: Current role in antimicrobial therapy. Pharmacotherapy 8: 334-50,1988.

Cunha BA. Pseudomonas aeruginosa: Resistance and therapy. Semin Respir Infect 17:231-9, 2002.

Edson RS, Terrel CL. The Aminoglycosides. Mayo Clin Proc 74:519-28, 1999.

Karakoc B, Gerceker AA. In-vitro activities of various antibiotics, alone and in combination with amikacin against Pseudomonas aeruginosa. Int J Antimicrob Agents 18:567-70, 2001.

Amoxicillin (Amoxil, A-cillin, Polymox, Trimox, Wymox)

Drug Class: Aminopenicillin
Usual Dose: 1 gm (PO) q8h

Pharmacokinetic Parameters:
Peak serum level: 14 mcg/mL
Bioavailability: 90%
Excreted unchanged: 60%
Serum half-life (normal/ESRD): 1.3/16 hrs
Plasma protein binding: 20%
Volume of distribution (V_d): 0.26 L/kg

Primary Mode of Elimination: Renal

Dosage Adjustments*

CrCl ~ 30-60 mL/min	500 mg (PO) q8h
CrCl ~ 10–30 mL/min	500 mg (PO) q12h
CrCl < 10 mL/min	500 mg (PO) q24h
Post–HD or post-PD	500 mg
CVVH dose	500 mg (PO) q12h
Moderate or severe hepatic insufficiency	No change

Drug Interactions: Allopurinol (↑ risk of rash)
Adverse Effects: Drug fever/rash, ↑SGOT/SGPT
Allergic Potential: High
Safety in Pregnancy: B
Comments: No irritative diarrhea with 1 gm (PO) q8h dose due to nearly complete proximal GI absorption. Na⁺ content = 2.7 mEq/g

Cerebrospinal Fluid Penetration:
Non-inflamed/inflamed meninges = 1%/8%

Bile Penetration: 3000%

REFERENCES:
[No authors listed]. Acute otitis media in children: amoxicillin remains the standard antibiotic, but justified in certain situations only. Prescrire Int. 12:184-9, 2003.

Cunha BA. The aminopenicillins. Urology 40:186-190,1992.

Curtin-Wirt C, Casey JR, Murray PC, et al. Efficacy of penicillin vs. amoxicillin in children with group A beta hemolytic streptococcal tonsillopharyngitis. Clin Pediatr (Phila). 42:219-25, 2003.

Donowitz GR, Mandell GL. Beta-lactam antibiotics. N Engl J Med 318:419-26 and 318:490-500, 1993.

Piglansky L, Leibovitz E, Raiz S, et al. Bacteriologic and clinical efficacy of high dose amoxicillin for therapy of acute otitis media in children. Pediatr Infect Dis J. 22:405-13, 2003.

Website: www.pdr.net

"Usual dose" assumes normal renal/hepatic function. * For renal insufficiency, give usual dose x 1 followed by maintenance dose per CrCl. For dialysis patients, dose the same as for CrCl < 10 mL/min and give supplemental (post-HD/PD dose) immediately after dialysis. CrCl = creatinine clearance; CVVH = continuous veno-venous hemo-filtration; HD/PD = hemodialysis/peritoneal dialysis. See pp. 293-297 for explanations, p. 1 for abbreviations

Amoxicillin/Clavulanic Acid (Augmentin)

Drug Class: Aminopenicillin/β-lactamase inhibitor combination
Usual Dose: 500/125 mg (PO) q8h or 875/125 mg (PO) q12h for severe infections or respiratory tract infections
Pharmacokinetic Parameters:
Peak serum level: 10.0/2.2 mcg/mL
Bioavailability: 90/60%
Excreted unchanged: 80/40%
Serum half-life (normal/ESRD): [1.3/16]/[1/2] hrs
Plasma protein binding: 18/25%
Volume of distribution (V_d): 0.26/0.3 L/kg
Primary Mode of Elimination: Renal
Dosage Adjustments* (based on 500 mg q8h):

CrCl ~ 40–60 mL/min	500/125 mg (PO) q12h
CrCl ~ 10–40 mL/min	500/125 mg (PO) q24h
CrCl < 10 mL/min	250/125 mg (PO) q24h
Post–HD dose	250/125 mg (PO)
Post–PD dose	None
CVVH dose	500/125 mg (PO) q24h
Moderate or severe hepatic insufficiency	No change

Drug Interactions: Allopurinol (↑ risk of rash)
Adverse Effects: Drug fever/rash, diarrhea, ↑ SGOT/SGPT. Rash same as ampicillin
Allergic Potential: High
Safety in Pregnancy: B
Comments: 875/125 mg formulation should not be used in patients with CrCl < 30 mL/min
Cerebrospinal Fluid Penetration:
Non-inflamed meninges = 1%
Inflamed meninges = 1%
Bile Penetration: 3000%

REFERENCES:
Cunha BA. Amoxicillin/clavulanic acid in respiratory infections: microbiologic and pharmacokinetic considerations. Clinical Therapeutics 14:418-25, 1992.
Donowitz GR, Mandell GL. Beta-lactam antibiotics. N Engl J Med 318:419-26 and 318:490-500, 1993.
Easton J, Noble S, Perry CM. Amoxicillin/clavulanic acid: a review of its use in the management of paediatric patients with acute otitis media. Drugs. 63:311-40, 2003.
Fernandez-Sabe N, Carratala J, Dorca J, et al. Efficacy and safety of sequential amoxicillin-clavulanate in the treatment of anaerobic lung infections. Eur J Clin Microbiol Infect Dis. 22:185-7, 2003.
Klein JO. Amoxicillin/clavulanate for infections in infants and children: past, present and future. Pediatr Infect Dis J. 22:S139-48, 2003.
Scaglione F, Caronzolo D, Pintucci JP, et al. Measurement of cefaclor and amoxicillin-clavulanic acid levels in middle-ear fluid in patients with acute otitis media. Antimicrob Agents Chemother. 47:2987-9, 2003.
Wright AJ, Wilkowske CJ. The penicillins. Mayo Clin Proc 66:1047-63, 1991.
Website: www.augmentin.com

Amoxicillin/Clavulanic Acid ES-600 (Augmentin ES-600)

Drug Class: Aminopenicillin/β-lactamase inhibitor combination
Usual Dose: 90 mg/kg/day oral suspension in 2 divided doses (see comments)
Pharmacokinetic Parameters:
Peak serum level: 15.7/1.7 mcg/mL
Bioavailability: 90/60%
Excreted unchanged: 70/40%
Serum half-life (normal/ESRD): [1.4/16]/[1.1/2] hrs
Plasma protein binding: 18%/25%
Volume of distribution (V_d): 0.26/0.3 L/kg
Primary Mode of Elimination: Renal
Dosage Adjustments*

CrCl < 30 mL/min	Avoid
Moderate or severe hepatic insufficiency	Use with caution

Drug Interactions: Allopurinol (↑ risk of rash)
Adverse Effects: Drug fever/rash, diarrhea, ↑ SGOT/SGPT. Rash potential same as ampicillin
Allergic Potential: High
Safety in Pregnancy: B
Comments: 5 mL contains 600 mg amoxicillin and 42.9 mg clavulanatic acid. Use in children > 3 months. Take at start of meal to minimize GI

"Usual dose" assumes normal renal/hepatic function. * For renal insufficiency, give usual dose x 1 followed by maintenance dose per CrCl. For dialysis patients, dose the same as for CrCl < 10 mL/min and give supplemental (post-HD/PD dose) immediately after dialysis. CrCl = creatinine clearance; CVVH = continuous veno-venous hemofiltration; HD/PD = hemodialysis/peritoneal dialysis. See pp. 293-297 for explanations, p. 1 for abbreviations

upset. Do not subsitute 400 mg or 200 mg/5 mL formulation for ES-600. Not for children < 3 months or > 40 kg. Contains phenylalanine

Volume of ES-600 to provide 90 mg/kg/day:

Weight	Volume (q12h)	Weight	Volume (q12h)
8 kg	3.0 mL	24 kg	9.0 mL
12 kg	4.5 mL	28 kg	10.5 mL
16 kg	6.0 mL	32 kg	12.0 mL
20 kg	7.5 mL	36 kg	13.5 mL

Cerebrospinal Fluid Penetration:
Non-inflamed meninges = 1%
Inflamed meninges = 1%
Bile Penetration: 3000%

REFERENCES:
Dagan R, Hoberman A, Johnson C, et al. Bacteriologic and clinical efficacy of high dose amoxicillin/clavulanate in children with acute otitis media. Pediatr Infect Dis J 20:829-37, 2001.
Easton J, Noble S, Perry CM. Amoxicillin/clavulanic acid: a review of its use in the management of paediatric patients with acute otitis media. Drugs 63:311-40, 2003.
Ghaffar F, Muniz LS, Katz K, et al. Effects of large dosages of amoxicillin/clavulanate or azithromycin on nasopharyngeal carriage of Streptococcus pneumoniae, Haemophilus influenzae, nonpneumococcal alpha-hemolytic streptococci, and Staphylococcus aureus in children with acute otitis media. Clin Infect Dis 34:1301-9, 2002.
Website: www.augmentin.com

Amoxicillin/Clavulanic Acid XR (Augmentin XR)

Drug Class: Aminopenicillin/β-lactamase inhibitor combination
Usual Dose: 2 tablets (PO) q12h (see comments)
Pharmacokinetic Parameters:
Peak serum level: 17/2 mcg/mL
Bioavailability: 90/60%
Excreted unchanged: 70/40%
Serum half-life (normal/ESRD): [1.3/16]/[1/2] hrs
Plasma protein binding: 18/25%
Volume of distribution (V_d): 0.26/0.3 L/kg
Primary Mode of Elimination: Renal
Dosage Adjustments*

CrCl ~ 30–60 mL/min	No change
CrCl < 30 mL/min	Avoid
Post–HD/PD dose	Avoid
CVVH dose	Avoid
Moderate or severe hepatic insufficiency	Use with caution

Drug Interactions: Allopurinol (↑ risk of rash); may ↓ effectiveness of oral contraceptives
Adverse Effects: Drug fever, rash, diarrhea, ↑ SGOT/SGPT, nausea, abdominal pain
Allergic Potential: High
Safety in Pregnancy: B
Comments: Amoxicillin/clavulanic acid XR is a time-released formulation. Do not crush tablets. XR formulation contains a different ratio of amoxicillin/clavulanic acid so other formulations cannot be interchanged. 2 tablets (1000/62.5 mg per tablet) = 2000/125 mg per dose. Take with food (not high fat meal) to increase absorption
Cerebrospinal Fluid Penetration:
Non-inflamed meninges = 1%
Inflamed meninges = 1%
Bile Penetration: 3000%

REFERENCES:
[No authors listed]. Augmentin XR. Med Lett Drugs Ther. 45:5-6, 2003.
Benninger MS. Amoxicillin/clavulanate potassium extended release tablets: a new antimicrobial for the treatment of acute bacterial sinusitis and community-acquired pneumonia. Expert Opin Pharmacother. 4:1839-46, 2003.
File Jr TM, Jacobs M, Poole M, et al. Outcome of treatment of respiratory tract infections due to Streptococcus pneumoniae, including drug-resistant strains, with pharmacokinetically enhanced amoxicillin/clavulatate. International J Antimicrobial Agents 20:235-247, 2002.
Kaye C, Allen A, Perry S, et al. The clinical pharmacokinetics of a new pharmacokinetically enhanced formulation of amoxicillin/clavulatate. Clin Therapeutics 23:578-584, 2001.
Website: www.augmentin.com

Amphotericin B (Fungizone)

Drug Class: Antifungal
Usual Dose: 0.5-0.8 mg/kg (IV) q24h
Pharmacokinetic Parameters:
Peak serum level: 1-2 mcg/mL
Bioavailability: Not applicable
Excreted unchanged: 5%
Serum half-life (normal/ESRD): 15/48 days
Plasma protein binding: 90%
Volume of distribution (V_d): 4 L/kg
Primary Mode of Elimination: Metabolized
Dosage Adjustments*

CrCl ~ 40–60 mL/min	No change
CrCl ~ 10–40 mL/min	No change
CrCl < 10 mL/min	0.5-0.8 mg/kg (IV) q36h
Post–HD or post-PD	None
CVVH dose	None
Moderate or severe hepatic insufficiency	No change

Drug Interactions: Adrenocorticoids (hypokalemia); aminoglycosides, cyclosporine, polymyxin B (↑ nephrotoxicity); digoxin (↑ digitalis toxicity due to hypokalemia); flucytosine (↑ flucytosine levels if amphotericin B produces renal dysfunction); neuromuscular blocking agents (↑ neuromuscular blockade due to hypokalemia)
Adverse Effects: Fevers/chills, flushing thrombophlebitis, bradycardia, seizures, hypotension, distal renal tubular acidosis (↓ K⁺/↓ Mg⁺⁺), anemia. If renal insufficiency is secondary to amphotericin, either ↓ daily dose by 50%, give amphotericin every other day, or switch to an amphotericin lipid formulation
Allergic Potential: Low
Safety in Pregnancy: B
Comments: Higher doses (1-1.5 mg/kg q24h) may be needed in severe life-threatening situations. Reconstitute in sterile water, not in dextrose, saline, or bacteriostatic water. Do not co-administer in same IV with other drugs. Give by slow IV infusion over 2 hours initially. Test dose unnecessary. Amphotericin B with granulocyte colony stimulating factor (GCSF) may result in ARDS. Amphotericin B with pentamidine may cause acute tubular necrosis in HIV/AIDS patients. Fevers/chills may be reduced by meperidine, aspirin, NSAIDs, hydrocortisone or acetaminophen, if given 30-60 minutes before infusion. For bladder irrigation, use 50 mg/L until cultures are negative.
Meningeal dose = usual dose plus 0.5 mg 3-5x/week (IT) via Ommaya reservoir
Cerebrospinal Fluid Penetration: < 10%

REFERENCES:
Arikan S, Lozano-Chiu M, Paetznick V, et al. In vitro synergy of caspofungin and amphotericin B against Aspergillus and Fusarium spp. Antimicrob Agents Chemother 46:245-7, 2002.
Cagnoni PJ. Liposomal amphotericin B versus conventional amphotericin B in the empirical treatment of persistently febrile neutropenic patients. J Antimicrob Chemother 49 Suppl 1:81-6, 2002.
Chocarro Martinez A, Gonzalez A, Garcia I. Caspofungin versus amphotericin B for the treatment of Candidal esophagitis. Clin Infect Dis 35:107; discussion 107-8, 2002.
Cruz JM, Peacock JE Jr., Loomer L, et al. Rapid intravenous infusion of Amphotericin B: A pilot study. Am J Med 93:123-30, 1992.
Deray G. Amphotericin B nephrotoxicity. J Antimicrob Chemother 49 Suppl 1:37-41, 2002.
Dupont B. Overview of the lipid formulations of amphotericin B. J Antimicrob Chemother 49 Suppl 1:31-6, 2002.
Ellis D. Amphotericin B: spectrum and resistance. J Antimicrob Chemother 49 Suppl 1:7-10, 2002.
Gallis HA, Drew RH, Pickard WW. Amphotericin B: 30 years of clinical experience. Rev Infect Dis 12:308-29, 1990.
Grim SA, Smith KM, Romanelli F, et al. Treatment of azole-resistant oropharyngeal candidiasis with topical amphotericin B. Ann Pharmacother 36:1383-6, 2002.
Lyman CA, Walsh TJ. Systemically administered antifungal agents: A review of their clinical pharmacology and therapeutic applications. Drugs 44:9-35, 1992.
Menzies D, Goel K, Cunha BA. Amphotericin B. Antibiotics for Clinicians 2:73-6, 1998.
Moosa MY, Alangaden GJ, Manavathu E. Resistance to amphotericin B does not emerge during treatment for invasive aspergillosis. J Antimicrob Chemother 49:209-13, 2002.
Website: www.pdr.net

Amphotericin B Lipid Complex (Abelcet) ABLC

Drug Class: Antifungal (see p. 297)
Usual Dose: 5 mg/kg (IV) q24h
Pharmacokinetic Parameters:
Peak serum level: 1.7 mcg/mL
Bioavailability: Not applicable
Excreted unchanged: 5%
Serum half-life (normal/ESRD): 173/173 hrs
Plasma protein binding: 90%
Volume of distribution (V_d): 131 L/kg
Primary Mode of Elimination: Metabolized
Dosage Adjustments*

CrCl ~ 40–60 mL/min	No change
CrCl < 40 mL/min	No change
Post–HD/PD dose	None
CVVH dose	None
Moderate or severe hepatic insufficiency	No change

Drug Interactions: Adrenocorticoids (hypokalemia); aminoglycosides, cyclosporine, polymyxin B (↑ nephrotoxicity); digoxin (↑ digitalis toxicity due to hypokalemia); flucytosine (↑ flucytosine effect); neuromuscular blocking agents (↑ neuromuscular blockade due to hypokalemia)
Adverse Effects: Fevers/chills, flushing thrombophlebitis, bradycardia, seizures, hypotension, distal renal tubular acidosis (↓ K^+/↓ Mg^{++}), anemia. Fewer/less severe side effects and less nephrotoxicity than amphotericin B. Renal toxicity is dose-dependent (use caution)
Allergic Potential: Low
Safety in Pregnancy: B
Comments: See p. 297. Useful in patients unable to tolerate amphotericin B or in patients with amphotericin B nephrotoxicity. Infuse at 2.5 mg/kg/hr
Cerebrospinal Fluid Penetration: < 10%

REFERENCES:
Arikan S, Rex JH. Lipid-based antifungal agents: current status. Curr Pharm Des 7:393-415, 2001.

Dupont B. Overview of the lipid formulations of amphotericin B. J Antimicrob Chemother 49 Suppl 1:31-6, 2002.

Hiemenz JW, Walsh TJ. Lipid formulations of Amphotericin B: Recent progress and future directions. Clin Infect Dis 2:133-144, 1996.

Kauffman CA, Carver PL. Antifungal agents in the 1990s: Current status and future developments. Drugs 53:539-49, 1997.

Slain D. Lipid-based Amphotericin B for the treatment of fungal infections. Pharmacotherapy 19:306-23, 1999.

Trouet A. The amphotericin B lipid complex or abelcet: its Belgian connection, its mode of action and specificity: a review. Acta Clin Belg 57:53-7, 2002.

Website: www.pdr.net

Amphotericin B Liposomal (AmBisome) L-AmB

Drug Class: Antifungal (see p. 297)
Usual Dose: 3-6 mg/kg (IV) q24h
Pharmacokinetic Parameters:
Peak serum level: 17-83 mcg/mL
Bioavailability: Not applicable
Excreted unchanged: 5%
Serum half-life (normal/ESRD): 153 hrs/no data
Plasma protein binding: 90%
Volume of distribution (V_d): 131 L/kg
Primary Mode of Elimination: Metabolized
Dosage Adjustments*

CrCl ~ 40–60 mL/min	No change
CrCl < 40 mL/min	No change
Post–HD/PD dose	None
CVVH dose	None
Moderate or severe hepatic insufficiency	No change

Drug Interactions: Adrenocorticoids (hypokalemia); aminoglycosides, cyclosporine, polymyxin B (↑ nephrotoxicity); digoxin (↑ digitalis toxicity due to hypokalemia); flucytosine (↑ flucytosine effect); neuromuscular blocking agents (↑ neuromuscular blockade due to hypokalemia)
Adverse Effects: Fevers/chills, flushing, thrombophlebitis, bradycardia, seizures,

---

hypotension, distal renal tubular acidosis
($\downarrow K^+/\downarrow Mg^{++}$), anemia
Allergic Potential: Low
Safety in Pregnancy: B
Comments: See p. 297. Less nephrotoxicity
than amphotericin B and other amphotericin
lipid preparations. For empiric therapy of
fungemia, 3 mg/kg (IV) q24h can be used. For
suspected/ known Aspergillus infection, use 5
mg/kg (IV) q24h. For cryptococcal meningitis in
HIV, use
6 mg/kg (IV) q24h
Cerebrospinal Fluid Penetration: < 10%

REFERENCES:

Adler-Moore J, Proffitt RT. AmBisome: liposomal
formulation, structure, mechanism of action and
preclinical experience. J Antimicrob Chemother 49
Suppl 1:211-30, 2002.
Chopra R. AmBisome in the treatment of fungal
infections: the UK experience. J Antimicrob Chemother
49 Suppl 1:43-7, 2002.
De Marie S. Clinical use of liposomal and lipid-
complexed amphotericin-B. J Antimicrob Chemother
33:907-16, 1994.
Hiemenz JW, Walsh TJ. Lipid formulations of
amphotericin B: Recent progress and future
directions. Clin Infect Dis 2:133-44, 1996.
Lequaglie C. Liposomal amphotericin B (AmBisome):
efficacy and safety of low-dose therapy in pulmonary
fungal infections. J Antimicrob Chemother 49 Suppl
1:49-50, 2002.
Slain D. Lipid-based amphotericin B for the treatment of
fungal infections. Pharmacotherapy 19:306-23, 1999.
Website: www.ambisome.com

Amphotericin B Cholesteryl Sulfate Complex (Amphotec), ABCD (amphotericin B colloidal dispersion)

Drug Class: Antifungal (see p. 297)
Usual Dose: 3-4 mg/kg (IV) q24h
Pharmacokinetic Parameters:
Peak serum level: 2.9 mcg/mL
Bioavailability: Not applicable
Excreted unchanged: 5%
Serum half-life (normal/ESRD): 39/29 hrs

Plasma protein binding: 90%
Volume of distribution (V_d): 4 L/kg
Primary Mode of Elimination: Metabolized
Dosage Adjustments*

CrCl ~ 40–60 mL/min	No change
CrCl < 40 mL/min	No change
Post–HD/PD dose	None
CVVH dose	None
Moderate or severe hepatic insufficiency	No change

Drug Interactions: Adrenocorticoids
(hypokalemia); aminoglycosides, cyclosporine,
polymyxin B (↑ nephrotoxicity); digoxin (↑
digitalis toxicity due to hypokalemia); flucytosine
(↑ flucytosine effect); neuromuscular blocking
agents (↑ neuromuscular blockade due to
hypokalemia)
Adverse Effects: Fevers/chills, flushing,
thrombophlebitis, bradycardia, seizures,
hypotension, distal renal tubular acidosis
($\downarrow K^+/\downarrow Mg^{++}$), anemia. Fewer/less severe side
effects/less nephrotoxicity vs. amphotericin B
Allergic Potential: Low
Safety in Pregnancy: B
Comments: See p. 297. Reconstitute in sterile
water, not dextrose, saline or bacteriostatic
water. Do not co-administer with in same IV line
with other drugs. Give by slow IV infusion over 2
hours
(1 mg/kg/hr). Test dose unnecessary
Cerebrospinal Fluid Penetration: < 10%

REFERENCES:

De Marie S. Clinical use of liposomal and lipid-
complexed amphotericin B. J Antimicrob Chemother
33:907-16, 1994.
Kline S, Larsen TA, Fieber L, et al. Limited toxicity of
prolonged therapy with high doses of amphotericin B
lipid complex. Clin Infect Dis 21:1154-8, 1995.
Rapp RP, Gubbins PO, Evans ME. Amphotericin B lipid
complex. Ann Pharmacother 31:1174-86, 1997.
Website: www.pdr.net

"Usual dose" assumes normal renal/hepatic function. * For renal insufficiency, give usual dose x 1 followed by
maintenance dose per CrCl. For dialysis patients, dose the same as for CrCl < 10 mL/min and give supplemental
(post-HD/PD dose) immediately after dialysis. CrCl = creatinine clearance; CVVH = continuous veno-venous hemo-
filtration; HD/PD = hemodialysis/peritoneal dialysis. See pp. 293-297 for explanations, p. 1 for abbreviations

Ampicillin (various)

Drug Class: Aminopenicillin
Usual Dose: 2 gm (IV) q4h, 500 mg (PO) q6h
Pharmacokinetic Parameters:
Peak serum level: 48 (IV) / 5 (PO) mcg/mL
Bioavailability: 50%
Excreted unchanged: 90%
Serum half-life (normal/ESRD): 0.8/10 hrs
Plasma protein binding: 20%
Volume of distribution (V_d): 0.25 L/kg
Primary Mode of Elimination: Renal
Dosage Adjustments*

CrCl ~ 50–60 mL/min	1 gm (IV) q4h 500 mg (PO) q6h
CrCl ~ 10–50 mL/min	1 gm (IV) q8h 250 mg (PO) q8h
CrCl < 10 mL/min	1 gm (IV) q12h 250 mg (PO) q12h
Post–HD dose	1 gm (IV) 500 mg (PO)
Post–PD dose	250 mg (PO)
CVVH dose	1 gm (IV) q8h 250 mg (PO) q12h
Moderate or severe hepatic insufficiency	No change

Drug Interactions: Allopurinol (↑ frequency of rash); warfarin (↑ INR)
Adverse Effects: Drug fever/rash, nausea, GI upset, irritative diarrhea, h SGOT/SGPT, ↑ incidence of rash vs. penicillin in patients with EBV, HIV, lymphocytic leukemias, or allopurinol, C. difficile diarrhea/colitis
Allergic Potential: High
Safety in Pregnancy: B
Comments: Incompatible in solutions containing amphotericin B, heparin, corticosteroids, erythromycin, aminoglycosides, or metronidazole. Na^+ content = 2.9 mEq/g. Meningeal dose = 2 gm (IV) q4h
Cerebrospinal Fluid Penetration:
Non-inflamed meninges = 1%
Inflamed meninges = 10%

Bile Penetration: 3000%

REFERENCES:
Donowitz GR, Mandell GL. Beta-lactam antibiotics. N Engl J Med 318:419-26 and 318:490-500, 1993.
Wright AJ. The penicillins. Mayo Clin Proc 74:290-307, 1999.
Wright AJ, Wilkowske CJ. The penicillins. Mayo Clin Proc 66:1047-63, 1991.

Ampicillin/sulbactam (Unasyn)

Drug Class: Aminopenicillin/β-lactamase inhibitor combination
Usual Dose: 1.5-3 gm (IV) q6h (see comments)
Pharmacokinetic Parameters:
Peak serum level: 109-150/48-88 mcg/mL
Bioavailability: Not applicable
Excreted unchanged: 80/80%
Serum half-life (normal/ESRD): [1/9]/[1/9] hrs
Plasma protein binding: 28/38%
Volume of distribution (V_d): 0.25/0.38 L/kg
Primary Mode of Elimination: Renal/hepatic
Dosage Adjustments* (based on 3 gm q6h):

CrCl ~ 40–60 mL/min	1.5 gm (IV) q6h
CrCl ~ 15–30 mL/min	1.5 gm (IV) q12h
CrCl < 15 mL/min	1.5 gm (IV) q24h
Post–HD dose	1.5 gm (IV)
Post–PD dose	None
CVVH dose	1.5 gm (IV) q12h
Moderate or severe hepatic insufficiency	No change

Drug Interactions: Probenecid (↑ ampicillin/sulbactam levels)
Adverse Effects: Drug fever/rash, ↑ SGOT/SGPT, C. difficile diarrhea/colitis
Allergic Potential: High
Safety in Pregnancy: B
Comments: For mild/moderate infection, 1.5 gm (IV) q6h may be used. Pseudoresistance with E. coli/Klebsiella (resistant in-vitro, not in-vivo). Na^+ content = 4.2 mEq/g

---

"Usual dose" assumes normal renal/hepatic function. * For renal insufficiency, give usual dose x 1 followed by maintenance dose per CrCl. For dialysis patients, dose the same as for CrCl < 10 mL/min and give supplemental (post-HD/PD dose) immediately after dialysis. CrCl = creatinine clearance; CVVH = continuous veno-venous hemofiltration; HD/PD = hemodialysis/peritoneal dialysis. See pp. 293-297 for explanations, p. 1 for abbreviations

Cerebrospinal Fluid Penetration: < 10%

REFERENCES:

Itokazu GS, Danziger LH. Ampicillin-sulbactam and ticarcillin-clavulanic acid: A comparison of their in vitro activity and review of their clinical efficacy. Pharmacotherapy 11:382-414, 1991.

Sensakovic JW, Smith LG. Beta-lactamase inhibitor combinations. Med Clin North Am 79:695-704, 1995.

Wood GC, Hanes SD, Croce MA, et al. Comparison of ampicillin-sulbactam and imipenem-cilastatin for the treatment of Acinetobacter ventilator-associated pneumonia. Clin Infect Dis 34:1425-30, 2002.

Wright AJ. The penicillins. Mayo Clin Proc 73:290-307,1999.

Website: www.pdr.net

Amprenavir (Agenerase)

Drug Class: Antiretroviral protease inhibitor
Usual Adult Dose: 1200 mg (PO) q12h (capsules) or 1400 mg (PO) q12h (solution); age 13‑16 years < 50 kg or pediatrics 4-12 years: 20 mg/kg (PO) q12h (capsules) or 1.5 ml/kg (PO) q12h (15 mg/mL solution). Maximum dose 2400 mg/d (capsules), 2800 mg/d (oral solution)
Pharmacokinetic Parameters:
Peak serum level: 7.6 mcg/mL
Bioavailability: No data
Excreted unchanged: 1%
Serum half-life (normal/ESRD): 7-10/7-10 hrs
Plasma protein binding: 90%
Volume of distribution (V_d): 6.1 L/kg
Primary Mode of Elimination: Hepatic
Dosage Adjustments*

CrCl ~ 40–60 mL/min	No information
CrCl < 40 mL/min	No information
Post–HD/PD dose	No information
CVVH dose	No information
Moderate hepatic insufficiency	450 mg (PO) q12h (capsules)
Severe hepatic insufficiency	300 mg (PO) q12h (capsules)

Antiretroviral Dosage Adjustments:

Delavirdine	Avoid
Didanosine buffered solution	Take amprenavir 1 hour before or after
Efavirenz	No information
Indinavir	No information
Lopinavir/ritonavir	No information
Nelfinavir	No information
Nevirapine	No information
Ritonavir	Limited data for amprenavir 600 mg q12h + ritonavir 100 mg q12h (or amprenavir 1200 mg q24h + ritonavir 200 mg q24h)
Saquinavir	No information
Rifampin	Avoid combination
Rifabutin	Rifabutin 150 mg q24h or 300 mg 2-3x/week

Drug Interactions: Antiretrovirals, rifabutin, rifampin (see dose adjustment grid, above); bepridil, cisapride, ergotamine, statins, benzodiazepines, St. John's wort, pimozide, sildenafil, methadone (avoid if possible); carbamazepine, phenobarbital, phenytoin (may ↓ amprenavir levels, monitor anticonvulsant levels)
Adverse Effects: Rash, Stevens-Johnson syndrome (rare), GI upset, headache, depression, taste perversion, diarrhea, perioral paresthesias, hyperglycemia (including worsening diabetes, new-onset diabetes, DKA), ↑ cholesterol/triglycerides (evaluate risk for coronary disease/pancreatitis), fat redistribution, ↑ SGOT/SGPT, possible increased bleeding in hemophilia
Allergic Potential: High. Amprenavir is a sulfonamide; use with caution in sulfa allergy

---

"Usual dose" assumes normal renal/hepatic function. * For renal insufficiency, give usual dose x 1 followed by maintenance dose per CrCl. For dialysis patients, dose the same as for CrCl < 10 mL/min and give supplemental (post-HD/PD dose) immediately after dialysis. CrCl = creatinine clearance; CVVH = continuous veno-venous hemofiltration; HD/PD = hemodialysis/peritoneal dialysis. See pp. 293-297 for explanations, p. 1 for abbreviations

Safety in Pregnancy: C
Comments: Can be taken with or without food, but avoid high fat meals (may ↓ absorption). High vitamin E content. Capsules and solution are not interchangeable on a mg per mg basis. Decrease dosage in moderate or severe liver disease; use with caution. Oral solution contains propylene glycol: avoid in pregnancy, hepatic/renal failure, patients taking disulfiram or metronidazole, or children < 4 years old. Effective antiretroviral therapy consists of three antiretrovirals (same/different classes)

REFERENCES:
Adkins JC, Faulds D. Amprenavir. Drugs 55:837-42,1998.
Go J, Cunha BA. Amprenavir. Antibiotics for Clinicians 4:49-55, 2000.
Kaul DR, Cinti SK, Carver PL, et al. HIV protease inhibitors: Advances in therapy and adverse reactions, including metabolic complications. Pharmacotherapy 19:281-98, 1999.
Panel on Clinical Practices for Treatment of HIV Infection. Guidelines for the use of antiretroviral agents in HIV-infected adults and adolescents. Department of Health and Human Services. www.aidsinfo.nih.gov/guidelines/. November 10, 2003.
Website: www.TreatHIV.com

Atazanavir (Reyataz)

Drug Class: Antiretroviral protease inhibitor
Usual Dose: 400 mg (PO) q24h
Pharmacokinetic Parameters:
Peak serum level: 3152 ng/mL
Bioavailability: No data
Excreted unchanged (urine/feces): 7%/20%
Serum half-life (normal/ESRD): 7 hrs/no data
Plasma protein binding: 86%
Volume of distribution (V_d): No data
Primary Mode of Elimination: Hepatic
Dosage Adjustments*

CrCl < 40-60 mL/min	No data
Post–HD or PD dose	No data
CVVH dose	No data

Moderate hepatic insufficiency	300 mg (PO) q24h
Severe hepatic insufficiency	Avoid

Antiretroviral Dosage Adjustments:

Delavirdine	No information
Didanosine	Give atazanavir 2 hrs before or 1 hr after didanosine buffered formulations
Efavirenz	Atazanavir 300 mg + ritonavir 100 + efavirenz 600 mg as single daily dose with food
Indinavir	Avoid combination
Lopinavir/ritonavir	No information
Nelfinavir	No information
Nevirapine	No information
Ritonavir	Atazanavir 300 mg/d +ritonavir 100 mg/d as single daily dose with food
Saquinavir	↑ saquinavir (soft-gel) levels; no information
Rifampin	Avoid combination
Rifabutin	150 mg q48h or 3x/week

Drug Interactions: Antacids or buffered medications (↓ atazanavir levels; give atazanavir 2 hours before or 1 hour after); H2-receptor blockers (↓ atazanavir levels; separate administration by 12 hours); antiarrhythmics (↑ amiodarone, systemic lidocaine, quinidine levels; monitor antiarrhythmic levels); antidepressants (↑ tricyclic antidepressant levels; monitor levels); calcium channel blockers (↑ calcium channel blocker levels, additive ↑ PR interval; ↓ diltiazem dose by 50%; use with caution; consider ECG monitoring); clarithromycin (↑ clarithromycin and atazanavir levels; consider 50% dose reduction; consider alternate agent for infections not caused by MAI); cyclosporine, sirolimus, tacrolimus (↑ immunosuppressant levels; monitor levels); ethinyl estradiol, norethindrone (↑ oral contraceptive levels; use lowest effective oral contraceptive dose); lovastatin, simvastatin (↑ risk of myopathy, rhabdomyolysis; avoid combination); sildenafil (↑ sildenafil levels; give sildenafil at 25 mg q48h and monitor for side effects); St. John's wort (avoid combination); warfarin (↑ warfarin levels; monitor INR). *Drugs that should not be co-administered with atazanavir* include cisapride, pimozide, rifampin, irinotecan, midazolam, triazolam, lovastatin, simvastatin, bepridil, some ergot derivatives, indinavir, proton pump inhibitors, St. John's wort, drugs that use CYP3A

Adverse Effects: Asymptomatic, dose-dependent ↑ PR interval (~ 24 msec). Use with caution with drugs that ↑ PR interval (e.g., beta blockers, verapamil, digoxin). May ↑ risk of hyperglycemia/diabetes. May ↑ risk of bleeding in hemophilia (types A + B). Reversible, asymptomatic ↑ in indirect (unconjugated) bilirubin may occur

Allergic Potential: Low

Safety in Pregnancy: B

Comments: Monitor LFTs in patients with HBV, HCV. Take 400 mg (2 200-mg capsules) once daily with food

REFERENCES:

Colonno RJ, Thiry A, Limoli K, Parkin N. Activities of atazanavir (BMS-232632) against a large panel of Human Immunodeficiency Virus Type 1 clinical isolates resistant to one or more approved protease inhibitors. Antimicrob Agents Chemother 47:1324-33, 2003.

Haas DW, Zala C, Schrader S, et al. Therapy with atazanavir plus saquinavir in patients failing highly active antiretroviral therapy: a randomized comparative pilot trial. AIDS 17:1339-1349,2003.

Panel on Clinical Practices for Treatment of HIV Infection. Guidelines for the Use of Antiretroviral Agents in HIV-Infected Adults and Adolescents. Department of Health and Human Services. www.aidsinfo.nih.gov/guidelines/. November 10, 2003.

Piliero PJ. Atazanavir: a novel HIV-1 protease inhibitor.

Expert Opin Investig Drugs 11:1295-301, 2002.

Sanne I, Piliero P, Squires K, et al. Results of a phase 2 clinical trial at 48 weeks (AI424-007): a dose-ranging, safety, and efficacy comparative trial of atazanavir at three doses in combination with didanosine and stavudine in antiretroviral-naive subjects. J Acquir Immune Defic Syndr 32:18-29, 2003.

Wang F, Ross J. Atazanavir: a novel azapeptide inhibitor of HIV-1 protease. Formulary 38:691-702, 2003.

Website: www.reyataz.com

Atovaquone (Mepron)

Drug Class: Antiprotozoal

Usual Dose: 750 mg (PO) q12h with food (treatment of PCP); 1500 mg (PO) q24h with food (prophylaxis)

Pharmacokinetic Parameters:

Peak serum level: 12-24 mcg/mL

Bioavailability: 30% (47% with food; food ↑ bioavailability by 2-fold)

Excreted unchanged (feces): > 94%

Serum half-life (normal/ESRD): 2.9/2.9 days

Plasma protein binding: 99.9%

Volume of distribution (V_d): 0.6 L/kg

Primary Mode of Elimination: Hepatic

Dosage Adjustments*

CrCl ~ 40–60 mL/min	No change
CrCl < 40 mL/min	No change
Post–HD/PD	No information
CVVH dose	No information
Moderate or severe hepatic insufficiency	No information

Drug Interactions: Rifabutin, rifampin (↓ atovaquone effect); zidovudine (↑ zidovudine levels). Rifampin decreases atovaquone levels by 50%.

Adverse Effects: Rash, nausea, headache, fever, cough, neurovascular, diarrhea, anemia, leukopenia, ↑ SGOT/SGPT

Allergic Potential: Low

Safety in Pregnancy: C

Comments: Active against T. gondii, P. carinii, Plasmodia, and Babesia. Take with food

---

"Usual dose" assumes normal renal/hepatic function. * For renal insufficiency, give usual dose x 1 followed by maintenance dose per CrCl. For dialysis patients, dose the same as for CrCl < 10 mL/min and give supplemental (post-HD/PD dose) immediately after dialysis. CrCl = creatinine clearance; CVVH = continuous veno-venous hemo-filtration; HD/PD = hemodialysis/peritoneal dialysis. See pp. 293-297 for explanations, p. 1 for abbreviations

REFERENCES:
Artymowicz RJ, James VE. Atovaquone: A new anti-pneumocystis agent. Clin Pharmacol 12:563-70, 1993.
Baggish AL, Hill DR. Antiparasitic agent atovaquone. Antimicrob Agents Chemother 46:1163-73, 2002.
Bonoan JT, Johnson DH, Schoch PE, Cunha BA. Life threatening babesiosis treated by exchange transfusion with azithromycin and atovaquone. Heart & Lung 27:42-8, 1998.
Chan C, Montaner J, LeFebvre BA, et al. Atovaquone suspension compared with aerosolized pentamidine for prevention of Pneumocystis carinii pneumonia in human immunodeficiency virus infected subsets intolerant of trimethoprim or sulfamethoxazole. J Infect Dis 180:369-376, 1999.
Haile LG, Flaherty JF. Atovaquone: A review. Ann Pharmacother 27:1488-94, 1993.
Van Riemsdijk MM, Sturkenboom MC, Ditters JM, et al. Atovaquone plus chloroguanide versus mefloquine for malaria prophylaxis: A focus on neuropsychiatric adverse events. Clin Pharmacol Ther 72:294-301, 2002.

Atovaquone + proguanil (Malarone)

Drug Class: Antimalarial
Usual Dose: Malarone tablet = 250 mg atovaquone + 100 mg proguanil. Usual dose = 1 tablet (PO) q24h (see comments)
Pharmacokinetic Parameters:
Peak serum level: 38 mcg/mL
Bioavailability: 23/90%
Excreted unchanged: 94/50%
Serum half-life (normal/ESRD): [60/60]/[21/no data] hrs
Plasma protein binding: 99/75%
Volume of distribution (V_d): 3.5/42 L/kg
Primary Mode of Elimination: Metabolized

Dosage Adjustments*

CrCl ~ 30–60 mL/min	No change
CrCl ~ 10–30 mL/min	Avoid
CrCl < 10 mL/min	Avoid
Post–HD/PD dose	No information
CVVH dose	No information

Moderate or severe hepatic insufficiency	No change

Drug Interactions: Chloroquine (↑ incidence of mouth ulcers); metoclopramide, rifabutin, rifampin, tetracycline (↓ atovaquone + proguanil effect); ritonavir (↑ or ↓ atovaquone + proguanil effect); typhoid vaccine (↓ typhoid vaccine effect)
Adverse Effects: Headache, dizziness, nausea, vomiting, diarrhea, abdominal pain, anorexia, myalgias, fever
Allergic Potential: Low
Safety in Pregnancy: C
Comments: Effective against chloroquine sensitive/resistant strains of P. falciparum, but not P. ovale, P. vivax, or P. malariae.
<u>Malaria prophylaxis:</u> 1 tablet (PO) q24h for 2 days before entering endemic area, daily during exposure, and daily x 1 week post-exposure
<u>Therapy:</u> 4 tablets (PO) as single dose x 3 days

REFERENCES:
Atovaquone/proguanil (Malarone) for malaria. Med Lett Drugs Ther 42:109-11, 2000.
Looareesuwan S, Chulay JD, Canfield CJ. Malarone (atovaquone and proguanil hydrochloride): a review of its clinical development for treating malaria. Malarone clinical trials study group. Am J Trop Med Hyg 60:533-41, 1999.
Marra F, Salzman JR, Ensom MH. Atovaquone-proguanil for prophylaxis and treatment of malaria. Ann Pharmacother. 37:1266-75, 2003.
McKeage K, Scott L. Atovaquone/proguanil: a review of its use for the prophylaxis of Plasmodium falciparum malaria. Drugs. 63:597-623, 2003.
Nosten F. Prophylactic effect of malarone against malaria: all good news? Lancet 356:1864-5, 2000.
Thapar MM, Ashton M, Lindegardh N, et al. Time-dependent pharmacokinetics and drug metabolism of atovaquone plus proguanil (Malarone) when taken as chemoprophylaxis. Eur J Clin Pharmacol 15:19-27, 2002.
Website: www.pdr.net

"Usual dose" assumes normal renal/hepatic function. * For renal insufficiency, give usual dose x 1 followed by maintenance dose per CrCl. For dialysis patients, dose the same as for CrCl < 10 mL/min and give supplemental (post-HD/PD dose) immediately after dialysis. CrCl = creatinine clearance; CVVH = continuous veno-venous hemofiltration; HD/PD = hemodialysis/peritoneal dialysis. See pp. 293-297 for explanations, p. 1 for abbreviations

Azithromycin (Zithromax)

Drug Class: Macrolide (Azolide)
Usual Dose: 500 mg (IV/PO) x 1 dose, then 250 mg (IV/PO) q24h
Pharmacokinetic Parameters:
Peak serum level: 1.1 (IV)/0.2 (PO) mcg/mL
Bioavailability: 35%
Excreted unchanged: 6%
Serum half-life (normal/ESRD): 68/68 hrs
Plasma protein binding: 50%
Volume of distribution (V_d): 31 L/kg
Primary Mode of Elimination: Hepatic
Dosage Adjustments*

CrCl ~ 40–60 mL/min	No change
CrCl ~ 10–40 mL/min	No change
CrCl < 10 mL/min	Use caution
Post–HD/PD dose	None
CVVH dose	None
Moderate or severe hepatic insufficiency	No information

Drug Interactions: Carbamazepine, cisapride, clozapine, corticosteroids, midazolam, triazolam, valproic acid (not studied/not reported); cyclosporine (↑ cyclosporine levels with toxicity); digoxin (↑ digoxin levels); pimozide (may ↑ QT interval, torsade de pointes)
Adverse Effects: Nausea, GI upset, diarrhea
Allergic Potential: Low
Safety in Pregnancy: B
Comments: May ↑ QT_c interval. Bioavailability is decreased by food. For C. trachomatis urethritis, use 1 gm (PO) x 1 dose. For N. gonorrhoea urethritis, use 2 gm (PO) x 1 dose. For MAI prophylaxis, use 1200 mg (PO) weekly. For MAI therapy, use 600 mg (PO) q24h
Cerebrospinal Fluid Penetration: < 10%
Bile/serum ratio: > 3000%

REFERENCES:
Alvarez-Elcoro S, Enzler MJ. The macrolides: Erythromycin, clarithromycin and azithromycin. Mayo Clin Proc 74:613-34, 1999.
Cunha BA. Macrolides, doxycycline, and fluoroquinolones in the treatment of Legionnaires' Disease. Antibiotics for Clinicians 2:117-8, 1998.
Ioannidis JP, Contopoulos-Ioannidis DG, Chew P, Lau J. Meta-analysis of randomized controlled trials on the comparative efficacy and safety of azithromycin against other antibiotics for upper respiratory tract infections. J Antimicrob Chemother 48:677-89, 2001.
Paradisi F, Corti G. Azithromycin. Antibiotics for Clinicians 3:1-8, 1999.
Phillips P, Chan K, Hogg R, et al. Azithromycin prophylaxis for Mycobacterium avium complex during the era of highly active antiretroviral therapy: evaluation of a provincial program. Clin Infect Dis 34:371-8, 2002.
Pichichero ME, Hoeger WJ, Casey JR. Azithromycin for the treatment of pertussis. Pediatr Infect Dis J. 22:847-9, 2003.
Plouffe JF, Breiman RF, Fields BS, et al. Azithromycin in the treatment of Legionella pneumonia requiring hospitalization. Clin Infect Dis. 37:1475-80, 2003.
Saiman L, Marshall BC, Mayer-Hamblett N, et al. Azithromycin in patients with cystic fibrosis chronically infected with Pseudomonas aeruginosa: a randomized controlled trial. JAMA. 290:1749-5, 2003..
Schlossberg D. Azithromycin and clarithromycin. Med Clin N Amer 79:803-816, 1995.
Wolter J, Seeney S, Bell S, et al. Effect of long term treatment with azithromycin on disease parameters in cystic fibrosis: a randomised trial. Thorax 57:212-6, 2002.
Website: www.zithromax.com

Aztreonam (Azactam)

Drug Class: Monobactam
Usual Dose: 1-2 gm (IV) q8h
Pharmacokinetic Parameters:
Peak serum level: 204 mcg/mL
Bioavailability: Not applicable
Excreted unchanged: 60-70%
Serum half-life (normal/ESRD): 1.7/7 hrs
Plasma protein binding: 56%
Volume of distribution (V_d): 0.2 L/kg
Primary Mode of Elimination: Renal
Dosage Adjustments* (based on 2 gm q8h):

CrCl ~ 30–60 mL/min	2 gm (IV) q8h
CrCl ~ 10–30 mL/min	1 gm (IV) q8h
CrCl < 10 mL/min	500 mg (IV) q8h
Post–HD dose	250 mg (IV)

"Usual dose" assumes normal renal/hepatic function. * For renal insufficiency, give usual dose x 1 followed by maintenance dose per CrCl. For dialysis patients, dose the same as for CrCl < 10 mL/min and give supplemental (post-HD/PD dose) immediately after dialysis. CrCl = creatinine clearance; CVVH = continuous veno-venous hemofiltration; HD/PD = hemodialysis/peritoneal dialysis. See pp. 293-297 for explanations, p. 1 for abbreviations

Post–PD dose	500 mg (IV)
CVVH dose	1 gm (IV) q8h
Moderate hepatic insufficiency	No change
Severe hepatic insufficiency	No change

Drug Interactions: None
Adverse Effects: None
Allergic Potential: Low
Safety in Pregnancy: B
Comments: Incompatible in solutions containing vancomycin or metronidazole. No cross allergenicity with penicillins, β–lactams; safe to use in penicillin allergic patients. Meningeal dose = 2 gm (IV) q6h
Cerebrospinal Fluid Penetration:
Non-inflamed meninges = 1%
Inflamed meninges = 40%
Bile Penetration: 300%

REFERENCES:
Brogden RN, Heal RC. Aztreonam: A review of its antibacterial activity, pharmacokinetic properties, and therapeutic use. Drugs 31:96-130, 1986.
Critchley IA, Sahm DF, Kelly LJ, et al. In vitro synergy studies using aztreonam and fluoroquinolone combinations against six species of Gram-negative bacilli. Chemotherapy. 49:44-8, 2003.
Cunha BA. Cross allergenicity of penicillin with carbapenems and monobactams. J Crit Illness 13:344, 1998.
Cunha BA. Aztreonam: A review. Urology 41:249-58, 1993.
Fleming DR, Ziegler C, Baize T, et al. Cefepime versus ticarcillin and clavulanate potassium and aztreonam for febrile neutropenia therapy in high-dose chemotherapy patients. Am J Clin Oncol. 26:285-8, 2003.
Hellinger WC, Brewer NS. Carbapenems and monobactams: Imipenem, meropenem, and aztreonam. Mayo Clin Proc 74:420-34, 1999.
Johnson C, Cunha BA. Aztreonam. Med Clin North Am 79:733-43, 1995.
Pendland SL, Messick CR, Jung R. In vitro synergy testing of levofloxacin, ofloxacin, and ciprofloxacin in combination with aztreonam, ceftazidime, or piperacillin against Pseudomonas aeruginosa. Diagn Microbiol Infect Dis 42:75-8, 2002.
Sader HS, Huynh HK, Jones RN. Contemporary in vitro

synergy rates for aztreonam combined with newer fluoroquinolones and beta-lactams tested against gram-negative bacilli. Diagn Microbiol Infect Dis 47(3): 547-50, 2003.
Website: www.elan.com/Products/

Capreomycin (Capastat)

Drug Class: Anti–TB drug
Usual Dose: 1 gm (IM) q24h
Pharmacokinetic Parameters:
Peak serum level: 30 mcg/mL
Bioavailability: Not applicable
Excreted unchanged: 50%
Serum half-life (normal/ESRD): 5/30 hrs
Plasma protein binding: No data
Volume of distribution (V_d): 0.4 L/kg
Primary Mode of Elimination: Renal
Dosage Adjustments*

CrCl ~ 40–60 mL/min	500 mg (IM) q24h
CrCl ~ 10–40 mL/min	500 mg (IM) q48h
CrCl < 10 mL/min	500 mg (IM) q72h
Post–HD dose	500 mg (IM)
Post–PD dose	None
CVVH dose	500 mg (IM) q48h
Moderate hepatic insufficiency	No change
Severe hepatic insufficiency	No change

Drug Interactions: None
Adverse Effects: Eosinophilia, leukopenia, drug fever/rash, ototoxicity (vestibular), nephrotoxicity (glomerular/tubular)
Allergic Potential: Moderate
Safety in Pregnancy: C
Comments: Pain/phlebitis at IM injection site. Additive toxicity with aminoglycosides/viomycin
Cerebrospinal Fluid Penetration: < 10%

REFERENCES:
Davidson PT, Le HQ. Drug treatment of tuberculosis - 1992. Drugs 43:651-73, 1992.
Drugs for tuberculosis. Med Lett Drugs Ther 35:99-

"Usual dose" assumes normal renal/hepatic function. * For renal insufficiency, give usual dose x 1 followed by maintenance dose per CrCl. For dialysis patients, dose the same as for CrCl < 10 mL/min and give supplemental (post-HD/PD dose) immediately after dialysis. CrCl = creatinine clearance; CVVH = continuous veno-venous hemofiltration; HD/PD = hemodialysis/peritoneal dialysis. See pp. 293-297 for explanations, p. 1 for abbreviations

101, 1993.
Iseman MD. Treatment of multidrug resistant tuberculosis. N Engl J Med 329:784-91, 1993.
Website: www.pdr.net

Caspofungin (Cancidas)

Drug Class: Echinocandin antifungal
Usual Dose: 70 mg (IV) x 1 dose, then 50 mg (IV) q24h
Pharmacokinetic Parameters:
Peak serum level:
70 mg: 12.1/14.83 mcg/mL (multiple dose)
50 mg: 7.6/8.7 mcg/mL (multiple dose)
Bioavailability: Not applicable
Excreted unchanged: 1.4%
Serum half-life (normal/ESRD): 10/10 hrs
Plasma protein binding: 97%
Volume of distribution (V_d): No data
Primary Mode of Elimination: Hepatic
Dosage Adjustments*

CrCl ~ 40–60 mL/min	No change
CrCl < 40 mL/min	No change
Post–HD/PD dose	None
CVVH dose	None
Moderate hepatic insufficiency	35 mg (IV) q24h (maintenance dose)
Severe hepatic insufficiency	No information

Drug Interactions: Carbamazepine, rifampin, dexamethasone, efavirenz, nelfinavir, nevirapine, phenytoin (↓ caspofungin levels; ↑ caspofungin maintenance dose to 70 mg/day); cyclosporine (↑ caspofungin levels, ↑ SGOT/SGPT); tacrolimus (↓ tacrolimus levels, ↑ SGOT/SGPT)
Adverse Effects: Drug fever/rash
Allergic Potential: Low
Safety in Pregnancy: C
Comments: Administer by slow IV infusion over 1 hour; do not give IV bolus. Do not mix/co-infuse with glucose solutions. If co-administered with drugs that ↓ caspofungin levels or for highly-resistant organisms, then 70 mg (IV) q24h dosing may be used. For esophageal candidiasis,

therapy is initiated with 50 mg (70 mg loading dose has not been studied)
Cerebrospinal Fluid Penetration: No data

REFERENCES:
Andriole VT. Current and future antifungal therapy: New targets for antifungal agents. J Antimicrob Chemother 44:151-62, 1999.
Arathoon EG, Gotuzzo E, Noriega LM, et al. Randomized, double-blind, multicenter study of caspofungin versus amphotericin B for treatment of oropharyngeal and esophageal candidiasis. Antimicrob Agents Chemother 46:451-7, 2002.
Bachmann SP, VandeWalle K, Ramage G, et al. In vitro activity of caspofungin against Candida albicans biofilms. Antimicrob Agents Chemother 46:3591-3596, 2002.
Barchiesi F, Schimizzi AM, Fothergill AW, et al. In vitro activity of the new echinocandin antifungal against common and uncommon clinical isolates of Candida species. Eur J Clin Microbiol Infect Dis 18:302-4, 1999.
Deresinski SC, Stevens DA. Caspofungin. Clin Infect Dis 36:1445-57, 2003.
Grau S, Mateu-De Antonio J. Caspofungin acetate for treatment of invasive fungal infections. Ann Pharmacother. 37:1919, 2003.
Keating G, Figgitt D. Caspofungin: a review of its use in esophageal candidiasis, invasive candidiasis and invasive aspergillosis. Drugs 63:2235-63, 2003.
Lomaestro BM. Caspofungin. Hospital Formulary 36:527-36, 2001.
Mora-Duarte J, Betts R, Rotstein C, et al. Comparison of caspofungin and amphotericin B for invasive candidiasis. N Engl J Med 347:2020-9, 2002.
Pacetti SA, Gelone SP. Caspofungin acetate for treatment of invasive fungal infections. Ann Pharmacother 37:90-8, 2003.
Pfaller MA, Messer SA, Boyken L, et al. Caspofungin activity against clinical isolates of fluconazole-resistant Candida. J Clin Microbiol 2003;41:5729-31.
Rubin MA, Carroll KC, Cahill BC. Caspofungin in combination with itraconazole for the treatment of invasive aspergillosis in humans. Clin Infect Dis 34:1160-1, 2002.
Stone EA, Fung HB, Hirschenbaum HL. Caspofungin: an echinocandin antifungal agent. Clin Ther 24:351-77, 2002.
Website: www.cancidas.com

Cefaclor (Ceclor)

Drug Class: 2nd generation oral cephalosporin
Usual Dose: 500 mg (PO) q8h
Pharmacokinetic Parameters:

"Usual dose" assumes normal renal/hepatic function. * For renal insufficiency, give usual dose x 1 followed by maintenance dose per CrCl. For dialysis patients, dose the same as for CrCl < 10 mL/min and give supplemental (post-HD/PD dose) immediately after dialysis. CrCl = creatinine clearance; CVVH = continuous veno-venous hemofiltration; HD/PD = hemodialysis/peritoneal dialysis. See pp. 293-297 for explanations, p. 1 for abbreviations

Peak serum level: 13 mcg/mL
Bioavailability: 80%
Excreted unchanged: 60-85%
Serum half-life (normal/ESRD): 0.8/3 hrs
Plasma protein binding: 25%
Volume of distribution (V_d): 0.30 L/kg
Primary Mode of Elimination: Renal
Dosage Adjustments*

CrCl ~ 40–60 mL/min	No change
CrCl < 40 mL/min	No change
Post–HD/PD dose	No information
CVVH dose	No change
Moderate or severe hepatic insufficiency	No change

Drug Interactions: None
Adverse Effects: Drug fever/rash
Allergic Potential: High
Safety in Pregnancy: B
Comments: Limited penetration into respiratory secretions. Ceclor CD 500 mg (PO) q12h is equivalent to ceclor 250 mg (PO) q8h, not ceclor 500 mg (PO) q8h. Ceclor CD (500 mg q12h) is equivalent to 250 mg q8h of Ceclor. Give with food
Cerebrospinal Fluid Penetration: < 10%.
Bile Penetration: 60%

REFERENCES:
Cazzola M, Di Perna F, Boveri B. Interrelationship between the pharmacokinetics and pharmacodynamics of cefaclor advanced formulation in patients with acute exacerbation of chronic bronchitis. J Chemother 12:216-22, 2000.
Mazzei T, Novelli A, Esposito S, et al. New insight into the clinical pharmacokinetics of cefaclor: Tissue penetration. J Chemother 12:53-62, 2000.
Meyers BR. Cefaclor revisited. Clin Ther 22:154-66, 2000.
Website: www.pdr.net

Cefadroxil (Duricef, Ultracef)

Drug Class: 1st generation oral cephalosporin
Usual Dose: 1000 mg (PO) q12h

Pharmacokinetic Parameters:
Peak serum level: 16 mcg/mL
Bioavailability: 99%
Excreted unchanged: 90%
Serum half-life (normal/ESRD): 0.5/22 hrs
Plasma protein binding: 20%
Volume of distribution (V_d): 0.31 L/kg
Primary Mode of Elimination: Renal
Dosage Adjustments*

CrCl ~ 25-50 mL/min	500 mg (PO) q12h
CrCl ~ 10–25 mL/min	500 mg (PO) q24h
CrCl < 10 mL/min	500 mg (PO) q36h
Post–HD dose	500 mg (PO)
Post–PD dose	250 mg (PO)
CVVH dose	500 mg (PO) q24h
Moderate hepatic insufficiency	No change
Severe hepatic insufficiency	No change

Drug Interactions: None
Adverse Effects: Drug fever/rash
Allergic Potential: High
Safety in Pregnancy: B
Comments: Penetrates oral/respiratory secretions well
Cerebrospinal Fluid Penetration: < 10%
Bile Penetration: 20%

REFERENCES:
Bucko AD, Hunt BJ, Kidd SL, et al. Randomized, double-blind, multicenter comparison of oral cefditoren 200 or 400 mg BID with either cefuroxime 250 mg BID or cefadroxil 500 mg BID for the treatment of uncomplicated skin and skin-structure infections. Clin Ther 24:1134-47, 2002.
Cunha BA. Antibiotics selection for the treatment of sinusitis, otitis media, and pharyngitis. Infect Dis Pract 7:S324-S326, 1998.
Donowitz GR, Mandell GL. Beta-lactam antibiotics. N Engl J Med 318:419-26 and 318:490-500, 1993.
Gustaferro CA, Steckelberg JM. Cephalosporins: Antimicrobic agents and related compounds. Mayo Clin Proc 66:1064-73, 1991.
Smith GH. Oral cephalosporins in perspective. DICP

"Usual dose" assumes normal renal/hepatic function. * For renal insufficiency, give usual dose x 1 followed by maintenance dose per CrCl. For dialysis patients, dose the same as for CrCl < 10 mL/min and give supplemental (post-HD/PD dose) immediately after dialysis. CrCl = creatinine clearance; CVVH = continuous veno-venous hemo-filtration; HD/PD = hemodialysis/peritoneal dialysis. See pp. 293-297 for explanations, p. 1 for abbreviations

24:45-51, 1990.
Website: www.pdr.net

Cefamandole (Mandol)

Drug Class: 2nd generation cephalosporin
Usual Dose: 2 gm (IV) q6h
Pharmacokinetic Parameters:
Peak serum level: 240 mcg/mL
Bioavailability: Not applicable
Excreted unchanged: 85%
Serum half-life (normal/ESRD): 1/11 hrs
Plasma protein binding: 76%
Volume of distribution (V_d): 0.29 L/kg
Primary Mode of Elimination: Renal
Dosage Adjustments* (based on 2 gm q6h):

CrCl ~ 25-50 mL/min	1 gm (IV) q6h
CrCl ~ 10–25 mL/min	1 gm (IV) q6h
CrCl < 10 mL/min	1 gm (IV) q12h
Post–HD dose	1 gm (IV)
Post–PD dose	None
CVVH dose	1 gm (IV) q6h
Moderate or severe hepatic insufficiency	No change

Drug Interactions: Alcohol (disulfiram-like reaction); antiplatelet agents, heparin, thrombolytics, warfarin (↑ risk of bleeding)
Adverse Effects: Drug fever/rash, ↑ INR
Allergic Potential: High
Safety in Pregnancy: B
Comments: Incompatible in solutions with Mg^{++} or Ca^{++}. Contains MTT side chain, but no increase in clinical bleeding. Na$^+$ content = 3.3 mEq/g

Cerebrospinal Fluid Penetration: < 10%
Bile Penetration: 300%

REFERENCES:
Cunha BA, Klimek JJ, Qunitiliani R. Cefamandole nafate in respiratory and urinary tract infections. Curr Ther Res 25:584-9, 1971.
Gentry LO, Zeluff BJ, Cooley DA. Antibiotic prophylaxis in open-heart surgery: A comparison of cefamandole, cefuroxime, and cefazolin. Ann Thorac Surg 46:167-
71, 1988.
Peterson CD, Lake KD, Arom KV. Antibiotic prophylaxis in open-heart surgery patients: Comparison of cefamandole and cefuroxime. Drug Intell Clin Pharmacol 21:728-32, 1987.

Cefazolin (Ancef, Kefzol)

Drug Class: 1st generation cephalosporin
Usual Dose: 1 gm (IV) q8h
Pharmacokinetic Parameters:
Peak serum level: 185 mcg/mL
Bioavailability: Not applicable
Excreted unchanged: 96%
Serum half-life (normal/ESRD): 1.8/40 hrs
Plasma protein binding: 85%
Volume of distribution (V_d): 0.2 L/kg
Primary Mode of Elimination: Renal
Dosage Adjustments*

CrCl ~ 35-55 mL/min	No change
CrCl ~ 10–34 mL/min	500 mg (IV) q12h
CrCl < 10 mL/min	500 mg (IV) q24h
Post–HD dose	No information
Post–PD dose	None
CVVH dose	500 mg (IV) q12h
Moderate or severe hepatic insufficiency	No change

Drug Interactions: None
Adverse Effects: Drug fever/rash
Allergic Potential: High
Safety in Pregnancy: B
Comments: Incompatible in solutions containing erythromycin, aminoglycosides, cimetidine, theophylline. Na$^+$ content = 2 mEq/g
Cerebrospinal Fluid Penetration: < 10%
Bile Penetrations: 300%

REFERENCES:
Gentry LO, Zeluff BJ, Cooley DA. Antibiotic prophylaxis in open-heart surgery: A comparison of cefamandole, cefuroxime, and cefazolin. Ann Thorac Surg 46:167-71, 1988.
Cunha BA, Gossling HR, Pasternak HS, et al. Penetration of cephalosporins into bone. Infection

---

"Usual dose" assumes normal renal/hepatic function. * For renal insufficiency, give usual dose x 1 followed by maintenance dose per CrCl. For dialysis patients, dose the same as for CrCl < 10 mL/min and give supplemental (post-HD/PD dose) immediately after dialysis. CrCl = creatinine clearance; CVVH = continuous veno-venous hemo-filtration; HD/PD = hemodialysis/peritoneal dialysis. See pp. 293-297 for explanations, p. 1 for abbreviations

12:80-4, 1984.

Kelkar PS, Li JTC. Cephalosporin allergy. N Engl J Med 345:804-809, 2001.

Khairullah Q, Provenzano R, Tayeb J, et al. Comparison of vancomycin versus cefazolin as initial therapy for peritonitis in peritoneal dialysis patients. Perit Dial Int 22:339-44, 2002.

Marshall WF, Blair JE. The cephalosporins. Mayo Clin Proc 74:187-95, 1999.

Nightingale CH, Klimek JJ, Quintiliani R. Effect of protein binding on the penetration of nonmetabolized cephalosporins into atrial appendage and pericardial fluids in open-heart surgical patients. Antimicrob Agents Chemother 17:595-8, 1980.

Quintiliani R, Nightingale CH. Cefazolin. Ann Intern Med 89:650-6, 1978.

Cefdinir (Omnicef)

Drug Class: 3rd generation oral cephalosporin
Usual Dose: 600 mg (PO) q24h
Pharmacokinetic Parameters:
Peak serum level: 2.9 mcg/mL
Bioavailability: 16% (tab) / 25% (suspension)
Excreted unchanged: 11.6%
Serum half-life (normal/ESRD): 1.7/3 hrs
Plasma protein binding: 70%
Volume of distribution (V_d): 0.35 L/kg
Primary Mode of Elimination: Renal
Dosage Adjustments*

CrCl ~ 30–60 mL/min	No change
CrCl < 30 mL/min	300 mg (PO) q24h
Post–HD dose	300 mg (PO)
Post–PD dose	None
CVVH dose	600 mg (PO) q24h
Moderate or severe hepatic insufficiency	No change

Drug Interactions: Probenecid (↑ cefdinir levels)
Adverse Effects: Drug fever/rash
Allergic Potential: High
Safety in Pregnancy: B
Comments: Good activity against bacterial respiratory pathogens. Available as capsules or suspension. Treat community-acquired pneumonia with 300 mg (PO) q12h; for other respiratory pathogens, use 600 mg (PO) q24h
Cerebrospinal Fluid Penetration: No data

REFERENCES:

Cefdinir: A new oral cephalosporin. Med Lett Drugs Therap 40:85-7, 1998.

Fogarty CM, Bettis RB, Griffin TJ, et al. Comparison of a 5 day regimen of cefdinir with a 10 day regimen of cefprozil for treatment of acute exacerbations of chronic bronchitis. J Antimicrob Chemother 45:851-8, 2000.

Guay DR. Cefdinir: an advanced-generation, broad-spectrum oral cephalosporin. Clin Ther 24:473-89, 2002.

Nemeth MA, Gooche WM 3rd, Hedrick J, et al. Comparison of cefdinir and penicillin for the treatment of pediatric streptococcal pharyngitis. Clin Ther 21:1525-32, 1999.

Website: www.omnicef.com

Cefditoren (Spectracef)

Drug Class: 3rd generation oral cephalosporin
Usual Dose: 400 mg (PO) q12h
Pharmacokinetic Parameters:
Peak serum level: 1.8 mcg/mL
Bioavailability: 16%
Excreted unchanged: 20%
Serum half-life (normal/ESRD): 1.5/5 hrs
Plasma protein binding: 88%
Volume of distribution (V_d): 0.13 L/kg
Primary Mode of Elimination: Renal
Dosage Adjustments*

CrCl ~ 50–60 mL/min	No change
CrCl ~ 30-50 mL/min	200 mg (PO) q12h
CrCl < 30 mL/min	200 mg (PO) q24h
Post–HD/PD dose	No information
CVVH dose	No information
Moderate or severe hepatic insufficiency	No change

Drug Interactions: H₂ receptor antagonists, Al⁺⁺, Mg⁺⁺ antacids (↓ absorption of cefditoran); Probenecid (↓ elimination of cefditoran)
Adverse Effects: Drug fever/rash
Allergic Potential: Low
Safety in Pregnancy: B

Comments: Serum concentrations increased ~ 50% if taken without food. ↑ elimination of carnitine; do not use in carnitine deficiency or hereditary carnitine metabolism disorder. Contains Na⁺ caseinate; avoid in patients with protein hypersensitivity

Cerebrospinal Fluid Penetration: No data

REFERENCES:

Balbisi EA. Cefditoren, a new aminothiazolyl cephalosporin. Pharmacotherapy 22:1278-93, 2002.

Chow J, Russel M, Bolk S. et al. Efficacy of cefditoren pivoxil vs. amoxicillin-clavulanic in acute maxillary sinusitis. Presented at the 40th Interscience Conference on Antimicrobial Agents and Chemotherapy; Abstract 835, Toronto, ON 2000.

Clark CL, Nagai K, Dewasse BE, et al. Activity of cefditoren against respiratory pathogens. J Antimicrob Chemother 50:33-41, 2002.

Darkes MJ, Plosker GL. Cefditoren pivoxil. Drugs 62:319-36, 2002.

Guay DR. Review of cefditoren, an advanced-generation, broad-spectrum oral cephalosporin. Clin Ther 23:1924-37, 2002.

Website: www.pdr.net

Cefepime (Maxipime)

Drug Class: 4th generation cephalosporin
Usual Dose: 1-2 gm (IV) q12h (see comments)
Pharmacokinetic Parameters:
Peak serum level: 163 mcg/mL
Bioavailability: Not applicable
Excreted unchanged: 85%
Serum half-life (normal/ESRD): 2.2/18 hrs
Plasma protein binding: 20%
Volume of distribution (V_d): 0.29 L/kg
Primary Mode of Elimination: Renal
Dosage Adjustments* (based on 2 gm q12h):

CrCl ~ 30–60 mL/min	2 gm (IV) q24h
CrCl ~ 11–29 mL/min	1 gm (IV) q24h
CrCl < 11 mL/min	500 mg (IV) q24h
Hemodialysis	1 gm on day 1, then 500 mg (IV) q24h; on HD days, give after HD
CAPD	2 gm (IV) q48h
CVVH dose	1 gm (IV) q24h
Moderate or severe hepatic insufficiency	No change

Drug Interactions: None
Adverse Effects: Drug fever/rash
Allergic Potential: Moderate
Safety in Pregnancy: B
Comments: For proven serious systemic P. aeruginosa infections, febrile neutropenia, or cystic fibrosis, use 2 gm (IV) q8h. Effective against most strains of ceftazidime-resistant P. aeruginosa. Meningeal dose: 2 gm (IV) q8h
Cerebrospinal Fluid Penetration:
Non-inflamed meninges = 1%
Inflamed meninges = 15%
Bile Penetration: 10%

REFERENCES:

Ambrose PF, Owens RC Jr, Garvey MJ, et al. Pharmacodynamic considerations in the treatment of moderate to severe pseudomonal infections with cefepime. J Antimicrob Chemother 49:445-53, 2002.

Badaro R, Molinar F, Seas C, et al. A multicenter comparative study of cefepime versus broad-spectrum antibacterial therapy in moderate and severe bacterial infections. Braz J Infect Dis 6:206-18, 2002.

Boselli E, Breilh D, Duflo F, et al. Steady-state plasma and intrapulmonary concentrations of cefepime administered in continuous infusion in critically ill patients with severe nosocomial pneumonia. Crit Care Med 31: 2102-6, 2003.

Chapman TM, Perry CM. Cefepime: a review of its use in the management of hospitalized patients with pneumonia. Am J Respir Med 2: 75-107, 2003.

Cornely OA, Bethe U, Seifert H, et al. A randomized monocentric trial in febrile neutropenic patients: ceftriaxone and gentamicin vs cefepime and gentamicin. Ann Hematol 81:37-43, 2002.

Cunha BA, Gill MV. Cefepime. Med Clin North Am 79:721-32, 1995.

Cunha BA. Pseudomonas aeruginosa: Resistance and therapy. Semin Respir Infect 17:231-9, 2002.

Fleming DR, Ziegler C, Baize T, et al. Cefepime versus ticarcillin and clavulanate potassium and aztreonam for febrile neutropenia therapy in high-dose chemotherapy patients. Am J Clin Oncol 26: 285-8, 2003.

Fritsche TR, Sader HS, Jones RN. Comparative activity and spectrum of broad-spectrum beta-lactams (cefepime, ceftazidime, ceftriaxone, piperacillin/tazobactam) tested against 12,295 staphylococci and streptococci: report from the SENTRY antimicrobial surveillance program (North America: 2001-2002). Diagn Microbiol Infect Dis 47: 435-40, 2003.

Montalar J, Segura A, Bosch C, et al. Cefepime monotherapy as an empirical initial treatment of patients with febrile neutropenia. Med Oncol 19:161-6, 2002.

Paradisi F, Corti G, Strohmeyer M. Cefepime. Antibiotics for Clinicians 3:41-50, 1999.

Tam VH, McKinnon PS, Akins RL, et al. Pharmacodynamics of cefepime in patients with gram-negative infections. J Antimicrob Chemother 50:425-8, 2002.

Tam VH, McKinnon PS, Akins RL, et al. Pharmacokinetics and pharmacodynamics of cefepime in patients with various degrees of renal function. Antimicrob Agents Chemother 47: 1853-61, 2003.

Toltzis P, Dul M, O'Riordan MA, et al. Cefepime use in a pediatric intensive care unit reduces colonization with resistant bacilli. Pediatr Infect Dis J. 22:109-14, 2003.
Website: www.elan.com/Products/

Cefixime (Suprax)

Drug Class: 3rd generation oral cephalosporin
Usual Dose: 400 mg (PO) q12h or 200 mg (PO) q12h
Pharmacokinetic Parameters:
Peak serum level: 3.7 mcg/mL
Bioavailability: 50%
Excreted unchanged: 50%
Serum half-life (normal/ESRD): 3.1/11 hrs
Plasma protein binding: 65%
Volume of distribution (V_d): 0.1 L/kg
Primary Mode of Elimination: Renal
Dosage Adjustments*

CrCl ~ 20–60 mL/min	300 mg (PO) q24h
CrCl < 20 mL/min	200 mg (PO) q24h
Post–HD dose	None
Post–PD dose	200 mg (PO)
CVVH dose	200 mg (PO) q12h
Moderate hepatic insufficiency	No change

Severe hepatic insufficiency	No change

Drug Interactions: Carbamazepine (↑ carbamazepine levels)
Adverse Effects: Drug fever/rash, diarrhea
Allergic Potential: High
Safety in Pregnancy: B
Comments: Little/no activity against S. aureus (MSSA)
Cerebrospinal Fluid Penetration: < 10%
Bile Penetration: 800%

REFERENCES:
Markham A, Brogden RN. Cefixime: A review of its therapeutic efficacy in lower respiratory tract infections. Drugs 49:1007-22, 1995.

Marshall WF, Blair JE. The cephalosporins . Mayo Clin Proc 74:187-95, 1999.

Quintiliani R. Cefixime in the treatment of patients with lower respiratory tract infections: Results of US clinical trials. Clinical Therapeutics 18:373-90, 1996.
Website: www.pdr.net

Cefoperazone (Cefobid)

Drug Class: 3rd generation cephalosporin
Usual Dose: 2 gm (IV) q12h
Pharmacokinetic Parameters:
Peak serum level: 240 mcg/mL
Bioavailability: Not applicable
Excreted unchanged: 20%
Serum half-life (normal/ESRD): 2.4/2.4 hrs
Plasma protein binding: 90%
Volume of distribution (V_d): 0.17 L/kg
Primary Mode of Elimination: Hepatic
Dosage Adjustments*

CrCl ~ 40–60 mL/min	No change
CrCl ~ 10–40 mL/min	No change
CrCl < 10 mL/min	No change
Post–HD dose	None
Post–PD dose	None
CVVH dose	None

"Usual dose" assumes normal renal/hepatic function. * For renal insufficiency, give usual dose x 1 followed by maintenance dose per CrCl. For dialysis patients, dose the same as for CrCl < 10 mL/min and give supplemental (post-HD/PD dose) immediately after dialysis. CrCl = creatinine clearance; CVVH = continuous veno-venous hemo-filtration; HD/PD = hemodialysis/peritoneal dialysis. See pp. 293-297 for explanations, p. 1 for abbreviations

Moderate hepatic insufficiency	No change
Severe hepatic insufficiency	1 gm (IV) q12h

Drug Interactions: Alcohol (disulfiram-like reaction); antiplatelet agents, heparin, thrombolytics, warfarin (↑ risk of bleeding)
Adverse Effects: Drug fever/rash. ↑ INR due to MTT side chain, but no increase in clinical bleeding. Prophylactic vitamin K unnecessary
Allergic Potential: Low
Safety in Pregnancy: B
Comments: One of the few antibiotics to penetrate into an obstructed biliary tract. May be administered IM. Concentration dependent serum half life. Na^+ content = 1.5 mEq/g.
Meningeal dose = 2 gm (IV) q8h
Cerebrospinal Fluid Penetration:
Non-inflamed meninges = 1%
Inflamed meninges = 10%
Bile Penetration: 1200%

REFERENCES:
Cunha BA: 3rd generation cephalosporins: A review. Clin Ther 14:616-52, 1992.
Klein NC, Cunha BA. Third-generation cephalosporins. Med Clin North Am 79:705-19, 1995.
Marshall WF, Blair JE. The cephalosporins. Mayo Clin Proc 74:187-95, 1999.
Website: www.pdr.net

Cefotaxime (Claforan)

Drug Class: 3rd generation cephalosporin
Usual Dose: 2 gm (IV) q6h
Pharmacokinetic Parameters:
Peak serum level: 214 mcg/mL
Bioavailability: Not applicable
Excreted unchanged: 60%
Serum half-life (normal/ESRD): 1/15 hrs
Plasma protein binding: 37%
Volume of distribution (V_d): 0.25 L/kg
Primary Mode of Elimination: Renal
Dosage Adjustments*

CrCl ~ 20–60 mL/min	No change
CrCl < 20 mL/min	1 gm (IV) q6h

Post–HD dose	1 gm (IV)
Post–PD dose	None
CVVH dose	2 gm (IV) q8h
Moderate hepatic insufficiency	No change
Severe hepatic insufficiency	No change

Drug Interactions: None
Adverse Effects: Drug fever/rash
Allergic Potential: Moderate
Safety in Pregnancy: B
Comments: Incompatible in solutions containing sodium bicarbonate, metronidazole, or aminoglycosides. Desacetyl metabolite ($t_{1/2}$ = 1.5 hrs) synergistic with cefotaxime against S. aureus/B. fragilis. Na^+ content = 2.2 mEq/g.
Meningeal dose = 3 gm (IV) q6h
Cerebrospinal Fluid Penetration:
Non-inflamed meninges = 1%
Inflamed meninges = 10%
Bile Penetration: 75%

REFERENCES:
Brogden RN, Spencer CM. Cefotaxime: A reappraisal of its antibacterial activity and pharmacokinetic properties and a review of its therapeutic efficacy when administered twice daily for the treatment of mild to moderate infections. Drugs 53:483-510, 1987.
Klein NC, Cunha BA. Third-generation cephalosporins. Med Clin North Am 79:705-19, 1995.
Marshall WF, Blair JE. The cephalosporins. Mayo Clin Proc 74:187-95, 1999.
Patel KB, Nicolau DP, Nightingale CH, et al. Comparative serum bactericidal activities of ceftizoxime and cefotaxime against intermediately penicillin-resistant Streptococcus pneumoniae. Antimicrob Agents Chemother 40:2805-8, 1996.
Website: www.pdr.net

Cefotetan (Cefotan)

Drug Class: 2nd generation cephalosporin (Cephamycin)
Usual Dose: 2 gm (IV) q12h
Pharmacokinetic Parameters:

"Usual dose" assumes normal renal/hepatic function. * For renal insufficiency, give usual dose x 1 followed by maintenance dose per CrCl. For dialysis patients, dose the same as for CrCl < 10 mL/min and give supplemental (post-HD/PD dose) immediately after dialysis. CrCl = creatinine clearance; CVVH = continuous veno-venous hemo-filtration; HD/PD = hemodialysis/peritoneal dialysis. See pp. 293-297 for explanations, p. 1 for abbreviations

Peak serum level: 237 mcg/mL
Bioavailability: Not applicable
Excreted unchanged: 51-81%
Serum half-life (normal/ESRD): 4/10 hrs
Plasma protein binding: 88%
Volume of distribution (V_d): 0.17 L/kg
Primary Mode of Elimination: Renal
Dosage Adjustments* (based on 2 gm q12h):

CrCl ~ 30–60 mL/min	2 gm (IV) q12h
CrCl ~ 10–30 mL/min	2 gm (IV) q24h
CrCl < 10 mL/min	2 gm (IV) q48h
Post–HD dose	1 gm (IV)
Post–PD dose	1 gm (IV)
CVVH dose	1 gm (IV) q12h
Moderate or severe hepatic insufficiency	No change

Drug Interactions: Alcohol (disulfiram-like reaction); antiplatelet agents, heparin, thrombolytics, warfarin (↑ risk of bleeding)
Adverse Effects: Drug fever/rash, hemolytic anemia. ↑ INR due to MTT side chain, but no increase in clinical bleeding
Allergic Potential: Low
Safety in Pregnancy: B
Comments: Less effective than cefoxitin against B. fragilis D.O.T strains. Na^+ content = 3.5 mEq/g
Cerebrospinal Fluid Penetration: < 10%
Bile Penetration: 20%

REFERENCES:
Moes GS, MacPherson BR. Cefotetan-induced hemolytic anemia: A case report and a review of the literature. Arch Pathol Lab Med 124:1344-6, 2000.
Ray EK, Warkentin TE, O'Hoski PL. Delayed onset of life-threatening immune hemolysis after perioperative antimicrobial prophylaxis with cefotetan. Can J Surg 43:461-2, 2000.
Stroncek D, Procter JL, Johnson J. Drug-induced hemolysis: Cefotetan-dependent hemolytic anemia mimicking an acute intravascular immune transfusion reaction. Am J Hematol 64:67-70, 2000.
Website: www.pdr.net

Cefoxitin (Mefoxin)

Drug Class: 2nd generation cephalosporin (Cephamycin)
Usual Dose: 2 gm (IV) q6h
Pharmacokinetic Parameters:
Peak serum level: 221 mcg/mL
Bioavailability: Not applicable
Excreted unchanged: 85%
Serum half-life (normal/ESRD): 1/21 hrs
Plasma protein binding: 75%
Volume of distribution (V_d): 0.12 L/kg
Primary Mode of Elimination: Renal
Dosage Adjustments*

CrCl ~ 30–50 mL/min	1 gm (IV) q8h
CrCl ~ 10–30 mL/min	1 gm (IV) q12h
CrCl < 10 mL/min	1 gm (IV) q24h
Post–HD dose	1 gm (IV)
Post–PD dose	1 gm (IV)
CVVH dose	2 gm (IV) q12h
Moderate hepatic insufficiency	No change
Severe hepatic insufficiency	No change

Drug Interactions: None
Adverse Effects: Drug fever/rash
Allergic Potential: Low
Safety in Pregnancy: B
Comments: Effective against B. fragilis, including D.O.T. strains B. distasonis, B. ovatus, B. thetiaotamicron. Na^+ content = 2.3 mEq/g
Cerebrospinal Fluid Penetration: < 10%
Bile Penetration: 250%

REFERENCES:
Hansen EA, Cunha BA. Cefoxitin. Antibiotics for Clinicians 5:33-41, 2001.
Donowitz GR, Mandell GL. Beta-lactam antibiotics. N Engl J Med 318:419-26 and 318:490-500, 1993.
Marshall WF Blair JE. The cephalosporins. Mayo Clin Proc 74:187-95, 1999.
Website: www.pdr.net

"Usual dose" assumes normal renal/hepatic function. * For renal insufficiency, give usual dose x 1 followed by maintenance dose per CrCl. For dialysis patients, dose the same as for CrCl < 10 mL/min and give supplemental (post-HD/PD dose) immediately after dialysis. CrCl = creatinine clearance; CVVH = continuous veno-venous hemofiltration; HD/PD = hemodialysis/peritoneal dialysis. See pp. 293-297 for explanations, p. 1 for abbreviations

Cefpodoxime (Vantin)

Drug Class: 3rd generation oral cephalosporin
Usual Dose: 200 mg (PO) q12h
Pharmacokinetic Parameters:
Peak serum level: 2.3 mcg/mL
Bioavailability: 50%
Excreted unchanged: 30%
Serum half-life (normal/ESRD): 2.3/9.8 hrs
Plasma protein binding: 21-33%
Volume of distribution (V_d): 0.9 L/kg
Primary Mode of Elimination: Renal
Dosage Adjustments*

CrCl ~ 30–60 mL/min	No change
CrCl ~ 10–30 mL/min	200 mg (PO) q24h
CrCl < 10 mL/min	200 mg (PO) q24h
Post–HD dose	200 mg (PO)
Post–PD dose	200 mg (PO)
CVVH dose	200 mg (PO) q12h
Moderate hepatic insufficiency	No change
Severe hepatic insufficiency	No change

Drug Interactions: None
Adverse Effects: Drug fever/rash, pulmonary infiltrates with eosinophilia, hepatotoxicity
Allergic Potential: High
Safety in Pregnancy: B
Comments: Only oral 3rd generation cephalosporin active against S. aureus (MSSA)
Cerebrospinal Fluid Penetration: < 10%
Bile Penetration: 100%

REFERENCES:
Adam D, Bergogne-Berezin E, Jones RN. Symposium on cefpodoxime proxetil: A new third generation oral cephalosporin. Drugs 42:1-66, 1991.
Cohen R. Clinical efficacy of cefpodoxime in respiratory tract infection. J Antimicrob Chemother 50(Suppl):23-7, 2002.
Cohen R. Clinical experience with cefpodoxime proxetil in acute otitis media. Pediatr Infect Dis J 14:S12-8, 1995.
Liu P, Muller M, Grant M, et al. Interstitial tissue concentrations of cefpodoxime. J Antimicrob Chemother 50(Suppl):19-22, 2002.
Schatz BS, Karavokiros KT, Taeubel MA, et al. Comparison of cefprozil, cefpodoxime proxetil, loracarbef, cefixime, and ceftibuten. Ann Pharmacother 30:258-68, 1996.
Website: www.pdr.net

Cefprozil (Cefzil)

Drug Class: 2nd generation oral cephalosporin
Usual Dose: 500 mg (PO) q12h
Pharmacokinetic Parameters:
Peak serum level: 10 mcg/mL
Bioavailability: 95%
Excreted unchanged: 60%
Serum half-life (normal/ESRD): 1.3/5.9 hrs
Plasma protein binding: 36%
Volume of distribution (V_d): 0.23 L/kg
Primary Mode of Elimination: Renal
Dosage Adjustments*

CrCl ~ 30–60 mL/min	No change
CrCl ~ 10–30 mL/min	250 mg (PO) q12h
CrCl < 10 mL/min	250 mg (PO) q12h
Post–HD dose	500 mg (PO)
Post–PD dose	None
CVVH dose	500 mg (PO) q24h
Moderate hepatic insufficiency	No change
Severe hepatic insufficiency	No change

Drug Interactions: None
Adverse Effects: Drug fever/rash
Allergic Potential: Low
Safety in Pregnancy: B
Comments: Penetrates oral/respiratory secretions well
Cerebrospinal Fluid Penetration: < 10%

REFERENCES:
Cunha BA. New antibiotics for the treatment of acute exacerbations of chronic bronchitis. Adv Ther 13:313-23, 1996.

"Usual dose" assumes normal renal/hepatic function. * For renal insufficiency, give usual dose x 1 followed by maintenance dose per CrCl. For dialysis patients, dose the same as for CrCl < 10 mL/min and give supplemental (post-HD/PD dose) immediately after dialysis. CrCl = creatinine clearance; CVVH = continuous veno-venous hemo-filtration; HD/PD = hemodialysis/peritoneal dialysis. See pp. 293-297 for explanations, p. 1 for abbreviations

Gainer RB 2nd. Cefprozil: A new cephalosporin; its use in various clinical trials. South Med J 88:338-46, 1995.

Marshall WF Blair JE. The cephalosporins. Mayo Clin Proc 74:187-95, 1999.

Schatz BS, Karavokiros KT, Taeubel MA, et al. Comparison of cefprozil, cefpodoxime, proxetil, loracarbef, cefixime, and ceftibuten. Ann Pharmacother 30:258-68, 1996.

Website: www.pdr.net

Ceftazidime (Fortaz, Tazicef, Tazidime)

Drug Class: 3rd generation cephalosporin
Usual Dose: 2 gm (IV) q8h
Pharmacokinetic Parameters:
Peak serum level: 170 mcg/mL
Bioavailability: Not applicable
Excreted unchanged: 82%
Serum half-life (normal/ESRD): 1.9/21 hrs
Plasma protein binding: 10%
Volume of distribution (V_d): 0.36 L/kg
Primary Mode of Elimination: Renal
Dosage Adjustments*

CrCl ~ 31–50 mL/min	1 gm (IV) q12h
CrCl ~ 16–30 mL/min	1 gm (IV) q24h
CrCl ~ 6-15 mL/min	500 mg (IV) q24h
CrCl < 5 mL/min	500 mg (IV) q48h
Post–HD dose	1 gm (IV)
Post–PD dose	500 mg (IV)
CVVH dose	1 gm (IV) q12h
Moderate hepatic insufficiency	No change
Severe hepatic insufficiency	No change

Drug Interactions: None
Adverse Effects: Drug fever/rash
Allergic Potential: High
Safety in Pregnancy: B
Comments: Incompatible in solutions containing vancomycin or aminoglycosides. Use increases prevalence of MRSA. Inducer of E.

coli/Klebsiella ESBLs. Na$^+$ content = 2.3 mEq/g.
Meningeal dose = 2 gm (IV) q8h
Cerebrospinal Fluid Penetration:
Non-inflamed meninges = 1%
Inflamed meninges = 20%
Bile Penetration: 50%

REFERENCES:
Berkhout J, Visser LG, van den Broek PJ, et al. Clinical pharmacokinetics of cefamandole and ceftazidime administered by continuous intravenous infusion. Antimicrob Agents Chemother. 47:1862-6, 2003.

Briscoe-Dwyer L. Ceftazidime. Antibiotics for Clinicians 1:41-8, 1997.

Klein NC, Cunha BA. Third-generation cephalosporins. Med Clin North Am 79:705-19, 1995.

Marshall WF, Blair JE. The cephalosporins. Mayo Clin Proc 74:187-95, 1999.

Nicolau DP, Nightingale CH, Banevicius MA, et al. Serum bactericidal activity of ceftazidime: Continuous infusion versus intermittent injections. Antimicrob Agents Chemother 40:61-4, 1996.

Owens JC, Jr, Ambrose PG, Quintiliani R. Ceftazidime to cefepime formulary switch: Pharmacodynamic rationale. Conn Med 61:225-7, 1997.

Rains CP, Bryson HM, Peters DH. Ceftazidime: An update of its antibacterial activity, pharmacokinetic properties, and therapeutic efficacy. Drugs 49:577-617, 1995.

Website: www.pdr.net

Ceftibuten (Cedax)

Drug Class: 3rd generation oral cephalosporin
Usual Dose: 400 mg (PO) q24h
Pharmacokinetic Parameters:
Peak serum level: 18 mcg/mL
Bioavailability: 80%
Excreted unchanged: 56%
Serum half-life (normal/ESRD): 2.4/22 hrs
Plasma protein binding: 65%
Volume of distribution (V_d): 0.2 L/kg
Primary Mode of Elimination: Renal
Dosage Adjustments*

CrCl ~ 50–60 mL/min	400 mg (PO) q24h
CrCl ~ 30–49 mL/min	200 mg (PO) q24h
CrCl < 30 mL/min	100 mg (PO) q24h
Post–HD dose	400 mg (PO)

"Usual dose" assumes normal renal/hepatic function. * For renal insufficiency, give usual dose x 1 followed by maintenance dose per CrCl. For dialysis patients, dose the same as for CrCl < 10 mL/min and give supplemental (post-HD/PD dose) immediately after dialysis. CrCl = creatinine clearance; CVVH = continuous veno-venous hemo-filtration; HD/PD = hemodialysis/peritoneal dialysis. See pp. 293-297 for explanations, p. 1 for abbreviations

Post–PD dose	No information
CVVH dose	200 mg (PO) q24h
Moderate hepatic insufficiency	No change
Severe hepatic insufficiency	No change

Drug Interactions: None
Adverse Effects: Drug fever/rash
Allergic Potential: High
Safety in Pregnancy: B
Comments: Least anti–S. pneumoniae activity among oral 3rd generation cephalosporins
Cerebrospinal Fluid Penetration: < 10%

REFERENCES:
Guay DR. Ceftibuten: A new expanded-spectrum oral cephalosporin. Ann Pharmacother 31:1022-33, 1997.
Owens RC Jr, Nightingale CH, Nicolau DP. Ceftibuten: An overview. Pharmacother 17:707-20, 1997.
Wiseman LR, Balfour JA. Ceftibuten: A review of its antibacterial activity, pharmacokinetic properties and clinical efficacy. Drugs 47:784-808, 1994.
Website: www.pdr.net

Ceftizoxime (Cefizox)

Drug Class: 3rd generation cephalosporin
Usual Dose: 2 gm (IV) q8h
Pharmacokinetic Parameters:
Peak serum level: 132 mcg/mL
Bioavailability: Not applicable
Excreted unchanged: 90%
Serum half-life (normal/ESRD): 1.7/35 hrs
Plasma protein binding: 30%
Volume of distribution (V_d): 0.32 L/kg
Primary Mode of Elimination: Renal
Dosage Adjustments*

CrCl ~ 40–60 mL/min	1 gm (IV) q8h
CrCl ~ 10–40 mL/min	1 gm (IV) q12h
CrCl < 10 mL/min	1 gm (IV) q24h
Post–HD dose	500 mg (IV)
Post–PD dose	500 mg (IV)

CVVH dose	1 gm (IV) q12h
Moderate hepatic insufficiency	No change
Severe hepatic insufficiency	No change

Drug Interactions: None
Adverse Effects: Drug fever/rash
Allergic Potential: High
Safety in Pregnancy: B
Comments: Na^+ content = 2.6 mEq/g.
Meningeal dose = 3 gm (IV) q6h
Cerebrospinal Fluid Penetration:
Non-inflamed meninges = 1%
Inflamed meninges = 10%
Bile Penetration: 50%

REFERENCES:
Klein NC, Cunha BA. Third-generation cephalosporins. Med Clin North Am 79:705-19, 1995.
Donowitz GR, Mandell GL. Beta-lactam antibiotics. N Engl J Med 318:419-26 and 318:490-500, 1993.
Marshall WF Blair JE. The cephalosporins. Mayo Clin Proc 74:187-95, 1999.
Website: www.pdr.net

Ceftriaxone (Rocephin)

Drug Class: 3rd generation cephalosporin
Usual Dose: 1-2 gm (IV) q24h
Pharmacokinetic Parameters:
Peak serum level: 151-257 mcg/mL
Bioavailability: Not applicable
Excreted unchanged: 33-67%
Serum half-life (normal/ESRD): 8/16 hrs
Plasma protein binding: 90%
Volume of distribution (V_d): 0.08-0.3 L/kg
Primary Mode of Elimination: Renal/hepatic
Dosage Adjustments*

CrCl ~ 40–60 mL/min	No change
CrCl ~ 10–40 mL/min	No change
CrCl < 10 mL/min	No change
Post–HD dose	None
Post–PD dose	None

"Usual dose" assumes normal renal/hepatic function. * For renal insufficiency, give usual dose x 1 followed by maintenance dose per CrCl. For dialysis patients, dose the same as for CrCl < 10 mL/min and give supplemental (post-HD/PD dose) immediately after dialysis. CrCl = creatinine clearance; CVVH = continuous veno-venous hemofiltration; HD/PD = hemodialysis/peritoneal dialysis. See pp. 293-297 for explanations, p. 1 for abbreviations

CVVH dose	No change
Moderate hepatic insufficiency	No change
Severe hepatic insufficiency	No change

Drug Interactions: None
Adverse Effects: Drug fever/rash, irritative diarrhea, pseudo-biliary lithiasis, may interfere with platelet aggregation
Allergic Potential: High
Safety in Pregnancy: B. Avoid near term in 3rd trimester (↑ incidence of kernicterus in newborns)
Comments: Useful to treat penicillin-resistant S. pneumoniae in CAP/CNS. CSF breakpoints for ceftriaxone are S (sensitive) ≤ 0.5 mcg/mL, I (intermediate) = 1 mcg/mL, and R (resistant) ≥ 2 mcg/mL. Non-meningeal breakpoints are S ≤ 1 mcg/mL, I = 2 mcg/mL, and R ≥ 4 mcg/mL. Ceftriaxone 1-2 gm (IV) q24h is useful for intra-abdominal/pelvic sepsis in combination with metronidazole 1 gm (IV) q24h. Ceftriaxone also has excellent activity against Group A streptococci and S. aureus (MSSA), making it useful for skin/soft tissue infections. May be given IV or IM. Incompatible in solutions containing vancomycin. Na+ content = 2.6 mEq/g. Meningeal dose = 2 gm (IV) q12h
Cerebrospinal Fluid Penetration:
Non-inflamed meninges = 1%
Inflamed meninges = 10%
Bile Penetration: 500%

REFERENCES:
Cunha BA, Klein NC. The selection and use of cephalosporins: A review. Adv Ther 12:83-101, 1995.
Dietrich ES, Bieser U, Frank U, et al. Ceftriaxone versus other cephalosporins for perioperative antibiotic prophylaxis: a meta analysis of 43 randomized controlled trials. Chemotherapy 48:49-56, 2002.
Freeman CD, Nightingale CH, Nicolau DP, et al. Serum bactericidal activity of ceftriaxone plus metronidazole against common intra-abdominal pathogens. Am J Hosp Pharm 51:1782-7, 1994.
Grassi C. Ceftriaxone. Antibiotics for Clinicians 2:49-57, 1998.
Karlowsky JA, Jones ME. Importance of using current NCCLS breakpoints to interpret cefotaxime and

ceftriaxone MICs for Streptococcus pneumoniae. J Antimicrob Chemother. 51:467-8, 2003.
Klein NC, Cunha BA. Third -generation cephalosporins. Med Clin North Am 79:705-19, 1995.
Lamb HM, Ormrod D, Scott LJ, et al. Ceftriazone: an update of its use in the management of community-acquired and nosocomial infections. Drugs 62:1041-89, 2002.
Marshall WF, Blair JE. The cephalosporins. Mayo Clin Proc 74:187-95, 1999.
Schaad UB, Suter S, Gianella-Borradori A, et al. A comparison of ceftriaxone and cefuroxime for the treatment of bacterial meningitis in children. N Engl J Med 322:141-7, 1990.
Woodfield JC, Van Rij AM, Pettigrew RA, et al. A comparison of the prophylactic efficacy of ceftriaxone and cefotaxime in abdominal surgery. Am J Surg. 185:45-9, 2003.
Website: www.rocheusa.com/products/rocephin

Cefuroxime (Kefurox, Zinacef, Ceftin)

Drug Class: 2nd generation IV/oral cephalosporin
Usual Dose: 1.5 gm (IV) q8h; 500 mg (PO) q12h
Pharmacokinetic Parameters:
Peak serum level: 100 (IV) / 7 (PO) mcg/mL
Bioavailability: 52%
Excreted unchanged: 50%
Serum half-life (normal/ESRD): 1.2/17 hrs
Plasma protein binding: 50%
Volume of distribution (V_d): 0.15 L/kg
Primary Mode of Elimination: Renal
Dosage Adjustments*

CrCl ~ 20–60 mL/min	750 mg (IV) q8h 250 mg (PO) q12h
CrCl ~ 10–20 mL/min	750 mg (IV) q12h 250 mg (PO) q12h
CrCl < 10 mL/min	750 mg (IV) q24h 250 mg (PO) q24h
Post–HD dose	750 mg (IV) 250 mg (PO)
Post–PD dose	No information

"Usual dose" assumes normal renal/hepatic function. * For renal insufficiency, give usual dose x 1 followed by maintenance dose per CrCl. For dialysis patients, dose the same as for CrCl < 10 mL/min and give supplemental (post-HD/PD dose) immediately after dialysis. CrCl = creatinine clearance; CVVH = continuous veno-venous hemo-filtration; HD/PD = hemodialysis/peritoneal dialysis. See pp. 293-297 for explanations, p. 1 for abbreviations

CVVH dose	1.5 gm (IV) q12h 500 mg (PO) q12h
Moderate hepatic insufficiency	No change
Severe hepatic insufficiency	No change

Drug Interactions: None
Adverse Effects: Drug fever/rash
Allergic Potential: High
Safety in Pregnancy: B
Comments: Oral preparation penetrates oral/respiratory secretions well. Na^+ content (IV preparation) = 2.4 mEq/g. Do not use for meningitis prophylaxis (H. influenzae bacteremia) or therapy
Cerebrospinal Fluid Penetration: < 10%

REFERENCES:
Bucko AD, Hunt BJ, Kidd SL, et al. Randomized, double-blind, multicenter comparison of oral cefditoren 200 or 400 mg BID with either cefuroxime 250 mg BID or cefadroxil 500 mg BID for the treatment of uncomplicated skin and skin-structure infections. Clin Ther 24:1134-47, 2002.
Gentry LO, Zeluff BJ, Cooley DA. Antibiotic prophylaxis in open-heart surgery: A comparison of cefamandole, cefuroxime, and cefazolin. Ann Thorac Surg 46:167-71, 1988.
Marshall WF, Blair JE. The cephalosporins. Mayo Clin Proc 74:187-95, 1999.
Perry Cm, Brogden RN. Cefuroxime axetil. A review of its antibacterial activity, pharmacokinetic properties, and therapeutic efficacy. Drugs 52:125-58, 1996.
Website: www.pdr.net

Cephalexin (Keflex)

Drug Class: 1st generation oral cephalosporin
Usual Dose: 500 mg (PO) q6h
Pharmacokinetic Parameters:
Peak serum level: 18 mcg/mL
Bioavailability: 99%
Excreted unchanged: > 90%
Serum half-life (normal/ESRD): 0.7/16 hrs
Plasma protein binding: 10%
Volume of distribution (V_d): 0.35 L/kg
Primary Mode of Elimination: Renal

Dosage Adjustments*

CrCl ~ 40–60 mL/min	No change
CrCl ~ 10–40 mL/min	250 mg (PO) q8h
CrCl < 10 mL/min	250 mg (PO) q12h
Post–HD dose	No information
Post–PD dose	No information
CVVH dose	250 mg (PO) q8h
Moderate hepatic insufficiency	No change
Severe hepatic insufficiency	No change

Drug Interactions: None
Adverse Effects: Drug fever/rash
Allergic Potential: High
Safety in Pregnancy: B
Comments: Highly active against S. aureus (MSSA) and Group A streptococci. Limited activity against H. influenzae
Cerebrospinal Fluid Penetration: < 10%
Bile Penetration: 200%

REFERENCES:
Chow M, Quintiliani R, Cunha BA, et al. Pharmacokinetics of high dose oral cephalosporins. J Pharmacol 19:185-194, 1979.
Donowitz GR, Mandell GL. Beta-lactam antibiotics. N Engl J Med 318:419-26 and 318:490-500, 1993.
Marshall WF Blair JE. The cephalosporins. Mayo Clin Proc 74:187-95, 1999.
Smith GH. Oral cephalosporins in perspective. DICP 24:45-51, 1990.
Website: www.pdr.net

Chloramphenicol (Chloromycetin)

Drug Class: Does not belong to specific class
Usual Dose: 500 mg (IV/PO) q6h
Pharmacokinetic Parameters:
Peak serum level: 9 mcg/mL
Bioavailability: 90%
Excreted unchanged: 10%
Serum half-life (normal/ESRD): 2.5/3 hrs

"Usual dose" assumes normal renal/hepatic function. * For renal insufficiency, give usual dose x 1 followed by maintenance dose per CrCl. For dialysis patients, dose the same as for CrCl < 10 mL/min and give supplemental (post-HD/PD dose) immediately after dialysis. CrCl = creatinine clearance; CVVH = continuous veno-venous hemo-filtration; HD/PD = hemodialysis/peritoneal dialysis. See pp. 293-297 for explanations, p. 1 for abbreviations

Plasma protein binding: 50%
Volume of distribution (V_d): 1 L/kg
Primary Mode of Elimination: Hepatic
Dosage Adjustments*

CrCl ~ 40–60 mL/min	No change
CrCl < 40 mL/min	No change
Post–HD/PD dose	None
CVVH dose	No change
Moderate or severe hepatic insufficiency	No change

Drug Interactions: Barbiturates (↑ barbiturate effect, ↓ chloramphenicol effect); cyclophosphamide (↑ cyclophosphamide toxicity); cyanocobalamin, iron (↓ response to interacting drug); warfarin (↑ INR); phenytoin (↑ phenytoin toxicity); rifabutin, rifampin (↓ chloramphenicol levels); sulfonylureas (↑ sulfonylurea effect, hypoglycemia)

Adverse Effects:
<u>Dose–related bone marrow suppression</u>
Reversible. Bone marrow aspirate shows vacuolated WBCs ("chloramphenicol effect," not toxicity). Does not precede aplastic anemia
<u>Idiosyncratic bone marrow toxicity</u>
Irreversible aplastic anemia. May occur after only one dose; monitoring with serial CBCs is useless. Very rare. Usually associated with IM, intraocular, or oral administration. Rarely, if ever, with IV chloramphenicol

Allergic Potential: Low
Safety in Pregnancy: C
Comments: Incompatible in solutions containing diphenylhydantoin, methylprednisone, aminophylline, ampicillin, gentamicin, erythromycin, vancomycin. Dose-related marrow suppression is common, but reversible. Hepatic toxicity related to prolonged/high doses (> 4 gm/d). Oral administration results in higher serum levels than IV administration. Do not administer IM. Chloramphenicol is inactivated in bile. Urinary concentrations are therapeutically ineffective. Na^+ content = 2.25 mEq/g.
Meningeal dose = usual dose

Cerebrospinal Fluid Penetration:
Non-inflamed meninges = 90%
Inflamed meninges = 90%

REFERENCES:
Cunha BA. New uses of older antibiotics. Postgrad Med 100:68-88, 1997.
Feder HM Jr, Osier C, Maderazo EG. Chloramphenicol: A review of its use in clinical practice. Rev Infect Dis 3:479- 91, 1981.
Kasten MJ. Clindamycin, metronidazole, and chloramphenicol. Mayo Clin Proc 74:825-33, 1999.
Safdar A, Bryan CS, Stinson S, et al. Prosthetic valve endocarditis due to vancomycin-resistant Enterococcus faecium: treatment with chloramphenicol plus minocycline. Clin Infect Dis 34:61-3, 2002.
Smilack JD, Wilson WE, Cocerill FR 3rd. Tetracycline, chloramphenicol, erythromycin, clindamycin, and metronidazole. Mayo Clin Proc 66:1270-80, 1991.
Tunkel AR, Wispelwey B, Scheld M. Bacterial meningitis: Recent advances in pathophysiology and treatment. Ann Intern Med 112:610-23, 1990.
Wareham DW, Wilson P. Chloramphenicol in the 21st century. Hosp Med 63:157-61, 2002.

Ciprofloxacin (Cipro)

Drug Class: Fluoroquinolone
Usual Dose: 400 mg (IV) q8-12h; 500-750 mg (PO) q12h
Pharmacokinetic Parameters:
Peak serum level: 4.6 (IV)/2.9 (PO) mcg/mL
Bioavailability: 70%
Excreted unchanged: 70%
Serum half-life (normal/ESRD): 4/8 hrs
Plasma protein binding: 20-40%
Volume of distribution (V_d): 2.5 L/kg
Primary Mode of Elimination: Renal
Dosage Adjustments*

CrCl ~ 30–50 mL/min	No change
CrCl ~ 5-29 mL/min	200-400 mg (IV) q18-24h 250-500 mg (PO) q18h
CrCl < 5 mL/min	200 mg (IV) q24h 250 mg (PO) q24h
Post–HD dose	200-400 mg (IV) 250-500 mg (PO)

"Usual dose" assumes normal renal/hepatic function. * For renal insufficiency, use usual dose x 1 followed by maintenance dose per CrCl. For dialysis patients, dose the same as for CrCl < 10 mL/min and give supplemental (post-HD/PD dose) immediately after dialysis. CrCl = creatinine clearance; CVVH = continuous veno-venous hemofiltration; HD/PD = hemodialysis/peritoneal dialysis. See pp. 293-297 for explanations, p. 1 for abbreviations

Post–PD dose	200 mg (IV) 250-500 mg (PO)
CVVH dose	200 mg (IV) q12h 250 mg (PO) q12h
Moderate hepatic insufficiency	No change
Severe hepatic insufficiency	No change

Drug Interactions: Al^{++}, Ca^{++}, Fe^{++}, Mg^{++}, Zn^{++} antacids, citrate/citric acid, dairy products (↓ absorption of ciprofloxacin only if taken together); caffeine, cyclosporine, theophylline (↑ interacting drug levels); cimetidine (↑ ciprofloxacin levels); foscarnet (↑ risk of seizures); oral hypoglycemics (slight ↑ or ↓ in blood glucose); NSAIDs (may ↑ risk of seizures/CNS stimulation); phenytoin (↑ or ↓ phenytoin levels); probenecid (↑ ciprofloxacin levels); warfarin (↑ INR)
Adverse Effects: Drug fever/rash, seizures, Achilles tendon rupture/tendinitis (class effect)
Allergic Potential: Low
Safety in Pregnancy: C
Comments: Enteral feeding decreases ciprofloxacin absorption ≥ 30%. Use with caution in patients with severe renal insufficiency or seizure disorder. Administer 2 hours before or after H_2 antagonists, omeprazole, sucralfate, calcium, iron, zinc, multivitamins, or aluminum/magnesium containing medications. Administer ciprofloxacin (IV) as an intravenous infusion over 1 hour
Cerebrospinal Fluid Penetration:
Non-inflamed meninges = 10%
Inflamed meninges = 26%
Bile Penetration: 3000%

REFERENCES:
Bellmann R, Egger P, Gritsch W, et al. Pharmacokinetics of ciprofloxacin in patients with acute renal failure undergoing continuous venovenous haemofiltration: influence of concomitant liver cirrhosis. Acta Med Austriaca 29:112-6, 2002.
Davis R, Markham A, Balfour JA. Ciprofloxacin: An updated review of its pharmacology, therapeutic efficacy, and tolerability. Drugs 51:1019-74, 1996.
Debon R, Breilh D, Boselli E, et al. Pharmacokinetic parameters of ciprofloxacin (500 mg/5mL) oral suspension in critically ill patients with severe bacterial pneumonia: a comparison of two dosages. J Chemother 14:175-80, 2002.
Peacock JE, Herrington DA, Wade JC, et al. Ciprofloxacin plus piperacillin compared with tobramycin plus piperacillin as empirical therapy in febrile neutropenic patients. A randomized, double-blind trial. Ann Intern Med 137:77-87, 2002.
Sanders CC. Ciprofloxacin: In vitro activity, mechanism of action, resistance. Rev Infect Dis 10:516-27, 1998.
Talan DA, Stamm WE, Hooton TM, et al. Comparison of ciprofloxacin (7 days) and trimethoprim-sulfamethoxazole (14 days) for acute uncomplicated pyelonephritis in women: a randomized trial. JAMA 283:1583-90, 2000.
Walker RC, Wright AJ. The fluoroquinolones. Mayo Clin Proc 66:1249-59, 1991.
Website: www.cipro.com

Ciprofloxacin Extended-Release (Cipro XR)

Drug Class: Fluoroquinolone
Usual Dose: 500 mg or 1000 mg (PO) q24h (see comments)
Pharmacokinetic Parameters (500/1000 mg):
Peak serum level: 1.59/3.11 mcg/mL
Bioavailability: 70%
Excreted unchanged: 35%
Serum half-life: 6.6/6.3 hrs
Plasma protein binding: 20-40%
Volume of distribution (V_d): 2.5 L/kg
Primary Mode of Elimination: Renal
Dosage Adjustments*

CrCl ~ 30–60 mL/min	No change
CrCl < 30 mL/min	No change for 500 mg dose; reduce 1000 mg dose to 500 mg (PO) q24h
Post–HD/PD dose	No information
CVVH dose	see CrCl < 30 mL/min
Moderate or severe hepatic insufficiency	No change

Drug Interactions: Al^{++}, Ca^{++}, Fe^{++}, Mg^{++}, Zn^{++} antacids, citrate/citric acid, dairy products,

---

"Usual dose" assumes normal renal/hepatic function. * For renal insufficiency, give usual dose x 1 followed by maintenance dose per CrCl. For dialysis patients, dose the same as for CrCl < 10 mL/min and give supplemental (post-HD/PD dose) immediately after dialysis. CrCl = creatinine clearance; CVVH = continuous veno-venous hemofiltration; HD/PD = hemodialysis/peritoneal dialysis. See pp. 293-297 for explanations, p. 1 for abbreviations

didanosine (↓ absorption of ciprofloxacin only if taken together); caffeine, cyclosporine, theophylline (↑ interacting drug levels); cimetidine (↑ ciprofloxacin levels); foscarnet (↑ risk of seizures); insulin, oral hypoglycemics (slight ↑ or ↓ in blood glucose); NSAIDs (may ↑ risk of seizures/CNS stimulation); phenytoin (↑ or ↓ phenytoin levels); probenecid (↑ ciprofloxacin levels); warfarin (↑ INR)

Adverse Effects: Drug fever/rash, seizures, Achilles tendon rupture/tendinitis (class effect)

Allergic Potential: Low

Safety in Pregnancy: C

Comments: Use 500 mg (PO) q 24h to treat uncomplicated UTI (acute cystitis); use 1000 mg (PO) q24h to treat complicated UTI or acute uncomplicated pyelonephritis. May be administered with or without food. Administer at least 2 hours before or 6 hours after H_2 antagonists, omeprazole, sucralfate, calcium, iron, zinc, multivitamins, or aluminum/magnesium containing medications

REFERENCES:
Website: www.ciproxr.com

Clarithromycin (Biaxin)

Drug Class: Macrolide
Usual Dose: 500 mg (PO) q12h
Pharmacokinetic Parameters:
Peak serum level: 1-4 mcg/mL
Bioavailability: 50%
Excreted unchanged: 20%
Serum half-life (normal/ESRD): 3-7/4 hrs
Plasma protein binding: 70%
Volume of distribution (V_d): 3 L/kg
Primary Mode of Elimination: Hepatic
Dosage Adjustments*

CrCl ~ 30–60 mL/min	No change
CrCl < 30 mL/min	250 mg (PO) q12h
Post–HD dose	None
Post–PD dose	None
CVVH dose	No change

Moderate hepatic insufficiency	No change
Severe hepatic insufficiency	No change

Drug Interactions: Amiodarone, procainamide, sotalol, astemizole, terfenadine, cisapride, pimozide (may ↑ QT interval, torsade de pointes); carbamazepine (↑ carbamazepine levels, nystagmus, nausea, vomiting, diarrhea); cimetidine, digoxin, ergot alkaloids, midazolam, triazolam, phenytoin, ritonavir, tacrolimus, valproic acid (↑ interacting drug levels); clozapine, corticosteroids (not studied); cyclosporine (↑ cyclosporine levels with toxicity); efavirenz (↓ clarithromycin levels); rifabutin, rifampin (↓ clarithromycin levels, ↑ interacting drug levels); statins (↑ risk of rhabdomyolysis); theophylline (↑ theophylline levels, nausea, vomiting, seizures, apnea); warfarin (↑ INR); zidovudine (↓ zidovudine levels)

Adverse Effects: Nausea, vomiting, GI upset, irritative diarrhea, abdominal pain. May ↑ QT_c; avoid with other medications that prolong the QT_c interval and in patients with cardiac arrhythmias/heart block

Allergic Potential: Low

Safety in Pregnancy: C

Comments: Peculiar taste of "aluminum sand" sensation on swallowing

Cerebrospinal Fluid Penetration: < 10%

Bile Penetration: 7000%

REFERENCES:
Alvarez-Elcoro S, Enzler MJ. The macrolides: Erythromycin, clarithromycin and azithromycin. Mayo Clin Proc 4:613- 34, 1999.

Benson CA, Williams PL, Cohn DL, and the ACTG 196/CPCRA 009 Study Team. Clarithromycin or rifabutin alone or in combination for primary prophylaxis of Mycobacterium avium complex disease in patients with AIDS: A randomized, double-blinded, placebo-controlled trial. J Infect Dis 181:1289-97, 2000.

Chaisson RE, Keiser P, Pierce M, et al. Clarithromycin and ethambutol with or without clofazimine for the treatment of bacteremic Mycobacterium avium complex disease in patients with HIV infection. AIDS 11:311-317, 1997.

Kraft M, Cassell AGH, Jpak J, et al. Mycoplasma

pneumoniae and Chlamydia pneumoniae in asthma: effect of clarithromycin. Chest 121:1782-8, 2002.

McConnell SA, Amsden GW. Review and comparison of advanced-generation macrolides clarithromycin and dirithromycin. Pharmacotherapy 19:404-15, 1999.

Periti P, Mazzei T. Clarithromycin: Pharmacokinetic and pharmacodynamic interrelationships and dosage regimen. J Chemother 11:11-27, 1999.

Portier H, Filipecki J, Weber P, et al Five day clarithromycin modified release versus 10 day penicillin V for group A streptococcal pharyngitis: a multi-centre, open-label, randomized study. J Antimicrob Chemother 49:337-44, 2002.

Rodvold KA. Clinical pharmacokinetics of clarithromycin. Clin Pharmacokinet 37:385-98, 1999.

Schlossberg D. Azithromycin and clarithromycin. Med Clin North Am 79:803-16, 1995.

Stein GE, Schooley S. Serum bactericidal activity of extended-release clarithromycin against macrolide-resistant strains of Streptococcus pneumoniae. Pharmacotherapy 22:593-6, 2002.

Svensson M, Strom M, Nelsson M et al. Pharmacodynamic effects of nitroimidazoles alone and in combination with clarithromycin on Helicobacter pylori. Antimicrob Agents Chemother 46:2244-8, 2002.

Tartaglione TA. Therapeutic options for the management and prevention of Mycobacterium avium complex infection in patients with acquired immunodeficiency syndrome. Pharmacotherapy 16:171-82, 1996.

Website: www.biaxin.com

Clarithromycin XL (Biaxin XL)

Drug Class: Macrolide
Usual Dose: 1 gm (PO) q24h
Pharmacokinetic Parameters:
Peak serum level: 3 mcg/mL
Bioavailability: 50%
Excreted unchanged: 20%
Serum half-life (normal/ESRD): 4/4 hrs
Plasma protein binding: 70%
Volume of distribution (V_d): 3 L/kg
Primary Mode of Elimination: Hepatic
Dosage Adjustments*

CrCl ~ 30–60 mL/min	500 mg (PO) q24h
CrCl < 30 mL/min	500 mg (PO) q48h
Post–HD dose	None
Post–PD dose	None
CVVH dose	No change
Moderate hepatic insufficiency	No change
Severe hepatic insufficiency	No change

Drug Interactions: Amiodarone, procainamide, sotalol, astemizole, terfenadine, cisapride, pimozide (may ↑ QT interval, torsade de pointes); carbamazepine (↑ carbamazepine levels, nystagmus, nausea, vomiting, diarrhea); cimetidine, digoxin, ergot alkaloids, midazolam, triazolam, phenytoin, ritonavir, tacrolimus, valproic acid (↑ interacting drug levels); clozapine, corticosteroids (not studied); cyclosporine (↑ cyclosporine levels with toxicity); efavirenz (↑ clarithromycin levels); rifabutin, rifampin (↓ clarithromycin levels, ↑ interacting drug levels); statins (↑ risk of rhabdomyolysis); theophylline (↑ theophylline levels, nausea, vomiting, seizures, apnea); warfarin (↑ INR); zidovudine (↓ zidovudine levels)
Adverse Effects: Few/no GI symptoms. May ↑ QT_c; avoid with other medications that prolong the QT_c interval and in patients with cardiac arrhythmias/heart block
Allergic Potential: Low
Safety in Pregnancy: C
Comments: Two 500 mg tablets of XL preparation permits once daily dosing and decreases GI intolerance
Cerebrospinal Fluid Penetration: < 10%
Bile Penetration: 7000%

REFERENCES:

Adler JL, Jannetti W, Schneider D, et al. Phase III, randomized, double-blind study of clarithromycin extended-release and immediate-release formulations in the treatment of patients with acute exacerbation of chronic bronchitis. Clin Ther 22:1410-20, 2000.

Anzueto A, Fisher CL Jr, Busman T. Comparison of the efficacy of extended-release clarithromycin tablets and amoxicillin/clavulanate tablets in the treatment of acute exacerbation of chronic bronchitis. Clin Ther 23:72-86, 2000.

Laine L, Estrada R, Trujillo M, et al. Once-daily therapy for H. pylori infection: Randomized comparison of

"Usual dose" assumes normal renal/hepatic function. * For renal insufficiency, give usual dose x 1 followed by maintenance dose per CrCl. For dialysis patients, dose the same as for CrCl < 10 mL/min and give supplemental (post-HD/PD dose) immediately after dialysis. CrCl = creatinine clearance; CVVH = continuous veno-venous hemofiltration; HD/PD = hemodialysis/peritoneal dialysis. See pp. 293-297 for explanations, p. 1 for abbreviations

four regimens. Am J Gastroenterol 94:962-6, 1999.

Nalepa P, Dobryniewska M, Busman T, et al. Short-course therapy of acute bacterial exacerbation of chronic bronchitis: a double-blind, randomized, multicenter comparison of extended-release versus immediate-release clarithromycin. Curr Med Res Opin. 19:411-20, 2003.

Website: biaxinxl.com

Clindamycin (Cleocin)

Drug Class: Lincosamide
Usual Dose: 600-900 mg (IV) q8h; 150-450 mg (PO) q6h
Pharmacokinetic Parameters:
Peak serum level: 2.5-10 mcg/mL
Bioavailability: 90%
Excreted unchanged: 10%
Serum half-life (normal/ESRD): 2.4/4 hrs
Plasma protein binding: 90%
Volume of distribution (V_d): 1 L/kg
Primary Mode of Elimination: Hepatic
Dosage Adjustments*

CrCl ~ 40–60 mL/min	No change
CrCl < 40 mL/min	No change
Post–HD/PD dose	None
CVVH dose	No change
Moderate or severe hepatic insufficiency	No change

Drug Interactions: Muscle relaxants, neuromuscular blockers (↑ apnea, respiratory paralysis); kaolin (↓ clindamycin absorption); theophylline (↑ theophylline levels, seizures)
Adverse Effects: C. difficile diarrhea/colitis, neuromuscular blockade
Allergic Potential: Low
Safety in Pregnancy: B
Comments: C. difficile diarrhea more common with PO vs. IV clindamycin. Anti-spasmodics contraindicated in C. difficile diarrhea
Cerebrospinal Fluid Penetration: < 10%
Bile Penetration: 300%

REFERENCES:

Coyle EA, Cha R, Rybak MJ. Influences of linezolid, penicillin, and clindamycin, alone and in combination, on streptococcal pyrogenic exotoxin a release. Antimicrob Agents Chemother. 47:1752-5, 2003.

Falagas ME, Gorbach SL. Clindamycin and metronidazole. Med Clin North Am 79:845-67, 1995.

Kasten MJ. Clindamycin, metronidazole, and chloramphenicol. Mayo Clin Proc 74:825-33, 1999.

Klepser ME, Nicolau DP, Quintiliani R, et al. Bactericidal activity of low-dose clindamycin administered at 8- and 12-hour intervals against Streptococcus pneumoniae and Bacteroides fragilis. Antimicrob Agents Chemotherap 41:630-5, 1997.

Lell B, Dremsner PG. Clindamycin as an antimalarial drug: review of clinical trials. Antimicrob Agents Chemother 46:2315-20, 2002.

Snydman DR, Jacobus NV, McDermott, et al. National survey on the susceptibility of Bacterolides Fragilis Group: report and analysis of trends for 1997-2000. Clin Infect Dis 35 (Supp. 1):S126-34, 2002.

Cycloserine (Seromycin)

Drug Class: Anti–TB drug
Usual Dose: 250 mg (PO) q12h
Pharmacokinetic Parameters:
Peak serum level: 20 mcg/mL
Bioavailability: 90%
Excreted unchanged: 65%
Serum half-life (normal/ESRD): 10-25 hrs/no data
Plasma protein binding: No data
Volume of distribution (V_d): 0.2 L/kg
Primary Mode of Elimination: Renal
Dosage Adjustments*

CrCl ~ 50–60 mL/min	No change
CrCl ~ 10–50 mL/min	250 mg (PO) q12-24h
CrCl < 10 mL/min	250 mg (PO) q24h
Post–HD dose	None
Post–PD dose	250 mg (PO)
CVVH dose	No change
Moderate or severe hepatic insufficiency	No change

Drug Interactions: Alcohol (seizures); ethambutol, ethionamide (drowsiness, dizziness); phenytoin (↑ phenytoin levels)
Adverse Effects: Peripheral neuropathy,

"Usual dose" assumes normal renal/hepatic function. * For renal insufficiency, give usual dose x 1 followed by maintenance dose per CrCl. For dialysis patients, dose the same as for CrCl < 10 mL/min and give supplemental (post-HD/PD dose) immediately after dialysis. CrCl = creatinine clearance; CVVH = continuous veno-venous hemo-filtration; HD/PD = hemodialysis/peritoneal dialysis. See pp. 293-297 for explanations, p. 1 for abbreviations

seizures (dose related), psychosis/delirium
Allergic Potential: Low
Safety in Pregnancy: C
Comments: Avoid in patients with seizures. Ethambutol, ethionamide, or ethanol may increase CNS toxicity.
Meningeal dose = usual dose
Cerebrospinal Fluid Penetration:
Non-inflamed meninges = 90%
Inflamed meninges = 90%

REFERENCES:
Davidson PT, Le HQ. Drug treatment of tuberculosis - 1992. Drugs 43:651-73, 1992.
Drugs for tuberculosis. Med Lett Drugs Ther 35:99-101,1993.
Iseman MD. Treatment of multidrug resistant tuberculosis. N Engl J Med 329:784-91, 1993.
Zhu M, Nix DE, Adam RD, et al. Pharmacokinetics of cycloserine under fasting conditions and with high-fat meal, orange juice, and antacids. Pharmacotherapy 21:891-7, 2001.

Dapsone

Drug Class: Antiparasitic (PABA antagonist)
Usual Dose: 100 mg (PO) q24h
Pharmacokinetic Parameters:
Peak serum level: 1.8 mcg/mL
Bioavailability: 85%
Excreted unchanged: 10%
Serum half-life (normal/ESRD): 25/30 hrs
Plasma protein binding: 80%
Volume of distribution (V_d): 1.2 L/kg
Primary Mode of Elimination: Hepatic/renal
Dosage Adjustments*

CrCl ~ 40–60 mL/min	No change
CrCl ~ 10–40 mL/min	No change
CrCl < 10 mL/min	No change
Post–HD dose	None
Post–PD dose	None
CVVH dose	No change
Moderate hepatic insufficiency	No change
Severe hepatic insufficiency	No information

Drug Interactions: Didanosine (↓ dapsone absorption); oral contraceptives (↓ oral contraceptive effect); pyrimethamine, zidovudine (↑ bone marrow suppression); rifabutin, rifampin (↓ dapsone levels); trimethoprim (↑ dapsone and trimethoprim levels, methemoglobinemia)
Adverse Effects: Drug fever/rash, nausea, vomiting, hemolytic anemia in G6PD deficiency, methemoglobinemia
Allergic Potential: High
Safety in Pregnancy: C
Comments: Useful in sulfa (SMX) allergic patients. Avoid, if possible, in G6PD deficiency or hemoglobin M deficiency
REFERENCES:
El-Sadr WM, Murphy RI, Yurik TM, et al. Atovaquone compared with dapsone to the prevention of Pneumocystis carinii in patients with HIV infection who cannot tolerate trimethoprim, sulfonamides, or both. N Engl J Med 339:1889-95, 1998.
Medina I, Mills J, Leoung G, et al. Oral therapy for Pneumocystis carinii pneumonia in the acquired immunodeficiency syndrome. A controlled trial of trimethoprim-sulfamethoxazole versus trimethoprim-dapsone. N Engl J Med 323:776-82, 1990.
Podzamczer D, Salazar A, Jiminez J, et al. Intermittent trimethoprim-sulfamethoxazole compared with dapsone-pyrimethamine for the simultaneous primary prophylaxis of Pneumocystis pneumonia and toxoplasmosis in patients infected with HIV. Ann Intern Med 122:755-61, 1995.
Website: www.pdr.net

Daptomycin (Cubicin)

Drug Class: Lipopeptide
Usual Dose: 4 mg/kg (IV) q24h
Pharmacokinetic Parameters:
Peak serum level: 4 mg/kg = 58 mcg/mL; 6 mg/kg = 99 mcg/mL
Bioavailability: Not applicable
Excreted unchanged: 53%
Serum half-life (normal/ESRD): 8.1/29.8 hrs
Plasma protein binding: 92%
Volume of distribution (V_d): 0.096 L/kg
Primary Mode of Elimination: Renal

"Usual dose" assumes normal renal/hepatic function. * For renal insufficiency, give usual dose x 1 followed by maintenance dose per CrCl. For dialysis patients, dose the same as for CrCl < 10 mL/min and give supplemental (post-HD/PD dose) immediately after dialysis. CrCl = creatinine clearance; CVVH = continuous veno-venous hemofiltration; HD/PD = hemodialysis/peritoneal dialysis. See pp. 293-297 for explanations, p. 1 for abbreviations

Dosage Adjustments*

CrCl ~ 30–60 mL/min	No change
CrCl < 30 mL/min, including hemodialysis or CAPD	4 mg/kg (IV) q48h
Post–HD dose	No information
Post–PD dose	No information
CVVH dose	No information
Moderate or severe hepatic insufficiency	No information

Drug Interactions: Warfarin/statin (no significant interaction in small number of volunteers; monitor INR for first several days after starting daptomycin and consider temporary suspension of statins during daptomycin use)

Adverse Effects: Constipation, nausea, headache. Dose/duration-dependent (transient) ↑ CPK. In clinical trials, the incidence of muscle pain or weakness with CPK > 4x ULN was very low (0.2%); symptoms resolved within 3 days and CPK elevation within 7-10 days after discontinuing treatment

Allergic Potential: No data

Safety in Pregnancy: B

Comments: Administer IV over 30 minutes in 0.9% in a 50 mL bag with NaCl. Not compatible with dextrose-containing diluents. Cannot be given IM. Unique mechanism of action: binds to bacterial cell and depolarizes membrane, inhibiting protein and DNA/RNA synthesis, which results in cell death. Monitor for muscle pain/weakness and CPK (weekly). Exhibits concentration-dependent killing and post-antibiotic effect of up to 6 hours

CSF Penetration: No data

REFERENCES:

Arbeit RD, et al. Daptomycin, a novel lipopeptide antibiotic in the treatment of complicated skin and soft tissue infections: combined results of 2 phase III studies. ICAAC Proceedings UL-10 (abstract), 2001.

Fuchs PC, Barry AL, Brown SD. In vitro bactericidal activity of daptomycin against staphylococci. J Antimicrob Chemother 49:467-70, 2002.

Goldstein EJ, Citron DM, Merriam CV, et al. In vitro activities of daptomycin, vancomycin, quinupristin-dalfopristin, linezolid, and five other antimicrobials against 307 gram-positive anaerobic and 31 Corynebacterium clinical isolates. Antimicrob Agents Chemother 47:337-41, 2003.

Sun HK, Kuti HI, Nicolau DP. Daptomycin: a novel lipopeptide antibiotic for the treatment of resistant gram-positive infections. Formulary 38:634-645, 2003.

Silverman JA, Perlmutter NG, Shapiro HM. Correlation of daptomycin bactericidal activity and membrane depolarization in Staphylococcus aureus. Antimicrob Agents Chemother 47:2538-44, 2003.

Vaudaux P, Francois P, Bisognano C, et al. Comparative efficacy of daptomycin and vancomycin in the therapy of experimental foreign body infection due to Staphylococcus aureus. J Antimicrob Chemother 52:89-95, 2003.

Wise R, et al. Activity of daptomycin against gram-positive pathogens: a comparison with other agents and determination of tentative breakpoints. J Antimicrob Chemother 48:563-67, 2001.

Website: www.cubist.com

Delavirdine (Rescriptor)

Drug Class: Antiretroviral NNRTI (non-nucleoside reverse transcriptase inhibitor)

Usual Dose: 400 mg (PO) q8h

Pharmacokinetic Parameters:
Peak serum level: 35 mcg/mL
Bioavailability: 85%
Excreted unchanged: 5%
Serum half-life (normal/ESRD): 5.8 hrs/no data
Plasma protein binding: 98%
Volume of distribution (V_d): 0.5 L/kg

Primary Mode of Elimination: Hepatic

Dosage Adjustments*

CrCl ~ 40–60 mL/min	No change
CrCl ~ 10–40 mL/min	No change
CrCl < 10 mL/min	No change
Post–HD dose	None
Post–PD dose	None
CVVH dose	No change
Moderate hepatic insufficiency	No information

"Usual dose" assumes normal renal/hepatic function. * For renal insufficiency, give usual dose x 1 followed by maintenance dose per CrCl. For dialysis patients, dose the same as for CrCl < 10 mL/min and give supplemental (post-HD/PD dose) immediately after dialysis. CrCl = creatinine clearance; CVVH = continuous veno-venous hemo-filtration; HD/PD = hemodialysis/peritoneal dialysis. See pp. 293-297 for explanations, p. 1 for abbreviations

Severe hepatic insufficiency	No information

Antiretroviral Dosage Adjustments:

Amprenavir	No information
Efavirenz	No information
Indinavir	Indinavir 600 mg q8h
Lopinavir/ritonavir	No information
Nelfinavir	No information (monitor for neutropenia)
Nevirapine	No information
Ritonavir	Delavirdine: no change; ritonavir: No information
Saquinavir soft-gel	Saquinavir soft-gel 800 mg q8h (monitor transaminases)
Rifampin, rifabutin	Avoid combination
Statins	Not recommended

Drug Interactions: Antiretrovirals, rifabutin, rifampin (see dose adjustment grid, above); astemizole, terfenadine, benzodiazepines, cisapride, H$_2$ blockers, proton pump inhibitors, ergot alkaloids, quinidine, statins (avoid if possible), carbamazepine, phenobarbital, phenytoin (may ↓ delavirdine levels, monitor anticonvulsant levels); clarithromycin, dapsone, nifedipine, warfarin (↑ interacting drug levels); sildenafil (do not exceed 25 mg in 48 hrs)
Adverse Effects: Drug fever/rash, Stevens–Johnson syndrome (rare), headache, nausea/vomiting, diarrhea, ↑ SGOT/SGPT
Allergic Potential: High
Safety in Pregnancy: C
Comments: May be taken with or without food, but food decreases absorption by 20%. May disperse 100 mg tablets in > 3 oz. water to produce slurry. Separate dosing with ddI or antacids by 1 hour. Effective antiretroviral therapy consists of at least 3 antiretrovirals

(same/different classes)
Cerebrospinal Fluid Penetration: 0.4%

REFERENCES:
Been-Tiktak AM, Boucher CA, Brun-Vezinet F, et al. Efficacy and safety of combination therapy with delavirdine and zidovudine: A European/Australian phase II trial. Intern J Antimcrob Agents 11:13-21, 1999.
Conway B. Initial therapy with protease inhibitor-sparing regimens: Evaluation of nevirapine and delavirdine. Clin Infect Dis 2:130-4, 2000.
Demeter LM, Shafer RW, Meehan PM, et al. Delavirdine susceptibilities and associated reverse transcriptase mutations in human immunodeficiency virus type 1 isolates from patients in a phase I/II trial of delavirdine monotherapy (ACTG260). Antimicrob Agents Chemother 44:794-7, 2000.
Panel on Clinical Practices for Treatment of HIV Infection. Guidelines for the use of antiretroviral agents in HIV-infected adults and adolescents. Department of Health and Human Services. www.aidsinfo.nih.gov/guidelines/. November 10, 2003.
Website: rescriptor.com

Didanosine (Videx) ddI

Drug Class: Antiretroviral NRTI (nucleoside reverse transcriptase inhibitor)
Usual Dose: > 60 kg: 200 mg (PO) q12h; < 60 kg: 125 mg (PO) q12h (see comments)
Pharmacokinetic Parameters:
Peak serum level: 29 mcg/mL
Bioavailability: 42%
Excreted unchanged: 60%
Serum half-life (normal/ESRD): 1.6/4.1 hrs
Plasma protein binding: ≤ 5%
Volume of distribution (V_d): 1.1 L/kg
Primary Mode of Elimination: Renal
Dosage Adjustments for Patients > 60 kg*

CrCl ~ 30–60 mL/min	200 mg (PO) q24h or 100 mg (PO) q12h
CrCl ~ 10–30 mL/min	150 mg (PO) q24h
CrCl < 10 mL/min	100 mg (PO) q24h
Post–HD dose	No information
Post–PD dose	100 mg (PO)

"Usual dose" assumes normal renal/hepatic function. * For renal insufficiency, give usual dose x 1 followed by maintenance dose per CrCl. For dialysis patients, dose the same as for CrCl < 10 mL/min and give supplemental (post-HD/PD dose) immediately after dialysis. CrCl = creatinine clearance; CVVH = continuous veno-venous hemo-filtration; HD/PD = hemodialysis/peritoneal dialysis. See pp. 293-297 for explanations, p. 1 for abbreviations

CVVH dose	150 mg (PO) q24h
Moderate hepatic insufficiency	No change
Severe hepatic insufficiency	No change

Drug Interactions: Alcohol, lamivudine, pentamidine, valproic acid (↑ risk of pancreatitis); dapsone, fluoroquinolones, ketoconazole, itraconazole, tetracyclines (↓ absorption of interacting drug; give 2 hours after didanosine); dapsone, INH, metronidazole, nitrofurantoin, stavudine, vincristine, zalcitabine, neurotoxic drugs or history of neuropathy (↑ risk of peripheral neuropathy); dapsone (↓ dapsone absorption, which increases risk of PCP); tenofovir (↑↑ didanosine levels; ↓ didanosine dose when given with tenofovir) ▾

Adverse Effects: Headache, depression, nausea, vomiting, GI upset/abdominal pain, diarrhea, drug fever/rash, anemia, leukopenia, thrombocytopenia, hepatotoxicity/hepatic necrosis, pancreatitis (may be fatal), hypertriglyceridemia, hyperuricemia, lactic acidosis, lipoatrophy, wasting, dose-dependent (≥ 0.06 mg/kg/d) peripheral neuropathy, hyperglycemia, lactic acidosis with hepatic steatosis (rare, but potentially life-threatening toxicity with use of NRTIs; *pregnant women taking didanosine + stavudine may be at increased risk*)

Allergic Potential: Low

Safety in Pregnancy: B

Comments: Available as tablets, buffered powder for oral solution, and enteric-coated extended-release capsules (Videx EC 400 mg PO q24h). Take 30 minutes before or 2 hours after meal (food decreases serum concentrations by 49%). Chew tablets thoroughly. Twice daily dosing is preferred, but once daily dosing (> 60 kg: 400 mg EC capsules; < 60 kg: 250 mg tablet or EC capsule) may be considered for patients requiring a simplified dosing schedule. Avoid in patients with alcoholic cirrhosis/history of pancreatitis. Use with caution with ribavirin. Na⁺ content = 11.5 mEq/g. Effective antiretroviral therapy consists of at least 3 antiretrovirals (same/different classes)

Cerebrospinal Fluid Penetration: 20%

REFERENCES:
Hirsch MS, D'Aquila RT. Therapy for human immunodeficiency virus infection. N Engl J Med 328:1686-95, 1993.

HIV Trialists' Collaborative Group. Zidovudine, didanosine, and zalcitabine in the treatment of HIV infection: Meta-analyses of the randomised evidence. Lancet 353:2014-2025, 1999.

Montaner JS, Reiss P, Cooper D, et al. A randomized, double-blind trial comparing combinations of nevirapine, didanosine, and zidovudine for HIV-infected patients: The INCAS trial. Italy, the Netherlands, Canada and Australia Study. J Am Med Assoc 279:930-937, 1998.

Panel on Clinical Practices for Treatment of HIV Infection. Guidelines for the use of antiretroviral agents in HIV-infected adults and adolescents. Department of Health and Human Services. www.aidsinfo.nih.gov/guidelines/. November 10, 2003.

Perry CM, Balfour JA. Didanosine: An update on its antiviral activity, pharmacokinetic properties, and therapeutic efficacy in the management of HIV disease. Drugs 52:928-62, 1996.

Rathbun RC, Martin ES 3ʳᵈ. Didanosine therapy in patients intolerant of or failing zidovudine therapy. Ann Pharmacother 26:1347-51, 1992.

Website: www.pdr.net

Doxycycline (Vibramycin, Vibra-tabs)

Drug Class: 2ⁿᵈ generation IV/PO tetracycline
Usual Dose: 100-200 mg (IV/PO) q12h or 200 mg (IV/PO) q24h (see comments)
Pharmacokinetic Parameters:
Peak serum level: 100/200 mg = 4/8 mcg/mL
Bioavailability: 93%
Excreted unchanged: 40%
Serum half-life (normal/ESRD): 18-22/18-22 hrs
Plasma protein binding: 93%
Volume of distribution (V_d): 0.75 L/kg
Primary Mode of Elimination: Hepatic
Dosage Adjustments*

CrCl < 60 mL/min	No change
Post–HD or PD dose	None

"Usual dose" assumes normal renal/hepatic function. * For renal insufficiency, give usual dose x 1 followed by maintenance dose per CrCl. For dialysis patients, dose the same as for CrCl < 10 mL/min and give supplemental (post-HD/PD dose) immediately after dialysis. CrCl = creatinine clearance; CVVH = continuous veno-venous hemofiltration; HD/PD = hemodialysis/peritoneal dialysis. See pp. 293-297 for explanations, p. 1 for abbreviations

CVVH dose	No change
Moderate or severe hepatic insufficiency	No change

Drug Interactions: Antacids, Al^{++}, Ca^{++}, Fe^{++}, Mg^{++}, Zn^{++}, multivitamins, sucralfate (↓ doxycycline absorption); barbiturates, carbamazepine, phenytoin (↓ doxycycline half-life); bicarbonate (↓ doxycycline absorption, ↑ doxycycline clearance); warfarin (↑ INR)
Adverse Effects: Nausea if not taken with food. Phlebitis if given IV in inadequate volume. Avoid in pregnancy and children < 8 years
Allergic Potential: Low
Safety in Pregnancy: D
Comments: Minimal potential for Candida overgrowth/diarrhea. Photosensitivity rare. Tablets better tolerated than capsules. Absorption minimally effected by iron, bismuth, milk, or antacids containing Ca^{++}, Mg^{++}, or Al^{++}. Serum half-life increases with multiple doses. For serious systemic infection, begin therapy with a loading dose of 200 mg (IV/PO) q12h x 3 days, then continue at same dose or decrease to 100 mg (IV/PO) q12h to complete therapy. Meningeal dose = 200 mg (IV/PO) q12h
Cerebrospinal Fluid Penetration:
Non-inflamed meninges = 25%
Inflamed meninges = 25%
Bile Penetration: 3000%

REFERENCES:
Cunha BA. Doxycycline. Antibiotics for Clinicians 3:21-33, 1999.
Cunha BA. Doxycycline for community-acquired pneumonia. Clin Infect Dis. 37:870, 2003.
Cunha BA. Doxycycline re-visited. Arch Intern Med 159:1006-7, 1999.
Cunha BA, Domenico PD, Cunha CB. Pharmacodynamics of doxycycline. Clin Micro Infect Dis 6:270-3, 2000.
Hoerauf A, Mand S, Fischer K, et al. Doxycycline as a novel strategy against bancroftian filariasis-depletion of Wolbachia endosymbionts from Wuchereria bancrofti and stop of microfilaria production. Med Microbiol Immunol (Berl). 192:211-6, 2003.
Johnson JR. Doxycycline for treatment of community-acquired pneumonia. Clin Infect Dis 35:632, 2002.
Shea KW, Ueno Y, Abumustafa F, et al. Doxycycline activity against Streptococcus pneumoniae. Chest 107:1775-6, 1995.

Efavirenz (Sustiva)

Drug Class: Antiretroviral NNRTI (non-nucleoside reverse transcriptase inhibitor)
Usual Dose: 600 mg (PO) q24h
Pharmacokinetic Parameters:
Peak serum level: 12.9 mcg/mL
Bioavailability: Increased with food
Excreted unchanged: 14-34%
Serum half-life (normal/ESRD): 40-55 hrs/no data
Plasma protein binding: 99%
Volume of distribution (V_d): No data
Primary Mode of Elimination: Hepatic
Dosage Adjustments*

CrCl < 60 mL/min	No change
Post–HD or PD dose	None
CVVH dose	No change
Moderate or severe hepatic insufficiency	No information

Antiretroviral Dosage Adjustments:

Amprenavir	No information
Delavirdine	No information
Indinavir	Indinavir 1000 mg q8h
Lopinavir/ritonavir (l/r)	Consider l/r 533/133 mg q12h in PI-experienced patients
Nelfinavir	No changes
Nevirapine	No information
Ritonavir	Ritonavir 600 mg q12h (500 mg q12h for intolerance)
Saquinavir	Avoid use as sole PI
Rifampin	No changes
Rifabutin	Rifabutin 450-600 mg q24h or 600 mg 2-3x/week if not on protease inhibitor

Drug Interactions: Antiretrovirals, rifabutin, rifampin (see dose adjustment grid, above);

astemizole, terfenadine, cisapride, ergotamine, midazolam, triazolam (avoid); carbamazepine, phenobarbital, phenytoin (monitor anticonvulsant levels; use with caution); caspofungin (↓ caspofungin levels, may ↓ caspofungin effect); methadone, telithromycin (↓ interacting drug levels; titrate methadone dose to effect)

Adverse Effects: Drug fever/rash, CNS symptoms (nightmares, dizziness, neuropsychiatric symptoms, difficulty concentrating, somnolence), ↑ SGOT/SGPT, E. multiforme/Stevens–Johnson syndrome (rare), false positive cannabinoid test

Allergic Potential: High

Safety in Pregnancy: C

Comments: Rash/CNS symptoms usually resolve spontaneously over 2-4 weeks. Take at bedtime. Avoid taking after high fat meals (levels ↑ 50%). Prolonged high peak serum concentrations avoids trough problems with antiretrovirals with short $t_{1/2}$. 600 mg dose available as single tablet. Effective antiretroviral therapy consists of at least 3 antiretrovirals

Cerebrospinal Fluid Penetration: 1%

REFERENCES:

Albrecht MA, Bosch RJ, Hammer SM, et al. Nelfinavir, efavirenz, or both after the failure of nucleoside treatment of HIV infection. N Engl J Med 345:398-407, 2001.

Go JC, Cunha BA. Efavirenz. Antibiotics for Clinicians 5:1-8, 2001.

Haas DW, Fessel WJ, Delapenha RA, et al. Therapy with efavirenz plus indinavir in patients with extensive prior nucleoside reverse-transcriptase inhibitor experience: A randomized, double-blind, placebo-controlled trial. J Infect Dis 183:392-400, 2001.

Marzolini C, Telenti A, Decosterd LA, et al. Efavirenz plasma levels can predict treatment failure and central nervous system side effects in HIV-1-infected patients. AIDS 15:71-5, 2001.

Negredo E, Cruz L, Paredes R, et al. Virological, immunological, and clinical impact of switching from protease inhibitors to nevirapine or to efavirenz in patients with human immunodeficiency virus infection and long-lasting viral suppression. Clin Infect Dis 34:504-510, 2002.

Panel on Clinical Practices for Treatment of HIV Infection. Guidelines for the use of antiretroviral agents in HIV-infected adults and adolescents. Department of Health and Human Services.

www.aidsinfo.nih.gov/guidelines/. November 10, 2003.
Website: www.sustiva.com

Emtricitabine (Emtriva) FTC

Drug Class: Antiretroviral NRTI (nucleoside reverse transcriptase inhibitor)

Usual Dose: 200 mg (PO) q24h

Pharmacokinetic Parameters:
Peak serum level: 1.8 mcg/mL
Bioavailability: 93%
Excreted unchanged: 86%
Serum half-life (normal/ESRD): 10 hrs/extended
Plasma protein binding: 4%

Primary Mode of Elimination: Renal

Dosage Adjustments*

CrCl ≥ 50 mL/min	200 mg (PO) q24h
CrCl ~ 30-49 mL/min	200 mg (PO) q48h
CrCl ~ 15-29 mL/min	200 mg (PO) q72h
CrCl < 15 mL/min	200 mg (PO) q96h
Post–HD dose	200 mg (PO) q96h
Post-PD dose	No information
CVVH dose	No information
Moderate or severe hepatic insufficiency	No change

Drug Interactions: No significant interactions with indinavir, stavudine, zidovudine, famciclovir, tenofovir

Adverse Effects: Headache, diarrhea, nausea, rash, lactic acidosis with hepatic steatosis (rare, but potentially life-threatening with NRTIs)

Allergic Potential: Low

Safety in Pregnancy: B

Comments: May be taken with or without food. Does not inhibit CYP450 enzymes. Mean intracellular half-live of 39 hours. Potential cross-resistance to lamivudine and zalcitabine. Low affinity for DNA polymerase-γ. Effective antiretroviral therapy consists of at least 3 antiretrovirals

---

"Usual dose" assumes normal renal/hepatic function. * For renal insufficiency, give usual dose x 1 followed by maintenance dose per CrCl. For dialysis patients, dose the same as for CrCl < 10 mL/min and give supplemental (post-HD/PD dose) immediately after dialysis. CrCl = creatinine clearance; CVVH = continuous veno-venous hemofiltration; HD/PD = hemodialysis/peritoneal dialysis. See pp. 293-297 for explanations, p. 1 for abbreviations

REFERENCES:
Panel on Clinical Practices for Treatment of HIV
Infection. Guidelines for the Use of Antiretroviral
Agents in HIV-Infected Adults and Adolescents.
Department of Health and Human Services.
www.aidsinfo.nih.gov/guidelines/. November 10,
2003.
Website: www.emtriva.com

Enfuvirtide (Fuzeon)

Drug Class: Antiretroviral fusion inhibitor
Usual Dose: 90 mg (SC) q12h
Pharmacokinetic Parameters:
Peak serum level: 4.9 mcg/mL
Bioavailability: 84.3%
Serum half-life (normal/ESRD): 3.8 hrs/no data
Plasma protein binding: 92%
Volume of distribution (V_d): 5.5 L
Primary Mode of Elimination: Metabolized
Dosage Adjustments*

CrCl ~ 35–60 mL/min	No change
CrCl ~ < 35 mL/min	No data
Post–HD dose	No data
Post–PD dose	No data
CVVH dose	No data
Moderate or severe hepatic insufficiency	No data

Drug Interactions: No clinically significant interactions with other antiretrovirals. Does not inhibit CYP450 enzymes
Adverse Effects: Local injection site reactions are common. Diarrhea, nausea, fatigue may occur. Laboratory abnormalities include mild/transient eosinophilia. Pneumonia may occur, but cause is unclear and may not be due to drug therapy
Allergic Potential: Hypersensitivity reactions may occur, including fever, chills, hypotension, rash, ↑ serum transaminases. Do not rechallenge following a hypersensitivity reaction
Safety in Pregnancy: B
Comments: Enfuvirtide interferes with entry of HIV-1 into cells by blocking fusion of HIV-1 and CD4 cellular membranes by binding to HR1 in the gp41 subunit of the HIV-1 envelope glycoprotein. Additive/synergistic with NRTIs, NNRTIs, and PIs, and no cross resistance to other antiretrovirals in cell culture. Compared to background regimen, enfuvirtide ↑ CD_4 (71 vs. 35 cells/mm^3) and ↓ HIV-1 RNA (−1.52 log$_{10}$ vs. −0.73 log$_{10}$ copies/mL) at 24 weeks. Reconstitute in 1.1 mL of sterile water. SC injection should be given into upper arm, anterior thigh, or abdomen. Rotate injection sites; do not inject into moles, scars, bruises. After reconstitution, use immediately or refrigerate and use within 24 hours (no preservatives added)

REFERENCES:
Coleman CI, Musial, BL, Ross, J. Enfuvirtide: the first
fusion inhibitor for the treatment of patients with HIV-
1 infection. Formulary 38:204-222, 2003.
Kilby JM, Lalezari JP, Eron JJ, et al. The safety, plasma
pharmacokinetics, and antiviral activity of
subcutaneous enfuvirtide (T-20), a peptide inhibitor of
gp41-mediated virus fusion, in HIV-infected adults.
AIDS Res Hum Retroviruses 18:685-93, 2002.
Lalezari JP, Henry K, O'Hearn M, et al. TORO 1 Study
Group. Enfuvirtide, an HIV-1 fusion inhibitor, for drug-
resistant HIV infection in North and South America. N
Engl J Med 348:2175-85, 2003.
Lalezari JP, Eron JJ, Carlson M, et al. A phase II clinical
study of the long-term safety and antiviral activity of
enfuvirtide-based antiretroviral therapy. AIDS 17:691-
8, 2003.
Lazzarin A, Clotet B, Cooper D, et al. TORO 2 Study
Group. Efficacy of enfuvirtide in patients infected with
drug-resistant HIV-1 in Europe and Australia. N Engl J
Med 348:2186-95, 2003.
Panel on Clinical Practices for Treatment of HIV
Infection. Guidelines for the Use of Antiretroviral
Agents in HIV-Infected Adults and Adolescents.
Department of Health and Human Services.
www.aidsinfo.nih.gov/guidelines/. November 10,
2003.
Website: www.fuzeon.com

Ertapenem (Invanz)

Drug Class: Carbapenem
Usual Dose: 1 gm (IV/IM) q24h
Pharmacokinetic Parameters:
Peak serum level: 150 mcg/mL
Bioavailability: 90% (IM)
Excreted unchanged: 38%
Serum half-life (normal/ESRD): 4/14 hrs
Plasma protein binding: 95%
Volume of distribution (V_d): 8 L/kg
Primary Mode of Elimination: Renal
Dosage Adjustments*

CrCl ~ 30–60 mL/min	No change
CrCl ~ 10–30 mL/min	500 mg (IV) q24h
CrCl < 10 mL/min	500 mg (IV) q24h
Post–HD dose	500 mg (IV) if within 6h of HD
Post–PD dose	No information
CVVH dose	No information
Moderate hepatic insufficiency	No change
Severe hepatic insufficiency	No change

Drug Interactions: Not a substrate/inhibitor of cytochrome P-450 enzymes; probenecid (↓ clearance of ertapenem)
Adverse Effects: Mild headache, infrequent nausea or diarrhea. Low seizure potential. Probenacid (significant ↓ clearance of ertapenem)
Allergic Potential: Low
Safety in Pregnancy: B
Comments: Concentration-dependent protein binding. Compared to imipenem, ertapenem has little activity vs. enterococci, Acinetobacter or P. aeruginosa. For deep muscle (IM) injection, mix 1 gm with 3.2 mL of 1% lidocaine. Na^+ content = 6 mEq/g

REFERENCES:
Aldridge KE. Ertapenem (MK-0826), a new carbapenem:

comparative in vitro activity against clinically significant anaerobes. Diagn Microbiol Infect Dis 44:181-6, 2002.
Curran M, Simpson D, Perry C. Ertapenem: a review of its use in the management of bacterial infections. Drugs 63:1855-78, 2003.
Graham DR, Lucasti C, Malafaia O, et al. Ertapenem once daily versus piperacillin-tazobactam 4 times per day for treatment of complicated skin and skin-structure infections in adults: results of a prospective, randomized, double-blind multicenter study. Clin Infect Dis 34:1460-8, 2002.
Livermore DM, Sefton AM, Scott GM. Properties and potential of ertapenem. J Antimicrob Chemother. 52:331-44, 2003.
Pelak BA, Bartizal K, Woods GL, et al. Comparative in vitro activities of ertapenem against aerobic and facultative bacterial pathogens from patients with complicated skin and skin structure infections. Diagn Microbiol Infect Dis 43:129-33, 2002.
Pelak BA, Woods GI, Teppler H. Comparative in-vitro activities of ertapenem against aerobic bacterial pathogens isolated from patients with complicated intra-abdominal infections. J Chemother 14:227-33, 2002.
Shah PM, Isaacs RD. Ertapenem, the first of a new group of carbapenems. J Antimicrob Chemother. 52:538-42, 2003.
Solomkin JS, Yellin AE, Rotstein OD, et al. Ertapenem versus piperacillin/tazobactam in the treatment of complicated intraabdominal infections: results of a double-blind, randomized comparative phase III trial. Ann Surg 237:235-45, 2003.
Vetter N, Cambronero-Hernandez E, Rohlf J, et al. A prospective, randomized, double-blind multicenter comparison of parenteral ertapenem and ceftriaxone for the treatment of hospitalized adults with community-acquired pneumonia. Clin Ther 24:1770-85, 2002.
Website: www.invanz.com

Erythromycin lactobionate, base (various)

Drug Class: Macrolide
Usual Dose: 1 gm (IV) q6h; 500 mg (PO) q6h
Pharmacokinetic Parameters:
Peak serum level: 12 (IV);1.2 (PO) mcg/mL
Bioavailability: 50%
Excreted unchanged: 5%
Serum half-life (normal/ESRD): 1.4/5.4 hrs
Plasma protein binding: 80%
Volume of distribution (V_d): 0.5 L/kg
Primary Mode of Elimination: Hepatic

Dosage Adjustments*

CrCl ~ 40–60 mL/min	No change
CrCl ~ 10–40 mL/min	No change
CrCl < 10 mL/min	500 mg (IV) q6h 250 mg (PO) q6h
Post–HD/PD dose	None
CVVH dose	No change
Moderate or severe hepatic insufficiency	No change

Drug Interactions: Amiodarone, procainamide, sotalol, astemizole, terfenadine, cisapride, pimozide (may ↑ QT interval, torsade de pointes); carbamazepine (↑ carbamazepine levels, nystagmus, nausea, vomiting, diarrhea; avoid combination); cimetidine, digoxin, ergot alkaloids, felodipine, midazolam, triazolam, phenytoin, ritonavir, tacrolimus, valproic acid (↑ interacting drug levels); clozapine (↑ clozapine levels; CNS toxicity); corticosteroids (↑ corticosteroid effect); cyclosporine (↑ cyclosporine levels with toxicity); efavirenz (↓ erythromycin levels); rifabutin, rifampin (↓ erythromycin levels, ↑ interacting drug levels); statins (↑ risk of rhabdomyolysis); theophylline (↑ theophylline levels, nausea, vomiting, seizures, apnea); warfarin (↑ INR); zidovudine (↓ zidovudine levels)

Adverse Effects: Nausea, vomiting, GI upset, irritative diarrhea, abdominal pain, phlebitis. May ↑ QT$_c$; avoid with other medications that prolong the QT$_c$ interval and in patients with cardiac arrhythmias/heart block

Allergic Potential: Low

Safety in Pregnancy: B

Comments: Do not mix erythromycin with B/C vitamins, glucose solutions, cephalothin, tetracycline, chloramphenicol, heparin, or warfarin. Increases GI motility. Monitor potential hepatotoxicity with serial SGOTs/SGPTs

Cerebrospinal Fluid Penetration: < 10%

REFERENCES:

Alvarez-Elcoro S, Enzler MJ. The macrolides: Erythromycin, clarithromycin and azithromycin. Mayo Clin Proc 74:613-34, 1999.

Amsden GW. Erythromycin, clarithromycin, and azithromycin: Are the differences real? Clinical Therapeutics 18:572, 1996.

Cunha BA. The virtues of doxycycline and the evils of erythromycin. Adv Ther 14:172-80, 1997.

Smilack JD, Wilson WE, Cocerill FR 3rd. Tetracycline, chloramphenicol, erythromycin, clindamycin, and metronidazole. Mayo Clin Proc 66:1270-80, 1991.

Website: www.pdr.net

Ethambutol (Myambutol) EMB

Drug Class: Anti–TB drug
Usual Dose: 15 mg/kg (PO) q24h
Pharmacokinetic Parameters:
Peak serum level: 2-5 mcg/mL
Bioavailability: 80%
Excreted unchanged: 50%
Serum half-life (normal/ESRD): 4/10 hrs
Plasma protein binding: 20%
Volume of distribution (V_d): 2 L/kg
Primary Mode of Elimination: Renal/hepatic
Dosage Adjustments*

CrCl ~ 40–60 mL/min	No change
CrCl < 40 mL/min	No change
Post–HD/PD dose	No information
CVVH dose	No change
Moderate or severe hepatic insufficiency	No change

Drug Interactions: Aluminum salts, didanosine buffer (↓ ethambutol and interacting drug absorption)

Adverse Effects: Drug fever/rash, ↓ visual acuity, central scotomata, color blindness (red–green), metallic taste, mental confusion, peripheral neuropathy, ↑ uric acid

Allergic Potential: Low

Safety in Pregnancy: B

Comments: Optic neuritis may occur with high doses (≥ 15 mg/kg/day).
Meningeal dose = 25 mg/kg (PO) q24h

Cerebrospinal Fluid Penetration:
Non-inflamed meninges = 1%

"Usual dose" assumes normal renal/hepatic function. * For renal insufficiency, give usual dose x 1 followed by maintenance dose per CrCl. For dialysis patients, dose the same as for CrCl < 10 mL/min and give supplemental (post-HD/PD dose) immediately after dialysis. CrCl = creatinine clearance; CVVH = continuous veno-venous hemofiltration; HD/PD = hemodialysis/peritoneal dialysis. See pp. 293-297 for explanations, p. 1 for abbreviations

Inflamed meninges = 40%

REFERENCES:
Chaisson RE, Keiser P, Pierce M, et al. Clarithromycin and ethambutol with or without clofazimine for the treatment of bacteremic Mycobacterium avium complex disease in patients with HIV infection. AIDS 11:311-317, 1997.
Davidson PT, Le HQ. Drug treatment of tuberculosis 1992. Drugs 43:651-73, 1992.
Drugs for tuberculosis. Med Lett Drugs Ther 35:99-101, 1993.
Van Scoy RE, Wilkowske CJ. Antituberculous agents. Mayo Clin Proc 67:179-87, 1992.

Ethionamide (Trecator)

Drug Class: Anti-TB drug
Usual Dose: 500 mg (PO) q12h
Pharmacokinetic Parameters:
Peak serum level: 5 mcg/mL
Bioavailability: Complete
Excreted unchanged: 1%
Serum half-life (normal/ESRD): 2/9 hrs
Plasma protein binding: 30%
Volume of distribution (V_d): No data
Primary Mode of Elimination: Renal/hepatic
Dosage Adjustments*

CrCl ~ 40–60 mL/min	No change
CrCl < 40 mL/min	No change
Post–HD/PD dose	No information
CVVH dose	No information
Moderate hepatic insufficiency	No change
Severe hepatic insufficiency	500 mg (PO) q24h

Drug Interactions: Cycloserine (↑ neurologic toxicity); ethambutol (↑ GI distress, neuritis, hepatotoxicity); INH (peripheral neuritis, hepatotoxicity); pyrazinamide, rifampin (hepatotoxicity)
Adverse Effects: ↑ SGOT/SGPT, headache, nausea/vomiting, abdominal pain, tremor, olfactory abnormalities, alopecia, gynecomastia, hypoglycemia, impotence, neurotoxicity

(central/peripheral neuropathy)
Allergic Potential: Low
Safety in Pregnancy: C
Comments: Additive toxicity with thiacetazone
Cerebrospinal Fluid Penetration: 100%

REFERENCES:
Davidson PT, Le HQ. Drug treatment of tuberculosis 1992. Drugs 43:651-73, 1992.
Drugs for tuberculosis. Med Lett Drugs Ther 35:99-101, 1993.
Iseman MD. Treatment of multidrug resistant tuberculosis. N Engl J Med 329:784-91, 1993.

Famciclovir (Famvir)

Drug Class: Antiviral
Usual Dose: HSV: 125 mg (PO) q12h;
VZV: 500 mg (PO) q8h
Pharmacokinetic Parameters:
Peak serum level: 3.3 mcg/mL
Bioavailability: 77%
Excreted unchanged: 60%
Serum half-life (normal/ESRD): 2.5/13 hrs
Plasma protein binding: 20%
Volume of distribution (V_d): 1.1 L/kg
Primary Mode of Elimination: Renal
Dosage Adjustments for HSV/VZV*

CrCl ~ 40–60 mL/min	No change 500 mg (PO) q12h
CrCl ~ 20–39 mL/min	125 mg (PO) q24h 500 mg (PO) q24h
CrCl < 20 mL/min	125 mg (PO) q24h 250 mg (PO) q24h
Post–HD dose	125 mg (PO) 250 mg (PO)
Post–PD dose	No information
CVVH dose	No information
Moderate hepatic insufficiency	No change
Severe hepatic insufficiency	No information

Drug Interactions: Digoxin (↑ digoxin levels)

"Usual dose" assumes normal renal/hepatic function. * For renal insufficiency, give usual dose x 1 followed by maintenance dose per CrCl. For dialysis patients, dose the same as for CrCl < 10 mL/min and give supplemental (post-HD/PD dose) immediately after dialysis. CrCl = creatinine clearance; CVVH = continuous veno-venous hemofiltration; HD/PD = hemodialysis/peritoneal dialysis. See pp. 293-297 for explanations, p. 1 for abbreviations

Adverse Effects: Headache, seizures/tremors (dose related), nausea
Allergic Potential: Low
Safety in Pregnancy: B
Comments: 99% converted to penciclovir in liver/GI tract.
Meningeal dose = VZV dose
Cerebrospinal Fluid Penetration: 50%

REFERENCES:
Alrabiah FA, Sacks SL. New anti-herpesvirus agents. Their targets and therapeutic potential. Drugs 52:17-32, 1996.
Bassett KL, Green CJ, Wright JM. Famciclovir and postherpetic neuralgia. Ann Intern Med 131:712-3, 1999.
Luber AD, Flaherty JF Jr. Famciclovir for treatment of herpesvirus infections. Ann Pharmacother 30:978-85, 1996.
Rayes N, Seehofer D, Hopf U, et al. Comparison of famciclovir and lamivudine in the long-term treatment of hepatitis B infection after liver transplantation. Transplantation 71:96-101, 2001.
Tyring S, Belanger R, Bezwoda W, et al. A randomized, double-blind trial of famciclovir versus acyclovir for the treatment of localized dermatomal herpes zoster in immunocompromised patients. Cancer Invest 19:13-22, 2001.
Yurdaydin C, Bozkaya H, Gurel S, et al. Famciclovir treatment of chronic delta hepatitis. J Hepatol 37:266-71, 2002.
Website: www.famvir.com

Fluconazole (Diflucan)

Drug Class: Antifungal
Usual Dose: 400 mg (IV/PO) x 1 dose, then 200 mg (IV/PO) q24h (see comments)
Pharmacokinetic Parameters:
Peak serum level: 6.7 mcg/mL
Bioavailability: 90%
Excreted unchanged: 80%
Serum half-life (normal/ESRD): 27/100 hrs
Plasma protein binding: 12%
Volume of distribution (V_d): 0.7 L/kg
Primary Mode of Elimination: Renal
Dosage Adjustments*

CrCl ~ 50–60 mL/min	No change
CrCl ~ 10–50 mL/min	100 mg (IV/PO) q24h
CrCl < 10 mL/min	100 mg (IV/PO) q24h
Post–HD dose	200 mg (IV/PO)
Post–PD dose	200 mg (IV/PO)
CVVH dose	No change
Moderate hepatic insufficiency	No change
Severe hepatic insufficiency	No change

Drug Interactions: Astemizole, cisapride, terfenadine (may ↑ QT interval, torsades de pointes); cyclosporine, oral hypoglycemics, tacrolimus, theophylline, zidovudine (↑ interacting drug levels with possible toxicity); hydrochlorothiazide (↑ fluconazole levels); phenytoin, rifabutin, rifampin (↓ fluconazole levels, ↑ interacting drug levels); warfarin (↑ INR)
Adverse Effects: ↑ SGOT/SGPT, hypokalemia
Allergic Potential: Low
Safety in Pregnancy: C
Comments: Usual dose for candidemia (C. albicans) = 400 mg (IV/PO) q24h after loading dose of 800 mg (IV/PO).
Meningeal dose = 400 mg (IV/PO) q24h
Cerebrospinal Fluid Penetration:
Non-inflamed meninges: = 80%
Inflamed meninges: = 80%

REFERENCES:
Goa KL, Barradell LB. Fluconazole: An update of its pharmacodynamics and pharmacokinetic properties and therapeutic use in superficial and systemic mycoses in immunocompromised patients. Drugs 50:658-90, 1995.
Kauffman CA, Carver PL. Antifungal agents in the 1990s: Current status and future developments. Drugs 53:539-49, 1997.
Koh LP, Kurup A, Goh YT, et al. Randomized trial of fluconazole versus low-dose amphotericin B in prophylaxis against fungal infections in patients undergoing hematopoietic stem cell transplantation. Am J Hematol 71:260-7, 2002.
Kowalsky SF, Dixon DM. Fluconazole: A new antifungal agent. Clin Pharmacol 10:179-94, 1991.
MacMillan ML, Goodman JL, DeFor Te, et al. Fluconazole to prevent yeast infections in bone marrow transplantation patients: a randomized trial of

high versus reduced dose and determination of the value of maintenance therapy. Am J Med 112:369-79, 2002.

Owens RC, Ambrose PG. Fluconazole. Antibiotics for Clinicians 1:109-117, 1997.

Rex JH, Pappas PG, Karchmer AW, et al. National Institute of Allergy and Infectious Diseases Mycoses Study Group. A randomized and blinded multicenter trial of high-dose fluconazole plus placebo versus fluconazole plus amphotericin B as therapy for candidemia and its consequences in nonneutropenic subjects. Clin Infect Dis. 36:1221-8, 2003.

Terrell CL. Antifungal agents: Part II. The azoles. Mayo Clin Proc 74:78-100, 1999.

Website: www.diflucan.com

Flucytosine (Ancobon) 5-FC

Drug Class: Antifungal
Usual Dose: 25 mg/kg (PO) q6h
Pharmacokinetic Parameters:
Peak serum level: 3.5 mcg/mL
Bioavailability: 80%
Excreted unchanged: 90%
Serum half-life (normal/ESRD): 4/85 hrs
Plasma protein binding: 4%
Volume of distribution (V_d): 0.6 L/kg
Primary Mode of Elimination: Renal
Dosage Adjustments*

CrCl ~ 40–60 mL/min	500 mg (PO) q12h
CrCl ~ 10–40 mL/min	500 mg (PO) q18h
CrCl < 10 mL/min	500 mg (PO) q24h
Post–HD dose	500 mg (PO)
Post–PD dose	500 mg (PO)
CVVH dose	500 mg (PO) q18h
Moderate or severe insufficiency	No change

Drug Interactions: Cytarabine (↓ flucytosine effect); zidovudine (neutropenia)
Adverse Effects: Leukopenia, anemia, thrombocytopenia, nausea, vomiting, abdominal pain, ↑ SGOT/SGPT, drug fever/rashes
Allergic Potential: High
Safety in Pregnancy: C
Comments: Always use in combination with amphotericin B for cryptococcal meningitis.
Na^+ content = 37.5 mEq/g.
Meningeal dose = usual dose
Cerebrospinal Fluid Penetration:
Non-inflamed meninges = 100%
Inflamed meninges = 100%

REFERENCES:
Lyman CA, Walsh TJ. Systemically administered antifungal agents. A review of their clinical pharmacology and therapeutic applications: Part I. Amphotericin B preparations and flucytosine. Mayo Clin Proc 73:1205-25, 1998.

Mosquera J, Shartt A, Moore CB, et al. In vitro interaction of terbinafine with itraconazole, fluconazole, amphotericin B and 5-flucytosine against Aspergillus spp. J Antimicrob Chemother 50:189-94, 2002.

Pfaller MA, Messer SA, Boyken L, et al. In vitro activities of 5-fluorocytosine against 8,803 clinical isolates of Candida spp.: Global assessment of primary resistance using National Committee for Clinical Laboratory Standards susceptibility testing methods. Antimicrob Agents Chemother 46:3518-3521, 2002.

Te Dorsthorst DT, Verweij PE, Meletidis J, et al. In vitro interaction of flucytosine combined with amphotericin B or fluconazole against thirty-five yeast isolates determined by both the fractional inhibitory concentration index and the response surface approach. Antimicrob Agents Chemother 46:2982-9, 2002.

Wintermeyer SM, Mahata MC. Stability of flucytosine in an extemporaneously compounded oral liquid. Am J Health Syst Pharm 53:407-9, 1996.

Website: www.pdr.net

Foscarnet (Foscavir)

Drug Class: Antiviral (HSV,CMV)
Usual Dose: <u>HSV</u>: 40 mg/kg (IV) q12h x 2-3 weeks; <u>CMV</u>: 90 mg/kg (IV) q12h x 2-3 weeks (induction dose), then 90 mg/kg (IV) q24h (maintenance dose) for life-long suppression
Pharmacokinetic Parameters:
Peak serum level: 150 mcg/mL
Bioavailability: Not applicable
Excreted unchanged: 85%
Serum half-life (normal/ESRD): 2-4/25 hrs
Plasma protein binding: 17%
Volume of distribution (V_d): 0.5 L/kg
Primary Mode of Elimination: Renal /hepatic

"Usual dose" assumes normal renal/hepatic function. * For renal insufficiency, give usual dose x 1 followed by maintenance dose per CrCl. For dialysis patients, dose the same as for CrCl < 10 mL/min and give supplemental (post-HD/PD dose) immediately after dialysis. CrCl = creatinine clearance; CVVH = continuous veno-venous hemofiltration; HD/PD = hemodialysis/peritoneal dialysis. See pp. 293-297 for explanations, p. 1 for abbreviations

Dosage Adjustments*

Induction (mg/kg)		
CrCl (mL/min/kg)	HSV	CMV
> 1.4	40 q12h	90 q12h
> 1.0 - 1.4	30 q12h	70 q12h
> 0.8 - 1.0	20 q12h	50 q12h
> 0.6 - 0.8	35 q24h	80 q24h
> 0.5 - 0.6	25 q24h	60 q24h
≥ 0.4 - 0.5	20 q24h	50 q24h
< 0.4	Not recommended	

CMV maintenance range (mg/kg)[†]		
CrCl > 1.4	90 q24h	120 q24h
> 1.0 - 1.4	70 q24h	90 q24h
> 0.8 - 1.0	50 q24h	65 q24h
> 0.6 - 0.8	80 q48h	105 q48h
> 0.5 - 0.6	60 q48h	80 q48h
≥ 0.4 - 0.5	50 q48h	65 q48h
< 0.4	Not recommended	
Post–HD dose	45 mg/kg (IV)	
Post–PD dose	40-80 mg/kg (IV)	
CVVH dose	60-105 mg/kg (IV) q48h	
Mod. hepatic insufficiency	No change	
Severe hepatic insufficiency	No change	

Infusion pump must be used. Adequate hydration is recommended to prevent renal toxicity
† *Higher doses may be considered for early reinduction due to progression of CMV retinitis, and for patients showing excellent tolerance*

Drug Interactions: Ciprofloxacin (↑ risk of seizures); amphotericin B, aminoglycosides, cis-platinum, cyclosporine, other nephrotoxic drugs (↑ nephrotoxicity); pentamidine IV (severe hypocalcemia reported; do not combine); zidovudine (↑ incidence/severity of anemia)
Adverse Effects: Major side effects include nephrotoxicity and tetany (from ↓ Ca^{++}). Others include anemia, nausea, vomiting, GI upset, headache, seizures, peripheral neuropathy, hallucinations, tremors, nephrogenic DI, ↓ Ca^{++}, ↓ Mg^{++}, ↓ PO$_4^-$, oral/genital ulcers
Allergic Potential: Low
Safety in Pregnancy: C
Comments: Renal failure prevented/minimized by adequate hydration. Administer by IV slow infusion ≤ 1 mg/kg/min using an infusion pump Meningeal dose = usual dose
Cerebrospinal Fluid Penetration:
Non-inflamed meninges = 90%
Inflamed meninges = 100%

REFERENCES:
Chrisp P, Clissold SP. Foscarnet: A review of its antiviral activity, pharmacokinetic properties, and therapeutic use in immunocompromised patients with cytomegalovirus retinitis. Drugs 41:104-29, 1991.
Derary G, Martinez F, Katlama C, et al. Foscarnet nephrotoxicity: Mechanism, Incidence and prevention. Am J Nephrol 9:316-21, 1989.
Whitley RJ, Jacobson MA, Friedberg DN, et al. Guidelines for the treatment of cytomegalovirus diseases in patients with AIDS in the era of potent antiretroviral therapy. Arch Intern Med 158:957-69, 1998.
Website: www.pdr.net

Fosamprenavir (Lexiva)

Drug Class: Antiretroviral protease inhibitor
Usual Dose: 1400 mg (PO) q12h (without ritonavir); in combination with ritonavir: either 1400 mg (PO) q24h plus ritonavir 200 mg (PO) q24h or 700 mg (PO) q12h plus ritonavir 100 mg (PO) q12h. For PI-experienced patients: 700 mg (PO) q12h plus ritonavir 100 mg (PO) q12h
Pharmacokinetic Parameters:
Peak serum level: 4.8 mcg/mL
Bioavailability: No data
Excreted unchanged (urine): 1%
Serum half-life (normal/ESRD): 7 hrs/no data

"Usual dose" assumes normal renal/hepatic function. * For renal insufficiency, give usual dose x 1 followed by maintenance dose per CrCl. For dialysis patients, dose the same as for CrCl < 10 mL/min and give supplemental (post-HD/PD dose) immediately after dialysis. CrCl = creatinine clearance; CVVH = continuous veno-venous hemo-filtration; HD/PD = hemodialysis/peritoneal dialysis. See pp. 293-297 for explanations, p. 1 for abbreviations

Plasma protein binding: 90%
Volume of distribution (V_d): 6.1 L/kg
Primary Mode of Elimination: Hepatic
Dosage Adjustments*

CrCl < 40-60 mL/min	No information
Post–HD or PD dose	No information
CVVH dose	No information
Mild-moderate hepatic insufficiency	700 mg (PO) q12h if given without ritonavir; no data with ritonavir
Severe hepatic insufficiency	Avoid

Antiretroviral Dosage Adjustments:

Delavirdine	Avoid combination
Efavirenz	Fosamprenavir 700 mg q12h + ritonavir 100 mg q12h + efavirenz; fosamprenavir 1400 mg q24h + ritonavir 200 mg q24h + efavirenz; no data for fosamprenavir 1400 mg q12h + efavirenz
Indinavir	No information
Lopinavir/ritonavir	No information
Nelfinavir	No information
Nevirapine	No information
Saquinavir	No information
Rifampin	Avoid combination
Rifabutin	Reduce usual rifabutin dose by 50% (or 75% if given with fosamprenavir plus ritonavir; max. 150 mg q48h)

Drug Interactions: Antiretrovirals (see dose adjustment grid, above). Contraindicated with: ergot derivatives, cisapride, midazolam, triazolam, pimozide, (flecainide and propafenone if administered with ritonavir). Do not coadminister with: rifampin, lovastatin, simvastatin, St. John's wort, delavirdine. Dose reduction (of other drug): atorvastatin, rifabutin, sildenafil, vardenafil, ketoconazole, itraconazole. Concentration monitoring (of other drug): amiodarone, systemic lidocaine, quinidine, warfarin (INR), tricyclic antidepressants, cyclosporin, tacrolimus, sirolimus
Adverse Effects: Rash, Stevens-Johnson syndrome (rare), GI upset, headache, depression, diarrhea, hyperglycemia (including worsening diabetes, new-onset diabetes, DKA), ↑ cholesterol/triglycerides (evaluate risk for coronary disease/pancreatitis), fat redistribution, ↑ SGOT/SGPT, possible increased bleeding in hemophilia
Allergic Potential: High. Fosamprenavir is a sulfonamide; use with caution if sulfa allergy
Safety in Pregnancy: C
Comments: Usually given in conjunction with ritonavir. May be taken with or without food. Fosamprenavir is rapidly hydrolyzed to amprenavir by gut epithelium during absorption. Amprenavir inhibits CYP3A4. Fosamprenavir contains a sulfonamide moiety

REFERENCES:
Lexiva (fosamprenavir) approved. AIDS Treat News 31;2, 2003.
Rodriguez-French A, Boghossian J, Gray GE, et al. The NEAT study: a 48-week open-label study to compare the antiviral efficacy and safety of GW433908 versus nelfinavir in antiretroviral therapy-naive HIV-1-infected patients. J Acquir Immune Defic Syndr 35: 22-32, 2004.
Website: www.TreatHIV.com

Fosfomycin (Monurol)

Drug Class: Urinary antiseptic
Usual Dose: 3 gm (PO) q24h
Pharmacokinetic Parameters:
Peak serum level: 26 mcg/mL
Bioavailability: 37%
Excreted unchanged: 56%
Serum half-life (normal/ESRD): 5.7/50 hrs
Plasma protein binding: 3%

"Usual dose" assumes normal renal/hepatic function. * For renal insufficiency, give usual dose x 1 followed by maintenance dose per CrCl. For dialysis patients, dose the same as for CrCl < 10 mL/min and give supplemental (post-HD/PD dose) immediately after dialysis. CrCl = creatinine clearance; CVVH = continuous veno-venous hemofiltration; HD/PD = hemodialysis/peritoneal dialysis. See pp. 293-297 for explanations, p. 1 for abbreviations

Volume of distribution (V_d): 2 L/kg
Primary Mode of Elimination: Renal
Dosage Adjustments*

CrCl ~ 40–60 mL/min	No change
CrCl ~ 10–40 mL/min	No information
CrCl < 10 mL/min	No information
Post–HD dose	No information
Post–PD dose	No information
CVVH dose	No information
Moderate or severe hepatic insufficiency	No change

Drug Interactions: Antacids, metoclopramide (↓ fosfomycin effect)
Adverse Effects: Nausea, vomiting, GI upset, diarrhea, ↑ SGOT/SGPT, thrombocytosis, eosinophilia
Allergic Potential: Low
Safety in Pregnancy: B
Comments: May be taken with or without food. Useful only for cystitis, not pyelonephritis/urosepsis. Treat UTIs x 3 days in males, as single dose in females.

REFERENCES:

Gosden PE, Reeves DS. Fosfomycin. Antibiotics for Clinicians 2:121-28, 1998.

Monden K, Ando E, Iida M, et al. Role of fosfomycin in a synergistic combination with ofloxacin against Pseudomonas aeruginosa growing in a biofilm. J Infect Chemother 8:218-26, 2002.

Okazaki M, Suzuki K, Asano N, et al. Effectiveness of fosfomycin combined with other antimicrobial agents against multidrug-resistant Pseudomonas aeruginosa isolates using the efficacy time index assay. J Infect Chemother 8:37-42, 2002.

Patel SS, Balfour JA, Bryson HM. Fosfomycin tromethamine: Pharmacokinetic properties and therapeutic efficacy as a single-dose oral treatment for acute uncomplicated low urinary tract infections. Drugs 53:637-56, 1997.

Shrestha NK, Chua JD, Tuohy MJ, et al. Antimicrobial susceptibility of vancomycin-resistant Enterococcus faecium: potential utility of fosfomycin. Scand J Infect Dis. 35:12-4, 2003.

Ungheri D, Albini E, Belluco G. In-vitro susceptibility of quinolone-resistant clinical isolates of Escherichia coli

to fosfomycin trometamol. J Chemother 14:237-40, 2002.
Website: www.pdr.net

Ganciclovir (Cytovene)

Drug Class: Antiviral, nucleoside inhibitor/analogue
Usual Dose: 5 mg/kg (IV) q12h x 3-6 weeks (induction), then 5 mg/kg (IV) q24h or 1 gm (PO) q8h (maintenance) for CMV retinitis (see comments)
Pharmacokinetic Parameters:
Peak serum level: 8.3 (IV)/1.2 (PO) mcg/mL
Bioavailability: 5%
Excreted unchanged: 90%
Serum half-life (normal/ESRD): 3.6/28 hrs
Plasma protein binding: 1%
Volume of distribution (V_d): 0.74 L/kg
Primary Mode of Elimination: Renal
Dosage Adjustments*

CrCl ~ 50–69 mL/min	2.5 mg/kg (IV) q12h (induction); 2.5 mg/kg (IV) q24h (maintenance); 500 mg (PO) q8h
CrCl ~ 25–49 mL/min	2.5 mg/kg (IV) q24h (induction); 1.25 mg/kg (IV) q24h (maintenance); 500 mg (PO) q12h
CrCl < 10-40 mL/min	1.25 mg/kg (IV) q24h (induction); 0.625 mg/kg (IV) q24h (maintenance); 500 mg (PO) q24h
CrCl < 10 mL/min	1.25 mg/kg (IV) 3x/week (induction); 0.625 mg/kg (IV) 3x/week (maintenance); 500 mg (PO) 3x/week
Post–HD dose	1.25 mg/kg (IV) (induction); 0.625 mg/kg (IV) (maintenance); 500 mg (PO)
Post–PD dose	None

CVVH dose	see CrCl ~ 10-40 mL/min
Moderate hepatic insufficiency	No change
Severe hepatic insufficiency	No change

Drug Interactions: Cytotoxic drugs (may produce additive toxicity: stomatitis, bone marrow depression, alopecia); imipenem (↑ risk of seizures); probenecid (↑ ganciclovir levels); zidovudine (↓ ganciclovir levels, ↑ zidovudine levels, possible neutropenia)
Adverse Effects: Headaches, hallucinations, seizures/tremor (dose related), drug fever/rash, diarrhea, nausea/vomiting, GI upset, leukopenia, thrombocytopenia, anemia, retinal detachment
Allergic Potential: High
Safety in Pregnancy: C
Comments: Induction doses are always given IV. Maintenance doses may be given IV or PO. For CMV encephalitis, use same dosing regimen as for CMV retinitis (CNS penetration = 70%). For CMV pneumonitis, give 2.5 mg/kg (IV) q8h x 20 doses plus IVIG 500 mg/kg (IV) q48h x 10 doses; then follow with 5 mg/kg (IV) 3-5x/week x 20 doses plus IVIG 500 mg/kg (IV) 2x/week x 8 doses. For CMV colitis/esophagitis, use same dose for CMV retinitis induction x 3-6 weeks. Continue maintenance doses for CMV retinitis, encephalitis, and colitis/esophagitis until CD₄ cell count > 100–200. Reduce dose with neutropenia/thrombocytopenia. Bioavailability increased with food: 5% fasting; 6-9% with food; 28-31% with fatty food. Na⁺ content = 4.0 mEq/g.
Meningeal dose = CMV retinitis dose
Cerebrospinal Fluid Penetration: 41%

REFERENCES:
Alraibah FA, Sacks SL. New antiherpesvirus agents: Their targets and therapeutic potential. Drugs 52:17-32,1996.
Czock D, Scholle C, Rasche FM, et al. Pharmacokinetics of valganciclovir and ganciclovir in renal impairment. Clin Pharmacol Ther 72:142-50, 2002.
Komanduri KV, Viswanathan MB, Wieder ED, et al. Restoration of cytomegalovirus-specific CD4+ T-lymphocyte responses after ganciclovir and highly active antiretroviral therapy in individuals infected with HIV-1. Nat Med 4:953-956, 1998.
Matthews T, Boehme R. Antiviral activity and mechanism of action of ganciclovir. Rev Infect Dis 10:490-4, 1988.
Paya CV, Wilson JA, Espy MJ, et al. Preemptive use of oral ganciclovir to prevent cytomegalovirus infection in liver transplant patients: a randomized, placebo-controlled trial J Infect Dis 185:861-7, 2002.
Singh N. Preemptive therapy for cytomegalovirus with oral ganciclovir after liver transplantation. Transplantation 73:1977-78, 2002.
Tokimasa S, Hara J, Osugi Y, et al. Ganciclovir is effective for prophylaxis and treatment of human herpesvirus-6 in allogeneic stem cell transplantation. Bone Marrow Transplant 29:595-8, 2002.
Whitley RJ, Jacobson MA, Friedberg DN, et al. Guidelines for the treatment of cytomegalovirus diseases in patients with AIDS in the era of potent antiretroviral therapy. Arch Intern Med 158:957-69, 1998.
Website: www.rocheusa.com/products/

Gatifloxacin (Tequin)

Drug Class: Fluoroquinolone
Usual Dose: 400 mg (IV/PO) q24h
Pharmacokinetic Parameters:
Peak serum level: 4.6 (IV)/4.2 (PO) mcg/mL
Bioavailability: 96%
Excreted unchanged: 70%
Serum half-life (normal/ESRD): 11/30 hrs
Plasma protein binding: 20%
Volume of distribution (V_d): 2 L/kg
Primary Mode of Elimination: Renal
Dosage Adjustments*

CrCl ~ 40–60 mL/min	No change
CrCl ~ 10–40 mL/min	200 mg (IV/PO) q24h
CrCl < 10 mL/min	200 mg (IV/PO) q24h
Post–HD dose	200 mg (IV/PO)
Post–PD dose	200 mg (IV/PO)
CVVH dose	200 mg (IV/PO) q24h
Moderate hepatic insufficiency	No change
Severe hepatic insufficiency	No information

Drug Interactions: Al^{++}, Fe^{++}, Mg^{++}, Zn^{++} antacids, citrate/citric acid, dairy products (↓ absorption of gatifloxacin only if taken together); amiodarone, procainamide, sotalol (may ↑ QT_c interval, torsade de pointes); digoxin (↑ digoxin levels 18-56%, ↑ digoxin effects); insulin, oral hypoglycemics (hypoglycemia); probenecid (↑ gatifloxacin levels); NSAIDs (CNS stimulation)

Adverse Effects: Headache, dizziness, nausea, diarrhea, vomiting, vaginitis, hypoglycemia > hyperglycemia

Allergic Potential: Low

Safety in Pregnancy: C

Comments: Nausea common GI side effect. Take 4 hours before aluminum/magnesium-containing antacids; not affected by calcium-containing antacids. Does not ↑ QT_c interval > 3 msec. C8-methoxy group increases activity and decreases resistance potential

Cerebrospinal Fluid Penetration: 36%

Bile Concentration: 500%

REFERENCES:

Arguedas A, Sher L, Lopez E, et al. Open label, multicenter study of gatifloxacin treatment of recurrent otitis media and acute otitis media treatment failure. Pediatr Infect Dis J. 22:949-56, 2003.

Correa JC, Badaro R, Bumroongkit C, et al. Randomized, open-label, parallel-group, multicenter study of the efficacy and tolerability of IV gatifloxacin with the option for oral stepdown gatifloxacin versus IV ceftriaxone (with or without erythromycin or clarithromycin) with the option for oral stepdown clarithromycin for treatment of patients with mild to moderate community-acquired pneumonia requiring hospitalization. Clin Ther. 25:1453-68, 2003.

Dawis MA, Isenberg HD, France KA, et al. In vitro activity of gatifloxacin alone and in combination with cefepime, meropenem, piperacillin and gentamicin against multidrug-resistant organisms. J Antimicrob Chemother. 51:1203-11, 2003.

Fish DN, North DS. Gatifloxacin, an advanced 8-methoxy fluoroquinolone. Pharmacotherapy 21:35-59, 2001.

Gatifloxacin and moxifloxacin: Two new fluoroquinolones. Med Lett Drugs Ther 42:1072:15, 2000.

Gradelski E, Kolek B, Bonner D, et al. Bactericidal mechanism of gatifloxacin compared with other quinolones. J Antimicrob Chemother 49:185-8, 2002.

Mignot A, Guillaume M, Gohler K, et al. Oral bioavailability of gatifloxacin in healthy volunteers under fasting and fed conditions. Chemotherapy 48:111-5, 2002.

Nicolau DP, Ambrose PG. Pharmacodynamic profiling of levofloxacin and gatifloxacin using Monte Carlo simulation for community-acquired isolates of Streptococcus pneumoniae. Am J Med 111 (Suppl 9A):13S-18S; discussion 36S-38S, 2001.

Nicholson SC, High KP, Gothelf S, Webb CD. Gatifloxacin in community-based treatment of acute respiratory tract infections in the elderly. Diagn Microbiol Infect Dis 44:109-16, 2002.

Nicholson SC, Webb CD, Andriole VT, et al. Haemophilus influenzae in respiratory tract infections in community-based clinical practice: therapy with gatifloxacin. Diagn Microbiol Infect Dis 44:101-7, 2002.

Perry CM, Ormrod D, Hurst M, et al. Gatifloxacin: a review of its use in the management of bacterial infections. Drugs 62:169-207, 2002.

Sethi S. Gatifloxacin in community-acquired respiratory tract infection. Expert Opin Pharmacother. 4:1847-55, 2003.

Sher LD, McAdoo MA, Bettis RB, et al. A multicenter, randomized, investigator-blinded study of 5- and 10-day gatifloxacin versus 10-day amoxicillin/clavulanate in patients with acute bacterial sinusitis. Clin Ther 24:269-81, 2002.

Tarshis GA, Miskin BM, Jones TM, et al. Once-daily oral gatifloxacin versus oral levofloxacin in treatment of uncomplicated skin and soft tissue infections: double-blind, multicenter, randomized study. Antimicrob Agents Chemother 45:2358-62, 2001.

White RL, Enzweiler KA, Friedrich LV, et al. Comparative activity of gatifloxacin and other antibiotics against 4009 clinical isolates of Streptococcus pneumoniae in the United States during 1999-2000. Diagn Microbiol Infect Dis 43:207-17, 2002.

Website: www.tequin.com

Gemifloxacin (Factive)

Drug Class: Fluoroquinolone

Usual Dose: 320 mg (PO) q24h

Pharmacokinetic Parameters:

Peak serum level: 1.6 mcg/mL

Bioavailability: 71%

Excreted unchanged: >60%

Serum half-life (normal/ESRD): 7/10 hrs

Plasma protein binding: 55-73%

Volume of distribution (V_d): 4.2 L/kg

Primary Mode of Elimination: Renal

"Usual dose" assumes normal renal/hepatic function. * For renal insufficiency, give usual dose x 1 followed by maintenance dose per CrCl. For dialysis patients, dose the same as for CrCl < 10 mL/min and give supplemental (post-HD/PD dose) immediately after dialysis. CrCl = creatinine clearance; CVVH = continuous veno-venous hemofiltration; HD/PD = hemodialysis/peritoneal dialysis. See pp. 293-297 for explanations, p. 1 for abbreviations

Dosage Adjustments*

CrCl ~ 41–60 mL/min	No change
CrCl ~ 10–40 mL/min	160 mg (PO) q24h
CrCl < 10 mL/min	160 mg (PO) q24h
Post–HD dose	No information
Post–PD dose	No information
Post–CVVH dose	No information
Moderate hepatic insufficiency	No change
Severe hepatic insufficiency	No change

Drug Interactions: Al^{++}, Fe^{++}, Mg^{++}, Zn^{++} antacids/multivitamins, didanosine, sucralfate (↓ gemifloxacin levels only if taken together); probenecid (↑ gemifloxacin levels); amiodarone, quinidine, procainamide, sotalol (may ↑ QT_c interval, torsade de pointes; avoid)

Adverse Effects: Rash, ↑ LFTs (doses > 320 mg/d)

Allergic Potential: Low

Safety in Pregnancy: C

Comments: Take at least 3 hours before or 2 hours after calcium/magnesium containing antacids. Take at least 2 hours before sucralfate. May ↑ QT_c interval > 3 msec.; avoid taking with other medications that prolong the QT_c interval, and in patients with prolonged QT interval/heart block. Do not exceed usual dose

Cerebrospinal Fluid Penetration: < 10%

REFERENCES:

Chagan L. Gemifloxacin for the treatment of acute bacterial exacerbation of chronic bronchitis and community-acquired pneumonia. P&T 28:769-79, 2003.

Goldstein EJ. Review of the in vitro activity of gemifloxacin against gram-positive and gram-negative anaerobic pathogens. J Antimicrob Chemother 45:55-65, 2000.

Hammerschlag MR. Activity of gemifloxacin and other new quinolones against Chlamydia pneumoniae: A review. J Antimicrob Chemother 45:35-9, 2000.

Santos J, Aguilar L, Garcia-Mendez E, et al. Clinical characteristics and response to newer quinolones in Legionella pneumonia: a report of 28 cases. J Chemother 15:461-5, 2003.

Saravolatz LD, Leggett J. Gatifloxacin, gemifloxacin, and moxifloxacin: the role of 3 newer fluoroquinolones. Clin Infect Dis 37:1210-5, 2003.

Waites KB, Crabb DM, Duffy LB. Inhibitory and bactericidal activities of gemifloxacin and other antimicrobials against Mycoplasma pneumoniae. Int J Antimicrob Agents 21:574-7, 2003.

Wilson R, Schentag JJ, Ball P, et al. A comparison of gemifloxacin and clarithromycin in acute exacerbations of chronic bronchitis and long-term clinical outcomes. Clin Ther 24:639-52, 2002.

Wilson R, Langan C, Ball P, et al. Oral gemifloxacin once daily for 5 days compared with sequential therapy with i.v. ceftriaxone/oral cefuroxime (maximum of 10 days) in the treatment of hospitalized patients with acute exacerbations of chronic bronchitis. Respir Med 97:242-9, 2003.

Website: www.factive.com

Gentamicin (Garamycin)

Drug Class: Aminoglycoside

Usual Dose: 5 mg/kg (IV) q24h or 240 mg (IV) q24h (preferred over q8h dosing)

Pharmacokinetic Parameters:
Peak serum levels: 4-8 mcg/mL (q8h dosing); 16-24 mcg/mL (q24h dosing)
Bioavailability: Not applicable
Excreted unchanged: 95%
Serum half-life (normal/ESRD): 2.5/48 hrs
Plasma protein binding: < 5%
Volume of distribution (V_d): 0.3 L/kg

Primary Mode of Elimination: Renal

Dosage Adjustments*

CrCl ~ 40–60 mL/min	2.5 mg/kg (IV) q24h or 120 mg (IV) q24h
CrCl ~ 20–40 mL/min	2.5 mg/kg (IV) q48h or 120 mg (IV) q48h
CrCl < 10 mL/min	1.25 mg/kg (IV) q48h or 60 mg (IV) q48h
Post–HD dose	1.25 mg/kg (IV) or 80 mg (IV)
Post–PD dose	0.6 mg/kg (IV) or 40 mg (IV)

"Usual dose" assumes normal renal/hepatic function. * For renal insufficiency, give usual dose x 1 followed by maintenance dose per CrCl. For dialysis patients, dose the same as for CrCl < 10 mL/min and give supplemental (post-HD/PD dose) immediately after dialysis. CrCl = creatinine clearance; CVVH = continuous veno-venous hemo-filtration; HD/PD = hemodialysis/peritoneal dialysis. See pp. 293-297 for explanations, p. 1 for abbreviations

CVVH dose	2.5 mg/kg (IV) or 120 mg (IV) q48h
Moderate hepatic insufficiency	No change
Severe hepatic insufficiency	No change

Drug Interactions: Amphotericin B, cephalothin, cyclosporine, enflurane, methoxyflurane, NSAIDs, polymyxin B, radiographic contrast, vancomycin ($\uparrow$ nephrotoxicity); cis-platinum ($\uparrow$ nephrotoxicity, $\uparrow$ ototoxicity); loop diuretics ($\uparrow$ ototoxicity); neuromuscular blocking agents, magnesium sulfate ($\uparrow$ apnea, prolonged paralysis); non-polarizing muscle relaxants ($\uparrow$ apnea)

Adverse Effects: Neuromuscular blockade with rapid infusion/absorption. Nephrotoxicity only with prolonged/extremely high serum trough levels; may cause reversible non-oliguric renal failure (ATN). Ototoxicity associated with prolonged/extremely high peak serum levels (usually irreversible): Cochlear toxicity (1/3 of ototoxicity) manifests as decreased high frequency hearing, but deafness is unusual. Vestibular toxicity (2/3 of ototoxicity) develops before ototoxicity, and typically manifests as tinnitus

Allergic Potential: Low
Safety in Pregnancy: C
Comments: Dose for synergy = 2.5 mg/kg (IV) q24h or 120 mg (IV) q24h. Single daily dosing greatly reduces nephrotoxic/ototoxic potential. Incompatible with solutions containing β–lactams, erythromycin, chloramphenicol, furosemide, sodium bicarbonate. IV infusion should be given slowly over 1 hour. May be given IM. Avoid intraperitoneal infusion due to risk of neuromuscular blockade. Avoid intratracheal/aerosolized intrapulmonary instillation, which predisposes to antibiotic resistance. V_d increases with edema/ascites, trauma, burns, cystic fibrosis; may require $\uparrow$ dose. V_d decreases with dehydration, obesity; may require $\downarrow$ dose. Renal cast counts are the best indicator of aminoglycoside nephrotoxicity, not serum creatinine. Dialysis removes ~ 1/3 of gentamicin from serum

Therapeutic Serum Concentrations:
Peak (q24h/q8h dosing) = 16-24/8-10 mcg/mL
Trough (q24h/q8h dosing) = 0/1-2 mcg/mL
Intrathecal (IT) dose = 5 mg (IT) q24h
Cerebrospinal Fluid Penetration:
Non-inflamed meninges = 0%
Inflamed meninges = 20%
Bile Penetration: 30%

REFERENCES:
Cornely OA, Bethe U, Seifert H, et al. A randomized monocentric trial in febrile neutropenic patients: ceftriaxone and gentamicin vs cefepime and gentamicin. Ann Hematol 81:37-43, 2002.
Cunha BA. Aminoglycosides: Current role in antimicrobial therapy. Pharmacotherapy 8:334-50, 1988.
Edson RS, Terrell CL. The aminoglycosides. Mayo Clin Proc 74:519-28, 1999.
Freeman CD, Nicolau DP, Belliveau PP, et al. Once-daily dosing of aminoglycosides: Review and recommendations for clinical practice. J Antimicrob Chemother 39:677-86, 1997.

Griseofulvin (Fulvicin, Grifulvin, Ultra, Gris-PEG, Grisactin)

Drug Class: Antifungal
Usual Dose: 500 mg-1 gm (PO) q24h (microsize); 330-375 mg (PO) q24h (ultramicrosize)
Pharmacokinetic Parameters:
Peak serum level: 1-2 mcg/mL
Bioavailability: 50%
Excreted unchanged: 1%
Serum half-life (normal/ESRD): 9/22 hrs
Plasma protein binding: 84%
Volume of distribution (V_d): No data
Primary Mode of Elimination: Hepatic
Dosage Adjustments*

CrCl < 40–60 mL/min	No change
Post-HD or PD dose	None
CVVH dose	No change

"Usual dose" assumes normal renal/hepatic function. * For renal insufficiency, give usual dose x 1 followed by maintenance dose per CrCl. For dialysis patients, dose the same as for CrCl < 10 mL/min and give supplemental (post-HD/PD dose) immediately after dialysis. CrCl = creatinine clearance; CVVH = continuous veno-venous hemo-filtration; HD/PD = hemodialysis/peritoneal dialysis. See pp. 293-297 for explanations, p. 1 for abbreviations

Moderate or severe hepatic insufficiency	No change

Drug Interactions: Alcohol (↑ griseofulvin toxicity); barbiturates (↓ griseofulvin levels); oral contraceptives, warfarin (↓ interacting drug levels)

Adverse Effects: Photosensitivity reactions, headache, nausea, vomiting, diarrhea, angular stomatitis, glossitis, leukopenia

Allergic Potential: Moderate

Safety in Pregnancy: C

Comments: May exacerbate SLE/acute intermittent porphyria. Take microsize griseofulvin with fatty meal to ↑ absorption to ~ 70%. Ultramicrosize griseofulvin is absorbed 1.5 times better than microsize griseofulvin

REFERENCES:

Trepanier EF, Amsden GW. Current issues in onychomycosis. Ann Pharmacotherapy 32:204-14, 1998.
Website: www.pdr.net

Imipenem/Cilastatin (Primaxin)

Drug Class: Carbapenem

Usual Dose: 500 mg (IV) q6h (see comments)

Pharmacokinetic Parameters:

Peak serum level: 21-58 mcg/mL (500 mg dose)
Bioavailability: Not applicable
Excreted unchanged: 70%
Serum half-life (normal/ESRD): 1/4 hrs
Plasma protein binding: 20% / 40% (cilastatin)
Volume of distribution (V_d): 0.2 L/kg

Primary Mode of Elimination: Renal

Dosage Adjustments* (based on 500 mg q6h and weight > 70 kg):

CrCl ~ 41–70 mL/min	500 mg (IV) q8h
CrCl ~ 21–40 mL/min	250 mg (IV) q6h
CrCl < 6–20 mL/min[†]	250 mg (IV) q12h
Post–HD dose	250 mg (IV)
Post–PD dose	250 mg (IV)

CVVH dose	250 mg (IV) q6h
Moderate hepatic insufficiency	No change
Severe hepatic insufficiency	No change

† Avoid if CrCl ≤ 5 mL/min unless dialysis is instituted within 48 hours

Drug Interactions: Cyclosporine (↑ cyclosporine levels); ganciclovir (↑ risk of seizures); probenecid (↑ imipenem levels)

Adverse Effects: Seizures, phlebitis

Allergic Potential: Low

Safety in Pregnancy: C

Comments: Imipenem:cilastatin (1:1). Infuse 500 mg (IV) over 20-30 minutes; 1 gm (IV) over 40-60 minutes. Imipenem is renally metabolized by dehydropeptidase I; cilastatin is an inhibitor of this enzyme, effectively preventing the metabolism of imipenem. Imipenem/cilastatin can be given IM (IM absorption: imipenem 75%; cilastatin 100%). For fully susceptible organisms, use 500 mg (IV) q6h; for moderately susceptible organisms (e.g., P. aeruginosa), use 1 gm (IV) q6-8h. Incompatible in solutions containing vancomycin or metronidazole. Seizures more likely in renal insufficiency/high doses (> 2 gm/d). Inhibits endotoxin release from gram-negative bacilli. Na[+] content = 3.2 mEq/gm

Cerebrospinal Fluid Penetration:

Non-inflamed meninges = 10%
Inflamed meninges = 15%

Bile Penetration: 1%

REFERENCES:

Balfour JA, Bryson HM, Brogden RN. Imipenem/cilastatin: An update of its antibacterial activity, pharmacokinetics, and therapeutic efficacy in the treatment of serious infections. Drugs 51:99-136, 1996.
Barza M. Imipenem: First of a new class of beta-lactam antibiotics. Ann Intern Med 103:552-60, 1985.
Bradley JS, Garau J, Lode H, et al. Carbapenems in clinical practice: a guide to their use in serious infection. Int J Antimicrob Agents 11:93-100, 1999.
Cunha BA. Cross allergenicity of penicillin with carbapenems and monobactams. J Crit Illness 13:344, 1998.
Helinger WC, Brewer NS. Carbapenems and

"Usual dose" assumes normal renal/hepatic function. * For renal insufficiency, give usual dose x 1 followed by maintenance dose per CrCl. For dialysis patients, dose the same as for CrCl < 10 mL/min and give supplemental (post-HD/PD dose) immediately after dialysis. CrCl = creatinine clearance; CVVH = continuous veno-venous hemofiltration; HD/PD = hemodialysis/peritoneal dialysis. See pp. 293-297 for explanations, p. 1 for abbreviations

monobactams: Imipenem, meropenem, and aztreonam. Mayo Clin Proc 74:420-34, 1999.

Ishihara S, Yamada T, Yokoi S, et al. Antimicrobial activity of imipenem against isolates from complicated urinary tract infections. Int J Antimicrob Agents 19:565-9, 2002.

Klastersky JA. Use of imipenem as empirical treatment of febrile neutropenia. Int J Antimicrob Agents 21:393-402, 2003.

Maravi-Poma E, Gener J, Alvarez-Lerma F, et al. Spanish Group for the Study of Septic Complications in Severe Acute Pancreatitis. Early antibiotic treatment (prophylaxis) of septic complications in severe acute necrotizing pancreatitis: a prospective, randomized, multicenter study comparing two regimens with imipenem-cilastatin. Intensive Care Med. 29:1974-80, 2003.

Website: www.pdr.net

Indinavir (Crixivan)

Drug Class: Antiretroviral protease inhibitor
Usual Dose: 800 mg (PO) q8h
Pharmacokinetic Parameters:
Peak serum level: 252 mcg/mL
Bioavailability: 65% (77% with food)
Excreted unchanged: < 20%
Serum half-life (normal/ESRD): 2 hrs/no data
Plasma protein binding: 60 %
Volume of distribution (V_d): No data
Primary Mode of Elimination: Hepatic
Dosage Adjustments*

CrCl ~ 40–60 mL/min	No change
CrCl ~ 10–40 mL/min	No change
CrCl < 10 mL/min	No change
Post–HD dose	None
Post–PD dose	None
CVVH dose	No change
Moderate hepatic insufficiency	600 mg (PO) q8h
Severe hepatic insufficiency	400 mg (PO) q8h

Antiretroviral Dosage Adjustments:

Amprenavir	No changes
Delavirdine	Indinavir 600 mg q8h
Efavirenz	Indinavir 1000 mg q8h
Lopinavir/ritonavir	Indinavir 600 mg q12h
Nelfinavir	Limited data for indinavir 1200 mg q12h + nelfinavir 1250 mg q12h
Nevirapine	Indinavir 1000 mg q8h
Ritonavir	Indinavir 800 mg q12h + ritonavir 100-200 mg q12h, or 400 mg q12h of each drug
Saquinavir	No information
Rifampin	Avoid combination
Rifabutin	Indinavir 1000 mg q8h; rifabutin 150 mg q24h or 300 mg 2-3x/week

Drug Interactions: Antiretrovirals, rifabutin, rifampin (see dose adjustment grid, above); astemizole, terfenadine, benzodiazepines, cisapride, ergot alkaloids, statins, St. John's wort (avoid if possible); calcium channel blockers (↑ calcium channel blocker levels); carbamazepine, phenobarbital, phenytoin (↓ indinavir levels, ↑ anticonvulsant levels; monitor);(↓ indinavir levels, ↑ tenofovir levels); clarithromycin, erythromycin, telithromycin (↑ indinavir and macrolide levels); didanosine (administer indinavir on empty stomach 2 hours apart); ethinyl estradiol, norethindrone (↑ interacting drug levels; no dosage adjustment); grapefruit juice (↓ indinavir levels); itraconazole, ketoconazole (↑ indinavir levels); sildenafil (↑ or ↓ sildenafil levels; do not exceed 25 mg in 48 hrs); theophylline (↓ theophylline levels)

"Usual dose" assumes normal renal/hepatic function. * For renal insufficiency, give usual dose x 1 followed by maintenance dose per CrCl. For dialysis patients, dose the same as for CrCl < 10 mL/min and give supplemental (post-HD/PD dose) immediately after dialysis. CrCl = creatinine clearance; CVVH = continuous veno-venous hemofiltration; HD/PD = hemodialysis/peritoneal dialysis. See pp. 293-297 for explanations, p. 1 for abbreviations

Adverse Effects: Nausea, vomiting, diarrhea, anemia, leukopenia, headache, insomnia, nephrolithiasis, hyperglycemia (including worsening diabetes, new-onset diabetes, DKA), ↑ SGOT/SGPT, ↑ indirect bilirubin (2° to drug-induced Gilbert's syndrome; inconsequential), fat redistribution, lipid abnormalities (evaluate risk of coronary disease/pancreatitis), abdominal pain, possible ↑ bleeding in hemophilia

Allergic Potential: Low

Safety in Pregnancy: C

Comments: Renal stone formation may be prevented/minimized by adequate hydration; ↑ risk of nephrolithiasis with alcohol. Take 1 hour before or 2 hours after meals (may take with skim milk or low fat meal). Separate dosing with ddl by 1 hour. Effective antiretroviral therapy consists of at least 3 antiretrovirals (same/different classes)

Cerebrospinal Fluid Penetration: 16%

REFERENCES:

Acosta EP, Henry K, Baken L, et al. Indinavir concentrations and antiviral effect. Pharmacotherapy 19:708-712, 1999.

Antinori A, Giancola MI, Griserri S, et al. Factors influencing virological response to antiretroviral drugs in cerebrospinal fluid of advanced HIV-1-infected patients. AIDS 16:1867-76, 2002.

Deeks SG, Smith M, Holodniy M, et al. HIV-1 protease inhibitors: A review for clinicians. JAMA 277:145-53, 1997.

Go J, Cunha BA. Indinavir: A review. Antibiotics for Clinicians 3:81-87, 1999.

Kopp JB, Falloon J, Filie A, et al. Indinavir-associated intestinal nephritis and urothelial inflammation: clinical and cytologic findings. Clin Infect Dis 34:1122-8, 2002.

Meraviglia P, Angeli E, Del Sorbo F, et al. Risk factors for indinavir-related renal colic in HIV patients: predicative value of indinavir dose-body mass index. AIDS 16:2089-2093, 2002.

McDonald CK, Kuritzkes DR. Human immunodeficiency virus type 1 protease inhibitors. Arch Intern Med 157:951-9, 1997.

Panel on Clinical Practices for Treatment of HIV Infection. Guidelines for the use of antiretroviral agents in HIV-infected adults and adolescents. Department of Health and Human Services. www.aidsinfo.nih.gov/guidelines/. November 10, 2003.

Website: www.crixivan.com

Isoniazid (INH)

Drug Class: Anti-TB drug
Usual Dose: 300 mg (PO) q24h
Pharmacokinetic Parameters:
Peak serum level: 7 mcg/mL
Bioavailability: 90%
Excreted unchanged: 50-70%
Serum half-life (normal/ESRD): 1/1 hr
Plasma protein binding: 15%
Volume of distribution (V_d): 0.75 L/kg
Primary Mode of Elimination: Hepatic
Dosage Adjustments*

CrCl ~ 40–60 mL/min	No change
CrCl ~ 10–40 mL/min	No change
CrCl < 10 mL/min	No change
Post–HD dose	None
Post–PD dose	None
CVVH dose	None
Moderate hepatic insufficiency	No change
Severe hepatic insufficiency	No change

Drug Interactions: Alcohol, rifampin (↑ risk of hepatic injury); alfentanil (↑ duration of alfentanil effect); aluminum salts (↓ isoniazid absorption); carbamazepine, phenytoin (↑ interacting drug levels); itraconazole (↓ itraconazole levels); warfarin (↑ INR)

Adverse Effects: ↑ SGOT/SGPT, drug fever/rash, age-dependent hepatotoxicity (after age 40), ↑ hepatotoxicity in slow acetylators, drug–induced ANA/SLE, hemolytic anemia, neuropsychiatric changes in the elderly

Allergic Potential: Low

Safety in Pregnancy: C

Comments: Administer with 50 mg of pyridoxine daily to prevent peripheral neuropathy. Increased blood pressure/rash with tyramine–containing products, e.g., cheese/wine.
Meningeal dose = usual dose

"Usual dose" assumes normal renal/hepatic function. * For renal insufficiency, give usual dose x 1 followed by maintenance dose per CrCl. For dialysis patients, dose the same as for CrCl < 10 mL/min and give supplemental (post-HD/PD dose) immediately after dialysis. CrCl = creatinine clearance; CVVH = continuous veno-venous hemofiltration; HD/PD = hemodialysis/peritoneal dialysis. See pp. 293-297 for explanations, p. 1 for abbreviations

Cerebrospinal Fluid Penetration:
Non-inflamed meninges = 90%
Inflamed meninges = 90%

REFERENCES:
Ahn C, Oh KH, Kim K, et al. Effect of peritoneal dialysis on plasma and peritoneal fluid concentrations of isoniazid, pyrazinamide, and rifampin. Perit Dial Int. 23:362-7, 2003.
Davidson PT, Le HQ. Drug treatment of tuberculosis 1992. Drugs 43:651-73, 1992. Drugs for tuberculosis. Med Lett Drugs Ther 35:99-101,1993.
Schaller A, Sun Z, Yang Y, et al. Salicylate reduces susceptibility of Mycobacterium tuberculosis to multiple antituberculosis drugs. Antimicrob Agents Chemother 46:2533-9, 2002.
Van Scoy RE, Wilkowske CJ. Antituberculous agents. Mayo Clin Proc 67:179-87, 1992.

Itraconazole (Sporanox)

Drug Class: Antifungal
Usual Dose: 200 mg (IV/PO) q24h; 200 mg capsules/solution (PO) q24h. Begin itraconazole for acute/severe infections with a loading regimen of 200 mg (IV) q12h x 2 days (4 doses), then give 200 mg (IV or PO) q24h maintenance dose. Each IV dose should be infused over 1 hour (see comments)
Pharmacokinetic Parameters:
Peak serum level: 2.8 mcg/mL
Bioavailability: 55%
Excreted unchanged: 35%
Serum half-life (normal/ESRD): 21-64/35 hrs
Plasma protein binding: 99.8%
Volume of distribution (V_d): 10 L/kg
Primary Mode of Elimination: Hepatic; metabolized predominantly by the cytochrome P450 3A4 isoenzyme system (CYP3A4)
Dosage Adjustments*

CrCl ~ 40–60 mL/min	No change
CrCl ~ 10–30 mL/min	No change
CrCl < 10 mL/min	No change
Post–HD dose	None
Post–PD dose	None
Post–CVVH dose	None
Moderate hepatic insufficiency	No change†
Severe hepatic insufficiency	No change†

† ↑ $t_{1/2}$ of itraconazole in patients with hepatic insufficiency should be considered when given with medications metabolized by P450 isoenzymes. Also see Adverse Effects for information regarding patients who develop liver dysfunction.

Drug Interactions: Itraconazole may ↑ plasma levels of: alfentanil, buspirone, busulfan, carbamazepine, cisapride, cyclosporine, digoxin, dihydropyridines, docetaxel, dofetilide, methylprednisolone, oral hypoglycemics (↑ risk of hypoglycemia), pimozide, quinidine, rifabutin, saquinavir, sirolimus, tacrolimus, trimetrexate, verapamil, vinca alkaloids, warfarin; alprazolam, diazepam, midazolam, triazolam (↑ sedative/hypnotic effects); atorvastatin, lovastatin, simvastatin (↑ risk of rhabdomyolysis); indinavir, ritonavir, saquinavir; coadministration of oral midazolam, triazolam, lovastatin, or simvastatin with itraconazole is contraindicated; coadministration of cisapride, pimozide, quinidine, or dofetilide with itraconazole is contraindicated due to the risk of ↑ QTc/life-threatening ventricular arrhythmias. Decreased itraconazole levels may occur with: antacids, carbamazepine, H_2-receptor antagonists, isoniazid, nevirapine, phenobarbital, phenytoin, proton pump inhibitors, rifabutin, rifampin; coadministration of rifampin with itraconazole is not recommended. Increased itraconazole levels may occur with: clarithromycin, erythromycin, indinavir, ritonavir

Adverse Effects: ≥ 2%: nausea, diarrhea, vomiting, headache, abdominal pain, bilirubinemia, rash, ↑ SGPT/SGOT, hypokalemia, ↑ serum creatinine. Rarely, itraconazole has been associated with serious hepatotoxicity (liver failure/death). If liver disease develops, discontinue treatment, perform liver function testing, and reevaluate risk/benefit of further treatment. Use itraconazole with caution in patients with ↑ liver enzymes, active liver disease, or previous drug-induced hepatotoxicity. Life-threatening ventricular arrhythmias/sudden death have occurred in patients using cisapride, pimozide, or quinidine concomitantly with itraconazole; coadministration of these drugs with itraconazole is contraindicated. Use itraconazole with caution in patients with ventricular dysfunction. IV itraconazole may cause transient, asymptomatic ↓ in ejection fraction for ≤ 12 hours. If CHF develops, consider discontinuation of itraconazole

Allergic Potential: Low

Safety in Pregnancy: C

Comments: *Oral itraconazole*: Requires gastric acidity for absorption. When antacids are required, administer ≥ 1 hour before or 2 hours after itraconazole capsules. Oral solution is better absorbed without food; capsules are better absorbed with food. Capsule bioavailability is food dependent: 40% fasting/90% post-prandial. For oral therapy, bioavailability of 10 mL of solution without food = 100 mg capsule with food. Administer with a cola beverage in patients with achlorhydria or taking H_2-receptor antagonists/other gastric acid suppressors. While oral solution and capsules can be interchanged for treatment of systemic disease if adequate blood levels are achieved, oral solution is preferred for oral/esophageal candidiasis where the local effect of the solution on the infection seems helpful. *IV itraconazole*: Hydroxypropyl-β-cyclodextrin stabilizer in IV formulation accumulates in renal failure. IV itraconazole should not be used in patients with CrCl < 30 mL/min; if possible, use the oral preparation. Infuse 60 mL of dilute solution (3.33 mg/mL = 200 mg itraconazole, pH ~ 4.8) IV over 60 minutes, using infusion set provided. After administration, flush the infusion set with 15-20 mL of normal saline injection. The compatibility of IV itraconazole with flush solutions other than normal saline is unknown.

Cerebrospinal Fluid Penetration: < 10%

REFERENCES:

Boogaerts M, Winston DJ, Bow EJ, et al. Intravenous and oral itraconazole versus intravenous amphotericin B deoxycholate as empirical antifungal therapy for persistent fever in neutropenic patients with cancer who are receiving broad-spectrum antibacterial therapy. A randomized controlled trial. Ann Intern Med 135:412-22, 2001.

Cleary JD, Taylor JW, Chapman SW. Itraconazole in antifungal therapy. Ann Pharmacother 26:502-9, 1992.

Go J, Cunha BA. Itraconazole. Antibiotics for Clinicians 3:61-70, 1999.

Grant SM, Clissoid SP. Itraconazole: A review of its pharmacodynamic and pharmacokinetic properties, and therapeutic use in superficial and systemic mycoses. Drugs 37:310-44, 1989.

Horousseau JL, Dekker AW, et al. Itraconazole oral solution for primary prophylaxis of fungal infections in patients with hematological malignancy and profound neutropenia: a randomized, double-blind, double-placebo, multicenter trial comparing itraconazole and amphotericin B. Antimicrob Agents Chemother 44:1887-93, 2000.

Kauffman CA, Carver PL. Antifungal agents in the 1990s: Current status and future developments. Drugs 53:539- 49, 1997.

Klein NC, Cunha BA. Antifungal therapy of the pulmonary mycoses. Chest 110:525-30, 1999.

Mosquera J, Shartt A, Moore CB, et al. In vitro interaction of terbinafine with itraconazole, fluconazole, amphotericin B and 5-flucytosine against Aspergillus spp. J Antimicrob Chemother 50:189-94, 2002.

Phillips EJ. Itraconazole was as effective as amphotericin B for fever and neutropenia in cancer and led to fewer adverse events. ACP J Club 136:58, 2002.

Rubin MA, Carroll KC, Cahill BC. Caspofungin in combination with itraconazole for the treatment of invasive aspergillosis in humans. Clin Infect Dis 34:1160-1, 2002.

Terrell CL. Antifungal agents Part II. The azoles. Mayo Clin Proc 74:78-100, 1999.

Winston DJ, Busuttil RW. Randomized controlled trial of oral itraconazole solution versus intravenous/oral fluconazole for prevention of fungal infections in liver transplant recipients. Transplantation 74:688-95, 2002.

Website: www.pdr.net

Ketoconazole (Nizoral)

Drug Class: Antifungal
Usual Dose: 200 mg (PO) q24h
Pharmacokinetic Parameters:
Peak serum level: 3.5 mcg/mL
Bioavailability: 82%
Excreted unchanged: 70%
Serum half-life (normal/ESRD): 6/20 hrs
Plasma protein binding: 99%
Volume of distribution (V_d): 2 L/kg
Primary Mode of Elimination: Hepatic
Dosage Adjustments*

CrCl ~ 40–60 mL/min	No change
CrCl < 40–40 mL/min	No change
Post–HD dose	None
Post–PD dose	None
CVVH dose	No change
Moderate hepatic insufficiency	No information
Severe hepatic insufficiency	Avoid

Drug Interactions: Astemizole, cisapride, terfenadine (may ↑ QT interval, torsades de pointes); carbamazepine, INH (↓ ketoconazole levels); cimetidine, famotidine, nizatidine, ranitidine, omeprazole, INH (↓ ketoconazole absorption); cyclosporine, digoxin, loratadine, tacrolimus (↑ interacting drug levels with possible toxicity); didanosine (↓ ketoconazole levels); midazolam, triazolam (↑ interacting drug levels, ↑ sedative effects); oral hypoglycemics (severe hypoglycemia); phenytoin, rifabutin, rifampin (↓ ketoconazole levels, ↑ interacting drug); statins (↑ statin levels; rhabdomyolysis reported); warfarin (↑ INR)
Adverse Effects: Nausea, vomiting, abdominal pain, pruritus
Allergic Potential: Low
Safety in Pregnancy: C
Comments: Dose-dependent reduction in gonadal (androgenic) function. Decreased cortisol production with doses ≥ 800 mg/day, but does not result in adrenal insufficiency. Give oral doses with citric juices
Cerebrospinal Fluid Penetration: < 10%

REFERENCES:
Allen LV. Ketoconazole oral suspension. US Pharm 18:98-9, 1993.
Como JA, Dismukes WE. Oral azole drugs as systemic antifungal therapy. N Engl J Med 330:263-72, 1993.
Lyman CA, Walsh TJ. Systemically administered antifungal agents : A review of their clinical pharmacology and therapeutic applications. Drugs 44:9-35, 1992.
Terrell CL. Antifungal agents: Part II. The azoles. Mayo Clin Proc 74:78-100, 1999.
Website: www.pdr.net

Lamivudine (Epivir) 3TC

Drug Class: Antiretroviral NRTI (nucleoside reverse transcriptase inhibitor); antiviral (HBV)
Usual Dose: 150 mg (PO) q12h or 300 mg (PO) q24h (HIV); 100 mg (PO) q24h (HBV)
Pharmacokinetic Parameters:
Peak serum level: 1.5 mcg/mL
Bioavailability: 86%
Excreted unchanged: 71%
Serum half-life (normal/ESRD): 5-7/20 hrs
Plasma protein binding: 36%
Volume of distribution (V_d): 1.3 L/kg
Primary Mode of Elimination: Renal
Dosage Adjustments*

CrCl ~ 30–49 mL/min	150 mg (PO) q24h
CrCl ~ 15–29 mL/min	100 mg (PO) q24h
CrCl ~ 5–14 mL/min	50 mg (PO) q24h
CrCl < 5 mL/min	25 mg (PO) q24h
Post–HD dose	No information
Post–PD dose	No information
CVVH dose	No information
Moderate hepatic insufficiency	No change
Severe hepatic insufficiency	No information

"Usual dose" assumes normal renal/hepatic function. * For renal insufficiency, give usual dose x 1 followed by maintenance dose per CrCl. For dialysis patients, dose the same as for CrCl < 10 mL/min and give supplemental (post-HD/PD dose) immediately after dialysis. CrCl = creatinine clearance; CVVH = continuous veno-venous hemo-filtration; HD/PD = hemodialysis/peritoneal dialysis. See pp. 293-297 for explanations, p. 1 for abbreviations

Drug Interactions: Didanosine, zalcitabine (↑ risk of pancreatitis); TMP-SMX (↑ lamivudine levels); tenofovir (↓ lamivudine levels); zidovudine (↑ zidovudine levels)

Adverse Effects: Drug fever/rash, abdominal pain/diarrhea, nausea, vomiting, anemia, leukopenia, photophobia, depression, cough, nasal complaints, headache, dizziness, peripheral neuropathy, pancreatitis, myalgias, lactic acidosis with hepatic steatosis (rare, but potentially life-threatening toxicity with NRTIs)

Allergic Potential: Low

Safety in Pregnancy: C

Comments: Potential cross resistance with didanosine. Prevents development of AZT resistance and restores AZT susceptibility. May be taken with or without food. Effective against HBV in HIV patients with 3-6 months of therapy, but HBV may reactivate after lamivudine therapy is stopped. Also a component of Combivir and Trizivir. Effective antiretroviral therapy consists of at least 3 antiretrovirals (same/different classes)

Cerebrospinal Fluid Penetration: 15%

REFERENCES:
Eron JJ, Benoit SL, Jemsek J, et al. Treatment with lamivudine, zidovudine, or both in HIV-positive patients with 200 to 500 CD4 cells per cubic millimeter. N Engl J Med 333:1662-9, 1995.
Lai Cl, Chien RN. Leung NW, et al. A one-year trial of lamivudine for chronic hepatitis B. N Engl J Med 339:61-8, 1998.
Lau GK, He ML, Fong DY, et al. Preemptive use of lamivudine reduces hepatitis B exacerbation after allogeneic hematopoietic cell transplantation. Hepatology 36:702-9, 2002.
Murphy RL, Brun S, Hicks C, et al. ABT-378/ritonavir plus stavudine and lamivudine for the treatment of antiretroviral-naive adults with HIV-1 infection: 48-week results. AIDS 15:F1-9, 2001.
Panel on Clinical Practices for Treatment of HIV Infection. Guidelines for the use of antiretroviral agents in HIV-infected adults and adolescents. Department of Health and Human Services. www.aidsinfo.nih.gov/guidelines/. November 10, 2003.
Perry CM, Faulds D. A review of its antiviral activity, pharmacokinetic properties and therapeutic efficacy in the management of HIV infection. Drugs 53:657-80, 1997.
Rivkina A, Rybalov S. Chronic hepatitis B: current and future treatment options. Pharmacotherapy 22:721-37, 2002.
Staszewski S, Morales-Ramirez J, Trashima KT, et al. Efavirenz plus zidovudine and lamivudine, efavirenz plus indinavir, and indinavir plus zidovudine and lamivudine in the treatment of HIV-1 infection in adults. N Engl J Med 341:1865-1873, 1999.
Website: www.TreatHIV.com

Lamivudine + zidovudine (Combivir)

Drug Class: Antiretroviral NRTIs combination
Usual Dose: Combivir tablet = 150 mg lamivudine + 300 mg zidovudine. Usual dose = 1 tablet (PO) q12h

Pharmacokinetic Parameters:
Peak serum level: 2.6/1.2 mcg/mL
Bioavailability: 82/60%
Excreted unchanged: 86/64%
Serum half-life (normal/ESRD): [6/1.1]/[20/2.2] hrs
Plasma protein binding: <36/<38%
Volume of distribution (V_d): 1.3/1.6 L/kg

Primary Mode of Elimination: Renal
Dosage Adjustments*

CrCl ~ 50–60 mL/min	No change
CrCl ~ 10–50 mL/min	Avoid
CrCl < 10 mL/min	Avoid
Post–HD dose	Avoid
Post–PD dose	Avoid
CVVH dose	Avoid
Moderate hepatic insufficiency	Avoid
Severe hepatic insufficiency	Avoid

Drug Interactions: Amprenavir, atovaquone (↑ zidovudine levels); stavudine (antagonist to stavudine; avoid combination); ganciclovir, doxorubicin (neutropenia); tenofovir (↓ lamivudine levels); TMP-SMX (↑ lamivudine and zidovudine levels)

Adverse Effects: Most common (>5%):

"Usual dose" assumes normal renal/hepatic function. * For renal insufficiency, give usual dose x 1 followed by maintenance dose per CrCl. For dialysis patients, dose the same as for CrCl < 10 mL/min and give supplemental (post-HD/PD dose) immediately after dialysis. CrCl = creatinine clearance; CVVH = continuous veno-venous hemofiltration; HD/PD = hemodialysis/peritoneal dialysis. See pp. 293-297 for explanations, p. 1 for abbreviations

nausea, vomiting, diarrhea, anorexia, insomnia, fever/chills, headache, malaise/fatigue. Others (less common): peripheral neuropathy, myopathy, steatosis, pancreatitis. Lab abnormalities: mild hyperglycemia, anemia, LFT elevations, hypertriglyceridemia, leukopenia

Allergic Potential: Low

Safety in Pregnancy: C

Comments: Avoid if history of pancreatitis.. Effective antiretroviral therapy consists of at least 3 antiretrovirals (same/different classes)

Cerebrospinal Fluid Penetration: Lamivudine = 12%; zidovudine = 60%

REFERENCES:
Drugs for AIDS and associated infections. Med Lett Drug Ther 35:79-86, 1993.

Hirsch MS, D'Aquila RT. Therapy for human immunodeficiency virus infection. N Engl J Med 328:1685-95, 1993.

McLeod GX, Hammer SM. Zidovudine: Five years later. Ann Intern Med 117:487-510, 1992.

Panel on Clinical Practices for Treatment of HIV Infection. Guidelines for the use of antiretroviral agents in HIV-infected adults and adolescents. Department of Health and Human Services. www.aidsinfo.nih.gov/guidelines/. November 10, 2003.

Staszewski S, Morales-Ramirez J, Trashima KT, et al. Efavirenz plus zidovudine and lamivudine, efavirenz plus indinavir, and indinavir plus zidovudine and lamivudine in the treatment of HIV-1 infection in adults. N Engl J Med 341:1865-1873, 1999.

Website: www.TreatHIV.com

Levofloxacin (Levaquin)

Drug Class: Fluoroquinolone

Usual Dose: 250-750 mg (IV/PO) q24h

Pharmacokinetic Parameters:
Peak serum level: 5-8 mcg/mL
Bioavailability: 99%
Excreted unchanged: 87%
Serum half-life (normal/ESRD): 7 hrs/prolonged
Plasma protein binding: 30%
Volume of distribution (V_d): 1.3 L/kg
Primary Mode of Elimination: Renal

Dosage Adjustments* (based on 500 mg q24h)

CrCl ~ 50–80 mL/min	No change
CrCl ~ 20–49 mL/min	250 mg (IV/PO) q24h
CrCl ~ 10-19 mL/min	250 mg (IV/PO) q48h
HD/CAPD	250 mg (PO) q48h
Post-HD dose	250 mg (IV/PO)
Post-PD dose	250 mg (IV/PO)
CVVH dose	No information
Moderate hepatic insufficiency	No change
Severe hepatic insufficiency	No change

Drug Interactions: Al^{++}, Fe^{++}, Mg^{++}, Zn^{++} antacids (↓ absorption of levofloxacin if taken together); NSAIDs (CNS stimulation); probenecid (↑ levofloxacin levels); warfarin (↑ INR)

Adverse Effects: Mild nausea, diarrhea, rash

Allergic Potential: Low

Safety in Pregnancy: C

Comments: Low incidence of GI side effects. Take 2 hours before or after aluminum/magnesium-containing antacids. Does not increase digoxin concentrations. Use 750 mg (IV/PO) for 5-day CAP regimen, nosocomial pneumonia, or complicated skin/soft tissue infection. May potentially lower seizure threshold or prolong the QTc interval, particularly in patients with predisposing conditions

Cerebrospinal Fluid Penetration: 16%

REFERENCES:
Croom KF, Goa KL. Levofloxacin: a review of its use in the treatment of bacterial infections in the United States. Drugs 63:2769-802, 2003.

Cunha BA. Community-acquired pneumonia: Diagnostic and therapeutic considerations. Med Clin North Am 85:43-77. 2001.

Cunha BA. Quinolones: Clinical aspects. Antibiotics for Clinicians 2:129-35, 1998.

Drago L, DeVecchi E, Mombelli L, et al. Activity of levofloxacin and ciprofloxacin against urinary pathogens. J. Antimicrobial Chemo 48: 37-45, 2001.

Dunbar LM, Wunderink RG, Habib MP, et al. High-dose, short-course levofloxacin for community-acquired pneumonia: a new treatment paradigm. Clin Infect Dis

---

"Usual dose" assumes normal renal/hepatic function. * For renal insufficiency, give usual dose x 1 followed by maintenance dose per CrCl. For dialysis patients, dose the same as for CrCl < 10 mL/min and give supplemental (post-HD/PD dose) immediately after dialysis. CrCl = creatinine clearance; CVVH = continuous veno-venous hemofiltration; HD/PD = hemodialysis/peritoneal dialysis. See pp. 293-297 for explanations, p. 1 for abbreviations

37:752-60, 2003.

Furlanut M, Brollo L, Lugatti E, et al. Pharmacokinetic aspects of levofloxacin 500 mg once daily during sequential intravenous/oral therapy in patients with lower respiratory tract infections. J Antimicrob Chemother 51:101-6, 2003.

Garrison MW. Comparative antimicrobial activity of levofloxacin and ciprofloxacin against Streptococcus pneumoniae. J Antimicrob Chemother 52:503-6, 2003.

Graham Dr, Taalan DA, Nichols RL. Once-daily, high-dose levofloxacin versus ticarcillin-clavulanate alone or followed by amoxicillin-clavulanate for complicated skin and skin-structure infections: a randomized, open label trial. Clin Infect Dis 35:381-9, 2002.

Marchetti F, Viale P. Current and future perspectives for levofloxacin in severe Pseudomonas aeruginosa infections. J Chemother 15:315-22, 2003.

Nicolau DP, Ambrose PG. Pharmacodynamic profiling of levofloxacin and gatifloxacin using Monte Carlo simulation for community-acquired isolates of Streptococcus pneumoniae. Am J Med 111(Suppl 9A):13S-18S, 2001.

Nightingale CH, Grant EM, Quintiliani R. Pharmacodynamics and pharmacokinetics of levofloxacin. Chemotherapy 46:6-14, 2000.

Pea F, Di Qual E, Cusenza A, et al. Pharmacokinetics and pharmacodynamics of intravenous levofloxacin in patients with early-onset ventilator-associated pneumonia. Clin Pharmacokinet 42:589-98, 2003.

Website: www.levaquin.com

Linezolid (Zyvox)

Drug Class: Oxazolidinone
Usual Dose: 600 mg (IV/PO) q12h
Pharmacokinetic Parameters:
Peak serum level: 15-21 mcg/mL
Bioavailability: 100% (IV and PO)
Excreted unchanged: 30%
Serum half-life (normal/ESRD): 6.4/7.1 hrs
Plasma protein binding: 31%
Volume of distribution (V_d): 0.64 L/kg
Primary Mode of Elimination:
Hepatic/metabolized
Dosage Adjustments*

CrCl ~ 40–60 mL/min	No change
CrCl ~ 10–40 mL/min	No change
CrCl < 10 mL/min	No change

Post–HD dose	200 mg (IV/PO)
Post–PD dose	None
CVVH dose	No change
Moderate hepatic insufficiency	No change
Severe hepatic insufficiency	No information

Drug Interactions: Pseudoephedrine, tyramine-containing foods (↑ risk of hypertensive crisis); serotonergic agents, e.g., SSRI's, tricyclic antidepressants (↑ risk of serotonin syndrome)
Adverse Effects: Mild, readily reversible thrombocytopenia, anemia, or leukopenia may occur after ≥ 2 weeks of therapy
Allergic Potential: Low
Safety in Pregnancy: C
Comments: May be taken with or without food. Ideal for IV-to-PO switch programs. Unlike vancomycin, linezolid does not increase VRE prevalence and is available orally for MRSA, MRSE, and E. faecalis infections. Unlike quinupristin/dalfopristin, linezolid is active against E. faecalis and is available orally for MRSA, MRSE, and E. faecium (VRE) infections. Meningeal dose = usual dose
Cerebrospinal Fluid Penetration: 70%

REFERENCES:

Andes D, van Ogtrop ML, Peng J, et al. In vivo pharmacodynamics of a new oxazolidinone (linezolid). Antimicrob Agents Chemother 46:3484-3489, 2002.

Cercenado E, Garcia-Garrote F, Bouza E. In vitro activity of linezolid against multiple resistant gram-positive clinical isolates. J Antimicrob Chemother 47:77-81, 2001.

Conte JE Jr, Golden JA, Dipps J, et al. Intrapulmonary pharmacokinetics of linezolid. Antimicrob Agents Chemother 46:1475-80, 2000.

Go J, Cunha BA. Linezolid: A review. Antibiotics for Clinicians 4:82-88, 2000.

Gunderson BW, Ibrahim KH, Peloquin CA, et al. Comparison of linezolid activities under aerobic and anaerobic conditions against methicillin-resistant Staphylococcus aureus and vancomycin-resistant Enterococcus faecium. Antimicrob Agents Chemother 47:398-9, 2003.

Hamel JC, Stapert D, Moerman JK, et al. Linezolid,

"Usual dose" assumes normal renal/hepatic function. * For renal insufficiency, give usual dose x 1 followed by maintenance dose per CrCl. For dialysis patients, dose the same as for CrCl < 10 mL/min and give supplemental (post-HD/PD dose) immediately after dialysis. CrCl = creatinine clearance; CVVH = continuous veno-venous hemo-filtration; HD/PD = hemodialysis/peritoneal dialysis. See pp. 293-297 for explanations, p. 1 for abbreviations

critical characteristics. Infection 28:60-4, 2000.

Hau T. Efficacy and safety of linezolid in the treatment of skin and soft tissue infections. Eur J Clin Microbiol Infect Dis 21:491-8, 2002.

Johnson JR. Linezolid versus vancomycin for methicillin-resistant Staphylococcus aureus infections. Clin Infect Dis. 36:236-7, 2003.

Kutscha-Lissberg F, Hebler U, Muhr G, et al. Linezolid penetration into bone and joint tissues infected with methicillin-resistant staphylococci. Antimicrob Agents Chemother. 47:3964-6, 2003.

Li JZ, Willke RJ, Rittenhouse BE, et al. Approaches to analysis of length of hospital stay related to antibiotic therapy in a randomized clinical trial: linezolid versus vancomycin for treatment of known or suspected methicillin-resistant Staphylococcus species infections. Pharmacotherapy 22(2 Pt 2):45S-54S, 2002.

Moylett EH, Pacheco SE, Brown-Elliott BA, et al. Clinical experience with linezolid for the treatment of nocardia infection.Clin Infect Dis. 36:313-8, 2003.

Paterson DL, Pasculle AW, McCurry K. Linezolid: the first oxazolidinone antimicrobial. Ann Intern Med. 139:863-4, 2003.

Plouffe JF. Emerging therapies for serious gram-positive bacterial infections: a focus on linezolid. Clin Infect Dis 4:144-9, 2000.

Ravindran V, John J, Kaye GC, et al. Successful use of oral linezolid as a single active agent in endocarditis unresponsive to conventional antibiotic therapy. J Infect. 47:164-6, 2003.

Saiman L, Goldfarb J, Kaplan SA, et al. Safety and tolerability of linezolid in children. Pediatr Infect Dis J. 22:S193-200, 2003.

San Pedro GS, Cammarata SK, Oliphant TH, Todisco T. Linezolid versus ceftriaxone/cefpodoxime in patients hospitalized for the treatment of Streptococcus pneumoniae pneumonia. Scand J Infect Dis 34:720-8, 2002.

Siegel RE. Linezolid to decrease length of stay in the hospital for patients with methicillin-resistant Staphylococcus aureus infection. Clin Infect Dis. 36:124-5, 2003.

Stalker DJ, Jungbluth GL. Clinical pharmacokinetics of linezolid, a novel oxazolidinone antibacterial. Clin Pharmacokinet. 42:1129-40, 2003.

Stevens DL, Herr D, Lampiris H, et al. Linezolid versus vancomycin for the treatment of methicillin-resistant Staphylococcus aureus infections. Clin Infect Dis 34:1481-90, 2002.

Villani P, Pegazzi MB, Marubbi F, et al. Cerebrospinal fluid linezolid concentrations in postneurosurgical central nervous system infections. Antimicrob Agents Chemother 46:936-7, 2002.

Wunderink RG, Rello J, Cammarata SK, et al. Linezolid vs vancomycin: analysis of two double-blind studies of patients with methicillin-resistant Staphylococcus aureus nosocomial pneumonia. Chest. 124:1789-97, 2003.

Website: www.zyvox.com

Lopinavir + ritonavir (Kaletra)

Drug Class: Antiretroviral protease inhibitor combination

Usual Dose: Kaletra capsule = 133.3 mg lopinavir + 33.3 mg ritonavir. Oral solution (per ml) = 80 mg lopinavir + 20 mg ritonavir. Usual dose = 3 capsules or 5 mL (PO) q12h with food

Pharmacokinetic Parameters:

Peak serum level: $9.6/\leq 1$ mcg/mL
Bioavailability: No data
Excreted unchanged: 3%
Serum half-life (normal/ESRD): 5-6/5-6 hrs
Plasma protein binding: 99%
Volume of distribution (V_d): No data/ 0.44 L/kg

Primary Mode of Elimination: Hepatic

Dosage Adjustments*

CrCl ~ 40–60 mL/min	No change
CrCl ~ 10–40 mL/min	No change
CrCl < 10 mL/min	No change
Post–HD dose	None
Post–PD dose	None
CVVH dose	No change
Moderate hepatic insufficiency	No change
Severe hepatic insufficiency	3 capsules (PO) q24h or 5 mL (PO) q24h

Antiretroviral Dosage Adjustments:

Amprenavir	Amprenavir 600-750 mg q12h
Delavirdine	No information

"Usual dose" assumes normal renal/hepatic function. * For renal insufficiency, give usual dose x 1 followed by maintenance dose per CrCl. For dialysis patients, dose the same as for CrCl < 10 mL/min and give supplemental (post-HD/PD dose) immediately after dialysis. CrCl = creatinine clearance; CVVH = continuous veno-venous hemo-filtration; HD/PD = hemodialysis/peritoneal dialysis. See pp. 293-297 for explanations, p. 1 for abbreviations

Efavirenz	Consider lopinavir/ritonavir 533/133 mg q12h in PI–experienced patients
Indinavir	Indinavir 600 mg q12h
Nelfinavir	No information
Nevirapine	Consider lopinavir/ritonavir 533/133 mg q12h in PI–experienced patients
Rifabutin	Max. dose of rifabutin 150 mg qod or 3 times per week
Saquinavir	Saquinavir 800 mg q12h

Drug Interactions: Antiretrovirals, rifabutin, (see dose adjustment grid, above); astemizole, terfenadine, benzodiazepines, cisapride, ergotamine, flecainide, pimozide, propafenone, rifampin, statins, St. John's wort (avoid if possible); tenofovir (↓ lopinavir levels, ↑ tenofovir levels). ↓ effectiveness of oral contraceptives. Insufficient data on other drug interactions listed for ritonavir alone
Adverse Effects: Diarrhea (very common), headache, nausea, vomiting, asthenia, ↑ SGOT/SGPT, abdominal pain, pancreatitis, paresthesias, hyperglycemia (including worsening diabetes, new-onset diabetes, DKA), ↑ cholesterol/triglycerides (evaluate risk for coronary disease, pancreatitis), ↑ CPK, ↑ uric acid, fat redistribution, possible increased bleeding in hemophilia. Oral solution contains 42.4% alcohol
Allergic Potential: Low
Safety in Pregnancy: C
Comments: Lopinavir serum concentrations with moderately fatty meals are increased 43% (capsules)/54% (oral solution). Refrigerated capsules stable until date on label; if stored at room temperature, capsules stable x 2 months. Ritonavir 100 mg is not an effective anti-HIV dose. Although Kaletra is a double drug combination, it should be regarded as equivalent to lopinavir monotherapy, requiring 2 additional

antiretroviral agents for effective antiretroviral therapy

REFERENCES:
Benson CA, Deeks SG, Brun SC, et al. Safety and antiviral activity at 48 weeks of lopinavir/ritonavir plus nevirapine and 2 nucleoside reverse-transcriptase inhibitors in human immunodeficiency virus type 1-infected protease inhibitor-experienced patients. J Infect Dis 185:599-607, 2002.
Fischl MA. Antiretroviral therapy in 1999 for antiretroviral-naive individuals with HIV infection. AIDS 13:49-59, 1999.
Panel on Clinical Practices for Treatment of HIV Infection. Guidelines for the use of antiretroviral agents in HIV-infected adults and adolescents. Department of Health and Human Services. www.aidsinfo.nih.gov/guidelines/. November 10, 2003.
Walmsley S, Bernstein B, King M, et al. Lopinavir-ritonavir versus nelfinavir for the initial treatment of HIV infection. N Engl J Med 346:2039-46, 2002.
Website: www.kaletra.com

Loracarbef (Lorabid)

Drug Class: 2nd generation oral cephalosporin
Usual Dose: 400 mg (PO) q12h
Pharmacokinetic Parameters:
Peak serum level: 14 mcg/mL
Bioavailability: 90%
Excreted unchanged: 90%
Serum half-life (normal/ESRD): 1.2/32 hrs
Plasma protein binding: 25%
Volume of distribution (V_d): 0.35 L/kg
Primary Mode of Elimination: Renal
Dosage Adjustments*

CrCl ~ 50–60 mL/min	400 mg (PO) q12h
CrCl ~ 10–49 mL/min	200 mg (PO) q12h
CrCl < 10 mL/min	200 mg (PO) q48h
Post–HD dose	400 mg (PO)
Post–PD dose	400 mg (PO)
CVVH dose	200 mg (PO) q12h
Moderate hepatic insufficiency	No change

"Usual dose" assumes normal renal/hepatic function. * For renal insufficiency, give usual dose x 1 followed by maintenance dose per CrCl. For dialysis patients, dose the same as for CrCl < 10 mL/min and give supplemental (post-HD/PD dose) immediately after dialysis. CrCl = creatinine clearance; CVVH = continuous veno-venous hemo-filtration; HD/PD = hemodialysis/peritoneal dialysis. See pp. 293-297 for explanations, p. 1 for abbreviations

Severe hepatic insufficiency	No change

Drug Interactions: None
Adverse Effects: Drug fever/rash, diarrhea
Allergic Potential: Low
Safety in Pregnancy: B
Comments: Take 1 hour before or 2 hours after meals
Cerebrospinal Fluid Penetration: < 10%

REFERENCES:
Bandak SI, Turnak MR, Allen BS, et al. Assessment of the susceptibility of Streptococcus pneumoniae to cefaclor and loracarbef in 13 cases. J Chemother 12:299-305, 2000.
Gooch WM 3rd, Adelglass J, Kelsey DK, et al. Loracarbef versus clarithromycin in children with acute otitis media with effusion. Clin her 21:711-22, 1999.
Paster RZ, McAdoo MA, Keyserling CH. A comparison of a five-day regimen of cefdinir with a seven-day regimen of loracarbef for the treatment of acute exacerbations of chronic bronchitis. Int J Clin Pract 64:293-9, 2000.
Vogel F, Ochs HR, Wettich K, et al. Effect of step-down therapy of ceftriazone plus loracarbef versus parenteral therapy of ceftriaxone on the intestinal microflora in patients with community-acquired pneumonia. Clin Microbiol Infect 7:376-9, 2001.
Website: www.pdr.net

Meropenem (Merrem)

Drug Class: Carbapenem
Usual Dose: 1 gm (IV) q8h
Pharmacokinetic Parameters:
Peak serum level: 49 mcg/mL
Bioavailability: Not applicable
Excreted unchanged: 70%
Serum half-life (normal/ESRD): 1/7 hrs
Plasma protein binding: 2%
Volume of distribution (V_d): 0.35 L/kg
Primary Mode of Elimination: Renal
Dosage Adjustments*

CrCl ~ 26–50 mL/min	1 gm (IV) q12h
CrCl ~ 10–25 mL/min	500 mg (IV) q12h
CrCl < 10 mL/min	500 mg (IV) q24h
Post–HD dose	No information
Post–PD dose	No information
CVVH dose	500 mg (IV) q12h
Moderate hepatic insufficiency	No change
Severe hepatic insufficiency	No change

Drug Interactions: Probenecid (↑ meropenem half-life by 40%)
Adverse Effects: Rarely, mild infusion site inflammation
Allergic Potential: Low
Safety in Pregnancy: B
Comments: No adverse effects with 2 gm (IV) q8h regimen. No cross allergenicity with penicillins/β-lactams; safe to use in penicillin allergic patients. Meropenem (1 gm) may be given by rapid IV infusion over 15-30 minutes (C_{max} = 49 mcg/mL) or as a bolus IV injection over 3-5 minutes (C_{max} = 112 mcg/mL). Inhibits endotoxin release from gram-negative bacilli. Na^+ content = 3.92 mEq/g.
Meningeal dose = 2 gm (IV) q8h
Cerebrospinal Fluid Penetration:
Non-inflamed meninges = 10%
Inflamed meninges = 15%

REFERENCES:
Cunha BA: The safety of meropenem in elderly and renally impaired patients. Intern J Antimcrob Ther 10:109-117, 1998.
Cunha BA. Cross allergenicity of penicillin with carbapenems and monobactams. J Crit Illness 13:344,1998.
Cunha BA. Pseudomonas aeruginosa: Resistance and therapy. Semin Respir Infect 17:231-9, 2002 .
Cunha BA. The use of meropenem in critical care. Antibiotics for Clinicians 4:59-66, 2000.
Erdem I, Kucukercan M, Ceran N. In vitro activity of combination therapy with cefepime, piperacillin-tazobactam, or meropenem with ciprofloxacin against multidrug-resistant Pseudomonas aeruginosa strains. Chemotherapy 2003;49:294-7.
Fish DN, Singletary TJ. Meropenem: A new carba-penem antibiotic. Pharmacotherapy 17:644-69, 1997.
Garcia-Rodriguez JA, Jones RN. Antimicrobial resistance in gram-negative isolates from European intensive care units: data from the Meropenem Yearly Susceptibility Test Information Collection (MYSTIC) programme. J

Chemother 2002;14:25-32.

Hellinger WC, Brewer NS. Carbapenems and monobactams: Imipenem, meropenem, and aztreonam. Mayo Clin Proc 74:420-34, 1999.

Kitzes-Cohen R, Farin D, Piva G, et al. Pharmacokinetics and pharmacodynamics of meropenem in critically ill patients. Int J Antimicrob Agents 19:105-10, 2002.

Perez-Simon JA, Garcia-Escobar I, Martinez J, et al. Antibiotic prophylaxis with meropenem after allogeneic stem cell transplantation. Bone Marrow Transplant 2004;33:183-7.

Rhomberg PR, Jones RN; MYSTIC Program (USA) Study Group. Antimicrobial spectrum of activity for meropenem and nine broad spectrum antimicrobials: report from the MYSTIC Program (2002) in North America. Diagn Microbiol Infect Dis 2003;47:365-72.

Website: www.MerremIV.com

Methenamine hippurate (Hiprex, Urex)
Methenamine mandelate (Mandelamine)

Drug Class: Urinary antiseptic
Usual Dose: 1 gm (PO) q6h (hippurate); 1 gm (PO) q6h (mandelate)
Pharmacokinetic Parameters:
Peak serum level: Not applicable
Bioavailability: 90%
Excreted unchanged: 90%
Serum half-life (normal/ESRD): 4 hrs/no data
Plasma protein binding: Not applicable
Volume of distribution (V_d): Not applicable
Primary Mode of Elimination: Renal
Dosage Adjustments*

CrCl ~ 40–60 mL/min	Avoid
CrCl ~ 10–40 mL/min	Avoid
CrCl < 10 mL/min	Avoid
Post–HD dose	Avoid
Post–PD dose	Avoid
CVVH dose	Avoid
Moderate hepatic insufficiency	No change
Severe hepatic insufficiency	Avoid

Drug Interactions: Acetazolamide, sodium bicarbonate, thiazide diuretics (↓ antibacterial effect due to ↑ urinary pH ≥ 5.5)
Adverse Effects: GI upset
Allergic Potential: Low
Safety in Pregnancy: C
Comments: Take with food to decrease GI upset. Effectiveness depends on maintaining an acid urine (pH ≤ 5.5) with acidifying agents (e.g., ascorbic acid). Useful only for catheter–associated bacteriuria, not UTIs. Forms formaldehyde in acid urine; resistance does not develop
REFERENCES:

Cunha BA, Comer JB. Pharmacokinetic considerations in the treatment of urinary tract infections. Conn Med 43:347-53, 1979.

Klinge D, Mannisto P, Mantyla R, et al. Pharmacokinetics of methenamine in healthy volunteers. J Antimicrob Chemother 9:209-16, 1982.

Musher DM, Griggith DP. Generation of formaldehyde from methenamine: Effect of pH and concentration, and antibacterial effect. Antimicobr Agents Chemother 6:708-11, 1974.

Musher DM, Griffith DP, Templeton GB. Further observations of the potentiation of the antibacterial effect of methenamine by acetohydroxamic acid. J Infect Dis 133:564-67, 1976.

Schiotz HA, Guttu K. Value of urinary prophylaxis with methenamine in gynecologic surgery. Acta Obstet Gynecol Scand 81:743-6, 2002.

Metronidazole (Flagyl)

Drug Class: Nitroimidazole antiparasitic/antibiotic
Usual Dose: 1 gm (IV) q24h; 500 mg (PO) q12h
Pharmacokinetic Parameters:
Peak serum level: 26 (IV)/12 (PO) mcg/mL
Bioavailability: 100%
Excreted unchanged: 20%
Serum half-life (normal/ESRD): 8/14 hrs
Plasma protein binding: 20%
Volume of distribution (V_d): 0.25-0.85 L/kg
Primary Mode of Elimination: Hepatic

"Usual dose" assumes normal renal/hepatic function. * For renal insufficiency, give usual dose x 1 followed by maintenance dose per CrCl. For dialysis patients, dose the same as for CrCl < 10 mL/min and give supplemental (post-HD/PD dose) immediately after dialysis. CrCl = creatinine clearance; CVVH = continuous veno-venous hemofiltration; HD/PD = hemodialysis/peritoneal dialysis. See pp. 293-297 for explanations, p. 1 for abbreviations

Dosage Adjustments*

CrCl ~ 40–60 mL/min	No change
CrCl ~ 10–40 mL/min	No change
CrCl < 10 mL/min	500 mg (IV) q24h 250 mg (PO) q12h
Post–HD dose	1 gm (IV) 500 mg (PO)
Post–PD dose	500 mg (IV) 250 mg (PO)
CVVH dose	No change
Moderate hepatic insufficiency	No change
Severe hepatic insufficiency	500 mg (IV/PO) q24h

Drug Interactions: Alcohol (disulfiram-like reaction); disulfiram (acute toxic psychosis); warfarin (↑ INR); phenobarbital, phenytoin (↑ metronidazole metabolism)
Adverse Effects: Disulfiram reaction (tachycardia/flushing) with alcohol, nausea, vomiting, GI upset, metallic taste
Allergic Potential: Low
Safety in Pregnancy: B (avoid in 1st trimester)
Comments: Q12h dosing is preferred to q6h dosing because of long half-life. May discolor urine brown. For C. difficile diarrhea, use 250 mg (PO) q6h. For C. difficile colitis, use 500 mg (IV or PO) q12h or 1 gm (IV) q24h.
Na⁺ content = 28 mEq/g.
Meningeal dose = usual dose
Cerebrospinal Fluid Penetration:
Non-inflamed meninges = 30%
Inflamed meninges = 100%

REFERENCES:

Bartlett JG. Clinical practice. Antibiotic-associated diarrhea. N Engl J Med 346:334-9, 2002.
Falagas ME, Gorbach SL. Clindamycin and metronidazole. Med Clin North Am 79:845-67, 1995.
Freeman CD, Klutman NE. Metronidazole: A therapeutic review and update. Drugs 54:679-708, 1997.
Freeman CD, Nightingale CH, Nicolau DP, et al. Serum bactericidal activity of ceftriaxone plus metronidazole against common intra-abdominal pathogens. Am J
Hosp Pharm 51:1782-7, 1994.
Ishikawa T, Okamura S, Oshimoto H, et al. Metronidazole plus ciprofloxacin therapy for active Crohn's disease. Intern Med. 42:318-21, 2003.
Kasten MJ. Clindamycin, metronidazole, and chloramphenicol. Mayo Clin Proc 74:825-33, 1999.
Vasa CV, Glatt AE. Effectiveness and appropriateness of empiric metronidazole for Clostridium difficile diarrhea. Am J Gastroenterol. 98:354-8, 2003.
Website: www.pdr.net

Mezlocillin (Mezlin)

Drug Class: Antipseudomonal penicillin
Usual Dose: 3 gm (IV) q6h
Pharmacokinetic Parameters:
Peak serum level: 300 mcg/mL
Bioavailability: Not applicable
Excreted unchanged: 65%
Serum half-life (normal/ESRD): 1.1/4 hrs
Plasma protein binding: 30%
Volume of distribution (V_d): 0.18 L/kg
Primary Mode of Elimination: Renal
**Dosage Adjustments*

CrCl ~ 30–60 mL/min	No change
CrCl ~ 10–30 mL/min	3 gm (IV) q8h
CrCl < 10 mL/min	2 gm (IV) q8h
Post–HD dose	3 gm (IV)
Post–PD dose	None
CVVH dose	3 gm (IV) q8h
Moderate hepatic insufficiency	No change
Severe hepatic insufficiency	3 gm (IV) q12h

Drug Interactions: Aminoglycosides (inactivation of mezlocillin in renal failure); warfarin (↑ INR); oral contraceptives (↓ oral contraceptive effect); cefoxitin (↓ mezlocillin effect)
Adverse Effects: Drug fever/rash, E. multiforme/Stevens–Johnson syndrome, anaphylactic reactions (hypotension, laryngospasm, bronchospasm), hives; serum

---

"Usual dose" assumes normal renal/hepatic function. * For renal insufficiency, give usual dose x 1 followed by maintenance dose per CrCl. For dialysis patients, dose the same as for CrCl < 10 mL/min and give supplemental (post-HD/PD dose) immediately after dialysis. CrCl = creatinine clearance; CVVH = continuous veno-venous hemofiltration; HD/PD = hemodialysis/peritoneal dialysis. See pp. 293-297 for explanations, p. 1 for abbreviations

sickness. Dose-dependent inhibition of platelet aggregation is minimal/absent (usual dose is less than carbenicillin)

Allergic Potential: Low

Safety in Pregnancy: B

Comments: Dose-dependent half-life ($t_{1/2}$). Na^+ content = 1.8 mEq/g

Cerebrospinal Fluid Penetration: < 10%

REFERENCES:

Donowitz GR, Mandell GL. Beta-lactam antibiotics. N Engl J Med 318:419-26 and 318:490-500, 1993.

Wright AJ, Wirkowske CJ. The penicillins. Mayo Clin Proc 66:1047-63, 1991.

Wright AJ. The penicillins. Mayo Clin Proc 74:290-307, 1999.

Website: www.pdr.net.

Minocycline (Minocin)

Drug Class: 2nd generation tetracycline

Usual Dose: 100 mg (IV/PO) q12h or 200 mg (IV/PO) q24h

Pharmacokinetic Parameters:

Peak serum level: 4 mcg/mL
Bioavailability: 95%
Excreted unchanged: 10%
Serum half-life (normal/ESRD): 15/18-69 hrs
Plasma protein binding: 75%
Volume of distribution (V_d): 1.5 L/kg

Primary Mode of Elimination: Hepatic

Dosage Adjustments*

CrCl ~ 40–60 mL/min	No change
CrCl ~ 10–40 mL/min	No change
CrCl < 10 mL/min	No change
Post–HD dose	None
Post–PD dose	None
CVVH dose	No change
Moderate hepatic insufficiency	No change
Severe hepatic insufficiency	100 mg (IV/PO) q24h

Drug Interactions: Antacids, Al^{++}, Ca^{++}, Fe^{++}, Mg^{++}, Zn^{++}, multivitamins, sucralfate (↓ minocycline absorption); isotretinoin (pseudotumor cerebri); warfarin (↑ INR)

Adverse Effects: Nausea, GI upset if not taken with food, hyperpigmentation of skin with prolonged use, vestibular toxicity (dizziness), photosensitivity rare

Allergic Potential: Low

Safety in Pregnancy: X

Comments: Infuse slowly over 1 hour. Dizziness due to high inner ear levels.
Meningeal dose = usual dose

Cerebrospinal Fluid Penetration:
Non-inflamed meninges = 50%
Inflamed meninges = 50%

Bile Penetration: 1000%

REFERENCES:

Cunha BA: Minocycline vs. doxycycline for the antimicrobial therapy of lyme neuroborreliosis. Clin Infect Dis 30:237-238, 2000.

Jonas M, Cunha BA. Minocycline. Therapeutic Drug Monitoring 4:137-45, 1982.

Klein NC, Cunha BA. New uses for older antibiotics. Med Clin North Am 85:125-32, 2001.

Lewis KE, Ebden P, Wooster SL, et al. Multi-system Infection with Nocardia farcinica-therapy with linezolid and minocycline. J Infect. 46:199-202, 2003.

Safdar A, Bryan CS, Stinson S, et al. Prosthetic valve endocarditis due to vancomycin-resistant Enterococcus faecium: treatment with chloramphenicol plus minocycline. Clin Infect Dis 34:E61-3, 2002.

Smilack JD, Wilson WE, Cocerill FR 3rd. Tetracycline, chloramphenicol, erythromycin, clindamycin, and metronidazole. Mayo Clin Proc 66:1270-80, 1991.

Website: www.pdr.net

Moxifloxacin (Avelox)

Drug Class: Fluoroquinolone

Usual Dose: 400 mg (IV/PO) q24h

Pharmacokinetic Parameters:

Peak serum level: 4.4 (IV)/4.5 (PO) mcg/mL
Bioavailability: 90%
Excreted unchanged: 45% (20% urine; 25% feces)
Serum half-life (normal/ESRD): 12/12 hrs
Plasma protein binding: 50%
Volume of distribution (V_d): 2.2 L/kg

Primary Mode of Elimination: Hepatic

"Usual dose" assumes normal renal/hepatic function. * For renal insufficiency, give usual dose x 1 followed by maintenance dose per CrCl. For dialysis patients, dose the same as for CrCl < 10 mL/min and give supplemental (post-HD/PD dose) immediately after dialysis. CrCl = creatinine clearance; CVVH = continuous veno-venous hemofiltration; HD/PD = hemodialysis/peritoneal dialysis. See pp. 293-297 for explanations, p. 1 for abbreviations

Dosage Adjustments*

CrCl ~ 40–60 mL/min	No change
CrCl ~ 10–40 mL/min	No change
CrCl < 10 mL/min	No change
Post–HD dose	None
Post–PD dose	None
CVVH dose	No change
Moderate hepatic insufficiency	No change
Severe hepatic insufficiency	No information

Drug Interactions: Al^{++}, Fe^{++}, Mg^{++}, Zn^{++} antacids, citrate/citric acid, dairy products (↓ absorption of fluoroquinolones only if taken together); amiodarone, procainamide, sotalol (may ↑ QTc interval, torsade de pointes)
Adverse Effects: May ↑ QT_c interval > 3 msec. (as with other quinolones); avoid taking with other medications that prolong the QT_c interval, and in patients with cardiac arrhythmias/heart block
Allergic Potential: Low
Safety in Pregnancy: C
Comments: Only quinolone with anti-B. fragilis activity. Metabolized to microbiologically-inactive glucuronide (M1)/sulfate (M2) conjugates. Take 4 hours before or 8 hours after calcium or magnesium containing antacids or didanosine. No interactions with oral hypoglycemics. C8-methoxy group increases activity and decreases resistance potential
Cerebrospinal Fluid Penetration: < 10%

REFERENCES:
Behra-Miellet J, Dubreuil L, Jumas-Bilak E. Antianaerobic activity of moxifloxacin compared with that of ofloxacin, ciprofloxacin, clindamycin, metronidazole and beta-lactams. Int J Antimicrob Agents 20:366-74, 2002.
Balfour JA, Wiseman LR. Moxifloxacin. Drugs 57:363-73, 1999.
Drummond MF, Becker DL, Hux M, et al. An economic evaluation of sequential i.v./po moxifloxacin therapy compared to i.v./po co-amoxiclav with or without clarithromycin in the treatment of community-acquired pneumonia. Chest. 124:526-35, 2003.
Klutman NE, Culley CM, Lacy ME, et al. Moxifloxacin. Antibiotics for Clinicians. 5:17-27, 2001.
Gatifloxacin and Moxifloxacin: Two new fluoroquinolones. Med Lett Drugs 1072:15-17, 2000.
Lode H, Grossman C, Choudhri S, et al. Sequential IV/PO moxifloxacin treatment of patients with severe community-acquired pneumonia. Respir Med. 97:1134-42, 2003.
Rijnders BJ. Moxifloxacin for community-acquired pneumonia. Antimicrob Agents Chemother 47:444-445, 2003.
Schentag JJ. Pharmacokinetic and pharmacodynamic predictors of antimicrobial efficacy: moxifloxacin and Streptococcus pneumoniae. J Chemother 14(Suppl 2):13-21, 2002.
Speciale A, Musumeci R, Blandino G, et al. Minimal inhibitory concentrations and time-kill determination of moxifloxacin against aerobic and anaerobic isolates. Int J Antimicrob Agents 19:111-8, 2002.
Torres A, Muir JF, Corris P, et al. Effectiveness of oral moxifloxacin in standard first-line therapy in community-acquired pneumonia. Eur Respir J. 21:135-43, 2003.
Website: www.avelox.com

Nafcillin (Unipen)

Drug Class: Antistaphylococcal penicillin
Usual Dose: 2 gm (IV) q4h
Pharmacokinetic Parameters:
Peak serum level: 80 mcg/mL
Bioavailability: Not applicable
Excreted unchanged: 35%
Serum half-life (normal/ESRD): 0.5/4 hrs
Plasma protein binding: 90%
Volume of distribution (V_d): 0.24 L/kg
Primary Mode of Elimination: Hepatic
Dosage Adjustments*

CrCl ~ 40–60 mL/min	No change
CrCl < 40 mL/min	No change
Post–HD/PD dose	None
CVVH dose	No change
Moderate or severe hepatic insufficiency	No change

Drug Interactions: Cyclosporine (↓

"Usual dose" assumes normal renal/hepatic function. * For renal insufficiency, give usual dose x 1 followed by maintenance dose per CrCl. For dialysis patients, dose the same as for CrCl < 10 mL/min and give supplemental (post-HD/PD dose) immediately after dialysis. CrCl = creatinine clearance; CVVH = continuous veno-venous hemofiltration; HD/PD = hemodialysis/peritoneal dialysis. See pp. 293-297 for explanations, p. 1 for abbreviations

cyclosporine levels); nifedipine, warfarin (↓ interacting drug effect)
Adverse Effects: Drug fever/rash, leukopenia
Allergic Potential: High
Safety in Pregnancy: B
Comments: Avoid oral formulation (not well absorbed/erratic serum levels). Na⁺ content = 3.1 mEq/g. Meningeal dose = usual dose
Cerebrospinal Fluid Penetration:
Non-inflamed meninges = 1%
Inflamed meninges = 20%
Bile Penetration: 100%

REFERENCES:
Donowitz GR, Mandell GL. Beta-lactam antibiotics. N Engl J Med 318:419-26 and 318:490-500, 1993.
Wright AJ. The penicillins. Mayo Clin Proc 74:290-307, 1999.
Website: www.pdr.net

Nelfinavir (Viracept)

Drug Class: Antiretroviral protease inhibitor
Usual Dose: 750 mg (PO) q8h or 1250 mg (PO) q12h
Pharmacokinetic Parameters:
Peak serum level: 35 mcg/mL
Bioavailability: 20-80%
Excreted unchanged: 23%
Serum half-life (normal/ESRD): 4 hrs/no data
Plasma protein binding: 98%
Volume of distribution (V_d): 5 L/kg
Primary Mode of Elimination: Hepatic
Dosage Adjustments*

CrCl ~ 40–60 mL/min	No change
CrCl ~ 10–40 mL/min	No change
CrCl < 10 mL/min	No change
Post–HD dose	None
Post-PD dose	None
CVVH dose	No change
Moderate hepatic insufficiency	No information

Severe hepatic insufficiency	No information

Antiretroviral Dosage Adjustments:

Amprenavir	No information
Delavirdine	No information (monitor for neutropenia)
Efavirenz	No changes
Indinavir	Limited data for nelfinavir 1250 mg q12h + indinavir 1200 mg q12h
Lopinavir/ritonavir	No information
Nevirapine	No information
Ritonavir	Nelfinavir 500-750 mg q12h + ritonavir 400 mg q12h
Saquinavir soft-gel	Saquinavir soft-gel 800 mg q8h or 1200 mg q12h
Rifampin	Avoid combination
Rifabutin	Nelfinavir 1250 mg q12h; rifabutin 150 mg q24h or 300 mg 2-3x/week

Drug Interactions: Antiretrovirals, rifabutin, rifampin (see dose adjustment grid, above); amiodarone, quinidine, astemizole, terfenadine, benzodiazepines, cisapride, ergot alkaloids, statins, St. John's wort (avoid if possible); carbamazepine, phenytoin, phenobarbital (↓ nelfinavir levels, ↑ anticonvulsant levels; monitor); caspofungin (↓ caspofungin levels, may ↓ caspofungin effect); clarithromycin, erythromycin, telithromycin (↑ nelfinavir and macrolide levels); didanosine (dosing conflict with food; give nelfinavir with food 2 hours before or 1 hour after didanosine); itraconazole, ketoconazole (↑ nelfinavir levels); lamivudine (↑ lamivudine levels); methadone (may require ↑

"Usual dose" assumes normal renal/hepatic function. * For renal insufficiency, give usual dose x 1 followed by maintenance dose per CrCl. For dialysis patients, dose the same as for CrCl < 10 mL/min and give supplemental (post-HD/PD dose) immediately after dialysis. CrCl = creatinine clearance; CVVH = continuous veno-venous hemofiltration; HD/PD = hemodialysis/peritoneal dialysis. See pp. 293-297 for explanations, p. 1 for abbreviations

methadone dose); oral contraceptives, zidovudine (↓ zidovudine levels); sildenafil (↑ or ↓ sildenafil levels; do not exceed 25 mg in 48 hrs)

Adverse Effects: Impaired concentration, nausea, abdominal pain, secretory diarrhea, ↑ SGOT/SGPT, rash, ↑ cholesterol/triglycerides (evaluate risk for coronary disease/pancreatitis), fat redistribution, hyperglycemia (including worsening diabetes, new-onset diabetes, DKA), possible increased bleeding in hemophilia

Allergic Potential: Low

Safety in Pregnancy: B

Comments: Take with food (absorption increased 300%). Effective antiretroviral therapy consists of at least 3 antiretrovirals (same/different classes)

Cerebrospinal Fluid Penetration: < 10%

REFERENCES:

Albrecht MA, Bosch RJ, Hammer SM, et al. Nelfinavir, efavirenz, or both after the failure of nucleoside treatment of HIV infection. N Engl J Med 345:398-407, 2001.

Clotet B, Ruiz L, Martinez-Picado J, et al. Prevalence of HIV protease mutations on failure of nelfinavir-containing HAART: a retrospective analysis of four clinical studies and two observational cohorts. HIV Clin Trials 3:316-23, 2002.

Deeks SG, Smith M, Holodniy M, et al. HIV-1 protease inhibitors: A review for clinicians. JAMA 277:145-53, 1997.

Go J, Cunha BA. Nelfinavir: A review. Antibiotics for Clinicians 4:17-23, 2000.

Kaul DR, Cinti SK, Carver PL, et al. HIV protease inhibitors: Advances in therapy and adverse reactions, including metabolic complications. Pharmacotherapy 19:281-98, 1999.

Panel on Clinical Practices for Treatment of HIV Infection. Guidelines for the use of antiretroviral agents in HIV-infected adults and adolescents. Department of Health and Human Services. www.aidsinfo.nih.gov/guidelines/. November 10, 2003.

Perry CM, Benfield P. Nelfinavir. Drugs 54:81-7, 1997.

Walmsley S, Bernstein B, King M, et al. Lopinavir-ritonavir versus nelfinavir for the initial treatment of HIV infection. N Engl J Med 346:2039-46, 2002.

Website: www.viracept.com

Nevirapine (Viramune)

Drug Class: Antiretroviral NNRTI (non-nucleoside reverse transcriptase inhibitor)

Usual Dose: 200 mg (PO) q24h x 2 weeks, then 200 mg (PO) q12h

Pharmacokinetic Parameters:
Peak serum level: 2.2 mcg/mL
Bioavailability: 90%
Excreted unchanged: 3%
Serum half-life (normal/ESRD): 30 hrs/no data
Plasma protein binding: 60%
Volume of distribution (V_d): 1.3 L/kg

Primary Mode of Elimination: Hepatic

Dosage Adjustments*

CrCl ~ 40–60 mL/min	No change
CrCl ~ 20–40 mL/min	No change
CrCl < 20 mL/min	No change; use caution
Post–HD dose	200 mg (PO)
Post–PD dose	None
CVVH dose	No change
Moderate hepatic insufficiency	Use caution
Severe hepatic insufficiency	Avoid

Antiretroviral Dosage Adjustments:

Amprenavir	No information
Delavirdine	No information
Efavirenz	No information
Indinavir	Indinavir 1000 mg q8h
Lopinavir/ritonavir (l/r)	Consider l/r 533/133 mg q12h in PI-experienced patients
Nelfinavir	No information
Ritonavir	No changes

"Usual dose" assumes normal renal/hepatic function. * For renal insufficiency, give usual dose x 1 followed by maintenance dose per CrCl. For dialysis patients, dose the same as for CrCl < 10 mL/min and give supplemental (post-HD/PD dose) immediately after dialysis. CrCl = creatinine clearance; CVVH = continuous veno-venous hemofiltration; HD/PD = hemodialysis/peritoneal dialysis. See pp. 293-297 for explanations, p. 1 for abbreviations

Saquinavir	No information
Rifampin	Not recommended
Rifabutin	No changes for non-PI-containing regimes

Drug Interactions: Antiretrovirals, rifabutin, rifampin (see dose adjustment grid, above); carbamazepine, phenobarbital, phenytoin (monitor anticonvulsant levels); caspofungin (↓ caspofungin levels, may ↓ caspofungin effect); ethinyl estradiol (↓ ethinyl estradiol levels; use additional/alternative method); ketoconazole (avoid); methadone (↓ metadone levels; titrate methadone dose to effect); tacrolimus (↓ tacrolimus levels)

Adverse Effects: Drug fever/rash (may be severe; usually occurs within 6 weeks), Stevens–Johnson syndrome, ↑ SGOT/SGPT, *fatal hepatitis*, headache, diarrhea, leukopenia, stomatitis, peripheral neuropathy, paresthesias

Allergic Potential: High

Safety in Pregnancy: C

Comments: Absorption not affected by food. Not to be used for post-exposure prophylaxis because of potential for fatal hepatitis. Effective antiretroviral therapy consists of at least 3 antiretrovirals (same/different classes)

Cerebrospinal Fluid Penetration: 45%

REFERENCES:

D'Aquila RT, Hughes MD, Johnson VA, et al. Nevirapine, zidovudine, and didanosine compared with zidovudine and didanosine in patients with HIV-1 infection. Ann Intern Med 124:1019-30, 1996.

Hammer SM, Kessler HA, Saag MS. Issues in combination antiretroviral therapy: A review. J Acquired Immune Defic Syndr 7:24-37, 1994.

Havlir DV. Lange JM. New antiretrovirals and new combinations. AIDS 12:165-74, 1998.

Johnson S, Chan J, Bennett CL. Hepatotoxicity after prophylaxis with a nevirapine-containing antiretroviral regimen. Ann Intern Med 137:146-7, 2002.

Montaner JS, Reiss P, Cooper D, et al. A randomized, double-blind trial comparing combinations of nevirapine, didanosine, and zidovudine for HIV-infected patients: The INCAS trial. Italy, the Netherlands, Canada and Australia Study. J Am Med Assoc 279:930-937, 1998.

Negredo E, Ribalta J, Paredes R, et al. Reversal of atherogenic lipoprotein profile in HIV-1 infected patients with lipodystrophy after replacing protease inhibitors by nevirapine. AIDS 16:1383-9, 2002.

Panel on Clinical Practices for Treatment of HIV Infection. Guidelines for the use of antiretroviral agents in HIV-infected adults and adolescents. Department of Health and Human Services. www.aidsinfo.nih.gov/guidelines/. November 10, 2003.

Weverling GJ, Lange JM, Jurriaans S, et al. Alternative multidrug regimen provides improved suppression of HIV-1 replication over triple therapy. AIDS 12:117-22, 1998.

Website: www.viramune.com

Nitrofurantoin (Macrodantin, Macrobid)

Drug Class: Urinary antiseptic
Usual Dose: 100 mg (PO) q12h
Pharmacokinetic Parameters:
Peak serum level: 1 mcg/mL
Bioavailability: 80%
Excreted unchanged: 25%
Serum half-life (normal/ESRD): 0.5/1 hrs
Plasma protein binding: 40%
Volume of distribution (V_d): 0.8 L/kg
Primary Mode of Elimination: Renal
Dosage Adjustments*

CrCl ~ 30–60 mL/min	100 mg (PO) q24h
CrCl ~ 10–30 mL/min	Avoid
CrCl < 10 mL/min	Avoid
Post–HD dose	Not applicable
Post–PD dose	Not applicable
CVVH dose	Not applicable
Moderate hepatic insufficiency	No change
Severe hepatic insufficiency	No change

Drug Interactions: Antacids, magnesium (↓ nitrofurantoin absorption); probenecid (↑ nitrofurantoin levels)
Adverse Effects:
Acute hypersensitivity reactions (reversible):

"Usual dose" assumes normal renal/hepatic function. * For renal insufficiency, give usual dose x 1 followed by maintenance dose per CrCl. For dialysis patients, dose the same as for CrCl < 10 mL/min and give supplemental (post-HD/PD dose) immediately after dialysis. CrCl = creatinine clearance; CVVH = continuous veno-venous hemo-filtration; HD/PD = hemodialysis/peritoneal dialysis. See pp. 293-297 for explanations, p. 1 for abbreviations

pneumonitis
Chronic reactions (irreversible): chronic hepatitis, peripheral neuropathy, interstitial fibrosis
Allergic Potential: Moderate
Safety in Pregnancy: B
Comments: For UTIs only, not systemic infection. GI upset minimal with microcrystalline preparations. No transplacental transfer. Chronic toxicities associated with prolonged use/renal insufficiency; avoid in severe renal insufficiency. Preferred antimicrobial for VRE catheter-associated bacteriuria

REFERENCES:
Cunha BA. Nitrofurantoin: A review. Adv Ther 6:213-36, 1989.
Cunha BA. Nitrofurantoin: An update. OB/GYN 44:399-406, 1989.
Cunha BA. Nitrofurantoin: Bioavailability and therapeutic equivalence. Adv Ther 5:54-63, 1988.
Duff P. Antibiotic selection in obstetrics: making cost-effective choices. Clin Obstet Gynecol 45:59-72, 2002.
Klein NC, Cunha BA. New uses for older antibiotics. Med Clin North Am 85:125-32, 2001.
Linden PK. Treatment options for vancomycin-resistant enterococcal infections. Drugs 62:425-41, 2002.
Nicolle LE. Urinary tract infection: traditional pharmacologic therapies. Am J Med 113(Suppl 1A):35S-44S, 2002.

Ofloxacin (Oflox)

Drug Class: Fluoroquinolone
Usual Dose: 400 mg (IV/PO) q12h
Pharmacokinetic Parameters:
Peak serum level: 5.5-7.2 mcg/mL
Bioavailability: 95%
Excreted unchanged: 90%
Serum half-life (normal/ESRD): 6/40 hrs
Plasma protein binding: 32%
Volume of distribution (V_d): 2 L/kg
Primary Mode of Elimination: Renal
Dosage Adjustments*

CrCl ~ 50–60 mL/min	400 mg (IV/PO) q12h
CrCl ~ 20–50 mL/min	400 mg (IV/PO) q24h
CrCl < 20 mL/min	200 mg (IV/PO) q24
Post–HD dose	200 mg (IV/PO)
Post–PD dose	200 mg (IV/PO)
CVVH dose	400 mg (IV/PO) q24h
Moderate hepatic insufficiency	No change
Severe hepatic insufficiency	400 mg (IV/PO) q24h

Drug Interactions: Al^{++}, Ca^{++}, Fe^{++}, Mg^{++}, Zn^{++} antacids, citrate/citric acid, dairy products (↓ absorption of ofloxacin only if taken together); cimetidine (↑ ofloxacin levels); cyclosporine (↑ cyclosporine levels); NSAIDs (CNS stimulation); probenecid (↑ ofloxacin levels); warfarin (↑ INR)
Adverse Effects: Drug fever/rash, mild neuroexcitatory symptoms
Allergic Potential: Low
Safety in Pregnancy: C
Comments: H_2 antagonist increases half-life by ~ 30%. Levofloxacin has improved pharmacokinetics/pharmacodynamics and greater antimicrobial activity. Take ofloxacin 2 hours before or after calcium/magnesium containing antacids
Cerebrospinal Fluid Penetration: < 10%
Bile Penetration: 1500%

REFERENCES:
Absalon J, Domenico PD, Ortega AM, Cunha, BA. The antibacterial activity of ofloxacin versus ciprofloxacin against Pseudomonas aeruginosa in human urine. Adv Ther 13:191-4, 1996.
Fuhrmann V, Schenk P, Thalhammer F. Ofloxacin clearance during continuous hemofiltration. Am J Kidney Dis. 42:1327-8, 2003.
Hooper JC, Wolfson JS. Fluoroquinolone antimicrobial agents. N Engl J Med. 324:384-94, 1991.
Monk JP, Campoli-Richards DM. Ofloxacin: A review of its antibacterial activity, pharmacokinetics properties, and therapeutic use. Drugs 33:346-91, 1987.
Pendland SL, Messick CR, Jung R. In vitro synergy testing of levofloxacin, ofloxacin, and ciprofloxacin in combination with aztreonam, ceftazidime, or piperacillin against Pseudomonas aeruginosa. Diagn Microbiol Infect Dis 42:75-8, 2002.
Schwartz M, Isenmann R, Weikert E, et al. Pharmacokinetic basis for oral perioperative prophylaxis with ofloxacin in general surgery. Infection 29:222-7, 2001.
Walker RC, Wright AJ. The fluoroquinolones. Mayo

"Usual dose" assumes normal renal/hepatic function. * For renal insufficiency, give usual dose x 1 followed by maintenance dose per CrCl. For dialysis patients, dose the same as for CrCl < 10 mL/min and give supplemental (post-HD/PD dose) immediately after dialysis. CrCl = creatinine clearance; CVVH = continuous veno-venous hemofiltration; HD/PD = hemodialysis/peritoneal dialysis. See pp. 293-297 for explanations, p. 1 for abbreviations

Clin Proc 66:1249-59, 1991.
Website: www.pdr.net

Oxacillin (Prostaphlin)

Drug Class: Antistaphylococcal penicillin
Usual Dose: 1-2 gm (IV) q4h
Pharmacokinetic Parameters:
Peak serum level: 43 mcg/mL
Bioavailability: Not applicable
Excreted unchanged: 96%
Serum half-life (normal/ESRD): 0.5/1 hrs
Plasma protein binding: 94%
Volume of distribution (V_d): 0.2 L/kg
Primary Mode of Elimination: Renal
Dosage Adjustments* (based on 2 gm q4h):

CrCl ~ 40–60 mL/min	No change
CrCl < 40 mL/min	No change
Post–HD dose	None
Post–PD dose	None
CVVH dose	No change
Moderate hepatic insufficiency	No change
Severe hepatic insufficiency	No change

Drug Interactions: Cyclosporine (↓ cyclosporine levels); nifedipine, warfarin (↓ interacting drug effect)
Adverse Effects: Drug fever/rash, leukopenia, ↑ SGOT/SGPT, interstitial nephritis
Allergic Potential: High
Safety in Pregnancy: B
Comments: Avoid oral formulation (not well absorbed/erratic serum levels). Na⁺ content = 3.1 mEq/g. Meningeal dose = usual dose
Cerebrospinal Fluid Penetration:
Non-inflamed meninges = 1%
Inflamed meninges = 10%
Bile Penetration: 25%

REFERENCES:
Al-Homaidhi H, Abdel-Haq NM, El-Baba M, et al. Severe hepatitis associated with oxacillin therapy. South Med J 95:650-2, 2002.

Donowitz GR, Mandell GL. Beta-lactam antibiotics. N Engl J Med 318:419-26 and 318:490-500, 1993.
Jensen AG, Wachmann CH, Espersen F, et al. Treatment and outcome of Staphylococcus aureus bacteremia: a prospective study of 278 cases. Arch Intern Med 162:25-32, 2002.
Jones ME, Mayfield DC, Thronsbery C, et al. Prevalence of oxacillin resistance in Staphylococcus aureus among inpatients and outpatients in the United States during 2000. Antimicrob Agents Chemother 46:3104-5, 2002.
Wright AJ. The penicillins. Mayo Clin Proc 74:290-307, 1999.
Website: www.pdr.net

Pegylated Interferon alfa-2a (Pegasys) + Ribavirin

Drug Class: Interferon/antiviral
Usual Dose: Pegasys: 180 mcg once weekly (SQ) x 48 weeks; ribivirin: 500 mg (< 75 kg) or 600 mg (> 75 kg) (PO) q12h x 48 weeks (see comments)
Pharmacokinetic Parameters:
Trough level: 16 ng/mL
Bioavailability: No data
Excreted unchanged: No data
Serum half-life (normal/ESRD): 80/100-120 hrs
Plasma protein binding: No data
Volume of distribution (V_d): No data
Primary Mode of Elimination: Renal
Dosage Adjustments*

CrCl ~ 40–60 mL/min	Pegasys: no change. Avoid ribavirin if CrCl < 50 mL/min
CrCl ~ 10–40 mL/min	Avoid ribavirin
CrCl < 10 mL/min	Pegasys: 135 mcg q week; avoid ribavirin
Post–HD dose	Pegasys: 135 mcg q week; avoid ribavirin
Post–PD dose	No information
CVVH dose	No information
Moderate hepatic insufficiency	135 mcg if ALT ↑

"Usual dose" assumes normal renal/hepatic function. * For renal insufficiency, give usual dose x 1 followed by maintenance dose per CrCl. For dialysis patients, dose the same as for CrCl < 10 mL/min and give supplemental (post-HD/PD dose) immediately after dialysis. CrCl = creatinine clearance; CVVH = continuous veno-venous hemofiltration; HD/PD = hemodialysis/peritoneal dialysis. See pp. 293-297 for explanations, p. 1 for abbreviations

Severe hepatic insufficiency	Avoid
Moderate depression	↓ Pegasys to 135 mcg (90 mcg in some); evaluate once weekly
Severe depression	Discontinue Pegasys; immediate psychiatric consult

Pegasys Adjustment for Hematologic Toxicity

Absolute neutrophil count < 750/ mm^3	↓ Pegasys to 135 mcg
Absolute neutrophil count < 500/ mm^3	Discontinue Pegasys until neutrophils > 1000/mm^3. Reinstitute at 90 mcg and monitor neutrophil count
Platelets < 50,000/ mm^3	↓ Pegasys to 90 mcg
Platelets < 25,000/ mm^3	Discontinue Pegasys

Ribavirin Adjustment for Hematologic Toxicity

Hgb < 10 gm/dL and no cardiac disease	↓ Ribavirin to 600 mg/day†
Hgb < 8.5 gm/dL and no cardiac disease	Discontinue ribavirin
Hgb ≥ 2 gm/dL ↓ during 4-week treatment period and stable cardiac disease	↓ Ribavirin to 600 mg/day*
Hgb < 12 gm/dL despite 4 weeks at reduced dose and stable cardiac disease	Discontinue ribavirin

* One 200-mg tablet in a.m. and two 200-mg tablets in p.m.

Drug Interactions: Inhibits CYP IA2. May ↑ theophylline levels
Adverse Effects: Flu-like symptoms, neuropsychiatric disturbances, bone marrow toxicity, nausea/vomiting/diarrhea, alopecia, hypothyroidism
Allergic Potential: Low
Safety in Pregnancy: Pegasys: C (ribavirin: X;

also avoid in partners of pregnant women)
Comments: Combination therapy is more effective than monotherapy. Avoid in autoimmune hepatitis and decompensated cirrhosis. Check CBC weekly. For genotypes 2 and 3, duration of therapy is 24 weeks and ribavirin dose is 400 mg (PO) q12h. Ribavirin should be taken with breakfast and dinner to ↑ bioavailability/↓ nausea. Ribavirin taken after dinner may cause insomnia. Ribavirin's long serum half-life allows q24h dosing, but ↑ nausea
Cerebrospinal Fluid Penetration: No data
Bile Penetration: No data

REFERENCES:
[No authors listed]. Peginterferon alfa-2a (Pegasys) for chronic hepatitis C. Med Lett Drugs Ther. 45:19-20, 2003.
Davis GL. Combination treatment with interferon and ribavirin for chronic hepatitis C. Clin Liver Dis 1:811-26,1999.
Ferenci P. Peginterferon alfa-2a (40KD) (Pegasys) for the treatment of patients with chronic hepatitis C. Int J Clin Pract. 57:610-5, 2003.
Fried MN, et al. Peg-interferon alfa-2a plus ribavirin for chronic hepatitis C virus infection. N Engl J Med 347:975-82, 2002.
Kamal SM, Et al. Peg-interferon alone or with ribavirin enhances HCV-specific CD4 T-helper responses in patients with chronic hepatitis C. Gastroenterology 123:1070-83, 2002.
Rajender Reddy K, Modi MW, Pedder S. Use of peginterferon alfa-2a (40 KD) (Pegasys) for the treatment of hepatitis C. Adv Drug Deliv Rev 54:571-86, 2002.
Rasenack J, Zeuzem S, Feinman SV, et al. Peginterferon alpha-2a (40KD) [Pegasys] improves HR-QOL outcomes compared with unmodified interferon alpha-2a [Roferon-A]: in patients with chronic hepatitis C. Pharmacoeconomics. 21:341-9, 2003.
Website: www.pegasys.com

Pegylated Interferon alfa-2b (Peg-Intron) + Ribavirin

Drug Class: Interferon/antiviral
Usual Dose: See pg 75
Pharmacokinetic Parameters:
Peak serum level: 30 IU/mL / 3680 ng/mL
Bioavailability: No data/64%
Excreted unchanged: No data/17%

"Usual dose" assumes normal renal/hepatic function. * For renal insufficiency, give usual dose x 1 followed by maintenance dose per CrCl. For dialysis patients, dose the same as for CrCl < 10 mL/min and give supplemental (post-HD/PD dose) immediately after dialysis. CrCl = creatinine clearance; CVVH = continuous veno-venous hemofiltration; HD/PD = hemodialysis/peritoneal dialysis. See pp. 293-297 for explanations, p. 1 for abbreviations

Serum half-life (normal/ESRD): [40 hrs/no data] / [298 hrs/no data]
Plasma protein binding: No data
Volume of distribution (V_d): No data/2825 L
Primary Mode of Elimination: Renal/renal
Dosage Adjustments*

CrCl ~ 50–60 mL/min	No change
CrCl ~ 10–50 mL/min	Avoid ribavirin
CrCl < 10 mL/min	Avoid ribavirin
Post–HD dose	No information
Post–PD dose	No information
CVVH dose	No information
Moderate hepatic insufficiency	None
Severe hepatic insufficiency	None
Moderate depression	↓ Peg-Intron by 50%; evaluate once weekly
Severe depression	Discontinue both drugs; immediate psychiatric consult

Dosage Adjustments for Hematologic Toxicity

Hgb < 10 gm/dL	↓ ribavirin by 200 mg/day
Hgb < 8.5 gm /dL	Permanently discontinue both drugs
WBC < 1.5 x 10⁹/L	↓ Peg-Intron by 50%
WBC < 1.0 x 10⁹/L	Permanently discontinue both drugs
Neutrophils < 0.75 x 10⁹/L	↓ Peg-Intron by 50%
Neutrophils < 0.5 x 10⁹/L	Permanently discontinue both drugs
Platelets < 80 x 10⁹/L	↓ Peg-Intron by 50%
Platelets < 50 x 10⁹/L	Permanently discontinue both drugs

Hgb ≥ 2 gm/dL ↓ during 4-week treatment period and stable cardiac disease	↓ Peg-Intron by 50% and ribavirin by 200 mg/day
Hgb < 12 gm/dL despite ribavirin dose reduction	Permanently discontinue both drugs

Drug Interactions: Nucleoside analogs: fatal/non-fatal lactic acidosis. May ↑ levels of theophylline. Overlapping toxicity with other bone marrow suppressants
Adverse Effects: Hemolytic anemia, psychological effects, cytopenias, pulmonary symptoms, pancreatitis, hypersensitivity reactions, ↑ triglycerides, flu-like symptoms, nausea/vomiting, alopecia, rash
Allergic Potential: Low
Safety in Pregnancy: Peg-Intron: C (ribavirin: X; also avoid in partners of pregnant women)
Comments: Avoid in autoimmune hepatitis. Check CBC pretreatment and at 2 and 4 weeks (must adjust doses for ↓ WBC, ↓ neutrophils, ↓ platelets, ↓ hemoglobin). Poorly tolerated in decompensated cirrhosis or recurrent hepatitis C after transplant
Cerebrospinal Fluid Penetration: No data
Bile Penetration: No data

REFERENCES:
Fried MN. Side effects of therapy of hepatitis C and their managment. Hepatology 36:S237-44, 2002.
Jaeckel E, Cornberg M, Wedemeyer H, et al. Treatment of acute hepatitis C with interferon alfa-2b. N Engl J Med 345:1452-7, 2001.
Wright TL. Treatment of patients with hepatitis C and cirrhosis. Hepatology 36:S185-91, 2002.
Website: www.pegintron.com

Penicillin G (various)

Drug Class: Natural penicillin
Usual Dose: 2-4 mu (IV) q4h
Pharmacokinetic Parameters:
Peak serum level: 20-40 mcg/mL
Bioavailability: Not applicable
Excreted unchanged: 60%
Serum half-life (normal/ESRD): 0.5/5.1 hrs
Plasma protein binding: 60%

"Usual dose" assumes normal renal/hepatic function. * For renal insufficiency, give usual dose x 1 followed by maintenance dose per CrCl. For dialysis patients, dose the same as for CrCl < 10 mL/min and give supplemental (post-HD/PD dose) immediately after dialysis. CrCl = creatinine clearance; CVVH = continuous veno-venous hemofiltration; HD/PD = hemodialysis/peritoneal dialysis. See pp. 293-297 for explanations, p. 1 for abbreviations

Volume of distribution (V_d): 0.3 L/kg
Primary Mode of Elimination: Renal
Dosage Adjustments*

CrCl ~ 50–60 mL/min	2–4 mu (IV) q4h
CrCl ~ 10–50 mL/min	1–2 mu (IV) q6h
CrCl < 10 mL/min	1 mu (IV) q6h
Post–HD dose	2 mu (IV)
Post–PD dose	2 mu (IV)
CVVH dose	2 mu (IV) q6h
Moderate hepatic insufficiency	No change
Severe hepatic insufficiency	No change

Drug Interactions: Probenecid (↑ penicillin G levels)
Adverse Effects: Drug fever/rash, E. multiforme/Stevens–Johnson syndrome; anaphylactic reactions (hypotension, laryngospasm, bronchospasm), hives, serum sickness
Allergic Potential: High
Safety in Pregnancy: B
Comments: Incompatible in solutions containing erythromycin, aminoglycosides, calcium bicarbonate, or heparin. Jarisch–Herxheimer reactions when treating spirochetal infections, e.g., Lyme disease, syphilis, yaws. Penicillin G (potassium): K^+ content = 1.7 mEq/g; Na^+ content = 0.3 mEq/g. Penicillin G (sodium): Na^+ content = 2 mEq/g. Meningeal dose = 4 mu (IV) q4h
Cerebrospinal Fluid Penetration:
Non-inflamed meninges ≤ 1%
Inflamed meninges = 5%
Bile Penetration: 500%

REFERENCES:
Donowitz GR, Mandell GL. Beta-lactam antibiotics. N Engl J Med 318:419-26 and 318:490-500, 1993.
Steininger C, Allerberger F, Gnaiger E. Clinical significance of inhibition kinetics for Streptococcus pyogenes in response to penicillin. J Antimicrob Chemother 50:517-23, 2002.
Wendel Jr GD, Sheffield JS, Hollier LM, et al. Treatment of syphilis in pregnancy and prevention of congenital syphilis. Clin Infect Dis 35(Suppl2):S200-9, 2002.
Wright AJ. The penicillins. Mayo Clin Proc 74:290-307, 1999.

Penicillin V (various)

Drug Class: Natural penicillin
Usual Dose: 500 mg (PO) q6h
Pharmacokinetic Parameters:
Peak serum level: 5 mcg/mL
Bioavailability: 60%
Excreted unchanged: 80%
Serum half-life (normal/ESRD): 0.5/8 hrs
Plasma protein binding: 70%
Volume of distribution (V_d): 0.5 L/kg
Primary Mode of Elimination: Renal
Dosage Adjustments*

CrCl ~ 40–60 mL/min	No change
CrCl ~ 10–40 mL/min	No change
CrCl < 10 mL/min	250-500 mg (PO) q8h
Post–HD dose	250 mg (PO)
Post–PD dose	250 mg (PO)
CVVH dose	500 mg (PO) q6h
Moderate hepatic insufficiency	No change
Severe hepatic insufficiency	No change

Drug Interactions: Probenecid (↑ penicillin V levels)
Adverse Effects: Drug fever/rash, E. multiforme/Stevens-Johnson syndrome, anaphylactic reactions (hypotension, laryngospasm, bronchospasm), hives, serum sickness
Allergic Potential: High
Safety in Pregnancy: B
Comments: Jarisch–Herxheimer reactions when treating spirochetal infections, e.g., Lyme disease, syphilis, yaws. Take 1 hour before or 2 hours after meals. K^+ content = 2.8 mEq/g
Cerebrospinal Fluid Penetration: < 10%

"Usual dose" assumes normal renal/hepatic function. * For renal insufficiency, give usual dose x 1 followed by maintenance dose per CrCl. For dialysis patients, dose the same as for CrCl < 10 mL/min and give supplemental (post-HD/PD dose) immediately after dialysis. CrCl = creatinine clearance; CVVH = continuous veno-venous hemo-filtration; HD/PD = hemodialysis/peritoneal dialysis. See pp. 293-297 for explanations, p. 1 for abbreviations

REFERENCES:

Bisno AL, Gerber MA, Swaltney JM, et al. Practice guidelines for the diagnosis and management of group A streptococcal pharyngitis. Infectious Diseases Society of America. Clin Infect Dis 35:113-25, 2002.

Donowitz GR, Mandell GL. Beta-lactam antibiotics. N Engl J Med 318:419-26 and 318:490-500, 1993.

Portier H, Filipecki J, Weber P, et al Five day clarithromycin modified release versus 10 day penicillin V for group A streptococcal pharyngitis: a multi-centre, open-label, randomized study. J Antimicrob Chemother 49:337-44, 2002.

Wright AJ. The penicillins. Mayo Clin Proc 74:290, 1999.

Pentamidine (Pentam 300, NebuPent)

Drug Class: Antiparasitic

Usual Dose: 4 mg/kg (IV) q24h

Pharmacokinetic Parameters:

Peak serum level: 0.6-1.5 mcg/mL
Bioavailability: Not applicable
Excreted unchanged: 50%
Serum half-life (normal/ESRD): 6.4/90 hrs
Plasma protein binding: 69%
Volume of distribution (V_d): 5 L/kg

Primary Mode of Elimination: Metabolized

Dosage Adjustments*

CrCl ~ 40–60 mL/min	No change
CrCl ~ 10–40 mL/min	No change
CrCl < 10 mL/min	No change
Post–HD dose	None
Post–PD dose	None
CVVH dose	No change
Moderate or severe hepatic insufficiency	No change

Drug Interactions: Alcohol, valproic acid (↑ risk of pancreatitis); foscarnet (severe hypocalcemia reported; do not combine); amphotericin B, aminoglycosides, capreomycin, cis-platinum, colistin, methoxyflurane, polymyxin B, vancomycin, other nephrotoxic drugs (↑ nephrotoxicity)

Adverse Effects: Rash, hypotension, hypocalcemia, hypoglycemia, h creatinine, pancreatitis, local injection site reactions, severe leukopenia, anemia, thrombocytopenia, may ↑ QT_c interval with IV administration

Allergic Potential: High

Safety in Pregnancy: C

Comments: Well absorbed IM, but painful. Administer IV slowly in D_5W over 1 hour, not saline. Inhaled pentamidine isethionate (NebuPent) 300 mg monthly via Respiragard II nebulizer can be used for PCP prophylaxis, but is less effective than IV/IM pentamidine and is not effective against extrapulmonary P. carinii. Adverse effects with aerosolized pentamidine include chest pain, arrhythmias, dizziness, wheezing, coughing, dyspnea, headache, anorexia, nausea, diarrhea, rash, pharyngitis. If PCP patient also has pulmonary TB, aerosolized pentamidine treatments may expose medical personnel to TB via droplet inhalation

Cerebrospinal Fluid Penetration: < 10%

REFERENCES:

Chan C, Montaner J, LeFebvre BA, et al. Atovaquone suspension compared with aerosolized pentamidine for prevention of Pneumocystis carinii pneumonia in human immunodeficiency virus infected subsets intolerant of trimethoprim or sulfamethoxazole. J Infect Dis 180:369-376, 1999.

Goa KL, Campoli-Richards GM. Pentamidine isethionate: A review of its antiprotozoal activity, pharmacokinetic properties and therapeutic use in Pneumocystis carinii pneumonia. Drugs 33:242-58, 1987.

Guerin PJ, Alar P, Sundar S, et al. Visceral leishmaniasis: current status of control, diagnosis and treatment, and a proposed research and development agenda. Lancet Infect Dis. 2:494-501, 2002.

Lionakis MS, Lewis RE, Samonis G, et al. Pentamidine is active in vitro against Fusarium species. Antimicrob Agents Chemother. 47:3252-9, 2003.

Monk JP, Benfield P. Inhaled pentamidine: An overview of its pharmacological properties and a review of its therapeutic use in Pneumocystis carinii pneumonia. Drugs 39:741-56, 1990.

Sattler FR, Cowam R, Nielsen DM, et al. Trimethoprim-sulfamethoxazole compared with pentamidine for treatment of Pneumocystis carinii pneumonia in the acquired immunodeficiency syndrome. Ann Intern Med 109:280-7, 1988.

Website: www.pdr.net

Piperacillin (Pipracil)

Drug Class: Antipseudomonal penicillin
Usual Dose: 3-4 gm (IV) q4-8h
Pharmacokinetic Parameters:
Peak serum level: 412 mcg/mL
Bioavailability: Not applicable
Excreted unchanged: 80%
Serum half-life (normal/ESRD): 1/3 hrs
Plasma protein binding: 16%
Volume of distribution (V_d): 0.24 L/kg
Primary Mode of Elimination: Renal
Dosage Adjustments* (based on 4 gm q8h):

CrCl ~ 40–60 mL/min	No change
CrCl ~ 20–40 mL/min	3 gm (IV) q8h
CrCl < 20 mL/min	3 gm (IV) q12h
Post–HD dose	1 gm (IV)
Post–PD dose	2 gm (IV)
CVVH dose	3 gm (IV) q8h
Moderate hepatic insufficiency	No change
Severe hepatic insufficiency	No change

Drug Interactions: Aminoglycosides (inactivation of piperacillin in renal failure); warfarin (↑ INR); oral contraceptives (↓ oral contraceptive effect); cefoxitin (↓ piperacillin effect)
Adverse Effects: Drug fever/rash, anaphylactic reactions (hypotension, laryngospasm, bronchospasm), hives, serum sickness, leukopenia
Allergic Potential: High
Safety in Pregnancy: B
Comments: 75% absorbed when given IM. Do not mix/administer with aminoglycosides. Most active antipseudomonal penicillin against P. aeruginosa. Na^+ content = 1.8 mEq/g. Meningeal dose = usual dose
Cerebrospinal Fluid Penetration:
Non-inflamed meninges = 1%
Inflamed meninges = 30%
Bile Penetration: 1000%

REFERENCES:
Donowitz GR, Mandell GL. Beta-lactam antibiotics. N Engl J Med 318:419-26 and 318:490-500, 1993.
Kim MK, Capitano B, Mattoes HM, et al. Pharmacokinetic and pharmacodynamic evaluation of two dosing regimens for piperacillin-susceptible organisms. Pharmacotherapy 22:569-77, 2002.
Peacock JE, Herrington DA, Wade JC, et al. Ciprofloxacin plus piperacillin compared with tobramycin plus piperacillin as empirical therapy in febrile neutropenic patients. A randomized, double-blind trial. Ann Intern Med 137:120, 2002.
Tan JS, File TM, Jr. Antipseudomonal penicillins. Med Clin North Am 79:679-93, 1995.
Wright AJ. The penicillins. Mayo Clin Proc 74:290, 1999.
Website: www.pdr.net

Piperacillin/tazobactam (Zosyn)

Drug Class: Antipseudomonal penicillin
Usual Dose: 4.5 gm (IV) q8h (see comments)
Pharmacokinetic Parameters:
Peak serum level: 400 mcg/mL
Bioavailability: Not applicable
Excreted unchanged: 70/80%
Serum half-life (normal/ESRD): [1.5/8] / [1/7] hrs
Plasma protein binding: 30/32%
Volume of distribution (V_d): 0.3/0.21 L/kg
Primary Mode of Elimination: Renal
Dosage Adjustments (see comments):

CrCl ~ 40–60 mL/min	3.375 gm (IV) q6h
CrCl ~ 20–40 mL/min	2.25 gm (IV) q6h
CrCl < 20 mL/min	2.25 gm (IV) q8h
Hemodialysis	2.25 gm (IV) q12h
Post–HD dose	0.75 gm (IV)
Post–PD dose	None
CVVH dose	2.25 gm (IV) q6h
Moderate or severe hepatic insufficiency	No change

Drug Interactions: Aminoglycosides (↓ aminoglycoside levels); vecuronium (↑ vecuronium effect)

"Usual dose" assumes normal renal/hepatic function. * For renal insufficiency, give usual dose x 1 followed by maintenance dose per CrCl. For dialysis patients, dose the same as for CrCl < 10 mL/min and give supplemental (post-HD/PD dose) immediately after dialysis. CrCl = creatinine clearance; CVVH = continuous veno-venous hemofiltration; HD/PD = hemodialysis/peritoneal dialysis. See pp. 293-297 for explanations, p. 1 for abbreviations

Adverse Effects: Drug fever/rash, leukopenia, insomnia, headache, constipation, nausea, hypertension
Allergic Potential: High
Safety in Pregnancy: B
Comments: Dose–dependent kinetics permit 4.5 gm (IV) q8h dosing. For nosocomial pneumonia, use 4.5 gm (IV) q6h for CrCl > 40 mL/min, 3.375 gm (IV) q6h for CrCl ~ 20-40 mL/min, 2.25 gm (IV) q8h for CrCl < 20 mL/min, and 2.25 gm (IV) q8h for HD or CAPD. Do not mix with Ringers lactate. Minimizes emergence of multi-drug resistant gram-negative rods and VRE. Na^+ content = 2.4 mEq/g
Cerebrospinal Fluid Penetration:
Non-inflamed meninges = 1%
Inflamed meninges = 30%
Bile Penetration: 6000%

REFERENCES:
Burgess DS, Waldrep T. Pharmacokinetics and pharmacodynamics of piperacillin/tazobactam when administered by continuous infusion and intermittent dosing. Clin Ther 24:1090-104, 2002.
Florea NR, Kotapati S, Kuti JL, et al. Cost analysis of continuous versus intermittent infusion of piperacillin-tazobactam: a time-motion study. Am J Health Syst Pharm. 60:2321-7, 2003.
Mattoes HM, Capitano B, Kim MK, et al. Comparative pharmacokinetic and pharmacodynamic profile of piperacillin/tazobactam 3.375 G Q4H and 4.5 G Q6H. Chemotherapy 458:59-63, 2002.
Minnaganti VR, Cunha BA. Piperacillin/tazobactam. Antibiotics for Clinicians 3:101-8, 1999.
Piperacillin/tazobactam. Med Lett Drugs Ther 36:7-9, 1994.
Sanders WE Jr, Sanders CC. Piperacillin/tazobactam: A critical review of the evolving clinical literature. Clin Infect Dis 22:107-23, 1996.
Schoonover LL, Occhipinti DJ, Rodvold KA, et al. Piperacillin/tazobactam: A new beta-lactam/beta-lactamase inhibitor combination. Ann Pharmacother 29:501-14, 1995.
Website: www.zosyn.com

Polymyxin B

Drug Class: Phospholipid cell membrane-altering antibiotic
Usual Dose: 0.75-1.25 mg/kg (IV) q12h (1 mg = 10,000 units)

Pharmacokinetic Parameters:
Peak serum level: 8 mcg/mL
Bioavailability: Not applicable
Excreted unchanged: 60%
Serum half-life (normal/ESRD): 6/48 hrs
Plasma protein binding: < 10%
Volume of distribution (V_d): No data
Primary Mode of Elimination: Renal
Dosage Adjustments*

CrCl ~ 20–60 mL/min	0.5-1 mg/kg (IV) q12h
CrCl ~ 5–20 mL/min	0.5 mg/kg (IV) q12h
CrCl < 10 mL/min	0.2 mg/kg (IV) q12h
Post–HD dose	No information
Post–PD dose	No information
CVVH dose	0.5 mg/kg (IV) q12h
Moderate hepatic insufficiency	No change
Severe hepatic insufficiency	No change

Drug Interactions: Amphotericin B, amikacin, gentamicin, tobramycin, vancomycin (↑ nephrotoxicity)
Adverse Effects: Renal failure. Neurotoxicity associated with very prolonged/high serum levels; neuromuscular blockade potential with renal failure/neuromuscular disorders
Allergic Potential: Low
Safety in Pregnancy: B
Comments: Inhibits endotoxin release from gram-negative bacilli. Avoid intraperitoneal infusion due to risk of neuromuscular blockade. Increased risk of reversible non–oliguric renal failure (ATN) when used with other nephrotoxic drugs. No ototoxic potential. May be given IM with procaine, but painful. Intrathecal (IT) polymyxin B dose = 5 mg (50,000 u) q24h x 3 days, then q48h x 2 weeks. Dissolve 50 mg (500,000 u) into 10 mL for IT administration
Cerebrospinal Fluid Penetration: < 10%

REFERENCES:
Evans ME, Feola DJ, Rapp RP. Polymyxin B sulfate and colistin: Old antibiotics for emerging multiresistant

---

"Usual dose" assumes normal renal/hepatic function. * For renal insufficiency, give usual dose x 1 followed by maintenance dose per CrCl. For dialysis patients, dose the same as for CrCl < 10 mL/min and give supplemental (post-HD/PD dose) immediately after dialysis. CrCl = creatinine clearance; CVVH = continuous veno-venous hemo-filtration; HD/PD = hemodialysis/peritoneal dialysis. See pp. 293-297 for explanations, p. 1 for abbreviations gram-negative bacteria. Ann Pharmacother 33:960-7, 1999.

Garnacho-Montero J, Ortiz-Leyba C, Jimenez-Jimenez FJ, et al. Treatment of multidrug-resistant Acinetobacter baumannii ventilator-associated pneumonia (VAP) with intravenous colistin: a comparison with imipenem-susceptible VAP. Clin Infect Dis. 36:1111-8, 2003.

Giamarellos-Bourboulis EJ, Sambatakou H, Galani I, et al. In vitro interaction of colistin and rifampin on multidrug-resistant Pseudomonas aeruginosa. J Chemother. 15:235-8, 2003.

Horton J, Pankey GA. Polymyxin B. Med Clin North Am 66:134-42, 1995.

Menzies D, Minnaganti VR, Cunha BA. Polymyxin B. Antibiotics for Clinicians 4:33-40, 2000.

Segal-Maurer S, Mariano N, Qavi A, et al. Successful treatment of ceftazidime-resistant Klebsiella pneumoniae ventriculitis with intravenous meropenem and intraventricular polymyxin B: Case report and review. Clin Infect Dis 28:1134-8, 1999.

Pyrazinamide (PZA)

Drug Class: Anti–TB drug
Usual Dose: 25 mg/kg (PO) q24h (max. 2 gm)
Pharmacokinetic Parameters:
Peak serum level: 30-50 mcg/mL
Bioavailability: 90%
Excreted unchanged: 10%
Serum half-life (normal/ESRD): 9/26 hrs
Plasma protein binding: 10%
Volume of distribution (V_d): 0.9 L/kg
Primary Mode of Elimination: Hepatic
Dosage Adjustments*

CrCl ~ 40–60 mL/min	No change
CrCl ~ 10–40 mL/min	No change
CrCl < 10 mL/min	No change
Post–HD dose	25 mg/kg (PO) or 1 gm (PO)
Post–PD dose	No change
CVVH dose	No information
Moderate hepatic insufficiency	No information
Severe hepatic insufficiency	Avoid

Drug Interactions: INH, rifabutin, rifampin (may ↑ risk of hepatoxicity)
Adverse Effects: Drug fever/rash, malaise, nausea, vomiting, anorexia, ↑ SGOT/SGPT, ↑ uric acid, sideroblastic anemia
Allergic Potential: Low
Safety in Pregnancy: C
Comments: Avoid in patients with gout (may precipitate acute attacks). May be administered as 4 gm (PO) 2x/week or 3 gm (PO) 3x/week. Meningeal dose = usual dose
Cerebrospinal Fluid Penetration: 100%

REFERENCES:

Ahn C, Oh KH, Kim K, et al. Effect of peritoneal dialysis on plasma and peritoneal fluid concentrations of isoniazid, pyrazinamide, and rifampin. Perit Dial Int. 23:362-7, 2003.

Davidson PT, Le HQ. Drug treatment of tuberculosis 1992. Drugs 43:651-73, 1992.

Drugs for tuberculosis. Med Lett Drugs Ther 35:99-101,1993.

Havlir DV, Barnes PF. Tuberculosis in patients with human immunodeficiency virus infection. N Engl J Med 340:367-73, 1999.

Iseman MD. Treatment of multidrug-resistant tuberculosis. N Engl J Med 329:784-91, 1993.

Van Scoy RE, Wilkowske CJ. Antituberculous agents. Mayo Clin Proc 67:179-87, 1992.

Pyrimethamine (Daraprim)

Drug Class: Antiparasitic
Usual Dose: 75 mg (PO) q24h (toxoplasmosis)
Pharmacokinetic Parameters:
Peak serum level: 0.4 mcg/mL
Bioavailability: 90%
Excreted unchanged: 25%
Serum half-life (normal/ESRD): 96/96 hrs
Plasma protein binding: 87%
Volume of distribution (V_d): 2.5 L/kg
Primary Mode of Elimination: Hepatic
Dosage Adjustments*

CrCl ~ 40–60 mL/min	No change
CrCl ~ 10–40 mL/min	No change

CrCl < 10 mL/min	No change; use caution
Post–HD/PD dose	None
CVVH dose	No change
Moderate hepatic insufficiency	No change
Severe hepatic insufficiency	No change; use caution

Drug Interactions: Folic acid (↓ pyrimethamine effect); lorazepam (↑ risk of hepatotoxicity); sulfamethoxazole, trimethoprim, TMP-SMX (↑ risk of thrombocytopenia, anemia, leukopenia)
Adverse Effects: Megaloblastic anemia, leukopenia, thrombocytopenia, ataxia, tremors, seizures
Allergic Potential: Low
Safety in Pregnancy: C
Comments: Antacids decrease absorption. Give folinic acid 50 mg (PO) q24h with pyrimethamine to prevent folic acid depletion
Cerebrospinal Fluid Penetration: No data

REFERENCES:
Bosch-Driessen LH, Verbraak FD, Suttorp-Schulten MS, et al. A prospective, randomized trial of pyrimethamine and azithromycin vs. pyrimethamine and sulfadiazine for the treatment of ocular toxoplasmosis. Am J Ophthalmol 134:34-40, 2002.
Chirgwin K, Hafner R, Leport C, et al. Randomized phase II trial of atovaquone with pyrimethamine or sulfadiazine for treatment of toxoplasmic encephalitis in patients with acquired immunodeficiency syndrome: ACTG 237/ANRS039 Study. AIDS Clinical Trials Group 237/Agence Nationale de Recherche sur le SIDA, Essai 039. Clin Infect Dis 34:1243-50, 2002.
Drugs for Parasitic Infections. Med Lett Drugs Ther 40:1-12, 2000.
Podzamczer D, Salazar A, Jiminez J, et al. Intermittent trimethoprim-sulfamethoxazole compared with dapsone-pyrimethamine for the simultaneous primary prophylaxis of Pneumocystis pneumonia and toxoplasmosis in patients infected with HIV. Ann Intern Med 122:755-61, 1995.
Porter SB, Sande MA. Toxoplasmosis of the central nervous system in the acquired-immunodeficiency syndrome. N Engl J Med 327:1643-8, 1992.
Website: www.pdr.net

Quinine sulfate

Drug Class: Antimalarial
Usual Dose: 600 mg (PO) q8h
Pharmacokinetic Parameters:
Peak serum level: 3.8 mcg/mL
Bioavailability: 80%
Excreted unchanged: 5%
Serum half-life (normal/ESRD): 7/14 hrs
Plasma protein binding: 95%
Volume of distribution (V_d): 3 L/kg
Primary Mode of Elimination: Renal/hepatic
Dosage Adjustments*

CrCl ~ 40–60 mL/min	No change
CrCl ~ 10–40 mL/min	600 mg (PO) q12h
CrCl < 10 mL/min	600 mg (PO) q12h
Post–HD dose	None
Post–PD dose	600 mg (PO)
CVVH dose	600 mg (PO) q12h
Moderate hepatic insufficiency	300 mg (PO) q8h; use caution
Severe hepatic insufficiency	300 mg (PO) q12h; use caution

Drug Interactions: Aluminum-based antacids (↓ quinidine absorption); astemizole, cisapride, terfenadine (↑ interacting drug levels, torsade de pointes; avoid); cimetidine, ritonavir (↑ quinidine toxicity: headache, deafness, blindness, tachycardia); cyclosporine (↓ cyclosporine levels); digoxin (↑ digoxin levels); dofetilide, flecainide (arrhythmias); mefloquine (seizures, may ↑ QT interval, torsade de pointes, cardiac arrest, ↓ mefloquine efficacy); metformin (↑ risk of lactic acidosis); pancuronium, succinylcholine, tubocurarine (neuromuscular blockade); warfarin (↑ INR)
Adverse Effects: Drug fever/rash, ↑ QT_c interval, arrhythmias, drug-induced SLE, lightheadedness, diarrhea, abdominal discomfort, nausea, vomiting, cinchonism with chronic use. Avoid in patients with G6PD deficiency

---

"Usual dose" assumes normal renal/hepatic function. * For renal insufficiency, give usual dose x 1 followed by maintenance dose per CrCl. For dialysis patients, dose the same as for CrCl < 10 mL/min and give supplemental (post-HD/PD dose) immediately after dialysis. CrCl = creatinine clearance; CVVH = continuous veno-venous hemo-filtration; HD/PD = hemodialysis/peritoneal dialysis. See pp. 293-297 for explanations, p. 1 for abbreviations

Allergic Potential: High
Safety in Pregnancy: D
Comments: Tablets (sulfate salt) (100 mg, 200 mg, 300 mg). Tablets are not crushable
Cerebrospinal Fluid Penetration: 2-5%

REFERENCES:
Croft AM, Herxheimer A. Tolerability of antimalaria drugs. Clin Infect Dis 34:1278; discussion 1278-9, 2002.
Drugs for Parasitic Infections. Med Letter. March, 2000.
Panisko DM, Keystone JS. Treatment of malaria. Drugs 39:160-89, 1990.
Wyler DJ. Malaria: Overview and update. Clin Infect Dis 16:449-56, 1993.

Quinupristin/dalfopristin (Synercid)

Drug Class: Streptogramin
Usual Dose: 7.5 mg/kg (IV) q8h
Pharmacokinetic Parameters:
Peak serum level: 3.2/8 mcg/mL
Bioavailability: Not applicable
Excreted unchanged: 15/19%
Serum half-life (normal/ESRD): [3.1/1]/[3.1/1] hrs
Plasma protein binding: 55/15%
Volume of distribution (V_d): 0.45/0.24 L/kg
Primary Mode of Elimination: Hepatic
Dosage Adjustments*

CrCl ~ 40–60 mL/min	No change
CrCl ~ 10–40 mL/min	No change
CrCl < 10 mL/min	No change
Post–HD dose	None
Post–PD dose	None
CVVH dose	No change
Moderate hepatic insufficiency	No change
Severe hepatic insufficiency	No information

Drug Interactions: Amlodipine (↑ amlodipine toxicity); astemizole, cisapride (may ↑ QT interval, torsades de pointes); carbamazepine (↑ carbamazepine toxicity: ataxia, nystagmus, diplopia, headache, seizures); cyclosporine, delavirdine, indinavir, nevirapine (↑ interacting drug levels); diazepam, midazolam (↑ interacting drug effect); diltiazem, felodipine, isradipine (↑ interacting drug toxicity: dizziness, hypotension, headache, flushing); disopyramide (↑ disopyramide toxicity: arrhythmias, hypotension, syncope); docetaxel (↑ interacting drug toxicity: neutropenia, anemia, neuropathy); lidocaine (↑ lidocaine toxicity: neurotoxicity, arrhythmias, seizures); methylprednisolone (↑ methylprednisolone toxicity: myopathy, diabetes mellitus, cushing's syndrome); nicardipine, nifedipine, nimodipine (↑ interacting drug toxicity: dizziness, hypotension, flushing, headache); statins (↑ risk of rhabdomyolysis)
Adverse Effects: Pain, inflammation, and swelling at infusion site, severe/prolonged myalgias, hyperbilirubinemia. Hepatic insufficiency increases concentration (AUC) of metabolites by 180%/50%
Allergic Potential: Low
Safety in Pregnancy: B
Comments: Administer in D_5W or sterile water, not in saline. Requires central IV line for administration. Does not cover E. faecalis
Cerebrospinal Fluid Penetration: < 10%

REFERENCES:
Abb J. Comparative activity of linezolid, quinupristin-dalfopristin and newer quinolones against Streptococcus pneumoniae. Int J Antimicrob Agents. 21:289-91, 2003.
Blondeau JM, Sanche Se. Quinupristin/dalfopristin. Expert Opin Pharmacother 3:1341-64, 2002.
Bryson HM, Spencer CM. Quinupristin/dalfopristin. Drugs 52:406-15, 1996.
Chant C, Ryback MH. Quinupristin/dalfopristin (RP 59500): A new streptogramin antibiotic. Ann Pharmacother 29:1022-7, 1995.
Goff DA, Sierawski SJ. Clinical experience of quinupristin-dalfopristin for the treatment of antimicrobial-resistant gram-positive infections. Pharmacotherapy 22:748-58, 2002.
Griswold MW, Lomaestro BM, Briceland LL. Quinupristin-dalfopristin (RP 59500): An injectable streptogramin combination. Am J Health Syst Pharm. 53:2045-53, 1996.
Kim MK, Nicolau DP, Nightingale CH, et al.

Quinupristin/dalfopristin: A treatment option for vancomycin-resistant enterococci. Conn Med 64:209-12, 2000.

Klastersky J. Role of quinupristin/dalfopristin in the treatment of Gram-positive nosocomial infections in haematological or oncological patients. Cancer Treat Rev. 29:431-40, 2003.

Nadler H, Dowzicky MJ, Feger C, et al. Quinupristin/dalfopristin: A novel selective-spectrum antibiotic for the treatment of multi-resistant and other gram-positive pathogens. Clin Microbiol Newslett 21:103-12, 1999.

Scotton PG, Rigoli R, Vaglia A. Combination of quinupristin/dalfopristin and glycopeptide in severe methicillin-resistant staphylococcal infections failing previous glycopeptide regimen. Infection 30:161-3, 2002.

Website: www.synercid.com

Ribavirin (Rebetol) (Copegus)

Drug Class: Antiviral
Usual Dose: 400 mg (PO) q12h
Pharmacokinetic Parameters:
Peak serum level: 0.07-0.28 mcg/mL
Bioavailability: 64%
Excreted unchanged: 40%
Serum half-life (normal/ESRD): 120 hrs/no data
Plasma protein binding: 0%
Volume of distribution (V_d): 10 L/kg
Primary Mode of Elimination: Hepatic
Dosage Adjustments*

CrCl ~ 50–60 mL/min	No change
CrCl ~ 10–50 mL/min	Avoid
CrCl < 10 mL/min	Avoid
Post–HD dose	Avoid
Post–PD dose	Avoid
CVVH dose	Avoid
Moderate hepatic insufficiency	No change
Severe hepatic insufficiency	No change

Drug Interactions: Zidovudine (↓ zidovudine

efficacy)
Adverse Effects: Drug fever/rash, nausea, vomiting, GI upset, leukopenia, hyperbilirubinemia, hemolytic anemia, ↑ uric acid
Allergic Potential: Low
Safety in Pregnancy: X
Comments: For chronic HCV patients ≥ 75 kg, give 600 mg (PO) q12h; for patients < 75 kg, give 1 gm (PO) q24h in 2 divided doses. Administer with pegylated interferon (see pg. 75)
Cerebrospinal Fluid Penetration: No data

REFERENCES:
Davis GL, Esteban-Mur R, Rustgi V, et al. Interferon Alfa-2b alone or in combination with ribavirin for the treatment of relapse of chronic hepatitis C: International hepatitis interventional therapy group. N Engl J Med 339:1493-9, 1998.

Keating MR. Antiviral agents. Mayo Clin Proc 67:160-78, 1992.

McHutchison JG, Gordon SC, Schiff ER, et al. Interferon Alfa-2b alone or in combination with ribavirin as initial treatment for chronic hepatitis C. International therapy group. N Engl J Med 339:1485-92, 1998.

Ottolini MG, Hemming VG. Prevention and treatment recommendations for respiratory syncytial virus infection: Background and clinical experience 40 years after discovery. Drugs 54:867-84, 1997.

Website: www.rocheusa.com/products/

Rifabutin (Mycobutin)

Drug Class: Anti-MAI drug
Usual Dose: 300 mg (PO) q24h
Pharmacokinetic Parameters:
Peak serum level: 0.38 mcg/mL
Bioavailability: 20-50%
Excreted unchanged: 10%
Serum half-life (normal/ESRD): 45/45 hrs
Plasma protein binding: 85%
Volume of distribution (V_d): 9.3 L/kg
Primary Mode of Elimination: Hepatic
Dosage Adjustments*

CrCl ~ 40–60 mL/min	No change
CrCl ~ 10–40 mL/min	No change
CrCl < 10 mL/min	No change

"Usual dose" assumes normal renal/hepatic function. * For renal insufficiency, give usual dose x 1 followed by maintenance dose per CrCl. For dialysis patients, dose the same as for CrCl < 10 mL/min and give supplemental (post-HD/PD dose) immediately after dialysis. CrCl = creatinine clearance; CVVH = continuous veno-venous hemofiltration; HD/PD = hemodialysis/peritoneal dialysis. See pp. 293-297 for explanations, p. 1 for abbreviations

Post–HD dose	None
Post–PD dose	None
CVVH dose	None
Moderate hepatic insufficiency	No change
Severe hepatic insufficiency	No change

Drug Interactions: Atovaquone, amprenavir, indinavir, nelfinavir, ritonavir, clarithromycin, erythromycin, telithromycin, fluconazole, itraconazole, ketoconazole (↓ interacting drug levels, ↑ rifabutin levels); beta-blockers, clofibrate, cyclosporine, enalapril, oral contraceptives, quinidine, sulfonylureas, tocainide, warfarin (↓ interacting drug effect); corticosteroids (↑ corticosteroid requirement); delavirdine (↓ delavirdine levels, ↑ rifabutin levels; avoid); digoxin, phenytoin, propafenone, theophylline, zidovudine (↓ interacting drug levels); methadone (↓ methadone levels, withdrawal); mexiletine (↑ mexiletine clearance); protease inhibitors (↓ protease inhibitor levels, ↑ rifabutin levels; caution)

Adverse Effects: Brown/orange discoloration of body fluids, ↑ SGOT/SGPT, leukopenia, anemia, thrombocytopenia, drug fever, rash, headache, nausea, vomiting

Allergic Potential: High

Safety in Pregnancy: C

Comments: Avoid in leukopenic patients with WBC ≤ 1000 cells/mm³. Always used as part of a multi-drug regimen, never as monotherapy. Meningeal dose = usual dose

Cerebrospinal Fluid Penetration: 50%

REFERENCES:

Benson CA, Williams PL, Cohn DL, and the ACTG 196/CPCRA 009 Study Team. Clarithromycin or rifabutin alone or in combination for primary prophylaxis of Mycobacterium avium complex disease in patients with AIDS: A randomized, double-blinded, placebo-controlled trial. J Infect Dis 181:1289-97, 2000.

Centers for Disease Control and Prevention. Notice to readers: Updated guidelines for the use of rifabutin or rifampin for the treatment and prevention of tuberculosis among HIV-infected patients taking protease inhibitors or nonnucleoside reverse transcriptase inhibitors. MMWR 49:183-189, 2000.

Drugs for AIDS and associated infections. Med Lett Drug Ther 35:79-86, 1993.

Finch CK, Chrisman CR, Baciewicz AM, et al. Rifampin and rifabutin drug interactions: an update. Arch Intern Med 162:985-92, 2002.

Hoy J, Mijch A, Sandland M, et al. Quadruple-drug therapy for Mycobacterium avium-intracellulare bacteremia in AIDS patients. J Infect Dis 161:801-5, 1990.

Nightingale SD, Cameron DW, Gordin FM, et al. Two controlled trials of rifabutin prophylaxis against Mycobacterium avium complex infection in AIDS. N Engl J Med 329:828-33, 1993.

Panel on Clinical Practices for Treatment of HIV Infection. Guidelines for the use of antiretroviral agents in HIV-infected adults and adolescents. Department of Health and Human Services. **www.aidsinfo.nih.gov/guidelines/.** November 10, 2003.

Website: www.pdr.net

Rifampin (Rifadin, Rimactane)

Drug Class: Antibiotic/anti-TB drug
Usual Dose: 600 mg (PO) q24h
Pharmacokinetic Parameters:
Peak serum level: 7 mcg/mL
Bioavailability: 95%
Excreted unchanged: 15%
Serum half-life (normal/ESRD): 3.5/11 hrs
Plasma protein binding: 80%
Volume of distribution (V_d): 0.93 L/kg
Primary Mode of Elimination: Hepatic
Dosage Adjustments*

CrCl ~ 40–60 mL/min	No change
CrCl ~ 10–40 mL/min	No change
CrCl < 10 mL/min	No change
Post–HD dose	None
Post–PD dose	None
CVVH dose	No change

"Usual dose" assumes normal renal/hepatic function. * For renal insufficiency, give usual dose x 1 followed by maintenance dose per CrCl. For dialysis patients, dose the same as for CrCl < 10 mL/min and give supplemental (post-HD/PD dose) immediately after dialysis. CrCl = creatinine clearance; CVVH = continuous veno-venous hemofiltration; HD/PD = hemodialysis/peritoneal dialysis. See pp. 293-297 for explanations, p. 1 for abbreviations

| Moderate hepatic insufficiency | No change; use caution |
| Severe hepatic insufficiency | Avoid |

Drug Interactions: Amprenavir, indinavir, nelfinavir (↑ rifampin levels); beta-blockers, clofibrate, cyclosporine, oral contraceptives, quinidine, sulfonylureas, tocainamide, warfarin (↓ interacting drug effect); caspofungin (↓ caspofungin levels, may ↓ caspofungin effect); clarithromycin, ketoconazole (↑ rifampin levels, ↓ interacting drug levels); corticosteroids (↑ corticosteroid requirement); delavirdine (↑ rifampin levels, ↓ delavirdine levels; avoid); disopyramide, itraconazole, phenytoin, propafenone, theophylline, methadone, nelfinavir, ritonavir, tacrolimus, drugs whose metabolism is induced by rifampin, e.g., ACE inhibitors, dapsone, diazepam, digoxin, diltiazem, doxycycline, fluconazole, fluvastatin, haloperidol, nifedipine, progestins, triazolam, tricyclics, zidovudine (↓ interacting drug levels); fluconazole, TMP-SMX (↑ rifampin levels); INH (INH converted into toxic hydrazine); mexiletine (↑ mexiletine clearance); nevirapine (↓ nevirapine levels; avoid)

Adverse Effects: Red/orange discoloration of body secretions, flu–like symptoms, ↑ SGOT/SGPT, drug fever, rash, thrombocytopenia

Allergic Potential: Moderate

Safety in Pregnancy: Probably safe

Comments: For anti–TB therapy, monitor potential hepatotoxicity with serial SGOT/SGPTs weekly x 3, then monthly x 3. Take 1 hour before or 2 hours after meals. As an anti-staphylococcal drug (with another anti-staph antibiotic), give as 300 mg (PO) q12h. Meningeal dose = usual dose

Cerebrospinal Fluid Penetration:
Non-inflamed meninges = 50%
Inflamed meninges = 50%

Bile Penetration: 7000%

REFERENCES:
Cascio A, Scarlata F, Giordano S, et al. Treatment of human brucellosis with rifampin plus minocycline. J Chemother. 15:248-52, 2003.
Centers for Disease Control and Prevention. Notice to readers: Updated guidelines for the use of rifabutin or rifampin for the treatment and prevention of tuberculosis among HIV-infected patients taking protease inhibitors or nonnucleoside reverse transcriptase inhibitors. MMWR 49:183-189, 2000.
Davidson PT, Le HQ. Drug treatment of tuberculosis 1992. Drugs 43:651-73, 1992.
Giamarellos-Bourboulis EJ, Sambatakou H, Galani I, et al. In vitro interaction of colistin and rifampin on multidrug-resistant Pseudomonas aeruginosa. J Chemother. 15:235-8, 2003.
Havlir DV, Barnes PF. Tuberculosis in patients with human immunodeficiency virus infection. N Engl J Med 340:367-73, 1999.
Krause PJ, Corrow CL, Bakken JS. Successful treatment of human granulocytic ehrlichiosis in children using rifampin. Pediatrics. 112:e252-3, 2003.
Lundstrom TS, Sobel JD. Vancomycin, trimethoprim - sulfamethoxazole, and rifampin. Infect Dis Clin North Am 91:747-67, 1995.
Panel on Clinical Practices for Treatment of HIV Infection. Guidelines for the use of antiretroviral agents in HIV-infected adults and adolescents. Department of Health and Human Services. www.aidsinfo.nih.gov/guidelines/. November 10, 2003.
Van Scoy RE, Wilkowske CJ. Antituberculous agents. Mayo Clin Proc 67:179-87, 1992.
Vesely JJ, Pien FD, Pien BC. Rifampin, a useful drug for nonmyocobacterial infections. Pharmacotherapy 18:345-57, 1998.
Website: www.pdr.net

Rimantadine (Flumadine)

Drug Class: Antiviral
Usual Dose: 100 mg (PO) q12h
Pharmacokinetic Parameters:
Peak serum level: 0.7 mcg/mL
Bioavailability: 90%
Excreted unchanged: 25%
Serum half-life (normal/ESRD): 25/38 hrs
Plasma protein binding: 40%
Volume of distribution (V_d): 4.5 L/kg
Primary Mode of Elimination: Hepatic
Dosage Adjustments*

CrCl ~ 40–60 mL/min	No change
CrCl ~ 10–40 mL/min	No change
CrCl < 10 mL/min	100 mg (PO) q24h

"Usual dose" assumes normal renal/hepatic function. * For renal insufficiency, give usual dose x 1 followed by maintenance dose per CrCl. For dialysis patients, dose the same as for CrCl < 10 mL/min and give supplemental (post-HD/PD dose) immediately after dialysis. CrCl = creatinine clearance; CVVH = continuous veno-venous hemofiltration; HD/PD = hemodialysis/peritoneal dialysis. See pp. 293-297 for explanations, p. 1 for abbreviations

Post–HD dose	None
Post–PD dose	None
CVVH dose	None
Moderate hepatic insufficiency	No change
Severe hepatic insufficiency	100 mg (PO) q24h

Drug Interactions: Alcohol (↑ CNS effects); benztropine, trihexyphenidyl, scopolamine (↑ interacting drug effect: dry mouth, ataxia, blurred vision, slurred speech, toxic psychosis); cimetidine (↓ rimantadine clearance); CNS stimulants (additive stimulation); digoxin (↑ digoxin levels); trimethoprim (↑ rimantadine and trimethoprim levels)
Adverse Effects: Dizziness, headache, insomnia, anticholinergic effects (blurry vision, dry mouth, orthostatic hypotension, urinary retention, constipation)
Allergic Potential: Low
Safety in Pregnancy: C
Comments: Less anticholinergic side effects than amantadine. Patients ≥ 60 years old or with a history of seizures should receive 100 mg (PO) q24h
Cerebrospinal Fluid Penetration: No data

REFERENCES:
Dolin R, Reichman RC, Madore HP, et al. A controlled trial of amantadine and rimantadine in the prophylaxis of Influenza A infection. N Engl J Med 307:580-4, 1982.
Keating MR. Antiviral agents. Mayo Clin Proc 67:160-78, 1992.
Gravenstein S, Davidson HE. Current strategies for management of influenza in the elderly population. Clin Infect Dis 35:729-37, 2002.
Wintermeyer SM, Nahata MC. Rimantadine: A clinical perspective. Ann Pharmacotherapy 29:299-310, 1995.
Website: www.pdr.net

Ritonavir (Norvir)

Drug Class: Antiretroviral protease inhibitor
Usual Dose: 600 mg (PO) q12h (see comments)

Pharmacokinetic Parameters:
Peak serum level: 11 mcg/mL
Bioavailability: No data
Excreted unchanged: 3.5%
Serum half-life (normal/ESRD): 4 hrs/no data
Plasma protein binding: 99%
Volume of distribution (V_d): 0.4 L/kg
Primary Mode of Elimination: Hepatic
Dosage Adjustments*

CrCl ~ 40–60 mL/min	No change
CrCl ~ 10–40 mL/min	No change
CrCl < 10 mL/min	No change
Post–HD dose	None
Post–PD dose	None
CVVH dose	None
Moderate hepatic insufficiency	No change
Severe hepatic insufficiency	No change; use caution

Antiretroviral Dosage Adjustments:

Amprenavir	Ritonavir 100 mg q12h (or 200 mg q24h) + amprenavir 600 mg q12h (or 1200 mg q24h)
Delavirdine	Delavirdine: no change; ritonavir: No information
Efavirenz	Ritonavir 600 mg q12h (500 mg q12h for intolerance)
Indinavir	Ritonavir 100-200 mg q12h + indinavir 800 mg q12h, or 400 mg q12h of each drug
Nelfinavir	Ritonavir 400 mg q12h + nelfinavir 500-750 mg q12h

Nevirapine	No changes
Saquinavir	Ritonavir 400 mg q12h + saquinavir 400 mg q12h
Ketoconazole	Caution; do not exceed ketoconazole 200 mg q24h
Rifampin	Avoid
Rifabutin	Rifabutin 150 mg q48h or 3x/week

Drug Interactions: Antiretrovirals, rifabutin, rifampin (see dose adjustment grid, above); alprazolam, diazepam, estazolam, flurazepam, midazolam, triazolam, zolpidem, meperidine, propoxyphene, piroxicam, quinidine, amiodarone, encainide, flecainide, propafenone, astemizole, bepridil, bupropion, cisapride, clorazepate, clozapine, pimozide, St. John's wort, terfenadine (avoid); alfentanil, fentanyl, hydrocodone, tramadol, disopyramide, lidocaine, mexiletine, erythromycin, clarithromycin, warfarin, dronabinol, ondansetron, metoprolol, pindolol, propranolol, timolol, amlodipine, diltiazem, felodipine, isradipine, nicardipine, nifedipine, nimodipine, nisoldipine, nitrendipine, verapamil, etoposide, paclitaxel, tamoxifen, vinblastine, vincristine, loratadine, tricyclic antidepressants, paroxetine, nefazodone, sertraline, trazodone, fluoxetine, venlafaxine, fluvoxamine, cyclosporine, tacrolimus, chlorpromazine, haloperidol, perphenazine, risperidone, thioridazine, clozapine, pimozide, methamphetamine (↑ interacting drug levels); telithromycin (↑ ritonavir levels); codeine, hydromorphone, methadone, morphine, ketoprofen, ketorolac, naproxen, diphenoxylate, oral contraceptives, theophylline (↓ interacting drug levels); carbamazepine, phenytoin, phenobarbital, clonazepam, dexamethasone, prednisone (↓ ritonavir levels, ↑ interacting drug levels; monitor anticonvulsant levels); metronidazole (disulfiram-like reaction); tenofovir, tobacco (↓ ritonavir levels); sildenafil (↑ or ↓ sildenafil levels; do not exceed 25 mg in 48 hrs)

Adverse Effects: Anorexia, anemia, leukopenia, hyperglycemia (including worsening diabetes, new-onset diabetes, DKA), ↑ cholesterol/triglycerides (evaluate risk for coronary disease/pancreatitis), fat redistribution, ↑ CPK, nausea, vomiting, diarrhea, abdominal pain, circumoral/extremity paresthesias, ↑ SGOT/SGPT, pancreatitis, taste perversion, possible increased bleeding in hemophilia
Allergic Potential: Low
Safety in Pregnancy: B
Comments: GI intolerance decreases over time. Take with food if possible (serum levels increase 15%, fewer GI side effects). Dose escalation regimen: day 1-2 (300 mg q12h), day 3-5 (400 mg q12h), day 6-13 (500 mg q12h), day 14 (600 mg q12h). Separate dosing from ddI by 2 hours. Refrigerate capsules, not oral solution. Effective antiretroviral therapy consists of at least 3 antiretrovirals (same/different classes)
Cerebrospinal Fluid Penetration: < 10%

REFERENCES:
Cameron DW, Japour AJ, Xu Y, et al. Ritonavir and saquinavir combination therapy for the treatment of HIV infection. AIDS 13:213-224, 1999.
Deeks SG, Smith M, Holodniy M, et al. HIV-1 protease inhibitors: A review for clinicians. JAMA 277:145-53, 1997.
Kaul DR, Cinti SK, Carver PL, et al. HIV protease inhibitors: Advances in therapy and adverse reactions, including metabolic complications. Pharmacotherapy 19:281-98, 1999.
Lea AP, Faulds D. Ritonavir. Drugs 52:541-6, 1996.
McDonald CK, Kuritzkes DR. Human immunodeficiency virus type 1 protease inhibitors. Arch Intern Med 157:951-9, 1997.
Panel on Clinical Practices for Treatment of HIV Infection. Guidelines for the use of antiretroviral agents in HIV-infected adults and adolescents. Department of Health and Human Services. www.aidsinfo.nih.gov/guidelines/. November 10, 2003.
Piliero PJ. Interaction between ritonavir and statins. Am J Med 112:510-1, 2002.
Rathbun RC, Rossi DR. Low-dose ritonavir for protease inhibitor pharmacokinetic enhancement. Ann Pharmacother 36:702-6, 2002.
Website: www.TreatHIV.com

"Usual dose" assumes normal renal/hepatic function. * For renal insufficiency, give usual dose x 1 followed by maintenance dose per CrCl. For dialysis patients, dose the same as for CrCl < 10 mL/min and give supplemental (post-HD/PD dose) immediately after dialysis. CrCl = creatinine clearance; CVVH = continuous veno-venous hemofiltration; HD/PD = hemodialysis/peritoneal dialysis. See pp. 293-297 for explanations, p. 1 for abbreviations

Saquinavir (Invirase/Fortovase)

Drug Class: Antiretroviral protease inhibitor
Usual Dose: Saquinavir soft-gel capsule (Fortovase): 1200 mg (PO) q8h; saquinavir hard-gel capsule (Invirase): 600 mg (PO) q8h. Take with a meal or within 2 hours after a meal.
Pharmacokinetic Parameters:
Peak serum level: 0.07 mcg/mL
Bioavailability: hard-gel (4%)/soft-gel (15%)
Excreted unchanged: 13%
Serum half-life (normal/ESRD): 7 hrs/no data
Plasma protein binding: 98%
Volume of distribution (V_d): 10 L/kg
Primary Mode of Elimination: Hepatic
Dosage Adjustments*

CrCl ~ 40–60 mL/min	No change
CrCl ~ 10–40 mL/min	No change
CrCl < 10 mL/min	No change
Post–HD dose	None
Post–PD dose	None
CVVH dose	No change
Moderate hepatic insufficiency	No change
Severe hepatic insufficiency	Use caution

Antiretroviral Dosage Adjustments:

Amprenavir	No information
Delavirdine	Saquinavir soft-gel 800 mg q8h (monitor transaminases)
Efavirenz	Avoid use as sole PI
Indinavir	No information
Lopinavir/ritonavir 3 casules q12h	Saquinavir 800 mg q12h
Nelfinavir	Saquinavir soft-gel 800 mg q8h or 1200 mg q12h
Nevirapine	No information
Ritonavir	Ritonavir 400 mg q12h + saquinavir 400 mg q12h
Rifampin	Avoid unless given with ritonavir, then use rifampin 600 mg q24h or 2-3x/week
Rifabutin	Avoid if possible. No changes unless given with ritonavir, then give rifabutin 150 mg 2-3x/week

Drug Interactions: Antiretrovirals, rifabutin, rifampin (see dose adjustment grid, above); astemizole, terfenadine, benzodiazepines, cisapride, ergotamine, statins, St. John's wort (avoid if possible); carbamazepine, phenytoin, phenobarbital, dexamethasone, prednisone (↓ saquinavir levels, ↑ interacting drug levels; monitor anticonvulsant levels); clarithromycin, erythromycin, telithromycin (↑ saquinavir and macrolide levels); grapefruit juice, itraconazole, ketoconazole (↑ saquinavir levels); sildenafil (↑ or ↓ sildenafil levels; do not give > 25 mg in 48 hrs)
Adverse Effects: Anorexia, headache, anemia, leukopenia, hyperglycemia (including worsening diabetes, new-onset diabetes, DKA), ↑ cholesterol/triglycerides (evaluate risk for coronary disease/pancreatitis), ↑ SGOT/SGPT, hyperuricemia, fat redistribution, possible increased bleeding in hemophilia
Allergic Potential: Low
Safety in Pregnancy: B
Comments: Increased GI absorption with soft-gel capsules. Take with a large meal or within 2 hours of a large meal. Avoid garlic supplements, which ↓ saquinavir levels ~ 50%. Fortovase and Invirase capsules are not bioequivalent and cannot be used interchangeably. When using saquinavir as part of an antiviral regimen, Fortovase is the recommended formulation. Effective antiretroviral therapy consists of at least 3 antiretrovirals
Cerebrospinal Fluid Penetration: < 1%

"Usual dose" assumes normal renal/hepatic function. * For renal insufficiency, give usual dose x 1 followed by maintenance dose per CrCl. For dialysis patients, dose the same as for CrCl < 10 mL/min and give supplemental (post-HD/PD dose) immediately after dialysis. CrCl = creatinine clearance; CVVH = continuous veno-venous hemo-filtration; HD/PD = hemodialysis/peritoneal dialysis. See pp. 293-297 for explanations, p. 1 for abbreviations

REFERENCES:
Borck C. Garlic supplements and saquinavir. Clin Infect Dis 35:343, 2002.

Cameron DW, Japour AJ, Xu Y, et al. Ritonavir and saquinavir combination therapy for the treatment of HIV infection. AIDS 13:213-224, 1999.

Cardiello PF, van Heeswijk RP, Hassink EA, et al. Simplifying protease inhibitor therapy with once-daily dosing of saquinavir soft-gelatin capsules/ritonavir (1600/100 mg): HIVNAT 001.3 study. J Acquir Immune Defic Syndr 29:464-70, 2002.

Hsu A, Granneman GR, Cao G, et al. Pharmacokinetic interactions between two human immunodeficiency virus protease inhibitors, ritonavir and saquinavir. Clin Pharmacol Ther 63:453-64, 1998.

Murphy RL, Brun S, Hicks C, et al. ABT-378/ritonavir plus stavudine and lamivudine for the treatment of antiretroviral-naive patients with HIV-1 infection: 48-week results. AIDS 15:F1-9, 2001.

Noble S, Faulds D. Saquinavir: A review of its pharmacology and clinical potential in the management of HIV infection. Drugs 52:93-112, 1996.

Perry CM, Noble S. Saquinavir soft-gel capsule formation: A review of its use in patients with HIV infection. Drugs 55;461-86, 1998.

Panel on Clinical Practices for Treatment of HIV Infection. Guidelines for the use of antiretroviral agents in HIV-infected adults and adolescents. Department of Health and Human Services. www.aidsinfo.nih.gov/guidelines/. November 10, 2003.

Vella S, Floridia M. Saquinavir: Clinical pharmacology and efficacy. Clin Pharmacokinet 34:189-201, 1998.

Website: www.fortovase.com

Spectinomycin (Spectam, Trobicin)

Drug Class: Aminocyclitol
Usual Dose: 2 gm (IM) x 1 dose
Pharmacokinetic Parameters:
Peak serum level: 100 mcg/mL
Bioavailability: Not applicable
Excreted unchanged: 80%
Serum half-life (normal/ESRD): 1.6/16 hrs
Plasma protein binding: 20%
Volume of distribution (V_d): 0.25 L/kg
Primary Mode of Elimination: Renal
Dosage Adjustments*

CrCl ~ 40–60 mL/min	No change
CrCl ~ 10–40 mL/min	No change
CrCl < 10 mL/min	No change
Post–HD dose	None
Post–PD dose	None
CVVH dose	None
Moderate hepatic insufficiency	No change
Severe hepatic insufficiency	No change

Drug Interactions: None
Adverse Effects: Local pain at injection site
Allergic Potential: Low
Safety in Pregnancy: B
Comments: Ineffective in pharyngeal GC (poor penetration into secretions)
Cerebrospinal Fluid Penetration: < 10%

REFERENCES:
Fiumara NJ. The treatment of gonococcal proctitis: An evaluation of 173 patients treated with 4 gm of spectinomycin. JAMA 239:735-7, 1978.

Holloway WJ. Spectinomycin. Med Clin North Am 66:169-173, 1995.

McCormack WM, Finland M. Spectinomycin. Ann Intern Med 84:712-16, 1976.

Tapsall J. Current concepts in the management of gonorrhoea. Expert Opin Pharmacother 3:147-57, 2002.

Website: www.pdr.net

Stavudine (Zerit) d4t

Drug Class: Antiretroviral NRTI (nucleoside reverse transcriptase inhibitor)
Usual Dose: ≥ 60 kg: 40 mg (PO) q12h; < 60 kg: 30 mg (PO) q12h
Pharmacokinetic Parameters:
Peak serum level: 42 mcg/mL
Bioavailability: 86%
Excreted unchanged: 40%
Serum half-life (normal/ESRD): 1.0/5.1 hrs
Plasma protein binding: 0%
Volume of distribution (V_d): 0.5 L/kg
Primary Mode of Elimination: Renal

"Usual dose" assumes normal renal/hepatic function. * For renal insufficiency, give usual dose x 1 followed by maintenance dose per CrCl. For dialysis patients, dose the same as for CrCl < 10 mL/min and give supplemental (post-HD/PD dose) immediately after dialysis. CrCl = creatinine clearance; CVVH = continuous veno-venous hemofiltration; HD/PD = hemodialysis/peritoneal dialysis. See pp. 293-297 for explanations, p. 1 for abbreviations

Dosage Adjustments* ≥ 60 kg / [≤ 60 kg]

CrCl ~ 50–60 mL/min	40 mg (PO) q12h [30 mg (PO) q12h]
CrCl ~ 26–50 mL/min	20 mg (PO) q12h [15 mg (PO) q12h]
CrCl ~ 10-25 mL/min	20 mg (PO) q24h [15 mg (PO) q24h]
Post–HD dose	20 mg (PO) [15 mg (PO)]
Post–PD dose	No information
CVVH dose	20 mg (PO) q24h [15 mg (PO) q24h]
Moderate hepatic insufficiency	No change
Severe hepatic insufficiency	No change

Drug Interactions: Dapsone, INH, other neurotoxic agents (↑ risk of peripheral neuropathy)
Adverse Effects: Drug fever/rash, nausea, vomiting, GI upset, diarrhea, headache, insomnia, dose dependent peripheral neuropathy, myalgias, pancreatitis, ↑ SGOT/SGPT, thrombocytopenia, leukopenia, lactic acidosis with hepatic steatosis (rare, but potentially life-threatening toxicity with use of NRTIs)
Allergic Potential: Low
Safety in Pregnancy: C
Comments: Pancreatitis may be severe/fatal. Avoid coadministration with AZT or ddC. Decrease dose in patients with peripheral neuropathy to 20 mg (PO) q12h. Pregnant women may be at increased risk for lactic acidosis/liver damage when stavudine is used with didanosine (ddI)
Effective antiretroviral therapy consists of at least 3 antiretrovirals (same/different classes)
Cerebrospinal Fluid Penetration: 30%

REFERENCES:
Berasconi E, Boubaker K, Junghans C, et al Abnormalities of body fat distribution in HIV-infected persons treated with antiretroviral drugs: The Swiss HIV Cohort Study. J Acquir Immune Defic Syndr 31:50-5, 2002.
Dudley MN, Graham KK, Kaul S, et al. Pharmacokinetics of stavudine in patients with AIDS and AIDS-related complex. J Infect Dis 166:480-5, 1992.
FDA notifications. FDA changes information for stavudine label. Aids Alert 17:67, 2002.
Joly V, Flandre P, Meiffredy V, et al. Efficacy of zidovudine compared to stavudine, both in combination with lamivudine and indinavir, in human immunodeficiency virus-infected nucleoside-experienced patients with no prior exposure to lamivudine, stavudine, or protease inhibitors (Novavir trial). Antimicrob Agents Chemother 46:1906-13, 2002.
Lea AP, Faulds D. Stavudine: A review of its pharmacodynamic and pharmacokinetic properties and clinical potential in HIV infection. Drugs 51:846-64, 1996.
Miller KD, Cameron M, Wood LV, et al. Lactic acidosis and hepatic steatosis associated with use of stavudine: Report of four cases. Ann Intern Med. 133:192-196, 2000.
Murphy RL, Brun S, Hicks C, et al. ABT-378/ritonavir plus stavudine and lamivudine for the treatment of antiretroviral-naive adults with HIV-1 infection: 48-week results. AIDS 15:F1-9, 2001.
Panel on Clinical Practices for Treatment of HIV Infection. Guidelines for the use of antiretroviral agents in HIV-infected adults and adolescents. Department of Health and Human Services. www.aidsinfo.nih.gov/guidelines/. November 10, 2003.
Website: www.zerit.com

Streptomycin

Drug Class: Aminoglycoside
Usual Dose: 15 mg/kg (IM) q24h or 1 gm (IM) q24h (see comments)
Pharmacokinetic Parameters:
Peak serum level: 25-50 mcg/mL
Bioavailability: Not applicable
Excreted unchanged: 90%
Serum half-life (normal/ESRD): 2.5/100 hrs
Plasma protein binding: 35%
Volume of distribution (V_d): 0.26 L/kg
Primary Mode of Elimination: Renal
Dosage Adjustments*

CrCl ~ 50–60 mL/min	No change

CrCl ~ 10–50 mL/min	15 mg/kg (IM) q48h or 1 gm (IM) q48h
CrCl < 10 mL/min	15 mg/kg (IM) q72h or 1 gm (IM) q72h
Post–HD dose	7.5 mg/kg (IM) or 500 mg (IM)
Post–PD dose	7.5 mg/kg (IM) or 500 mg (IM)
CVVH dose	15 mg/kg (IM) or 1 gm (IM) q48h
Moderate hepatic insufficiency	No change
Severe hepatic insufficiency	No change

Drug Interactions: Amphotericin B, cephalothin, cyclosporine, enflurane, methoxyflurane, NSAIDs, polymyxin B, radiographic contrast, vancomycin (↑ nephrotoxicity); cis-platinum (↑ nephrotoxicity, ↑ ototoxicity); loop diuretics (↑ ototoxicity); neuromuscular blocking agents (↑ apnea, prolonged paralysis); non-polarizing muscle relaxants (↑ apnea)
Adverse Effects: Most ototoxic aminoglycoside (usually vestibular ototoxicity); least nephrotoxic aminoglycoside
Allergic Potential: Low
Safety in Pregnancy: D
Comments: May be given IV slowly over 1 hour. Dose for tularemia = 1 gm (IV/IM) q12h. Dose for plague = 2 gm (IV/IM) q12h. Dose for TB = 1 gm (IM) q24h 2-3x/week
Cerebrospinal Fluid Penetration: 20%

REFERENCES:
Akaho E, Maekawa T, Uchinashi M. A study of streptomycin blood level information of patients undergoing hemodialysis. Biopharm Drug Dispos 23:47-52, 2002.
Davidson PT, Le HQ. Drug treatment of tuberculosis 1992. Drugs 43:651-73, 1992.
Kim-Sing A, Kays MB, Vivien EJ, et al. Intravenous streptomycin use in a patient infection with high-level gentamicin-resistant Streptococcus faecalis. Ann Pharmacother 27:712-4, 1993.

Morris JT, Cooper RH. Intravenous streptomycin: A useful route of administration. Clin Infect Dis 19:1150-1, 1994.
Van Scoy RE, Wilkowske CJ. Antituberculous agents. Mayo Clin Proc 67:179-87, 1992.
Ormerod P. The clinical management of the drug-resistant patient. Ann NY Acad Sci 953:185-91, 2001.

Telithromycin (Ketek)

Drug Class: Ketolide
Usual Dose: 800 mg (PO) q24h, taken as two 400-mg tablets at once q24h
Pharmacokinetic Parameters:
Peak serum level: 2.27 mcg/mL
Bioavailability: 57%
Excreted unchanged: 20%
Serum half-life (normal/ESRD): 9.8/11 hrs
Plasma protein binding: 65%
Volume of distribution (V_d): No data
Primary Mode of Elimination: Hepatic
Dosage Adjustments*

CrCl ~ 40–60 mL/min	No change
CrCl ~ 10–30 mL/min	400 mg (PO) q24h
CrCl < 10 mL/min	400 mg (PO) q24h
Post–HD dose	800 mg
Post–PD dose	None
CVVH dose	None
Moderate hepatic insufficiency	No change
Severe hepatic insufficiency	No change

Drug Interactions: Cisapride (may ↑ QT interval, torsade de pointes); digoxin (↑ interacting drug levels); ergot derivatives (acute ergot toxicity); itraconazole, ketoconazole (↑ telithromycin levels, ↓ interacting drug levels); midazolam, triazolam (↑ interacting drug levels, sedation); simvastatin (↑ risk of rhabdomyolysis); theophylline (additive nausea)
Adverse Effects: Nausea, diarrhea, dizziness
Resistance Potential: Low

"Usual dose" assumes normal renal/hepatic function. * For renal insufficiency, give usual dose x 1 followed by maintenance dose per CrCl. For dialysis patients, dose the same as for CrCl < 10 mL/min and give supplemental (post-HD/PD dose) immediately after dialysis. CrCl = creatinine clearance; CVVH = continuous veno-venous hemofiltration; HD/PD = hemodialysis/peritoneal dialysis. See pp. 293-297 for explanations, p. 1 for abbreviations

Allergic Potential: Low
Safety in Pregnancy: C
Comments: May take with or without food

REFERENCES:

Bhargava V, Lenfant B, Perret C. Lack of effect of food on the bioavailability of a new ketolide antibacterial, telithromycin. Scan J Inf 2002;34:823-826.

Cantalloube C, Bhargava V, Sultan E. Pharmacokinetics of the ketolide telithromycin after single and repeated doses in patients with renal impairment. Int J Antimicro Agents 2003;22:112-121.

Carbon C, Moola S, Velancsics I, et al. Telithromycin 800 mg once daily for seven to ten days is an effective and well-tolerated treatment for community-acquired pneumonia. Clin Microbiol Infect 9:691-703, 2003.

Clark JP, Langston E. Ketolides: a new class of antibacterial agents for treatment of community acquired respiratory tract infections in a primary care setting. Mayo Clin Proc 2003;78:1113-1124.

Doern GV, Brown SD. Antimicrobial susceptibility among community acquired respiratory pathogens in the USA: data from PROTEKT US 2000-01. J Inf 2004;48:56-65.

Felmingham D. Microbiological profile of telithromycin, the first ketolide antimicrobial. Clin Microbiol Infect 7:2-10, 2001.

Kohno S, Hoban D, et al. Comparative in vitro activity of telithromycin and beta-lactam antimicrobials against bacterial respiratory pathogens from community-acquired respiratory tract infections: data from the first year of PROTEKT (1999-2000). J Chemother 15:335-41, 2003.

Zervos MJ, Heyder AM, Leroy B. Oral telithromycin 800 mg once daily for 5 days versus cefuroxime axetil 500 mg twice daily for 10 days in adults with acute exacerbations of chronic bronchitis. J Int Med Res 31:157-69, 2003.

Website: www.ketek.com

Tenofovir Disoproxil Fumarate (Viread)

Drug Class: Antiretroviral (nucleotide analogue)
Usual Dose: 300 mg (PO) q24h
Pharmacokinetic Parameters:
Peak serum level: 0.29 mcg/mL
Bioavailability: 25%/39% (fasting/high fat meal)
Excreted unchanged: 32%
Serum half-life (normal/ESRD): 17 hrs/no data
Plasma protein binding: 0.7-7.2%
Volume of distribution (V_d): 1.3 L/kg
Primary Mode of Elimination: Renal
Dosage Adjustments*

CrCl ≥ 50 mL/min	No change
CrCl ~ 30–49 mL/min	300 mg (PO) q48h
CrCl ~ 10-29 mL/min	300 mg (PO) q72-96h
CrCl < 10 mL/min	No information
Post–HD dose	300 mg q7d or after 12 hours on HD
Post–PD dose	No information
CVVH dose	No information
Moderate hepatic insufficiency	No change
Severe hepatic insufficiency	No change

Drug Interactions: Didanosine (↑ didanosine levels); no clinically significant interactions with lamivudine, lopinavir/ritonavir, efavirenz, methadone, oral contraceptives. Not a substrate/inhibitor of cytochrome P-450 enzymes
Adverse Effects: Mild nausea, vomiting, GI upset, diarrhea, lactic acidosis with hepatic steatosis (rare, but potentially life-threatening with NRTIs)
Allergic Potential: Low
Safety in Pregnancy: B
Comments: Eliminated by glomerular filtration/tubular secretion. May be taken with or without food. When administered with didanosine, consider reducing dose of didanosine. Excellent safety profile; side effects are few/mild. Effective antiretroviral therapy consists of at least 3 antiretrovirals (same/different classes)
Cerebrospinal Fluid Penetration: No data

REFERENCES:

Guidelines for the Use of Antiretroviral Agents for HIV-1-infected Adults and Adolescents: recommendations of the Panel on Clinical Practices for Treatment of HIV Infection; www.aidsinfo.gov/guidelines/,

---

"Usual dose" assumes normal renal/hepatic function. * For renal insufficiency, give usual dose x 1 followed by maintenance dose per CrCl. For dialysis patients, dose the same as for CrCl < 10 mL/min and give supplemental (post-HD/PD dose) immediately after dialysis. CrCl = creatinine clearance; CVVH = continuous veno-venous hemofiltration; HD/PD = hemodialysis/peritoneal dialysis. See pp. 293-297 for explanations, p. 1 for abbreviations

November 10, 2003.

Terrault NA. Treatment of recurrent hepatitis B infection in liver transplant recipients. Liver Transpl 8(Suppl 1):S74-81, 2002.

Thomson CA. Prodrug of tenofovir diphosphate approved for combination HIV therapy. Am J Health Syst Pharm 59:18, 2002.

Website: www.viread.com

Terbinafine (Lamisil, Daskil)

Drug Class: Antifungal
Usual Dose: 250 mg (PO) q24h
Pharmacokinetic Parameters:
Peak serum level: 1 mcg/mL
Bioavailability: 70%
Excreted unchanged: 75%
Serum half-life (normal/ESRD): 24 hrs/no data
Plasma protein binding: 99%
Volume of distribution (V_d): 13.5 L/kg
Primary Mode of Elimination: Renal/hepatic
Dosage Adjustments*

CrCl ~ 50–60 mL/min	No change
CrCl < 50 mL/min	Avoid
Post–HD dose	Avoid
Post–PD dose	Avoid
CVVH dose	Avoid
Moderate or severe hepatic insufficiency	Avoid

Drug Interactions: Cimetidine (↓ terbinafine clearance, ↑ terbinafine levels); phenobarbital, rifampin (↑ terbinafine clearance, ↓ terbinafine levels)
Adverse Effects: Drug fever/rash, lymphopenia, leukopenia, ↑ SGOT/SGPT, visual disturbances, nausea, vomiting, GI upset
Allergic Potential: Low
Safety in Pregnancy: B
Comments: May cause green vision and changes in the lens/retina
Cerebrospinal Fluid Penetration: < 10%

REFERENCES:
Abdel-Rahman SM, Nahata MC. Oral terbinafine: A new antifungal agent. Ann Pharmacother 31:445-56, 1997.

Amichai B, Grunwald MH. Adverse drug reactions of the new oral antifungal agents - terbinafine, fluconazole, and itraconazole. Int J Dermatol 37:410-5, 1998.

Darkes MJ, Scott LJ, Goa KL. Terbinafine: a review of its use in onychomycosis in adults. Am J Clin Dermatol. 4:39-65, 2003.

Gupta AK, Shear NH. Terbinafine: An update. J Am Acad Dermatol 37:979-88, 1997.

Jain S, Sehgal VN. Itraconazole versus terbinafine in the management of onychomycosis: an overview. J Dermatolog Treat. 14:30-42, 2003.

Mosquera J, Shartt A, Moore CB, et al. In vitro interaction of terbinafine with itraconazole, fluconazole, amphotericin B and 5-flucytosine against Aspergillus spp. J Antimicrob Chemother 50:189-94, 2002.

Salo H, Pekurinen M. Cost effectiveness or oral terbinafine (Lamisil) compared with oral fluconazole (Diflucan) in the treatment of patients with toenail onychomycosis. Pharmacoeconomics 20:319-24, 2002.

Trepanier EF, Amsden GW. Current issues in onychomycosis. Ann Pharmacother 32:204-14, 1998.

Website: www.pdr.net

Tetracycline (various)

Drug Class: Tetracycline
Usual Dose: 500 mg (PO) q6h
Pharmacokinetic Parameters:
Peak serum level: 1.5 mcg/mL
Bioavailability: 60%
Excreted unchanged: 5%
Serum half-life (normal/ESRD): 8/108 hrs
Plasma protein binding: 5%
Volume of distribution (V_d): 0.7 L/kg
Primary Mode of Elimination: Renal
Dosage Adjustments*

CrCl ~ 50–60 mL/min	500 mg (PO) q8h
CrCl ~ 10–50 mL/min	500 mg (PO) q12h
CrCl < 10 mL/min	Avoid
Post–HD dose	Avoid
Post–PD dose	Avoid
CVVH dose	Avoid

Moderate hepatic insufficiency	No change
Severe hepatic insufficiency	≤ 1 gm (PO) q24h

Drug Interactions: Antacids, Al^{++}, Ca^{++}, Fe^{++}, Mg^{++}, Zn^{++}, multivitamins, sucralfate (↓ absorption of tetracycline); barbiturates, carbamazepine, phenytoin (↓ half-life of tetracycline); bicarbonate (↓ absorption and ↑ clearance of tetracycline); digoxin (↑ digoxin levels); insulin (↑ insulin effect); methoxyflurane (↑ nephrotoxicity)

Adverse Effects: Nausea, vomiting, GI upset, diarrhea, hepatotoxicity, vaginal candidiasis, photosensitizing reactions, benign intracranial hypertension (pseudotumor cerebri)

Allergic Potential: Low

Safety in Pregnancy: D

Comments: Hepatotoxicity dose dependent (≥ 2 gm/day), especially in pregnancy/renal failure. Avoid prolonged sun exposure

Cerebrospinal Fluid Penetration:
Non-inflamed meninges = 5%
Inflamed meninges = 5%

Bile Penetration: 1000%

REFERENCES:
Cunha BA, Comer J, Jonas M. The tetracyclines. Med Clin North Am 66:293-302, 1982.
Donovan BJ, Weber DJ, Rublein JC, et al. Treatment of tick-borne diseases. Ann Pharmacother 36:1590-1597, 2002.
Pugliese A, Cunha BA. Tetraclyclines. Int J Urogyn 5:221-7, 1994.
Smilack JD, Wilson WE, Cocerill Fr 3rd. Tetracycline, chloramphenicol, erythromycin, clindamycin, and metronidazole. Mayo Clin Proc 66:1270-80, 1991.

Ticarcillin (Ticar)

Drug Class: Antipseudomonal penicillin

Usual Dose: 3 gm (IV) q6h

Pharmacokinetic Parameters:
Peak serum level: 118-300 mcg/mL
Bioavailability: Not applicable
Excreted unchanged: 85%
Serum half-life (normal/ESRD): 1/5 hrs
Plasma protein binding: 45%
Volume of distribution (V_d): 0.2 L/kg
Primary Mode of Elimination: Renal

Dosage Adjustments*

CrCl ~ 30–60 mL/min	2 gm (IV) q4h
CrCl ~ 10–30 mL/min	2 gm (IV) q8h
CrCl < 10 mL/min	2 gm (IV) q12h
Post–HD dose	2 gm (IV)
Post–PD dose	3 gm (IV)
CVVH dose	2 gm (IV) q8h
Moderate hepatic insufficiency	No change
Severe hepatic insufficiency	No change

Drug Interactions: Aminoglycosides (inactivation of ticarcillin in renal failure); warfarin (↑ INR); oral contraceptives (↓ oral contraceptive effect); cefoxitin (↓ ticarcillin effect)

Adverse Effects: Drug fever/rash; E. multiforme/Stevens–Johnson syndrome, anaphylactic reactions (hypotension, laryngospasm, bronchospasm), hives, serum sickness. Dose-dependent inhibition of platelet aggregation is minimal/absent (usual dose is less than carbenicillin)

Allergic Potential: High

Safety in Pregnancy: B

Comments: Administer 1 hour before or after aminoglycoside. Na^+ content = 5.2 mEq/g. Meningeal dose = usual dose

Cerebrospinal Fluid Penetration:
Non-inflamed meninges = 1%
Inflamed meninges = 30%

REFERENCES:
Donowitz GR, Mandell GL. Beta-lactam antibiotics. N Engl J Med 318:419-26 and 318:490-500, 1993.
Tan JS, File TM, Jr. Antipseudomonal penicillins. Med Clin North Am 79:679-93, 1995.
Wright AJ. The penicillins. Mayo Clin Proc 74:290-307, 1999.

Ticarcillin/clavulanate (Timentin)

Drug Class: Antipseudomonal penicillin
Usual Dose: 3.1 gm (IV) q6h
Pharmacokinetic Parameters:
Peak serum level: 330 mcg/mL
Bioavailability: Not applicable
Excreted unchanged: 70/45%
Serum half-life (normal/ESRD): [1/13]/[1/2] hrs
Plasma protein binding: 45/25%
Volume of distribution (V_d): 0.2/0.3 L/kg
Primary Mode of Elimination: Renal
Dosage Adjustments*

CrCl ~ 30–60 mL/min	2 gm (IV q4h)
CrCl ~ 10–30 mL/min	2 gm (IV) q8h
CrCl < 10 mL/min	2 gm (IV) q12h
Post–HD dose	2 gm (IV)
Post–PD dose	3.1 gm (IV)
CVVH dose	3.1 gm (IV) q8h
Moderate hepatic insufficiency	If CrCl < 10 mL/min: 2 gm (IV) q24h
Severe hepatic insufficiency	If CrCl < 10 mL/min: 2 gm (IV) q24h

Drug Interactions: Aminoglycosides (↓ aminoglycoside levels); methotrexate (↑ methotrexate levels); vecuronium (↑ vecuronium effect)
Adverse Effects: Drug fever/rash, E. multiforme/Stevens–Johnson syndrome, anaphylactic reactions (hypotension, laryngospasm, bronchospasm), hives, serum sickness
Allergic Potential: High
Safety in Pregnancy: B
Comments: 20% of clavulanate removed by dialysis. Na^+ content = 4.75 mEq/g. K^+ content = 0.15 mEq/g
Cerebrospinal Fluid Penetration: < 10%

REFERENCES:
Donowitz GR, Mandell GL. Beta-lactam antibiotics. N Engl J Med 318:419-26 and 318:490-500, 1993.
Graham DR, Talan DA, Nichols RL, et al. Once-daily, high-dose levofloxacin versus ticarcillin-clavulanate alone or followed by amoxicillin-clavulanate for complicated skin and skin-structure infections: a randomized, open-label trial. Clin Infect Dis 35:381-9, 2002.
Itokazu GS, Danziger LH. Ampicillin-sulbactam and ticarcillin-clavulanic acid: A comparison of their in vitro activity and review of their clinical efficacy. Pharmacotherapy 11:382-414, 1991.
Wright AJ. The penicillins. Mayo Clin Proc 74:290-307, 1999.
Website: www.timentin.com

TMP–SMX (Bactrim, Septra)

Drug Class: Folate antagonist/sulfonamide
Usual Dose: 2.5-5 mg/kg (IV/PO) q6h
Pharmacokinetic Parameters:
Peak serum level: 2-8/40-80 mcg/mL
Bioavailability: 98%
Excreted unchanged: 67/30%
Serum half-life (normal/ESRD): (10/8)/40-80 hrs
Plasma protein binding: 44-70%
Volume of distribution (V_d): 1.8/0.3 L/kg
Primary Mode of Elimination: Renal
Dosage Adjustments*

CrCl ~ 30–60 mL/min	No change
CrCl ~ 15-30 mL/min	1.25-2.5 mg/kg (IV/PO) q6h
CrCl < 15 mL/min	Avoid
Post–HD dose	Avoid
Post–PD dose	Avoid
CVVH dose	Avoid
Moderate hepatic insufficiency	No change
Severe hepatic insufficiency	No change

Drug Interactions: *TMP component:* Azathioprine (leukopenia); amantadine, dapsone, digoxin, methotrexate, phenytoin, rifampin, zidovudine (↑ interacting drug levels, nystagmus with phenytoin); diuretics (↑ serum

K⁺ with K⁺-sparing diuretics, ↓ serum Na⁺ with thiazide diuretics); warfarin (↑ INR, bleeding). *SMX component*: Cyclosporine (↓ cyclosporine levels); phenytoin (↑ phenytoin levels, nystagmus, ataxia); methotrexate (↑ antifolate activity); sulfonylureas, thiopental (↑ interacting drug effect); warfarin (↑ INR, bleeding)

Adverse Effects:
TMP: Folate deficiency, hyperkalemia
SMX: Leukopenia, thrombocytopenia, hemolytic anemia ± G6PD deficiency, aplastic anemia, ↑ SGOT/SGPT, severe hypersensitivity reactions (E. multiforme/Stevens–Johnson syndrome)

Allergic Potential: Very high (SMX); none (TMP)

Safety in Pregnancy: X

Comments: Drug fever/rash increased in HIV/AIDS. Excellent bioavailability (IV = PO).
1 SS tablet = 80 mg TMP + 400 mg SMX.
1 DS tablet = 160 mg TMP + 800 mg SMX.
1 SS tablet (PO) q6h = 10 mg/kg (IV) q24h.
1 DS tablet (PO) q6h = 20 mg/kg (IV) q24h.
Meningeal dose = 5 mg/kg (IV/PO) q6h

Cerebrospinal Fluid Penetration:
Non-inflamed meninges = 40%
Inflamed meninges = 40%

Bile Penetration: 100%

REFERENCES:
Cockerill FR, Edson RS. Trimethoprim-sulfamethoxazole. Mayo Clin Proc 66:1260-9, 1991.
El-Sadr W, Luskin-Hawk R, Yurik TM, et al. A randomized trial of daily and thrice weekly trimethoprim-sulfamethoxazole for the prevention of Pneumocystis carinii pneumonia in HIV infected individuals. Clin Infect Dis 29:775-83, 1999.
Giannakopoulos G, Johnson ES. TMP-SMX. Antibiotics for Clinicians 1:63-9, 1997.
Lundstrom TS, Sobel JD. Vancomycin, trimethoprim-sulfamethoxazole, and rifampin. Infect Dis Clin North Am 9:747-67, 1995.
Nicolle LE. Urinary tract infection: traditional pharmacologic therapies. Am J Med 113(Suppl 1A):35S-44S, 2002.
Para MF, Dohn M, Frame P, et al, for the ACTG 268 dapsoneStudy Team. Reduced toxicity with gradual initiation of trimethoprim-sulfamethoxazole as primary prophylaxis for Pneumocystis carinii pneumonia: AIDS Clinical Trials Group 268. J Acquire Immune Defic Syndr 24:337-43, 2000.
Schaffer AJ. Empiric use of trimethoprim-

sulfamethoxazole (TMP-SMX) in the treatment of women with uncomplicated urinary tract infections, in a geographic area with a high prevalence of TMP-SMX-resistance uropathogens. J Urol 168 (4 Pt 1):1652-3, 2002.
Smith LG, Sensakovic J. Trimethoprim-sulfamethoxazole. Med Clin North Am 66:143-56, 1982.
Website: www.pdr.net

Tobramycin (Nebcin)

Drug Class: Aminoglycoside
Usual Dose: 5 mg/kg (IV) q24h or 240 mg (IV) q24h (preferred over q8h dosing)

Pharmacokinetic Parameters:
Peak serum levels: 4-8 mcg/mL (q8h dosing); 16-24 mcg/mL (q24h dosing)
Bioavailability: Not applicable
Excreted unchanged: 95%
Serum half-life (normal/ESRD): 2.5/56 hrs
Plasma protein binding: 10%
Volume of distribution (V_d): 0.24 L/kg

Primary Mode of Elimination: Renal
Dosage Adjustments*

CrCl ~ 40–60 mL/min	2.5 mg/kg (IV) q24h or 120 mg (IV) q24h
CrCl ~ 10–40 mL/min	2.5 mg/kg (IV) q48h or 120 mg (IV) q48h
CrCl < 10 mL/min	1.25 mg/kg (IV) q48h or 60 mg (IV) q48h
Post–HD dose	1.25 mg/kg (IV) or 80 mg (IV)
Post–PD dose	0.6 mg/kg (IV) or 40 mg (IV)
CVVH dose	2.5 mg/kg (IV) or 120 mg (IV) q48h
Moderate hepatic insufficiency	No change
Severe hepatic insufficiency	No change

Drug Interactions: Amphotericin B, cyclosporine, enflurane, methoxyflurane,

---

"Usual dose" assumes normal renal/hepatic function. * For renal insufficiency, give usual dose x 1 followed by maintenance dose per CrCl. For dialysis patients, dose the same as for CrCl < 10 mL/min and give supplemental (post-HD/PD dose) immediately after dialysis. CrCl = creatinine clearance; CVVH = continuous veno-venous hemo-filtration; HD/PD = hemodialysis/peritoneal dialysis. See pp. 293-297 for explanations, p. 1 for abbreviations

NSAIDs, polymyxin B, radiographic contrast, vancomycin (↑ nephrotoxicity); cis-platinum (↑ nephrotoxicity, ↑ ototoxicity); loop diuretics (↑ ototoxicity); neuromuscular blocking agents (↑ apnea, prolonged paralysis); non-polarizing muscle relaxants (↑ apnea)

Adverse Effects: Neuromuscular blockade with rapid infusion/absorption. Nephrotoxicity only with prolonged/extremely high serum trough levels; may cause reversible non–oliguric renal failure (ATN). Ototoxicity associated with prolonged/extremely high peak serum levels (usually irreversible): Cochlear toxicity (1/3 of ototoxicity) manifests as decreased high frequency hearing, but deafness is unusual. Vestibular toxicity (2/3 of ototoxicity) develops before ototoxicity, and typically manifests as tinnitus

Allergic Potential: Low

Safety in Pregnancy: C

Comments: Dose for synergy = 2.5 mg/kg (IV) q24h or 120 mg (IV) q24h. Single daily dosing greatly reduces nephrotoxic/ototoxic potential. Incompatible with solutions containing β–lactams, erythromycin, chloramphenicol, furosemide, sodium bicarbonate. IV infusion should be given slowly over 1 hour. May be given IM. Avoid intraperitoneal infusion due to risk of neuromuscular blockade. Avoid intratracheal/aerosolized intrapulmonary instillation, which predisposes to antibiotic resistance. V_d increases with edema/ascites, trauma, burns, cystic fibrosis; may require ↑ dose. V_d decreases with dehydration, obesity; may require ↓ dose. Renal cast counts are the best indicator of aminoglycoside nephrotoxicity, not serum creatinine. Dialysis removes ~ 1/3 of tobramycin from serum

Therapeutic Serum Concentrations:
Peak (q24h/q8h dosing) = 16-24/8-10 mcg/mL
Trough (q24h/q8h dosing) = 0/1-2 mcg/mL
Dose for synergy = 2.5 mg/kg (IV) q24h or 120 mg (IV) q24h
Intrathecal (IT) dose = 5 mg (IT) q24h

Cerebrospinal Fluid Penetration:
Non-inflamed meninges = 0%
Inflamed meninges = 20%

Bile Penetration: 30%

REFERENCES:
Begg EJ, Barclay ML. Aminglycosides - 50 years on. Br J Clin Pharmacol 39:597-603, 1995.
Buijk SE, Mouton JW, Gyssens IC, et al. Experience with a once-daily dosing program of aminoglycosides in critically ill patients. Intensive Care Med 28:936-42, 2002.
Cheer SM, Waugh J, Noble S. Inhaled tobramycin (TOBI): a review of its use in the management of Pseudomonas aeruginosa infections in patients with cystic fibrosis. Drugs. 63:2501-20, 2003.
Cunha BA. Aminoglycosides: Current role in antimicrobial therapy. Pharmacotherapy 8: 334-50, 1988.
Edson RS, Terrel CL. The aminoglycosides. Mayo Clin Proc 74:519-28, 1999.
Geller DE, Pistlick WH, Nardella PA, et al. Pharmacokinetics and bioavailability of aerosolized tobramycin in cystic fibrosis. Chest 122:219-26, 2002.
Gilbert DN. Once-daily aminoglycoside therapy. Antimicrob Agents Chemother 35:399-405, 1991.
Hustinx WN, Hoepelman IM. Aminoglycoside dosage regimens: Is once a day enough? Clin Pharmacokinet 25:427-32, 1993.
Kahler DA, Schowengerdt KO, Fricker FJ, et al. Toxic serum trough concentrations after administration of nebulized tobramycin. Pharmacotherapy. 23:543-5, 2003.
Lortholary O, Tod M, Cohen Y, et al. Aminoglycosides. Med Clin North Am 79:761-87, 1995.
McCormack JP, Jewesson PJ. A critical reevaluation of the "therapeutic range" of aminoglycosides. Clin Infect Dis 14:320-39, 1992.
Moss RB. Long-term benefits of inhaled tobramycin in adolescent patients with cystic fibrosis. Chest 121:55-63, 2002.
Whitehead A, Conway SP, Etherington C, et al. Once-daily tobramycin in the treatment of adult patients with cystic fibrosis. Eur Respir J 19:303-9, 2002.
Website: www.pdr.net

Trimethoprim (Proloprim, Trimpex)

Drug Class: Folate antagonist
Usual Dose: 100 mg (PO) q12h
Pharmacokinetic Parameters:
Peak serum level: 2-8 mcg/mL
Bioavailability: 98%
Excreted unchanged: 67%
Serum half-life (normal/ESRD): 8/24 hrs

"Usual dose" assumes normal renal/hepatic function. * For renal insufficiency, give usual dose x 1 followed by maintenance dose per CrCl. For dialysis patients, dose the same as for CrCl < 10 mL/min and give supplemental (post-HD/PD dose) immediately after dialysis. CrCl = creatinine clearance; CVVH = continuous veno-venous hemofiltration; HD/PD = hemodialysis/peritoneal dialysis. See pp. 293-297 for explanations, p. 1 for abbreviations

Plasma protein binding: 44%
Volume of distribution (V_d): 1.8L/kg
Primary Mode of Elimination: Renal
Dosage Adjustments*

CrCl ~ 30–60 mL/min	No change
CrCl ~ 15–30 mL/min	50 mg (PO) q12h
CrCl < 15 mL/min	Not recommended
Post–HD dose	100 mg (PO)
Post–PD dose	100 mg (PO)
CVVH dose	50 mg (PO) q12h
Moderate hepatic insufficiency	No change
Severe hepatic insufficiency	No change

Drug Interactions: Azathioprine (leukopenia); amantadine, dapsone, digoxin, methotrexate, phenytoin, rifampin, zidovudine (↑ interacting drug levels, nystagmus with phenytoin); diuretics (↑ serum K^+ with K^+-sparing diuretics, ↓ serum Na^+ with thiazide diuretics); warfarin (↑ INR, bleeding)
Adverse Effects: Folate deficiency
Allergic Potential: Low
Safety in Pregnancy: X
Comments: Useful in sulfa-allergic patients unable to take TMP-SMX.
Meningeal dose = 300 mg (PO) q6h
Cerebrospinal Fluid Penetration: 40%

REFERENCES:

Brogden RN, Carmine AA, Heel RC, et al. Trimethoprim: A review of its antibacterial activity, pharmacokinetics and therapeutic use in urinary tract infections. Drugs 23:405-30, 1982.

Friesen WT, Hekster YA, Vree TB. Trimethoprim: Clinical use and pharmacokinetics. Drug Intelligence & Clinical Pharmacy 15:325-30, 1981.

Neu HC. Trimethoprim alone for treatment of urinary tract infection. Rev Infect Dis 4:366-71, 1982.

Website: www.pdr.net

Trimethoprim-Sulfamethoxazole, see TMP–SMX (Bactrim, Septra)

Valacyclovir (Valtrex)

Drug Class: Antiviral (HSV, VZV)
Usual Dose: <u>VZV</u>: 1 gm (PO) q8h x 7 days; <u>HSV-genital, initial</u>: 1 gm (PO) q12h x 10 days; <u>HSV-genital, recurrence</u>: 500 mg (PO) q12h x 3 days; <u>HSV-genital, suppression</u>: 1 gm (PO) q24h (alternate dose of 500 mg [PO] q24h for ≤ 9 recurrences/year); <u>HSV-genital, reduce risk of transmission</u>: 500 mg (PO) q24h; <u>HSV-oral</u>: 2 gm (PO) q12h x 1 day; <u>HSV-genital, suppression in HIV patients</u>: 500 mg (PO) q12h
Pharmacokinetic Parameters:
Peak serum level: 3.3–5.7 mcg/mL
Bioavailability: 55%
Excreted unchanged: 1%
Serum half-life (normal/ESRD): 2.5-3.3/14 hrs
Plasma protein binding: 15%
Primary Mode of Elimination: Renal
Dosage Adjustments* (based on 1 gm q8h) (go to www.valtrex.com for dosage adjustments based on other treatment regimens):

CrCl ~ 30–49 mL/min	1 gm (PO) q12h
CrCl ~ 10-29 mL/min	1 gm (PO) q24h
CrCl < 10 mL/min	500 mg (PO) q24h
Post–HD dose	Give daily dose (based on CrCl) post-HD
Post–PD dose	No information
CVVH dose	Dose based on CrCl
Moderate or severe hepatic insufficiency	No change

Drug Interactions: Cimetidine, probenecid (↑ acyclovir levels in renal insufficiency)
Adverse Effects: Headache, nausea, abdominal pain, dizziness, vomiting. Fatigue, headache,

rash in HIV patients
Allergic Potential: Low
Safety in Pregnancy: B
Comments: Converted to acyclovir in intestine and/or liver.

REFERENCES:
Acost EP, Fletcher CV. Valacyclovir. Ann Pharmacotherapy 31:185-91, 1997.
Alrabiah FA, Sacks SL. New antiherpesvirus agents: Their targets and therapeutic potential. Drugs 52:17-32, 1996.
Baker DA. Valacyclovir in the treatment of genital herpes and herpes zoster. Expert Opin Pharmacother 3:51-8, 2002.
Corey L, Wald A, Patel R, et al. Once-daily valacyclovir to reduce the risk of transmission of genital herpes. N Engl J Med 350:11-20, 2004.
Fiddian P, Sabin CA, Griffiths PD. Valacyclovir provides optimum acyclovir exposure for prevention of cytomegalovirus and related outcomes after argan transplantation. J Infect Dis 186(Suppl 1):S110-5, 2002.
Geers TA, Isada CM. Update on antiviral therapy for genital herpes infection. Cleve Clinic J Med 67:567-73, 2000.
Leone PA, Trottier S, Miller JM. Valacyclovir for episodic treatment of genital herpes: a shorter 3-day treatment course compared with 5-day treatment. Clin Infect Dis 34:958-62, 2002.
Ljungman P, de La Camara R, Milpied N, et al. Randomized study of valacyclovir as prophylaxis against cytomegalovirus reactivation in recipients of allogeneic bone marrow transplants. Blood 99:3050-6, 2002.
Perry CM, Faulds D. Valacyclovir: A review of its antiviral activity, pharmacokinetic properties, and therapeutic efficacy in herpesvirus infections. Drugs 52:754-72, 1996.
Tyring SK, Baker D, Snowden W. Valacyclovir for herpes simplex virus infection: long-term safety and sustained efficacy after 20 years' experience with acyclovir. J Infect Dis 186(Suppl 1):S40-6, 2002.
Warkentin DI, Epstein JB, Campbell LM, et al. Val-acyclovir vs acyclovir for HSV prophylaxis in neutro-penic patients. Ann Pharmacother 36:1525-31, 2002.
Website: www.valtrex.com

Valganciclovir (Valcyte)

Drug Class: Antiviral, Nucleoside inhibitor/analogue
Usual Dose: 900 mg (PO) q12h x 21 days

(induction), then 900 mg (PO) q24h for life (maintenance)
Pharmacokinetic Parameters:
Peak serum level: 5.6 mcg/mL
Bioavailability: 59.4%
Excreted unchanged: 90%
Serum half-life (normal/ESRD): 4.1/67.5 hrs
Plasma protein binding: 1%
Volume of distribution (V$_d$): 15.3 L/kg
Primary Mode of Elimination: Renal
Dosage Adjustments*

CrCl ~ 40–59 mL/min	450 mg (PO) q12h (induction), then 450 mg (PO) q24h (maintenance)
CrCl ~ 25–39 mL/min	450 mg (PO) q24h (induction), then 450 mg (PO) q48h (maintenance)
CrCl ~ 10–24 mL/min	450 mg (PO) q48h (induction), then 450 mg (PO) 2x/week (maintenance)
CrCl < 10 mL/min	No information
Post–HD dose	Avoid
Post–PD dose	No information
CVVH dose	No information
Moderate hepatic insufficiency	No change
Severe hepatic insufficiency	No change

Drug Interactions: Cytotoxic drugs (may produce additive toxicity: stomatitis, bone marrow depression, alopecia); imipenem (↑ risk of seizures); probenecid (↑ valganciclovir levels); zidovudine (↓ valganciclovir levels, ↑ zidovudine levels, possible neutropenia)
Adverse Effects: Drug fever/rash, diarrhea, nausea, vomiting, GI upset, leukopenia, anemia, thrombocytopenia, paresthesias/peripheral neuropathy, retinal detachment, aplastic anemia
Allergic Potential: Low

"Usual dose" assumes normal renal/hepatic function. * For renal insufficiency, give usual dose x 1 followed by maintenance dose per CrCl. For dialysis patients, dose the same as for CrCl < 10 mL/min and give supplemental (post-HD/PD dose) immediately after dialysis. CrCl = creatinine clearance; CVVH = continuous veno-venous hemo-filtration; HD/PD = hemodialysis/peritoneal dialysis. See pp. 293-297 for explanations, p. 1 for abbreviations

Safety in Pregnancy: C

Comments: Valganciclovir exposures (AUC) larger than for IV ganciclovir. Tablets should be taken with food. Valganciclovir is rapidly hydrolyzed to ganciclovir. Indicated for induction/maintenance therapy of CMV retinitis/infection. Not interchangeable on a tablet-to-tablet basis with oral ganciclovir. Much higher bioavailability than ganciclovir capsules; serum concentration equivalent to IV ganciclovir. Meningeal dose = usual dose

Cerebrospinal Fluid Penetration: 70%

REFERENCES:
[No authors listed] Valganciclovir: new preparation. CMV retinitis: a simpler, oral treatment. Prescrire Int. 12:133-5, 2003.
Cocohoba JM, McNicholl IR. Valganciclovir: an advance in cytomegalovirus therapeutics. Ann Pharmacother 36:1075-9, 2002.
Czock D, Scholle C, Rasche FM, et al. Pharmacokinetics of valganciclovir and ganciclovir in renal impairment. Clin Pharmacol Ther 72:142-50, 2002.
Jung D, Dorr A. Single-dose pharmacokinetics of valganciclovir in HIV and CMV seropositive subjects. J Clin Pharmacol 39:800-804, 1999.
Martin DF, Sierra-Madero J, Walmsley S, et al. A controlled trial of valganciclovir as induction therapy for cytomegalovirus retinitis. N Engl J Med 346:1119-26, 2002.
Pescovitz MD, Rabkin J, Merion RM, et al. Valganciclovir results in improved oral absorption of ganciclovir in liver transplant recipients. Antimicrob Agents Chemother 44:2811-15, 2000.
Segarra-Newnham M, Salazar MI. Valganciclovir: A new oral alternative for cytomegalovirus retinitis in human immunodeficiency virus-seropositive individuals. Pharmacotherapy 22:1124-8, 2002.
Website: www.rocheusa.com/products/

Vancomycin (Vancocin)

Drug Class: Glycopeptide
Usual Dose: 1 gm (IV) q12h (see comments)
Pharmacokinetic Parameters:
Peak serum level: 63 mcg/mL
Bioavailability: IV (not applicable)/PO (0%)
Excreted unchanged: 90%
Serum half-life (normal/ESRD): 6/180 hrs
Plasma protein binding: 55%
Volume of distribution (V_d): 0.7 L/kg

Primary Mode of Elimination: Renal
Dosage Adjustments*

CrCl ~ 40–60 mL/min	500 mg (IV) q12h
CrCl ~ 10–40 mL/min	500 mg (IV) q24h
CrCl < 10 mL/min	1 gm (IV) qweek
Post–HD dose	None
Post–PD dose	None
CVVH dose	1 gm (IV) q24h
Moderate hepatic insufficiency	No change
Severe hepatic insufficiency	No change

Drug Interactions: Aminoglycosides, amphotericin B, polymyxin B (↑ nephrotoxicity)
Adverse Effects: "Red man/neck syndrome" with rapid IV infusion (histamine mediated), leukopenia, cardiac arrest, hypotension
Allergic Potential: Low
Safety in Pregnancy: C
Comments: Not nephrotoxic. "Red man/neck syndrome" can be prevented/minimized by infusing IV vancomycin slowly over 1–2 hours. Intraperitoneal absorption = 40%. IV vancomycin use increases prevalence of VRE. For C. difficile diarrhea, use oral vancomycin 125 mg (PO) q6h. Vancomycin (IV/PO) ineffective for C. difficile colitis. Intrathecal (IT) dose = 20 mg (IT) in preservative free NaCl

Therapeutic Serum Concentrations:
Peak = 25-40 mcg/mL
Trough = 5-12 mcg/mL
Potentially toxic peak levels: ≥ 80 mcg/mL

Cerebrospinal Fluid Penetration:
Non-inflamed meninges = 0%
Inflamed meninges = 25%

Bile Penetration: 50%

REFERENCES:
Cantu TG, Yamanaka-Yuen NA, Lietman PS. Serum vancomycin concentrations: Reappraisal of their clinical value. Clin Infect Dis 18:533-43, 1994.
Cohen E, Dadashev A, Drucker M, et al. Once-daily versus twice-daily intravenous administration of

vancomycin for infections in hospitalized patients. J
Antimicrob chemother 49:155-60, 2002.

Cunha BA, Deglin J, Chow M, et al. Pharmacokinetics of
vancomycin in patients undergoing chronic
hemodialysis. Rev Infect Dis 3:269-72, 1981.

Cunha BA. Vancomycin. Med Clin North Am 79:817-
31, 1995.

Hamilton-Miller JM. Vancomycin-resistant
Staphylococcus aureus: a real and present danger?
Infection 30:118-24, 2002.

Lacy MK, Tessier PR, Nicolau DP, et al. Comparison of
vancomycin pharmacodynamics (1 gm every 12 or 25
h) against methicillin-resistant staphylococci. Intern J
Antimicrob Agents 15:25-30, 2000.

Menzies D. Goel K, Cunha BA. Vancomycin. Antibiotics
for Clinicians 2:97-9, 1998.

Website: www.pdr.net

Voriconazole (Vfend)

Drug Class: Antifungal (triazole)
Usual Dose: IV dosing: Loading dose of 6
mg/kg (IV) q12h x 1 day, then maintenance
dose of 4 mg/kg (IV) q12h. Can switch to
weight-based PO maintenance dosing anytime
while on maintenance IV dose (see comments)
PO dosing: Weight ≥ 40 kg: Loading dose of
400 mg (PO) q12h x 1 day, then maintenance
dose of 200 mg (PO) q12h. Weight < 40 kg:
Loading dose of 200 mg (PO) x 1 day, then
maintenance dose of 100 mg (PO) q12h. For
chronic/non-life-threatening infections, loading
dose may be given PO (see comments)
Pharmacokinetic Parameters:
Peak serum level: 2.3-4.7 mcg/mL
Bioavailability: 96%
Excreted unchanged: 1.5%
Serum half-life (normal/ESRD): 6/6 hrs
Plasma protein binding: 58%
Volume of distribution (V_d): 4.6 L/kg
Primary Mode of Elimination: Hepatic
Dosage Adjustments*

CrCl ~ 50–60 mL/min	No change
CrCl ~ 10–50 mL/min	No change PO; do not use IV
CrCl < 10 mL/min	No change PO; do not use IV

Post–HD dose	None
Post–PD dose	No information
CVVH dose	No information
Moderate hepatic insufficiency	6 mg/kg (IV) q12h x 1 day or 200 mg (PO) q12h x 1 day, then 2 mg/kg (IV) q12h or 100 mg (PO) q12h (> 40 kg)
Severe hepatic insufficiency	No information

Drug Interactions: Benzodiazepines, vinca
alkaloids (↑ interacting drug levels);
carbamazepine, ergot alkaloids, rifampin,
rifabutin, sirolimus, long-acting barbiturates
(contraindicated with voriconazole);
cyclosporine, omeprazole (↑ interacting drug
levels, ↓ interacting drug dose by 50%);
tacrolimus (↑ tacrolimus levels, ↓ tacrolimus
dose by 66%); phenytoin (↓ voriconazole levels);
↑ voriconazole dosee from 4 mg/kg [IV] to 5
mg/kg [IV] and from 200 mg [PO] to 400 mg
[PO]; warfarin (↑ INR); statins (↑ risk of
rhabdomyolysis); dihydropyridine calcium
channel blockers (hypotension); sulfonylureas
(hypoglycemia). Voriconazole has not been
studied with protease inhibitors or NNRTI's, but
↑ voriconazole levels are predicted (↑
hepatotoxicity/adverse effects)
Adverse Effects: ↑ SGOT/SGPT; dose-
dependent arrhythmias, hepatotoxicity, visual
events (blurring vision, ↑ brightness, pain; effect
on vision is not know > 28 days of therapy) ↑
QT_c interval; 20% incidence of rash noted in
trials, including severe Stevens-Johnson
Syndrome; photosensitivity reactions (avoid
direct sunlight)
Allergic Potential: High
Safety in Pregnancy: D
Comments: Non-linear kinetics (doubling of
oral dose = 2.8-fold increase in serum levels).
10-15% of patients have serum levels > 6
mcg/mL. Food decreases bioavailability; take 1
hour before or after meals. Do not use IV
voriconazole if CrCl < 50 mL/min to prevent

"Usual dose" assumes normal renal/hepatic function. * For renal insufficiency, give usual dose x 1 followed by
maintenance dose per CrCl. For dialysis patients, dose the same as for CrCl < 10 mL/min and give supplemental
(post-HD/PD dose) immediately after dialysis. CrCl = creatinine clearance; CVVH = continuous veno-venous hemo-
filtration; HD/PD = hemodialysis/peritoneal dialysis. See pp. 293-297 for explanations, p. 1 for abbreviations

accumulation of voriconazole IV vehicle, sulphobutyl ether cyclodextrin (SBECD); instead use oral formulation, which has no SBECD. Loading dose may be given PO for chronic/non-life-threatening infections. If during usual oral maintenance dose, additional therapeutic effect is desired, increase dose from 200 mg (PO) q12h to 300 mg (PO) q12h for weight ≥ 40 kg, or from 100 mg (PO) q12h to 150 mg (PO) q12h for weight < 40 kg. Because of visual effects, do not drive or operate machinery. Monitor LFTs before and during therapy
Meningeal dose = usual dose
Cerebrospinal Fluid Penetration: 90%

REFERENCES:

Castiglioni B, Sutton DA, Rinaldi MG, et al. Pseudallescheria boydii (Anamorph Scedosporium apiospermum). Infection in solid organ transplant recipients in a tertiary medical center and review of the literature. Medicine (Baltimore) 81:333-48, 2002.

Chandrasekar PH, Manavathu E. Voriconazole. A second-generation triazole. Drugs for Today 37:135-48, 2001.

Denning DW, Ribaud P, Milpied N, et al. Efficacy and safety of voriconazole in the treatment of acute invasive aspergillosis. Clin Infect Dis 34:563-71, 2002.

Espinel-Ingroff A, Boyle K, Sheehan DJ. In vitro antifungal activities of voriconazole and reference agents as determined by NCCLS methods: Review of the literature. Mycopathologia 150:101-115, 2001.

Ghannoum MA, Kuhn DM. Voriconazole – better chances for patients with invasive mycoses. Eur J Med Res 7:242-256, 2002.

Herbrecht R, Denning DW, Patterson TF, et al. Voriconazole versus amphotericin B for primary therapy of invasive aspergillosis. N Engl J Med 347:408-15, 2002.

Hoffman HL, Rathbun RC. Review of the safety and efficacy of voriconazole. Expert Opin Investig Drugs 11:409-29, 2002.

Lazarus HM, Blumer JL, Yanovich, et al. Safety and pharmacokinetics of oral voriconazole in patients at risk of fungal infection: a dose escalation study. J Clin Pharmacol 42:395-402, 2002.

Powers JH, Dixon CA, Goldberger MJ. Voriconazole versus liposomal amphotericin B in patients with neutropenia and persistent fever. N Engl J Med 346:289-90, 2002.

Poza G, Montoya J, Redondo C, et al. Meningitis caused by Psedallescheria boydii treated with voriconazole. Clin Infect Dis 30:981-2, 2000.

Purkins L, Wood N, Ghahramani P, et al.

Pharmacokinetics and safety of voriconazole following intravenous- to oral-dose escalation regimens. Antimicrob Agents Chemother 46:2546-53, 2002.

Sabo JA, Abdel-Rahman SM. Voriconazole: A new antifungal. Ann Pharmacotherapy 34:1032-43, 2000.

Walsh TJ, Pappas P, Winston DJ, et al. Voriconazole compared with liposomal amphotericin B for empirical antifungal therapy in patients with neutropenia and persistent fever. N Engl J Med 346:225-34, 2002.

Website: www.vfend.com

Zalcitabine (HIVID) ddC

Drug Class: Antiretroviral NRTI (nucleoside reverse transcriptase inhibitor)
Usual Dose: 0.75 mg (PO) q8h
Pharmacokinetic Parameters:
Peak serum level: 0.08 mcg/mL
Bioavailability: 80%
Excreted unchanged: 75%
Serum half-life (normal/ESRD): 2/8.5 hrs
Plasma protein binding: 0%
Volume of distribution (V_d): 0.54 L/kg
Primary Mode of Elimination: Renal
Dosage Adjustments*

CrCl ~ 40–60 mL/min	No change
CrCl ~ 10–40 mL/min	0.75 mg (PO) q12h
CrCl < 10 mL/min	0.75 mg (PO) q24h
Post–HD dose	No information
Post–PD dose	No information
CVVH dose	0.75 mg (PO) q12h
Moderate hepatic insufficiency	No change
Severe hepatic insufficiency	No change

Drug Interactions: Cimetidine, probenecid, TMP-SMX (↑ zalcitabine levels); dapsone, didanosine, stavudine, INH, phenytoin, metronidazole, other neurotoxic agents or history of neuropathy (↑ risk of peripheral neuropathy); magnesium/aluminum containing

---

"Usual dose" assumes normal renal/hepatic function. * For renal insufficiency, give usual dose x 1 followed by maintenance dose per CrCl. For dialysis patients, dose the same as for CrCl < 10 mL/min and give supplemental (post-HD/PD dose) immediately after dialysis. CrCl = creatinine clearance; CVVH = continuous veno-venous hemofiltration; HD/PD = hemodialysis/peritoneal dialysis. See pp. 293-297 for explanations, p. 1 for abbreviations

antacids, metoclopramide (↓ bioavailability of zalcitabine); pentamidine IV, valproic acid, alcohol, other agents known to cause pancreatitis (↑ risk of pancreatitis)

Adverse Effects: Drug fever/rash, leukopenia, anemia, thrombocytopenia, hepatomegaly, hepatotoxicity/hepatic necrosis, peripheral neuropathy, pancreatitis, stomatitis, oral ulcers, dysphagia, arthritis, hyperglycemia, lipotrophy, wasting, lactic acidosis with hepatic steatosis (rare, but potentially life-threatening toxicity with use of NRTIs)

Allergic Potential: High

Safety in Pregnancy: C

Comments: Foscarnet may increase toxicity. Do not use with stavudine, didanosine, or lamivudine to avoid additive toxicities. Food decreases absorption by 39%. Effective antiretroviral therapy consists of at least 3 antiretrovirals (same/different classes)

Cerebrospinal Fluid Penetration: 25%

REFERENCES:

Drugs for AIDS and associated infections. Med Lett Drug Ther 35:79-86, 1993.

HIV Trialists' Collaborative Group. Zidovudine, didanosine, and zalcitabine in the treatment of HIV infection: Meta-analyses of the randomised evidence. Lancet 353:2014-2025, 1999.

Panel on Clinical Practices for Treatment of HIV Infection. Guidelines for the use of antiretroviral agents in HIV-infected adults and adolescents. Department of Health and Human Services. www.aidsinfo.nih.gov/guidelines/. November 10, 2003.

Shelton MJ, O'Donnell AM, Morse GD. Zalcitabine. Ann Pharmacotherapy 27:480-9, 1993.

Skowron G, Bozzette SA, Lim L, et al. Alternating and intermittent regimens of zidovudine and dideoxycytidine in patients with AIDS or AIDS-related complex. Ann Intern Med 118:321-30, 1993.

Website: www.rocheusa.com/products/

Zidovudine (Retrovir) ZDV Azidothymidine AZT

Drug Class: Antiretroviral NRTI (nucleoside reverse transcriptase inhibitor)

Usual Dose: 300 mg (PO) q12h (see comments)

Pharmacokinetic Parameters:
Peak serum level: 1.2 mcg/mL
Bioavailability: 64%
Excreted unchanged: 16%
Serum half-life (normal/ESRD): 1.1/1.4 hrs
Plasma protein binding: < 38%
Volume of distribution (V_d): 1.6 L/kg

Primary Mode of Elimination: Hepatic

Dosage Adjustments*

CrCl ~ 40–60 mL/min	No change
CrCl ~ 15–40 mL/min	No change
CrCl < 15 mL/min	300 mg (PO) q24h
HD/PD	100 mg (PO) q6-8h
Post–HD/PD dose	None
CVVH dose	300 mg (PO) q24h
Moderate or severe hepatic insufficiency	No information

Drug Interactions: Acetaminophen, atovaquone, fluconazole, methadone, probenecid, valproic acid (↑ zidovudine levels); clarithromycin, nelfinavir, rifampin, rifabutin (↓ zidovudine levels); dapsone, flucytosine, ganciclovir, interferon alpha, bone marrow suppressive/cytotoxic agents (↑ risk of hematologic toxicity); indomethacin (↑ levels of zidovudine toxic metabolite); phenytoin (↑ zidovudine levels, ↑ or ↓ phenytoin levels); ribavirin (↓ zidovudine effect; avoid)

Adverse Effects: Nausea, vomiting, GI upset, diarrhea, malaise, anorexia, leukopenia, anemia, macrocytosis, thrombocytopenia, headaches, ↑ SGOT/SGPT, myalgias, insomnia, blue/black nail discoloration, asthenia, lactic acidosis with hepatic steatosis (rare, but potentially life-threatening toxicity with use of NRTIs)

Allergic Potential: Low

Safety in Pregnancy: C

Comments: Antagonized by ganciclovir or ribavirin. Also a component of Combivir and Trizivir. Effective antiretroviral therapy consists of at least 3 antiretrovirals (same/different classes)

Cerebrospinal Fluid Penetration: 60%

"Usual dose" assumes normal renal/hepatic function. * For renal insufficiency, give usual dose x 1 followed by maintenance dose per CrCl. For dialysis patients, dose the same as for CrCl < 10 mL/min and give supplemental (post-HD/PD dose) immediately after dialysis. CrCl = creatinine clearance; CVVH = continuous veno-venous hemo-filtration; HD/PD = hemodialysis/peritoneal dialysis. See pp. 293-297 for explanations, p. 1 for abbreviations

REFERENCES:

Barry M, Mulcahy F, Merry C, et al. Pharmacokinetics and potential interactions amongst antiretroviral agents used to treat patients with HIV infection. Clin Pharmacol 36:289-304, 1999.

Been-Tiktak AM, Boucher CA, Brun-Vezinet F, et al. Efficacy and safety of combination therapy with delavirdine and zidovudine: A European/Australian phase II trial. Intern J Antimcrob Agents 11:13-21, 1999.

McDowell JA, Lou Y, Symonds WS, et al. Multiple-dose pharmacokinetics and pharmacodynamics of abacavir alone and in combination with zidovudine in human immunodeficiency virus-infected adults. Antimicrob Agents Chemother 44:2061-7, 2000.

Montaner JS, Reiss P, Cooper D, et al. A randomized, double-blind trial comparing combinations of nevirapine, didanosine, and zidovudine for HIV-infected patients: The INCAS trial. Italy, the Netherlands, Canada and Australia Study. J Am Med Assoc 279:930-937, 1998.

Panel on Clinical Practices for Treatment of HIV Infection. Guidelines for the use of antiretroviral agents in HIV-infected adults and adolescents. Department of Health and Human Services. www.aidsinfo.nih.gov/guidelines/. November 10, 2003.

Piscitelli SC, Gallicano KD. Interactions among drugs for HIV and opportunistic infections. N Engl J Med 344:984-996, 2001.

Simpson DM. Human immunodeficiency virus-associated dementia: A review of pathogenesis, prophylaxis, and treatment studies of zidovudine therapy. Clin Infect Dis 29:19-34, 1999.

Website: www.TreatHIV.com

REFERENCES AND SUGGESTED READINGS*

Ambrose P, Nightingale AT (eds). Principles of Pharmacodynamics. Marcel Dekker, Inc., New York, 2001.

Anderson RJ, Schrier RW (eds). Clinical Use of Drugs in Patients with Kidney and Liver Disease. W. B. Saunders Company, Philadelphia, 1981.

Bartlett JG (ed). The Johns Hopkins Hospital Guide to Medical Care of Patients with HIV Infection, 10th edition, Lippincott Williams & Wilkins, Philadelphia, 2002.

Bennet WM, Aronoff GR, Golper TA, Morrison G, Brater DC, Singer I (eds). Drug Prescribing in Renal Failure, 2nd Edition. American College of Physicians, Philadelphia, 2000.

Cunha BA. Antimicrobial side effects. Medical Clinics of North America 85:149-185, 2001.

Cunha BA (ed). Medical Clinics of North America: Antimicrobial Therapy I. W.B. Saunders Company, Philadelphia, 2000.

Cunha BA (ed). Medical Clinics of North America: Antimicrobial Therapy II. W.B. Saunders Company, Philadelphia, 2001.

Dolin R, Masur H, Saag MS (eds). AIDS Therapy, 2nd edition. Churchill Livingstone, New York, 2003.

Gorbach SL, Bartlett JG, Blacklow NR (eds). Infectious Diseases, 3rd Edition. W.B. Saunders Company, Philadelphia, 2003.

Guidelines for using antiretroviral agents among HIV-infected adults and adolescents: recommendations of the Panel on Clinical Practices for Treatment of HIV. www.aidsinfo.nih.gov/guidelines/. November 10, 2003.

Ieada CM, Keaten, Jr, BL, Goldman MP, Gray LD, Aberg JA (eds). Infectious Diseases Handbook, 4th Edition. Lexi-Comp, Inc., Hudson, 2001.

Kucers A, Crowe S, Grayson ML, Hoy J (eds). The Use of Antibiotics: A Clinical Review of Antibacterial, Antifungal, and Antiviral Drugs, 5th Edition. Butterworth-Heinemann, Oxford, 1997.

Mandell GL, Bennett JE, Dolin R (eds). Mandell, Douglas and Bennett's Principles and Practice of Infectious Disease, 5th Edition. Churchill Livingstone, Philadelphia, 2000.

O'Grady F, Lambert HP, Finch RG, Greenwood D (eds). Antibiotic and Chemotherapy, 2nd Edition. Churchill Livingstone, New York, 1997.

Physicians' Desk Reference, 57th Edition. Thompson PDR, Montvale, NJ, 2003.

Piscitelli SC, Rodvold KE (eds). Drug Interactions in Infectious Diseases. Humana Press, Totowa, 2001.

Piscitelli SC, Gallicano KD. Interactions among drugs for HIV and opportunistic infections. N Engl J Med 344:984-996, 2001.

Pratt WB, Fekety R (eds). The Antimicrobial Drugs, 1st Edition. Oxford University Press, New York, 1986.

Ristuccia AM, Cunha BA (eds). Antimicrobial Therapy. Raven Press, New York, 1984.

Root RK (ed). Clinical Infectious Diseases: A Practical Approach. Oxford University Press, New York, 1999.

Schlossberg D (ed). Current Therapy of Infectious Disease, 2nd Edition. Mosby-Yearbook, St. Louis, 2001.

Scholar EM, Pratt WB (eds). The Antimicrobial Drugs, 2nd Edition. Oxford University Press, New York, 2000.

Yoshikawa TT, Norman DC (eds). Antimicrobial Therapy in the Elderly. Marcel Dekker, New York, 1994.

Yu VL, Merigan, Jr. TC, Barriere SL (eds). Antimicrobial Therapy and Vaccines. Williams & Wilkens, Baltimore, 1999.

Zinner SH, Young LS, Acar JF, Ortiz-Neu C (eds). New Considerations for Macrolides, Azalides, Streptogramins, and Ketolides. Marcel Dekker, Inc., New York, 2000.

*   See drug summaries (Chapter 7) for additional references

INDEX

ANTIBIOTIC ESSENTIALS — ORDERING INFORMATION

Price (U.S. dollars)
1–9 copies:	$14.95 each
10–49 copies:	$13.95 each
50–100 copies:	$12.95 each
> 100 copies:	call

Shipping
<u>USA</u>: UPS Ground delivery
1–3 copies:	add $5
4–10 copies:	add $7
10–49 copies:	add $10
50–100 copies:	add $15
> 100 copies:	call

Call for next day, 2-day, or 3-day express delivery charges

<u>Outside USA</u>: Call, fax, or e-mail for delivery charges

Michigan residents: add 6%

4 Ways to Order:
By Internet:	www.physicianspress.com
By Phone:	(248) 616-3023
By Fax:*	(248) 616-3003
By Mail:*	Physicians' Press
	620 Cherry Street
	Royal Oak, Michigan 48073

*   Please print or type name, mailing address, credit card number and expiration date or purchase order number (if applicable), telephone number (important), fax number, and e-mail address. We accept VISA, MasterCard, and American Express.

Visit our website at www.physicianspress.com

- HIV Essentials
- ACS (Acute Coronary Syndrome) Essentials
- Hypertension Essentials
- Dyslipidemia Essentials
- Stroke Essentials

- Diabetes Essentials
- Essentials of Cardiovascular Medicine
- The Complete Guide to ECGs
- The ECG Criteria Book
- Other Titles, Quizzes, Reviews

PHYSICIANS' PRESS

Innovative Medical Publishing